Magnetic Resonance Imaging: Tools and Techniques

Magnetic Resonance Imaging: Tools and Techniques

Editor: Aaron Jackson

FOSTER ACADEMICS

www.fosteracademics.com

www.fosteracademics.com

FOSTER
ACADEMICS

Cataloging-in-Publication Data

Magnetic resonance imaging : tools and techniques / edited by Aaron Jackson.
p. cm.
Includes bibliographical references and index.
ISBN 978-1-63242-555-3
1. Magnetic resonance imaging. 2. Diagnostic imaging--Equipment and supplies.
3. Diagnostic imaging--Digital techniques. I. Jackson, Aaron.
RC78.7.N83 M34 2018
616.075 48--dc23

Foster Academics,
118-35 Queens Blvd., Suite 400,
Forest Hills, NY 11375, USA

ISBN 978-1-63242-555-3 (Hardback)

Printed and bound in China.

Contents

Preface IX

Chapter 1 **Active Ultrasound Pattern Injection System (AUSPIS) for Interventional Tool Guidance** 1
Xiaoyu Guo, Hyun-Jae Kang, Ralph Etienne-Cummings, Emad M. Boctor

Chapter 2 **Auditory Conflict Resolution Correlates with Medial–Lateral Frontal Theta/Alpha Phase Synchrony** 14
Samantha Huang, Stephanie Rossi, Matti Hämäläinen, Jyrki Ahveninen

Chapter 3 **High-Resolution Mechanical Imaging of Glioblastoma by Multifrequency Magnetic Resonance Elastography** 27
Kaspar-Josche Streitberger, Martin Reiss-Zimmermann., Florian Baptist Freimann, Simon Bayerl, Jing Guo, Felix Arlt, Jens Wuerfel, Jürgen Braun, Karl-Titus Hoffmann, Ingolf Sack

Chapter 4 **Hippocampal and Left Subcallosal Anterior Cingulate Atrophy in Psychotic Depression** 36
Kelly Rowe Bijanki, Brendan Hodis, Michael C. Brumm, Emily L. Harlynn, Laurie M. McCormick

Chapter 5 **Optimal Brain MRI Protocol for New Neurological Complaint** 43
William A. Mehan Jr., R. Gilberto González, Bradley R. Buchbinder, John W. Chen, William A. Copen, Rajiv Gupta, Joshua A. Hirsch, George J. Hunter, Scott Hunter, Jason M. Johnson, Hillary R. Kelly, Mykol Larvie, Michael H. Lev, Stuart R. Pomerantz, Otto Rapalino, Sandra Rincon, Javier M. Romero, Pamela W. Schaefer, Vinil Shah

Chapter 6 **Atlas-Based Quantification of Cardiac Remodeling due to Myocardial Infarction** 53
Xingyu Zhang, Brett R. Cowan, David A. Bluemke, J. Paul Finn, Carissa G. Fonseca, Alan H. Kadish, Daniel C. Lee, Joao A. C. Lima, Avan Suinesiaputra, Alistair A. Young, Pau Medrano-Gracia

Chapter 7 **The Functional Connectivity Landscape of the Human Brain** 66
Bratislav Mišić., Zainab Fatima, Mary K. Askren, Martin Buschkuehl, Nathan Churchill, Bernadine Cimprich, Patricia J. Deldin, Susanne Jaeggi, Misook Jung, Michele Korostil, Ethan Kross, Katherine M. Krpan, Scott Peltier, Patricia A. Reuter-Lorenz, Stephen C. Strother, John Jonides, Anthony R. McIntosh, Marc G. Berman

Chapter 8 **Decreased Fronto-Temporal Interaction during Fixation after Memory Retrieval** 87
Masaki Katsura, Satoshi Hirose, Hiroki Sasaki, Harushi Mori, Akira Kunimatsu, Kuni Ohtomo, Koji Jimura, Seiki Konishi

Chapter 9 **Episodic Future Thinking in Semantic Dementia: A Cognitive and fMRI Study** 98
Armelle Viard, Pascale Piolino, Serge Belliard, Vincent de La Sayette, Béatrice Desgranges, Francis Eustache

Chapter 10 **Comparison of Total Variation with a Motion Estimation based Compressed Sensing Approach for Self-Gated Cardiac Cine MRI in Small Animal Studies** 120
Juan F. P. J. Abascal, Paula Montesinos, Eugenio Marinetto, Javier Pascau, Manuel Desco

Chapter 11 **Deep White Matter in Huntington's Disease** 130
Owen Phillips, Ferdinando Squitieri, Cristina Sanchez-Castaneda, Francesca Elifani, Carlo Caltagirone, Umberto Sabatini, Margherita Di Paola

Chapter 12 **Greater BOLD Variability in Older Compared with Younger Adults during Audiovisual Speech Perception** 141
Sarah H. Baum, Michael S. Beauchamp

Chapter 13 **Distribution of Mesenchymal Stem Cells and Effects on Neuronal Survival and Axon Regeneration after Optic Nerve Crush and Cell Therapy** 151
Louise Alessandra Mesentier-Louro, Camila Zaverucha-do-Valle, Almir Jordão da Silva-Junior, Gabriel Nascimento-dos-Santos, Fernanda Gubert, Ana Beatriz Padilha de Figueirêdo, Ana Luiza Torres, Bruno D. Paredes, Camila Teixeira, Fernanda Tovar-Moll, Rosalia Mendez- Otero, Marcelo F. Santiago

Chapter 14 **Investigation of Cross-Species Translatability of Pharmacological MRI in Awake Nonhuman Primate – A Buprenorphine Challenge Study** 167
Stephanie Seah, Abu Bakar Ali Asad, Richard Baumgartner, Dai Feng, Donald S. Williams, Elaine Manigbas, John D. Beaver, Torsten Reese, Brian Henry, Jeffrey L. Evelhoch, Chih-Liang Chin

Chapter 15 **Identifying Predictors of Early Growth Response and Adverse Radiation Effects of Vestibular Schwannomas to Radiosurgery** 178
Soroush Larjani, Eric Monsalves, Houman Pebdani, Boris Krischek, Fred Gentili, Michael Cusimano, Normand Laperriere, Caroline Hayhurst, Gelareh Zadeh

Chapter 16 **IV t-PA Influences Infarct Volume in Minor Stroke** 185
Kersten Villringer, Ulrike Grittner, Lars-Arne Schaafs, Christian H. Nolte, Heinrich Audebert, Jochen B. Fiebach

Chapter 17 **Comparison of ^{99m}Tc-3PRGD2 Integrin Receptor Imaging with ^{99m}Tc-MDP Bone Scan in Diagnosis of Bone Metastasis in Patients with Lung Cancer** 192
Weibing Miao, Shan Zheng, Haojie Dai, Feng Wang, Xiaona Jin, Zhaohui Zhu, Bing Jia

Chapter 18 **MR Quantification of Total Liver Fat in Patients with Impaired Glucose Tolerance and Healthy Subjects** 199
Zhi Dong, Yanji Luo, Zhongwei Zhang, Huasong Cai, Yanbing Li, Tao Chan, Ling Wu, Zi-Ping Li, Shi-Ting Feng

Chapter 19 **Stochastic Tracking of Infection in a CF Lung** 206
Sara Zarei, Ali Mirtar, Forest Rohwer, Peter Salamon

Chapter 20 **Consensus between Pipelines in Structural Brain Networks** 215
Christopher S. Parker, Fani Deligianni, M. Jorge Cardoso, Pankaj Daga, Marc Modat, Michael Dayan, Chris A. Clark, Sebastien Ourselin, Jonathan D. Clayden

Permissions

List of Contributors

Index

Preface

Magnetic resonance imaging is used in developing images of human body. It uses magnetic field and pulses of radio wave energy to generate pictures of organs of the body. MRIs are performed to detect tumors, injuries, or infections. It can be performed on the head, chest, abdomen, bones and joints. This book presents the complex subject of magnetic resonance imaging in the most comprehensible and easy to understand language. It will prove to be immensely beneficial to students and researchers in this field.

After months of intensive research and writing, this book is the end result of all who devoted their time and efforts in the initiation and progress of this book. It will surely be a source of reference in enhancing the required knowledge of the new developments in the area. During the course of developing this book, certain measures such as accuracy, authenticity and research focused analytical studies were given preference in order to produce a comprehensive book in the area of study.

This book would not have been possible without the efforts of the authors and the publisher. I extend my sincere thanks to them. Secondly, I express my gratitude to my family and well-wishers. And most importantly, I thank my students for constantly expressing their willingness and curiosity in enhancing their knowledge in the field, which encourages me to take up further research projects for the advancement of the area.

Editor

Active Ultrasound Pattern Injection System (AUSPIS) for Interventional Tool Guidance

Xiaoyu Guo[1]*, Hyun-Jae Kang[2], Ralph Etienne-Cummings[1], Emad M. Boctor[2,3]

1 Dept. of Electrical and Computer Engineering, Johns Hopkins University, Baltimore, MD, United States of America, **2** Dept. of Computer Science, Johns Hopkins University, Baltimore, MD, United States of America, **3** Dept. of Radiology, Johns Hopkins University, Baltimore, MD, United States of America

Abstract

Accurate tool tracking is a crucial task that directly affects the safety and effectiveness of many interventional medical procedures. Compared to CT and MRI, ultrasound-based tool tracking has many advantages, including low cost, safety, mobility and ease of use. However, surgical tools are poorly visualized in conventional ultrasound images, thus preventing effective tool tracking and guidance. Existing tracking methods have not yet provided a solution that effectively solves the tool visualization and mid-plane localization accuracy problem and fully meets the clinical requirements. In this paper, we present an active ultrasound tracking and guiding system for interventional tools. The main principle of this system is to establish a bi-directional ultrasound communication between the interventional tool and US imaging machine within the tissue. This method enables the interventional tool to generate an active ultrasound field over the original imaging ultrasound signals. By controlling the timing and amplitude of the active ultrasound field, a virtual pattern can be directly injected into the US machine B mode display. In this work, we introduce the time and frequency modulation, mid-plane detection, and arbitrary pattern injection methods. The implementation of these methods further improves the target visualization and guiding accuracy, and expands the system application beyond simple tool tracking. We performed ex vitro and in vivo experiments, showing significant improvements of tool visualization and accurate localization using different US imaging platforms. An ultrasound image mid-plane detection accuracy of ±0.3 mm and a detectable tissue depth over 8.5 cm was achieved in the experiment. The system performance is tested under different configurations and system parameters. We also report the first experiment of arbitrary pattern injection to the B mode image and its application in accurate tool tracking.

Editor: Arrate Muñoz-Barrutia, University of Navarra, Spain

Funding: This work is supported by the internal funding of the Johns Hopkins University. The funder had no role in study design, data collection and analysis, decision to publish, or preparation of the manuscript.

Competing Interests: The authors have declared that no competing interests exist.

* Email: xguo9@jhu.edu

Introduction

Tool tracking/guidance techniques have broad utility in medical intervention and image-guided therapy. In medical interventions, including biopsy, ablative therapy, and cardiac catheterization, image guidance is the pivotal task and technology that determines operation success and guarantees clinical outcome. In literature, research shows that in many applications, intervention outcome can be greatly improved if an effective tool tracking method is introduced [1]. Various medical imaging modalities are used to recover the pose of the interventional tools [2]. Compared to CT and MRI, ultrasound (US) imaging has several advantages including low cost, safety, mobility and ease-of-use. Two major limitations, however, prevent conventional ultrasound imaging systems from providing effective tracking and guidance. The first one is the poor visualization of interventional tools. Ultrasonography reconstructs images from received echo ultrasound signals. In interventional procedures, many catheters or needles cannot be reliably visualized in ultrasound images due to the low echo signal amplitude, large reflection angle, strong tissue attenuation or the complicated image background [3]. The second limitation is the low localization accuracy in the elevational dimension. The acoustic beam width usually ranges from several millimeters to one centimeter, which means an object shown on a 2D ultrasound image has an inherent uncertainly of a few millimeters to one centimeter along the elevation axis.

In recent years, several approaches have been proposed to enable tool visualization and pose recovery, including beam steering, optical tracking, electromagnetic (EM) tracking, and passive/active ultrasound markers [4–11]. The beam steering method has been developed and validated by several research groups and currently is integrated into a commercial ultrasound scanner from SonoSite Inc. The basic principle is to steer the imaging beam directions to get the optimized reflection from the catheter. It has been proven effective when the catheter is in-plane of the US image. For cases where catheters simply intersect the imaging plane with a large angle, this method is not effective [4]. In the optical tracking approach, an optical marker is attached at the end of the tool and uses a stereo camera to capture the 3D position of the marker [5]. This approach suffers from several limitations, including high cost, calibration complexity, intrusive setup, needle bending error, and the need for clear line-of-sight from the camera to the tool. Electro Magnetic (EM) tracking approach was recently introduced and integrated into several commercial ultrasound scanners (GE LOGIQ E9, Ultrasonix

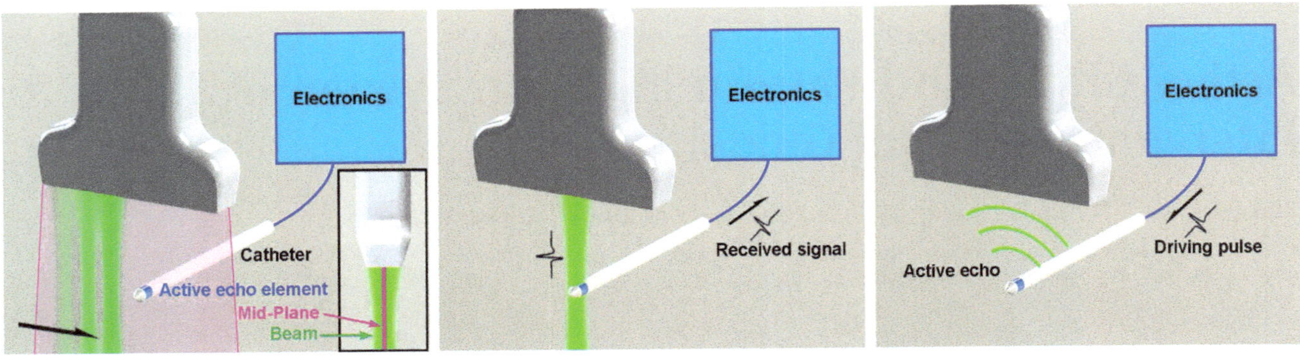

Figure 1. The configuration of the active reflector tracking system. Left: the imaging probe fires a serious of ultrasound beams scanning the image region. The center plane of the image region is the mid-plane. Middle: When an ultrasound beam intersects the active echo element, an electrical pulse is received by the electronics. Right: The received pulse triggers the electronics, a driving pulse is sent to the element to fire an active echo pulse.

GPS, etc.). In this approach, an EM field is generated by an EM emitter; EM sensors are implanted in both the catheter and the imaging probe. The relative pose of the catheter is estimated and injected as a graphic overlay to the B-mode image [6]. The EM tracking quickly became a commercialized technology due to its merits of excellence in off-plane detection capability. However, several disadvantages limit its applications to all interventions: the overall navigation accuracy can easily be worse than 2~3 mm; it requires specially designed imaging equipment; and any ferro-magnetic object in the operation region may affect the system accuracy. Another approach with a similar concept is to use ultrasound sensors instead of EM sensors. Several research groups have demonstrated the system in which an ultrasound receiver is attached to a catheter. The catheter localization is retrieved by measuring the timing of the ultrasound pulses from the imaging probe [8–10]. This method requires specialized US system and image processing software; thus its application is limited.

Other than detecting the tool spatial location, some researchers focus on the visualization enhancement of the catheter in B-mode images. One approach is to improve image quality by using passive ultrasound markers. In this method, ultrasound markers, sometimes in the form of scattering coatings, are integrated into the tool to improve the echo amplitude [7]. The major issue of this approach is that the visualization enhancement by scattering coating is limited; with markers, they are usually too bulky for small catheters. On the other hand, active ultrasound marker approach has also been proposed. F. Simonetti introduced the concept that using biopsy needles as ultrasound waveguide [11]. An ultrasound wave is injected from the end of the needle. It travels along the needle and leaks into the tissue, and is picked up by an external imaging probe working in passive mode. The limitation of this method is that the phase, waveform, timing and leaking position of the guided beam cannot be well controlled; It requires the ultrasound system to stop normal operation and work in passive mode, which is not a direct visualization enhancement; its performance highly relies on the mechanical property of the needle and cannot be generally applied to any surgery tools. B. Breyer and I. Cikes reported an active ultrasound marker system that fires an ultrasound signal from the catheter, which shows a visible pattern in the B-mode image [12]. The timing is acquired by receiving the imaging pulses from the ultrasound probe. This approach directly injects the marker in the B-mode image and does not require special designed imaging system. B. Breyer's and I. Cikes' work for the first time presented the active marker concept on the medical ultrasound imaging system. However, this method was not eventually used in clinics. Experiment results show that in the in-vivo B mode images, it is difficult to identify the active echo spot from the tissue texture. Even in the water tank environment, a simple receive and echo configuration does not provide enough feedback to the operator; the echo spot may show up within a large range of tool position, the elevation localization accuracy is poor.

In this paper we introduce a new technique called ultrasound active pattern injection, a further development of the active visualization enhancement approach. Unlike previous works, the tool visualization and localization is not simply achieved by introducing an ultrasound beam to the tissue or echoing the imaging pulses. The Active Ultrasound Pattern Injection System (AUSPIS) is composed of an interventional tool with one or multiple ultrasound elements (active echo element), ultrasound analog frontends, a signal processing system, and a pulser. The system receives the image beacon pulses, analyzes the acquired signal, and fires one or a series of active echo pulses from the same active echo element with a proper timing, frequency, duration and amplitude. Thus it enables us to inject any "virtual" pattern into the B-mode image. Unlike the image overlay technologies used in other tracking or image registrations, the pattern injected to the B mode image from the actively encoded ultrasound field in the tissue. The encoding is based on the B-mode ultrasound image forming mechanism, so it doesn't require any hardware or software modification to the ultrasound machine. It continuously measures the local acoustic signal amplitude, by which a sub-millimeter elevation localization accuracy can be achieved. By configuring the pattern formations, the technique can be used for tracking, tool guiding, and annotation. In this study, we 1) developed a hardware and firmware prototype of the AUSPIS; 2) performed the lab bench experiment to test the design idea and investigated the working conditions and limitations of the system; 3) tested the system performance in-vivo.

Methods

The basic principle of AUSPIS is shown in figure 1. When acquiring a B-mode image, one or a group of array elements is driven to fires an ultrasound pulse, which propagates along a transmission beam line. After the pulsing, the array is switched to receive mode to acquire the echo. Element groups are fired one by one until the entire image region is covered to reconstruct ultrasound Brightness mode (B-mode) from the multiple RF lines. In the active pattern injection system, a small ultrasound

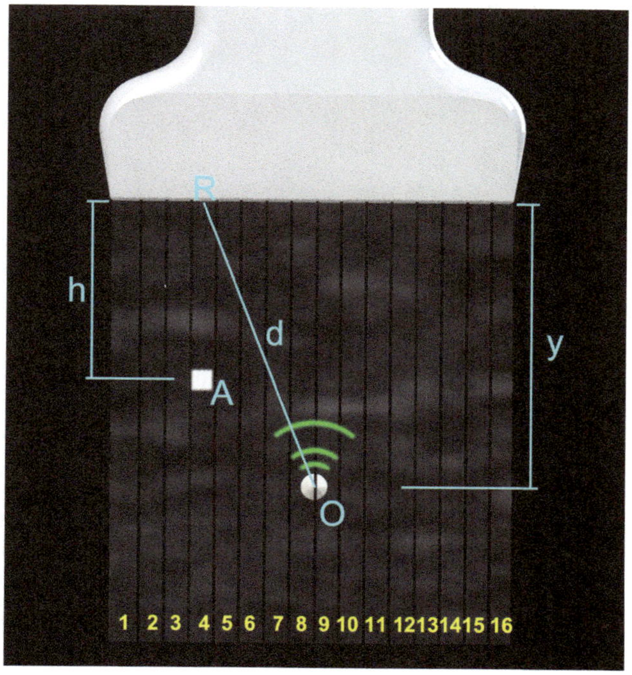

Figure 2. B-mode Pattern injection with a linear array. This picture illustrates how a single virtual pixel is injected to the B-mode image from an active echo element.

transducer (active echo element or AE element) is integrated with the catheter. When a transmission beam reaches the element, an electrical pulse signal is excited and sent to the electronics. To simply improve the tool visualization, the electronics drive the AE element immediately to send an ultrasound pulse back to the imaging probe. The receiving-transmitting delay is in nanoseconds and negligible for US imaging. The active ultrasound pulse is superimposed on the catheter echo wave, resulting in an enhanced echo pulse with a much higher amplitude, broader frequency range and wider emission angle. This pulse travels back to the imaging probe, and appears as a bright spot (AE spot) that indicates the AE element location in the B-mode image.

As described previously, simply echoing the imaging pulses is not very useful in many cases. However, based on the signal received by the AE element, more complex functions can be developed to improve the tracking performance.

1. Time modulation

In clinical or ex-vivo conditions, simple active echoing has very limited improvement in the visualization, because a static echo spot can barely be seen from a complex B-mode background. To overcome this problem, the signal processing unit periodically enables/disables the active echo feedback. As a result, the active echo spot blinks in the B mode image with the same period, making it distinct from the background B mode textures. The tissue phantom and in-vivo experiments proved a good improvement of catheter visualization and tracking using this method.

2. Frequency modulation

The signal processing unit can also control the echo pulse frequency and duration. Although the signal waveform is not shown in the B-mode image, in the raw ultrasound or beamformed RF signals, filtering method can be used to differentiate the background B-mode signal and the active echo signal, which has a different frequency or waveform characters than the imaging pulses. This can be used for the automatic tool guidance.

3. Mid-plane detection

In surgical interventions, even if the tool shows good visualization in B-mode image, it is difficult to determine whether it is well aligned with the image mid-plane due to the ultrasound beam width, as was previously described. To achieve high localization accuracy, a tracking system should be able to detect the image mid-plane, as shown in figure 1. In ultrasound imaging, the beam transmitted from an imaging probe has higher power intensity at the center, and lower intensity away from the center. Since the AE element is capable of measuring the local ultrasound pressure in real time, the beam intensity distribution can be utilized to localize the mid-plane. In the AUSPIS, when the AE element is well aligned with the mid-plane, the received beacon signal amplitude reaches its maximum, and when it moves away, the strength of beacon is decreased. Practically, the US beam intensity is determined by many factors including probe type, tissue attenuation, image depth, focusing point, etc. It is difficult to preset a trigger threshold that makes the AUSPIS only respond to the maximum US signal. However, we found that if the threshold is set to a relatively low value, the AUSPIS will be triggered multiple times in each image frame, and the trigger count, which is defined as the number of triggers received in each frame, reaches its maximum when the AE element is well aligned with the mid-plane. This is because when the US probe scans the FOV, each beacon beam has spatial overlapping with one or more of its neighboring beams. So the AE element receives US signal not only from the beam that intersects it, but also from the nearby beams, just with lower amplitude. When the AE element moves closer to the mid-plane, the received signal amplitude increases; as a result, more nearby beams exceed the threshold, so the trigger count increases. Since the trigger count indicates the alignment between AE element and mid-plane, it can be used for mid-plane detection. AUSPIS is able to read the trigger count and feedback to the operator in multiple ways, like a number displayed on the screen, a beeping sound with a frequency proportional to the trigger count, or an injected virtual pattern on the B-mode image, which will be discussed later.

4. Arbitrary pattern injection

The pattern injected into the image is not limited to the AE spot. As described previously, a B-mode image is formed by a series of A-mode lines. As shown in figure 2, suppose a B mode image is composed of 16 A-mode lines; the normal distance from the AE element to the probe is y. To generate a virtual spot on the point A, an ultrasound pulse should be received by the probe when the A-mode line #4 is being acquired, with a delay of

$$t_{delay} = \frac{2 \times h}{c}$$

where c is the speed of sound in this medium. The ultrasound pulse is generated from the AE element at position O, the distance between O and the center of the imaging elements R is d. The time for sound to travel from O to R is $t_{travel} = d/c$. So the timing that the element should send an ultrasound pulse is:

$$t = t_{delay} - t_{travel} = \frac{2 \times h - d}{c}$$

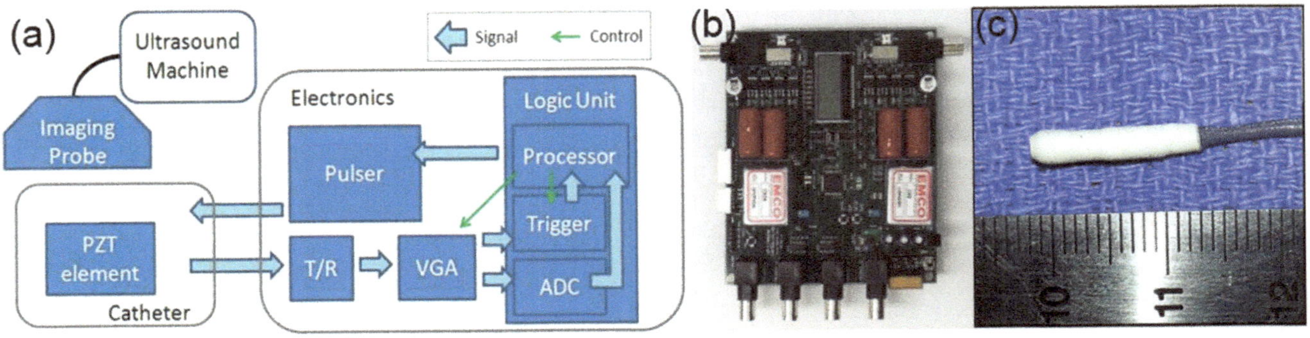

Figure 3. The prototype AUSPIS setup. a) The block diagram of the AUSPIS. b) The pulser and logic unit board. c) One of the prototype catheters; it has an active echo element very close to the tip.

In other words, if an ultrasound pulse is fired from the AE element t seconds after the probe starts acquiring the A mode line #4, it will be shown as a virtual spot at position A in the B-mode image.

Having these spots as "pixels", arbitrary patterns can be formed and injected to the image. The challenging issue is that the relative position between O and R is unknown in the real application scenario. Two methods can be used to overcome this problem. The first method can be used if the ultrasound system is able to output synchronization signals. Since the linear array size, the total number of A-mode lines, and the speed of sound are known parameters, d can be automatically determined from the delay between received signal and the synchronization signal. In this case the arbitrary pattern can be injected into any pre-defined position in the B-mode image, i.e., the injected pattern can be either at an absolute position in the image coordinate, or at a relevant position moving with the active element. The second method can be used when the synchronization signal is unavailable. In this case injecting a pattern to an absolute position in the image coordinate is not possible. However, since the AE element is able to receive multiple neighboring beacon pulses when the probe is acquiring the nearby A-lines, the A-line period can be acquired by the system. Using the received pulse as the synchronization signal, and calculating the desired time delay from the A-line period, virtual patterns can be injected into the B-mode image with the AE element coordinate. The implementations of both methods will be presented in the following paragraphs.

Prototype System

Figure 3a shows the block diagram of the AUSPIS prototype. A piezoelectric element for both ultrasound receiving and transmitting is integrated with a catheter. The element is connected to a customized electronic circuit, which consists of a transmit/receive (T/R) switch, a variable gain amplifier (VGA) with analog filters, triggering circuit, analog to digital converter (ADC), an embedded microprocessor, and a pulser. Figure 3b and 3c show the circuit board and the catheter tip. The T/R switch circuit is built with a TX810 8 channel integrated switch to protect the receiving circuit from the transmission driving voltage, which can go up to a hundred volts. Analog filters have a low and high cutoff frequency of 0.1 MHz and 20 MHz. The trigger circuit compares the absolute value of the signal amplitude and the threshold, and sends

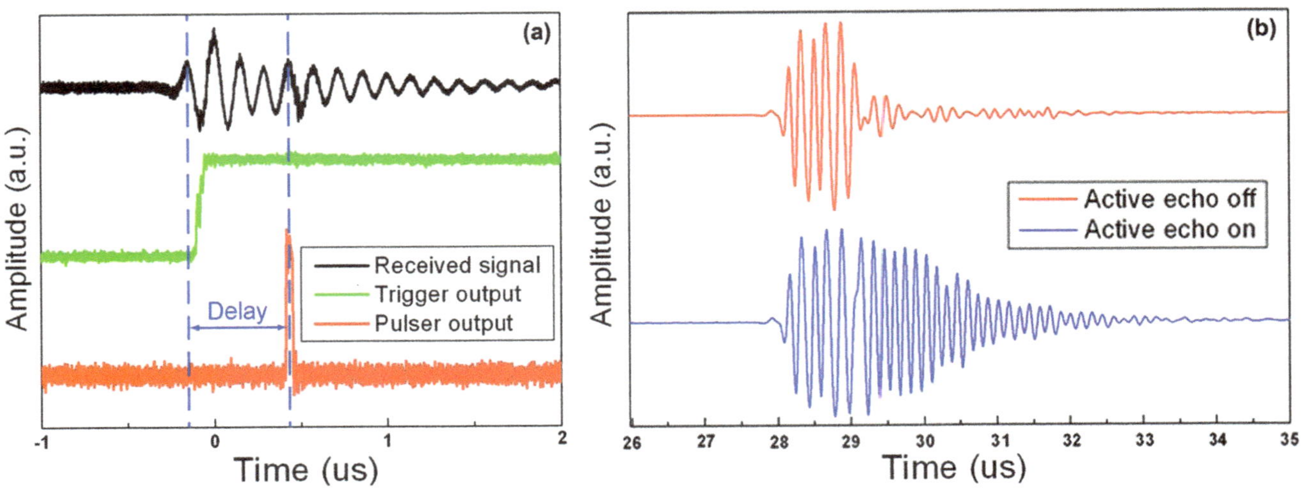

Figure 4. The system received and transmitted signals. a) The signal received by the active echo element (black), the output of the trigger unit (green), the output of the active echo driving pulse (red). b) A RF line received by the imaging probe with and without enabling the active echo system. The active echo adds a ringing tail after the original signal.

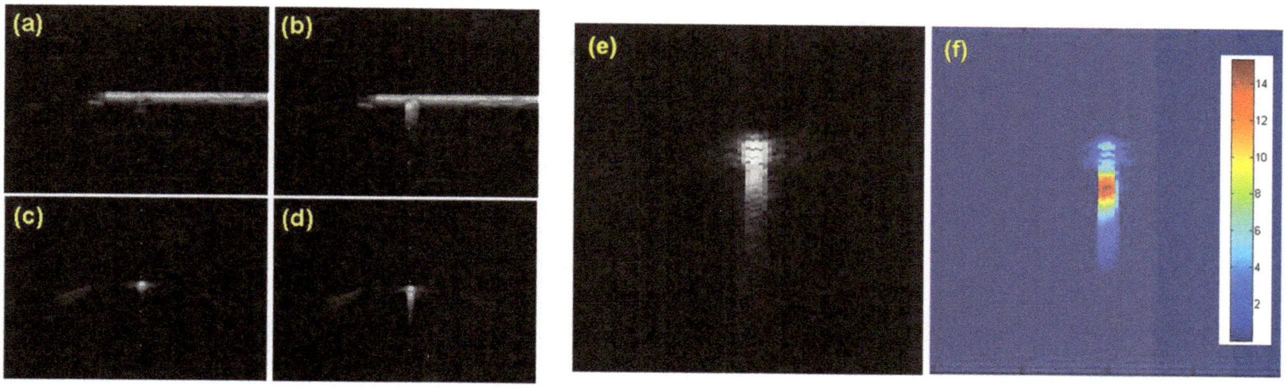

Figure 5. The active echo image in water tank. The catheter used in this experiment has an AE element integrated about 5 mm away from the tip. a)~d) The B-mode image of the catheter in water tank. a, b) the in-plane configuration, c, d) the off-plane configuration. The active echo is enabled in b) and d). e) The B mode image of the catheter with the active echo signal. f) The active echo signal extracted from the B mode image using the template filtering method. The color code represents the convolution value between the signal and template.

pulses out when it is higher than the threshold. Since the receiver and emitter are the same element, the trigger circuit has a latch and reset function to prevent oscillating triggering. The ADC converts the analog signal to digital. The control program runs on an embedded processor, which controls all the peripherals on the AUSPIS circuit. To drive the element, the pulser is able to generate pulses with a minimum duration of 12.5 ns and variable voltage from zero to ±150 V. The active echo element is a customized small tube made of PZT5-H material with an outer diameter of 2.08 mm, inner diameter of 1.47 mm, and length of 2 mm. The catheter has a sealing layer around the element, which makes the overall diameter of the catheter tip close to 3.0 mm. A Sonix RP and a Sonix Touch ultrasound systems (UltraSonix Co.) with L14-5W (128 element) linear probe and 4DL14-5/38 (128 element) 3D probe is used in the experiment. We've also tested the AUSPIS with SonoSite portable ultrasound system to verify the cross platform operation performance.

Results

1. Active echo validation

Figure 4a indicates that the prototype device has an overall electronic loop delay of 0.6 μs. Due to this delay, the active echo spot is about 0.3 mm away along the axial direction from the true element position in the B-mode image. Figure 4b shows the signal received by the imaging probe. The red waveform is the reflection from the catheter; the active echo system is not enabled. The blue line shows the received waveform when the active echo is enabled.

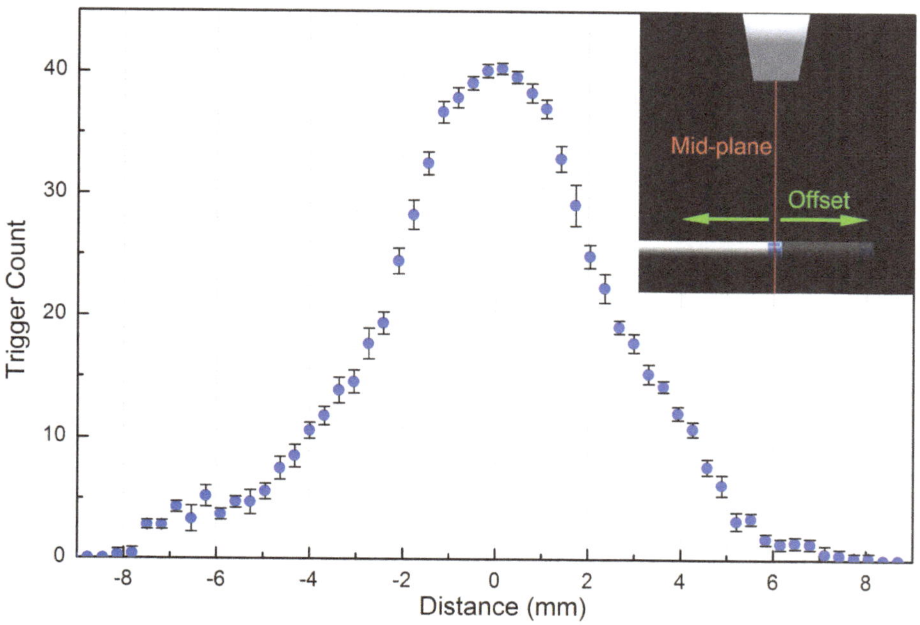

Figure 6. The trigger count versus the offset between the active element and the mid-plane. In this experiment the catheter is fixed in a water tank and perpendicular to the image plane. The probe is mounted on a translation stage, which moves perpendicular to the mid-plane. The error bar represents the standard deviation over 10 measurements, each time the translation stage moves from −9 mm to 9 mm, stops at the same sample positions and takes the trigger count reading.

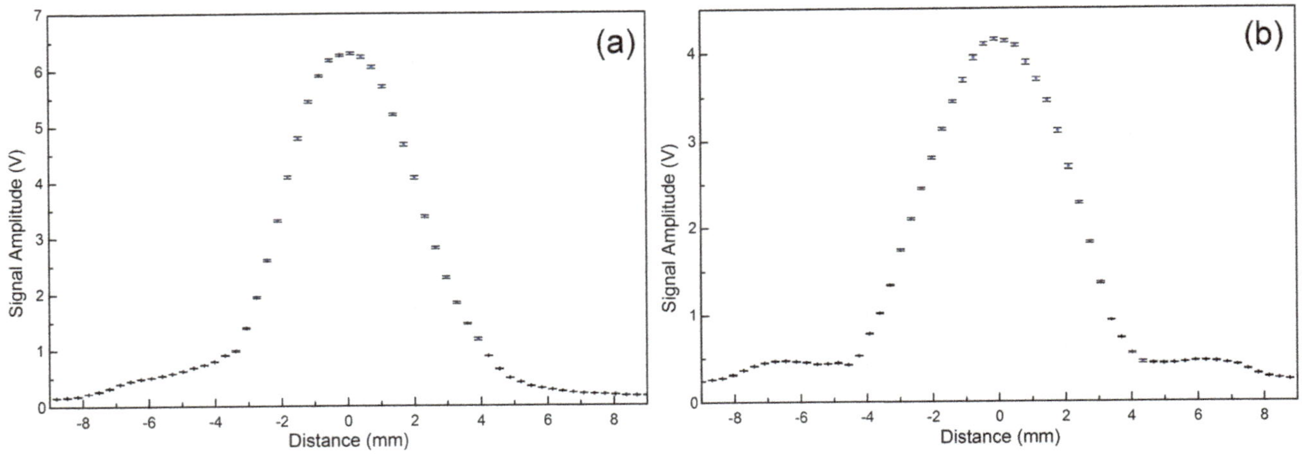

Figure 7. The local ultrasound amplitude measurement for mid-plane detection. a, b) the amplitude of the signal received by the active echo element verses the position of the probe. The depth of the US transmission beam focus is close to the catheter to probe distance, so the two plots are showing the signal distribution near the focus. a) The results with catheter perpendicular to the image plane (off-plane) b) catheter parallel to the image plane (in-plane). The error bar represents the standard deviation over 10 measurements, each time the translation stage moves from −9 mm to 9 mm, stops at the same sample positions and takes the signal amplitude reading.

From this plot we can clearly see that the active echo is fired after the reflection signal, with a delay of around 1 μs. The additional 0.4 μs delay may be due to the response of the prototype PZT element, which is relatively large in size. The active echo adds a ringing tail after the original signal. The frequency of the active echo is adjustable; in this plot, it has a slightly higher frequency than the original signal.

2. Frequency modulation

Figure 5 a)–d) shows the B-mode image with and without enabling the active echo. Due to the transmission signal ringing after the main pulse peak, the active echo spot has a tail away from the US probe. Longer ringing tail improves the active echo spot visualization; at the same time it may decrease the visual localization accuracy in some cases. An adjustable termination circuit can be used to control the ringing settling time. Figure 5 e)

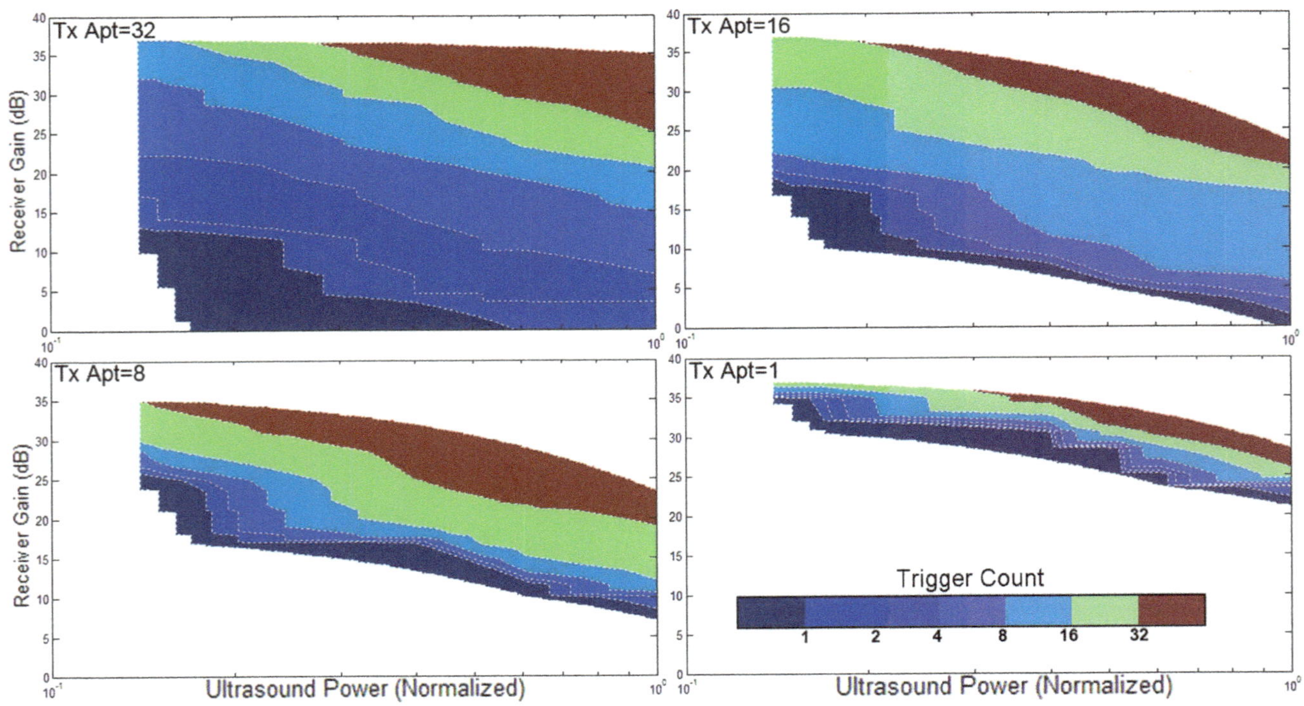

Figure 8. The trigger count versus ultrasound system settings. Catheter is perpendicular to the image plane. Ultrasound beams are focused to the catheter insertion depth.

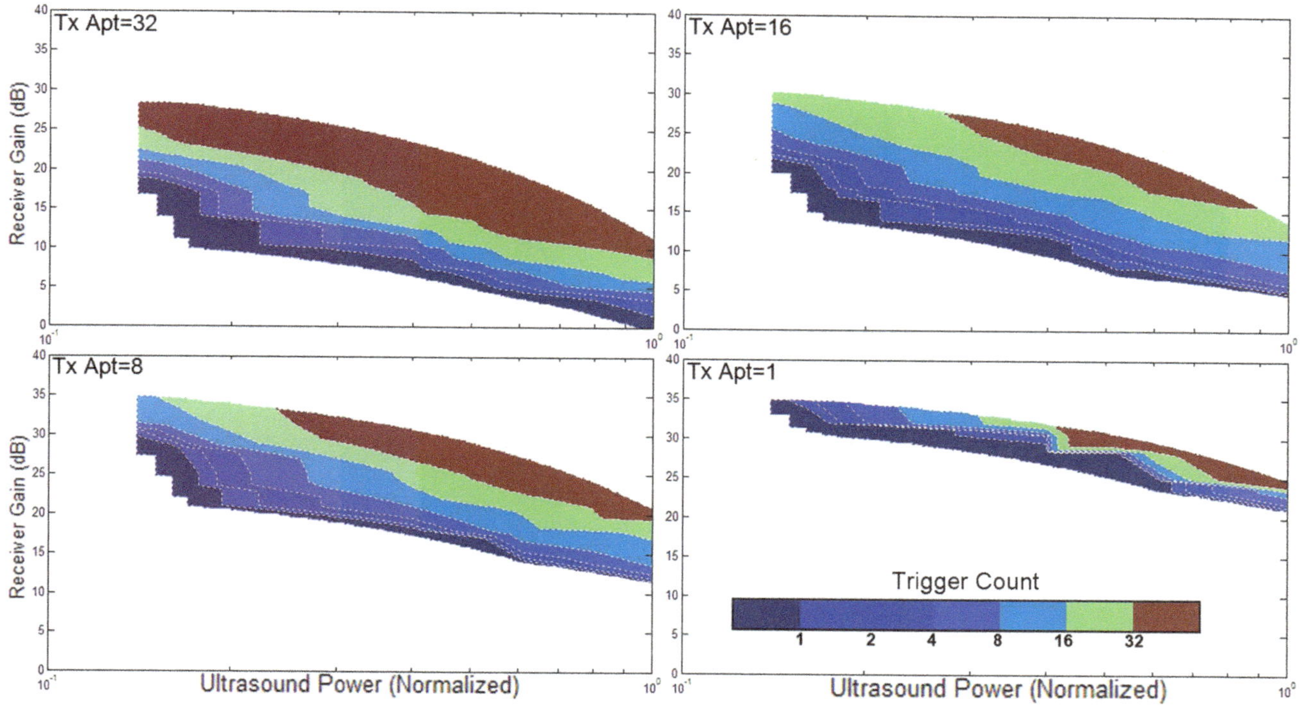

Figure 9. The trigger count versus ultrasound system settings. Catheter is perpendicular to the image plane. Ultrasound pulses are not focused.

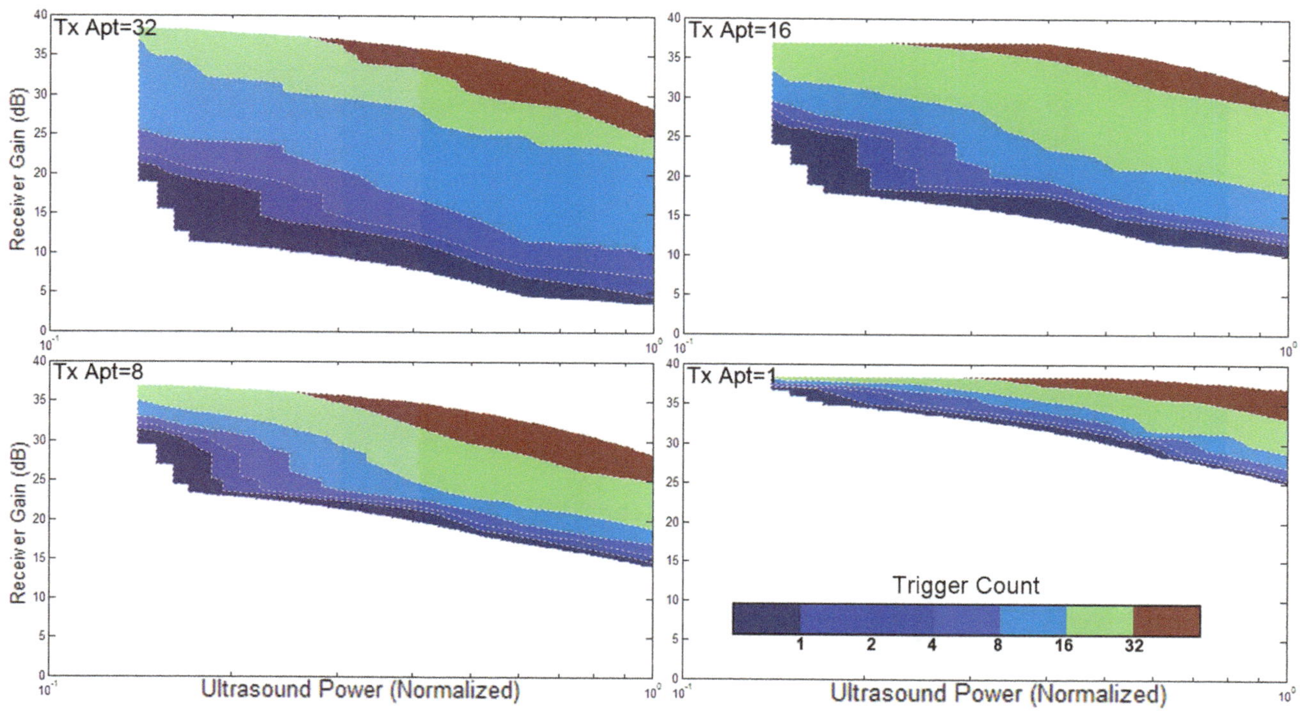

Figure 10. The trigger count versus ultrasound system settings. Catheter is parallel to the image plane. Ultrasound beams are focused to the catheter insertion depth.

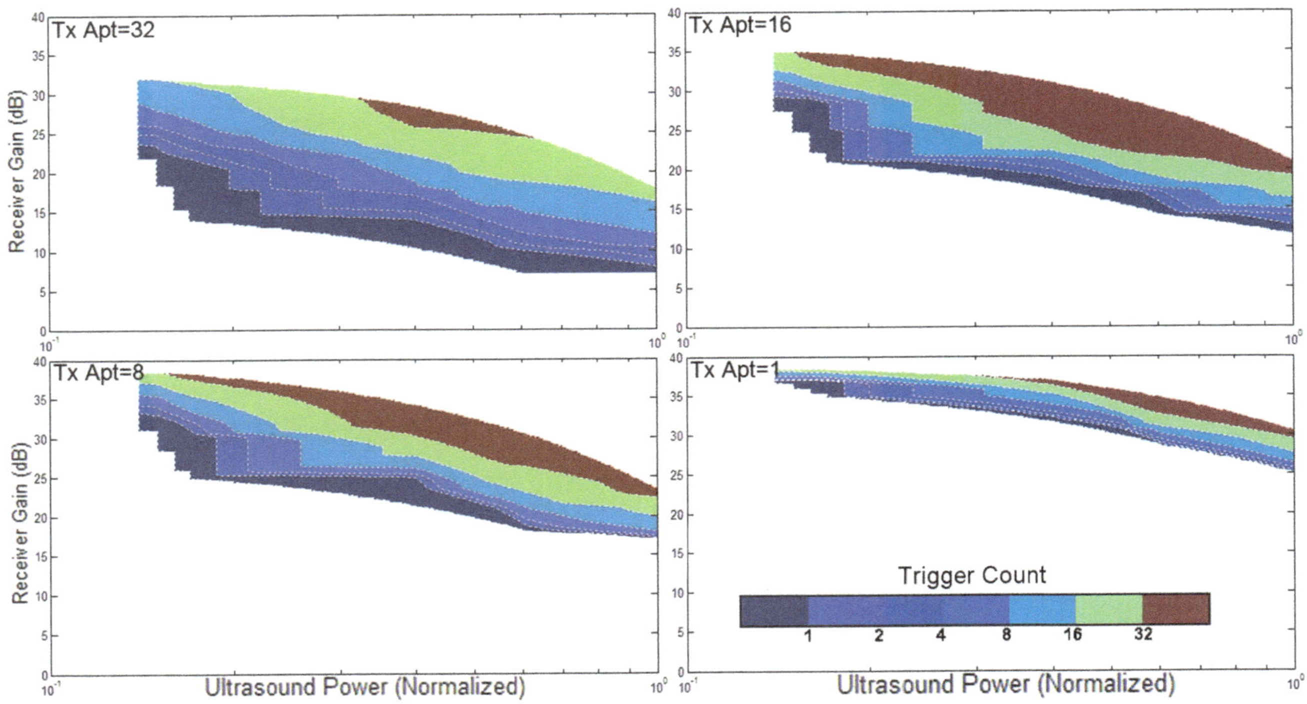

Figure 11. The trigger count versus ultrasound system settings. Catheter is parallel to the image plane. Ultrasound beams are not focused.

and f) shows the original active echo B-mode image and the result after template filtering. The waveform template of the active echo is acquired by subtracting the RF lines with and without active echo enabled.

3. Mid-plane detection

As discussed previously, either the peak signal amplitude or the trigger count can be used in mid-plane detection. Practically, in the trigger count method the AUSPIS starts to response the beacon pulse even if the AE element is not well aligned with the mid-plane, it provides a large detection range, which is useful for a quick target search before the accurate tool tip localization. Once

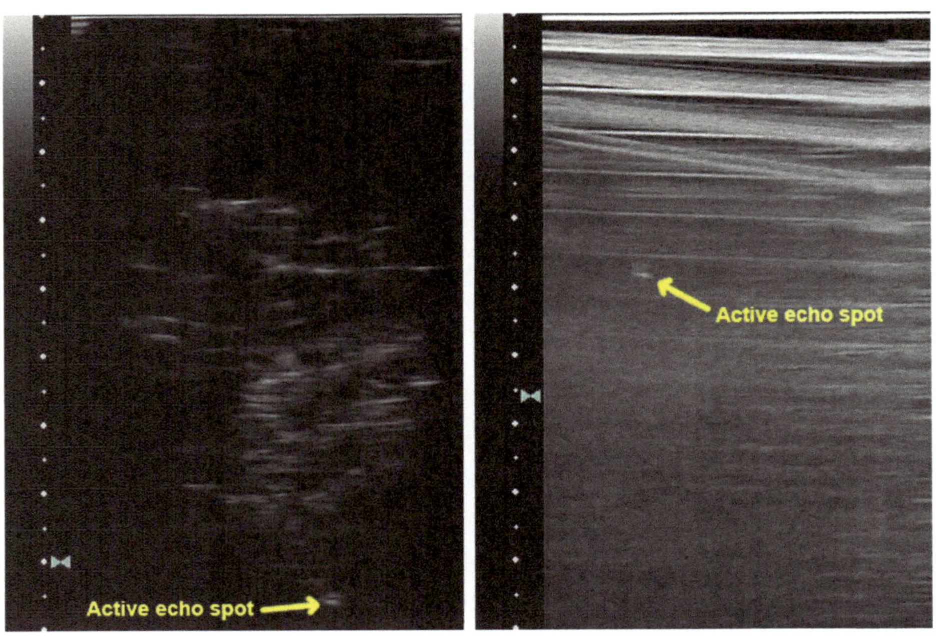

Figure 12. Large depth and impedance mismatching condition test result. Left: the active echo spot under 8.5 cm deep chicken breast tissue. Right: the active echo spot below a 1 inch thick aluminum plate.

the active echo signal is received, the peak signal amplitude method can be used for a more accurate alignment.

A typical trigger count versus AE element to mid-plane distance plot is shown in Figure 6. The data is acquired with a fixed AUSPIS receiver gain of 19 dB. The AE element is about 4 cm away from the probe. The US probe is running on its maximum transmission power with 32 element transmission aperture and 4 cm focus depth. In each frame the probe fires 256 RF lines. When the offset increases, the frame trigger count drops from the maximum 41 to 0 at an offset of 8 mm. The result indicates that, with these system parameter settings, the active echo detectable range is about ±8 mm from the mid-plane. The range can be increased or decreased by using higher or lower amplifier gain.

Once the AE element is triggered, the next step is to accurately align it to the mid-plane. Figure 7a, b shows the catheter received signal amplitude verses the imaging probe position. In the plot, the mid-plane position is indicated by the maximum of the signal amplitude. If the trigger level is set to a value close to the maximum, the active echo system can only be triggered when the element overlaps the mid-plane. For example, if a trigger is set to 90% of the maximum amplitude, a localizing accuracy of ±0.5 mm is expected from the Figure 7. In the water tank validation, the receiver gain is decreased until only one trigger per frame is achieved at the well aligned position. Then gradually move the catheter away from the mid-plane. At an offset of ±0.31 mm, the active echo spot disappears. The result is repeatable and stable over test runs. Using this method, a mid-plane localization accuracy of 0.3 mm can be achieved.

4. Insertion angle test

In the previous tests, the catheter is perpendicular to the imaging ultrasound beams. However, this condition is not always satisfied in clinical applications. An experiment is performed to validate the system performance when the catheter is inserted at an angle. Since the prototype active element has a cylindrical shape, the most sensitive configuration is the cylinder axis

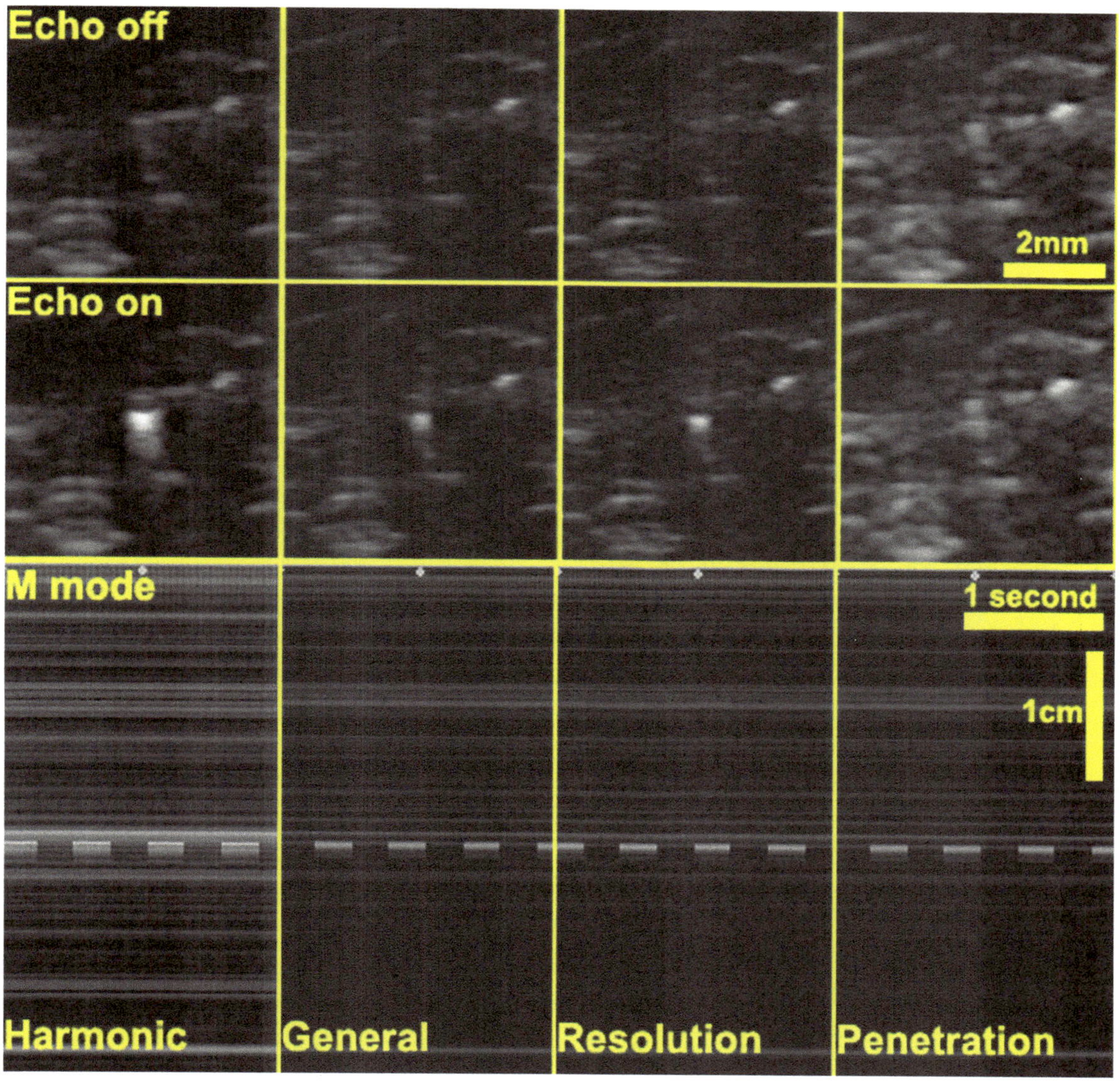

Figure 13. The B-mode and M-mode image of active echo spot using different imaging methods. The echo spot blinking can be clearly seen as a "dashed line" in the M-mode image. The blinking frequency is about 2 Hz.

Table 1. The SNR and CNR under different ultrasound imaging mode.

	Harmonic	General	Resolution	Penetration
CNR	5.93	4.65	5.10	1.92
SNR	5.66	4.35	4.77	1.78

perpendicular to the ultrasound beam, which is marked as 0° in the experiment. Keeping the element at the same location, the catheter rotates from −50° to 90° with 10° increment steps. Because the element is not an omnidirectional sensor, the received ultrasound pulse amplitude varies with the angle, so the receiver gain needs to be adjusted at different angles. The active echo performs properly at all angles we tested in the experiment. Because the catheter interferes with the ultrasound probe, we were not able to test at angles from −90 to −50 degrees.

5. Validation with different ultrasound powers, apertures, focuses, orientations, and gains

The triggering condition of the active echo system is mainly affected by two factors: the amount of acoustic power received by the active element, and the gain of the receiver. The former factor also relies on many parameters like the probe transmission power, transmission aperture, focusing, tissue attenuation, etc. An experiment is performed to investigate the working conditions of AUSPIS. In this experiment, the active echo element is aligned with the probe mid-plane in a water tank. An attenuation layer is placed between the probe and catheter to mimic tissue attenuation. The trigger count is recorded under different parameter settings. Shown in Figure 8–11, the color code indicates the trigger count per frame. Generally, to achieve the same trigger count, it requires more probe transmission power at lower receiver gain than at a higher gain. Larger transmission aperture delivers more acoustic power, thus resulting in a higher trigger count when other parameters are the same. Comparing the focusing and no focusing, the former one is relatively less sensitive to the receiver gain setting, i.e., the trigger count changes less when varying the gain. Take the figure 8 and 9 "Tx aperture = 32" as an example, the color bands between the contour lines are wider in 8a, which indicates that, within a larger range of receiver gain setting, the trigger count remains the same. This is because the focused beam has smaller beam width, when the ultrasound probe acquires a B-mode image frame, only the A-mode lines close to the element can trigger the active echo. Since the energy is spatially concentrated, less transmission power is required to trigger the active echo, so in the focused beam conditions, the functional zone (colored area) extends to lower gain area, as shown in figure 8. In the unfocused case, since the beams are wider and have more overlapping, the beams far away from the element may also trigger the echo, so the trigger count growths rapidly when increasing the gain. Similarly, smaller transmission aperture results in wider beam, the bands are narrower than that with the larger aperture. In the experiment, the data with a trigger count higher than 40 are discarded; that is why the colored area does not extend to the very high gain region in figure 8–11. Though it may be useful in the quick-tool-searching purpose, high gain with large trigger counts makes the active echo spot wide and distorted, which may result in an inaccurate tool indication in the original B-mode image.

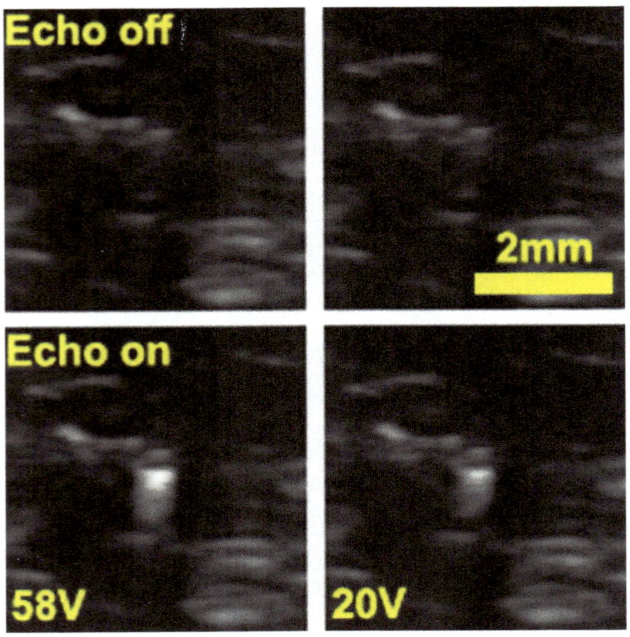

Figure 14. The active echo spot with different driving voltage. The left images are the active echo spot and the reference frame at 58 V driven voltage. In the right images, the driven voltage is reduced to 20 V. The echo intensity is dimmer on the right image; a lower SNR and CNR is expected.

6. Detection depth test

To further investigate the extreme functional conditions of the system, we performed two lab bench experiments. In the first one, we insert the catheter into ex vivo chicken breast tissue at 8.5 cm depth, which is close to the limit of the probe we use. This is to mimic the deep needle insertion in clinical operations. An ultrasound video is given in Video S1. In the second experiment, we placed a 1 inch thick aluminum plate in the water tank between the imaging probe and catheter to mimic the impedance of highly mismatched tissues like hard bone. As shown in figure 12, in both of the two experiments, the catheter can be effectively localized by the active echo spot. In the second test, since the speed of sound in the aluminum layer is much higher than that in water, the spot looks much closer than it actually is in the B-mode image.

7. Validation with different imaging modes

Most clinical ultrasound systems provide different imaging modes, like harmonic mode (or pulse inversion mode), high resolution mode, high penetration mode, etc., which also affect active echo system performance. Using the Sonix Touch system with a L14-5W linear probe, we tested the active echo under four modes: harmonic mode, general mode, resolution mode, and penetration mode. Videos of the ultrasound system display are given in Videos S2, S3, S4, and S5. In Harmonic mode, the ultrasound system transmits pulses with central frequency of 5 MHz, and reconstructs the B-mode image from the received

Table 2. The SNR and CNR with different driving pulse voltage.

	Pulse peak voltage = 58 V	Pulse peak voltage = 20 V
CNR	6.20	4.73
SNR	6.36	4.51

second harmonic (10 MHz) signals. In both general and resolution mode, the transmission frequency is 10 MHz; the difference is that in the resolution mode, the Rx frequency band is slightly higher than the general mode for better image resolution. In the penetration mode, the Tx frequency is reduced to 6.6 MHz to improve the penetration depth. We compared the signal to noise ratio (SNR) and contrast to noise ratio (CNR) of chicken breast tissue images using these imaging methods. The SNR is defined as:

$$SNR = \frac{DiffSignal_{avg}}{Background_{std}}$$

$$CNR = \frac{Signal_{avg} - SurroundingArea_{avg}}{Background_{std}}$$

where the "*DiffSignal*" is differential signal extracted by using the echo on frame subtracting the echo off frame, the "*background*" is the echo off frame, the "*SurroundingArea*" is a 50 by 50 pixel area around the active echo spot.

Comparing the B-mode images in figure 13, the harmonic-mode image has the most observable echo spot. This is expected since the harmonic imaging relies on the tissue harmonic echoes, the amplitude of which is much lower than that of the original pulses. The active echo element is configured to transmit at a frequency close to the second harmonic (10 MHz) in this experiment, so the active echo signal significantly stands out from the tissue harmonic background. The penetration-mode image has the least observable echo spot, in part because the active echo frequency (about 9 MHz) is out of the Rx frequency band in this mode. This observation is consistent with the SNR and CNR measurements, as shown in table 1. However, even in the penetration mode, though the active echo spot is not clear in the static images, it is easy for the human eye to capture the spot during the operation due to its blinking.

8. Validation with different AE transmission powers

Despite the imaging methods, the driving voltage of the element also affects the active echo spot visualization, since higher driving voltage results in stronger ultrasound. As shown in figure 14, with 20 V driving pulse, the echo spot is dimmer than that with 58 V driving pulse. However, since the B-mode image does not linearly represent the signal strength, we could not see the linear relationship in the CNR and SNR measurements, as shown in table 2.

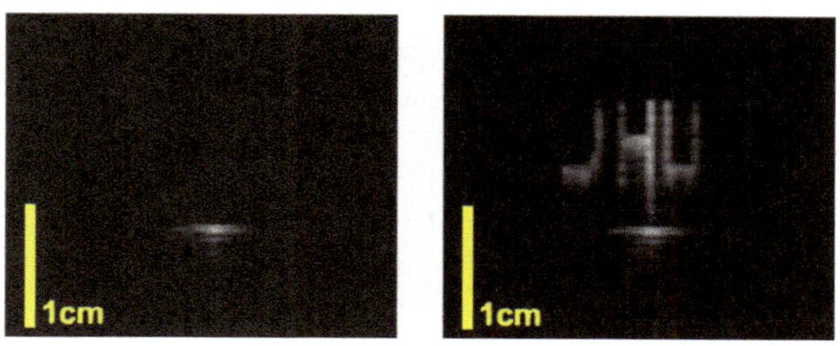

Figure 15. The B mode image of arbitrary pattern injection. The experiment is in a water tank with Sonix CEP machine and L12-5 linear probe. Left image is the reference without turning on the AUSPIS. On the right image, a virtual "JHU" pattern is injected to the image.

9. Arbitrary pattern Injection

Figure 15 shows an example of arbitrary pattern injection method. The left image is the reference, the B-mode image of the catheter in a water tank, and right is the image with the pattern injection system turned on. A virtual "JHU" pattern is shown in the B-mode image. A video is given in Video S6. In this image, the "pixel" that forms the pattern can be seen. Each pixel corresponds to one ultrasound pulse firing from the catheter. Method 1 mentioned in the pattern injection paragraph is used in this experiment. Ultrasound system synchronization trigger is utilized, and the pattern is injected into an absolute position in the image coordinate.

10. Mid-plane indication using pattern injection

In the previous paragraph, we introduced the method to detect the image mid-plane. The detection result can be directly displayed on the B-mode image using arbitrary pattern injection technique. As shown in figure 16, virtual bars that are proportional to the trigger count are injected into the image. With this real-time feedback, the operator can easily navigate the tool tip to the ultrasound image mid-plane, which is indicated by the maximum number of bars. Videos of this experiment are given in Videos S7, S8. This experiment is an implementation of method 2 mentioned in the pattern injection paragraph. Only the received signal is used for synchronization, and the pattern is injected into a relevant position moving with the active element in the image.

11. In vivo experiment

The in vivo experiment was performed on a pig. The catheter is inserted into the liver tissue. 3D Volumetric B-mode images are collected by a 3D wobbler probe 4DL14-5/38. Figure 17 shows the images of the liver tissue with the catheter inserted. In a) and b), the catheter incidents the B-mode image plane with a small angle. c) and d) has the catheter perpendicular with the image plane. Although the catheter is visible in these B-mode images due to its large diameter and small insertion angle, it is not very distinguishable from the tissue texture, as shown in figure 17 a). Also, it is difficult to identify the location of the element, especially in the condition of c). In figure 17 b) and d), the active echo is enabled. With the echo spot clearly shown in the image, it is easy to identify the catheter from the tissue, and locate the element position.

Discussion

The previous discussions are based on linear imaging arrays. For phased arrays, theoretically the active reflection, blinking and frequency modulation functions should have similar performance. The arbitrary pattern injection, however, works differently in the case of phased arrays or curved linear arrays due to the different image forming methods and parameters. How the system works with different type of probes is a future work to be investigated.

With single AE element, the AUSPIS provides 5 degrees of freedom to the probe, as shown in figure 18. It limits the image plane to intersect the AE element, which is a point. As a comparison, active beam-steering method constrains the image plane to intersect the catheter line, thus resulting in 4 degrees of

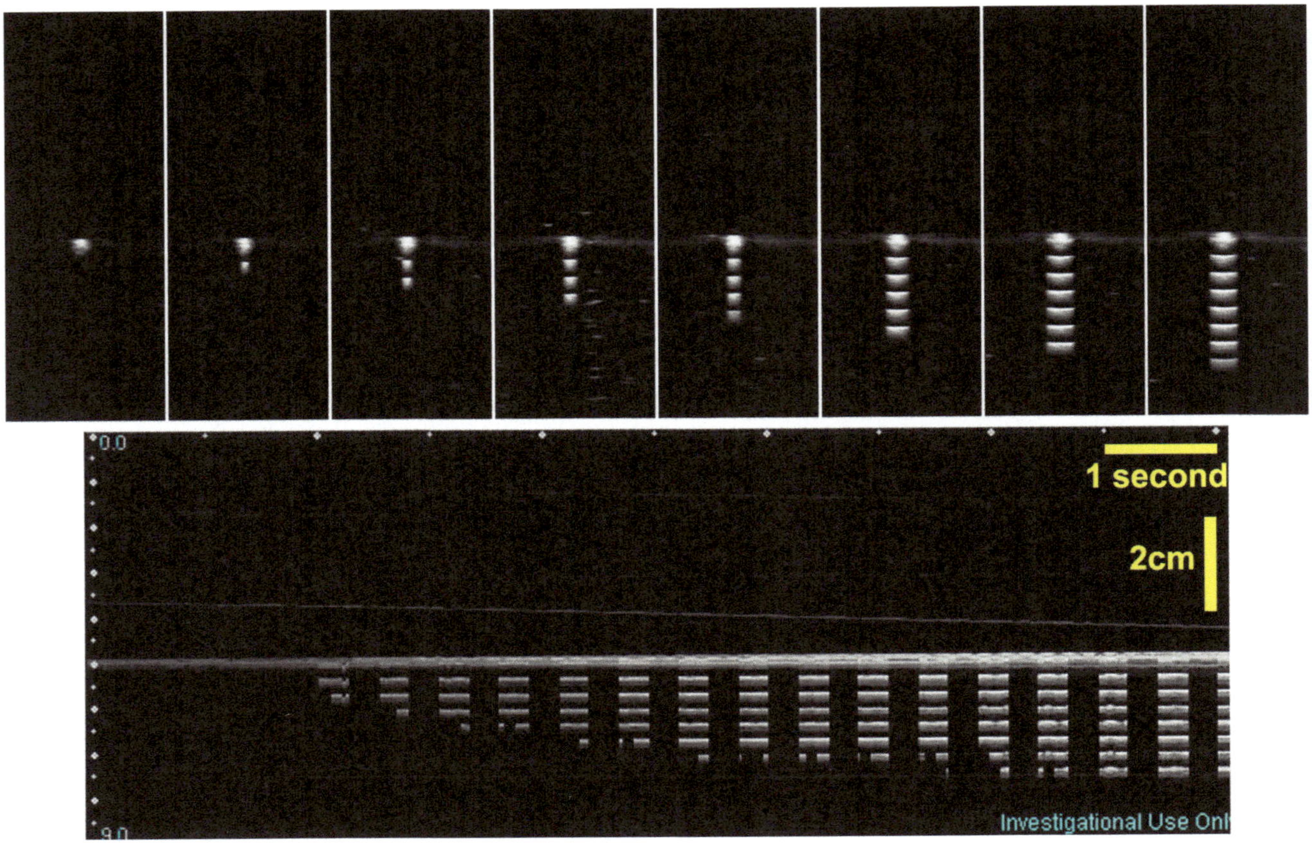

Figure 16. Mid-plane indication using the pattern injection method. The top column shows when the catheter moves closer to the mid-pane, the number of injected virtual bar increases. More bars means higher trigger count, thus indicating the catheter is closer to the mid-plane. The bottom picture shows an M-mode image acquired during the catheter moving in process.

freedom. In clinic, more DOFs mean less constraints on the probe position and orientation; this is especially important in applications like cardiac catheterization, in which doctors have to image from the very limited imaging window to avoid the ribs.

Like any other tracking system, AUSPIS has its limitations. This method is not able to localize the tool or project the insertion path when the AE element is far away from the ultrasound image plane. Using catheters with single AE element, the maximum detectable range in our experiments is around ± 12 mm from the mid-plane. However, for certain applications, it can be improved by integrating multiple AE elements at different locations of the tool. Moreover, using multiple active elements not only the tool position but also the pose can be tracked. Another limitation in the prototype system is the shape and size of the AE element. For easy assembling and wiring, the piezoelectric element we use is a 2×2 mm cylindrical tube. The localization accuracy is expected to improve by reducing the element size. Last but not least, the operation of AUSPIS is very different from existing tracking methods. Although we have demonstrated the concept in both ex

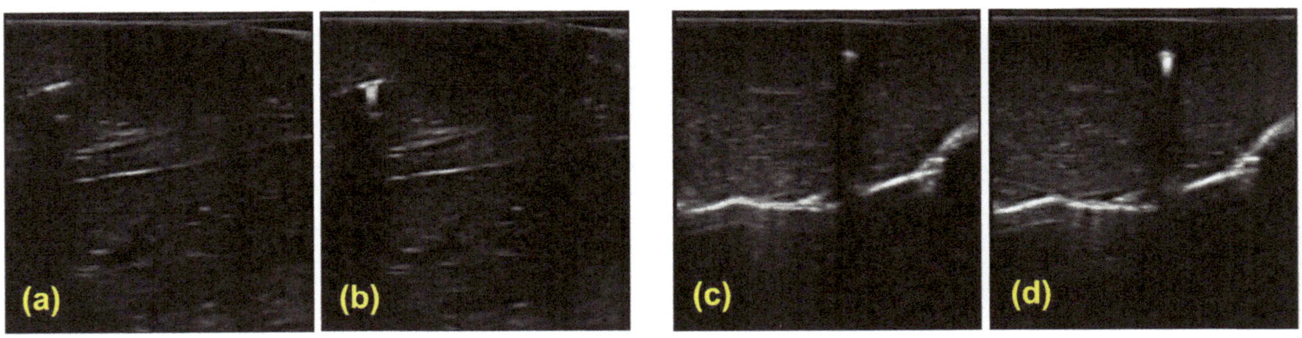

Figure 17. In vivo B-mode images extracted from the 3D volumetric data. The imaging array scans perpendicularly to the image plane with a step size of 0.5 mm. a–b) B mode images with the catheter in-plane. c–d) B mode images with the catheter perpendicular to the image plane. a) & c) Reference images with active element turned off. b) & d) images with the active echo spot.

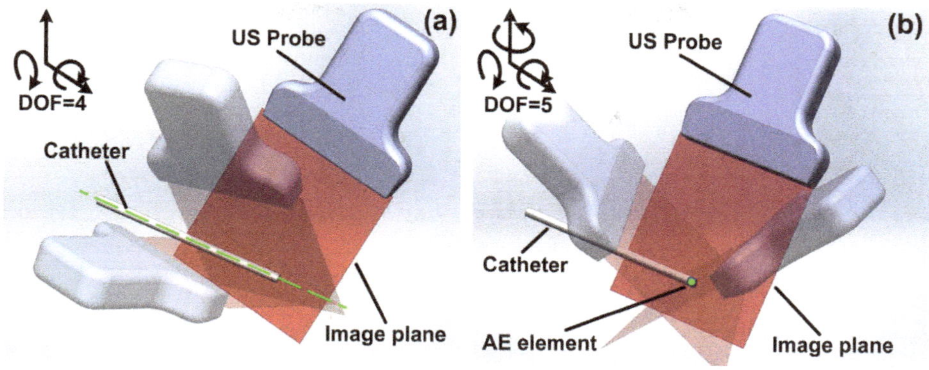

Figure 18. Degree of freedom (DOF) comparison between AUSPIS and beam steering method. a) Beam steering method requires the image plane to intersect the catheter line (the green line in figure a), the probe DOF is 4. b) The AUSPIS requires the image plane to intersect the AE element point (the green dot in figure b), the probe DOF is 5.

vivo and in vivo experiments, further study is needed to investigate how the technology can be integrated into the clinic workflow.

Conclusions

In summary, we introduced a new active ultrasound pattern injection method for interventional tool tracking, designed and built a prototype system, and performed preliminary ex vivo and in vivo experiment to prove feasibility. Significant visualization enhancement and highly accurate mid-plane localization have been achieved. Arbitrary pattern injection has been demonstrated. We also presented the study and analysis of the system operating under different configurations. Finally the limitations and future developments have been discussed.

Supporting Information

Video S1 The active echo spot under 8.5 cm deep chicken breast tissue.

Video S2 The active echo spot in the harmonic mode.

Video S3 The active echo spot in the general mode.

Video S4 The active echo spot in the resolution mode.

Video S5 The active echo spot in the penetration mode.

Video S6 A virtual "JHU" logo is injected into the B-mode image by a single active element on the catheter tip. The experiment is performed in a water tank.

Video S7 Using virtual pattern injection method to indicate the ultrasound mid-plane. The experiment is performed in a water tank.

Video S8 Using virtual pattern injection method to indicate the ultrasound mid-plane. The experiment is performed in ex vivo chicken breast tissue.

Acknowledgments

The authors thank Dr. Behnoosh Tavakoli and Alexis Cheng for technical assistance in the experiments.

Author Contributions

Conceived and designed the experiments: XG HK RE EB. Performed the experiments: XG HK RE EB. Analyzed the data: XG HK RE EB. Contributed reagents/materials/analysis tools: XG HK RE EB. Wrote the paper: XG HK RE EB.

References

1. Fishman JE, Milikowski C (2003) US-guided core-needle biopsy of the breast how many specimens are necessary. Radiology 226: 779–782.
2. Dodd GD III, Soulen MC, Kane RA, Livraghi T, Lees WR, et al. (2000) Minimally invasive treatment of malignant Hepatic Tumors: at the threshold of a major breakthrough. Radio Graphics 20: 9–27.
3. Harvey CJ, Albrecht T (2001) Ultrasound of focal liver lesions. Eur Radiol 11: 1578–1593.
4. Cheung S, Rohling R (2004) Enhancement of needle visibility in ultrasound-guided percutaneous procedures. Ultrasound in Med & Biol Vol. 30 No. 5 pp. 617–624.
5. Chan C, Lam F, Rohling R (2005) A needle tracking device for ultrasound guided percutaneous procedures. Ultrasound in Med & Biol Vol. 31 No. 11 pp. 1469–1483.
6. Krucker J, Xu S, Glossop N, Viswanathan A, Borgert J, et al. (2007) Electromagnetic tracking for thermal ablation and biopsy guidance: clinical evaluation of spatial accuracy. J Vasc Interv Radiol 18: 1141–1150.
7. Stoll J, Dupont P (2005) Passive Markers for Ultrasound Tracking of Surgical Instruments. MICCAI 2005 LNCS 3750 pp. 41–48.
8. Vilkomerson D, Lyons D (1997) A system for ultrasonic beacon-guidance of catheters and other minimally-invasive medical devices. IEEE Transactions on Ultrasonics, Ferroelectrics, and Frequency Control vol. 44 no. 1.
9. Merdes CL, Wolf PD (2001) Locating a catheter transducer in a three-dimensional ultrasound imaging field. IEEE Transactions on Biomedical Engineering vol. 48 no. 12.
10. Mung J, Vignon F, Jain A (2011) A Non-disruptive Technology for Robust 3D Tool Tracking for Ultrasound-Guided Interventions. MICCAI 2011 Part I LNCS 6891 pp. 153–160.
11. Simonetti F (2009) A guided wave technique for needle biopsy under ultrasound guidance. Proc of SPIE vol. 7261 726118-1.
12. Breyer B, Cikes I (1984) Ultrasonically marked catheter—A method for positive echo graphic catheter position identification. Med Biol Eng Comput vol. 22 pp. 268–271.

2

Auditory Conflict Resolution Correlates with Medial–Lateral Frontal Theta/Alpha Phase Synchrony

Samantha Huang[1]*, Stephanie Rossi[1], Matti Hämäläinen[1,2], Jyrki Ahveninen[1]

1 Harvard Medical School, Athinoula A. Martinos Center for Biomedical Imaging, Department of Radiology, Massachusetts General Hospital, Charlestown, Massachusetts, United States of America, 2 Harvard–MIT Division of Health Sciences and Technology, Cambridge, Massachusetts, United States of America

Abstract

When multiple persons speak simultaneously, it may be difficult for the listener to direct attention to correct sound objects among conflicting ones. This could occur, for example, in an emergency situation in which one hears conflicting instructions and the loudest, instead of the wisest, voice prevails. Here, we used cortically-constrained oscillatory MEG/EEG estimates to examine how different brain regions, including caudal anterior cingulate (cACC) and dorsolateral prefrontal cortices (DLPFC), work together to resolve these kinds of auditory conflicts. During an auditory flanker interference task, subjects were presented with sound patterns consisting of three different voices, from three different directions (45° left, straight ahead, 45° right), sounding out either the letters "A" or "O". They were asked to discriminate which sound was presented centrally and ignore the flanking distracters that were phonetically either congruent (50%) or incongruent (50%) with the target. Our cortical MEG/EEG oscillatory estimates demonstrated a direct relationship between performance and brain activity, showing that efficient conflict resolution, as measured with reduced conflict-induced RT lags, is predicted by theta/alpha phase coupling between cACC and right lateral frontal cortex regions intersecting the right frontal eye fields (FEF) and DLPFC, as well as by increased pre-stimulus gamma (60–110 Hz) power in the left inferior fontal cortex. Notably, cACC connectivity patterns that correlated with behavioral conflict-resolution measures were found during both the pre-stimulus and the pre-response periods. Our data provide evidence that, instead of being only transiently activated upon conflict detection, cACC is involved in sustained engagement of attentional resources required for effective sound object selection performance.

Editor: Lawrence M. Ward, University of British Columbia, Canada

Funding: This work was supported by National Institutes of Health Awards R01MH083744, R21DC010060, R21DC014134, R01HD040712, R01NS037462, and 5R01EB009048. This research was carried out at the Athinoula A. Martinos Center for Biomedical Imaging at the Massachusetts General Hospital, using resources provided by the Center for Functional Neuroimaging Technologies, P41EB015896, and a P41 Biotechnology Resource Grant supported by the National Institute of Biomedical Imaging and Bioengineering (NIBIB), National Institutes of Health. The research environment was additionally supported by National Center for Research Resources Shared Instrumentation Grants S10RR014978, S10RR021110, S10RR019307, S10RR014798, and S10RR023401. The funders had no role in study design, data collection and analysis, decision to publish, or preparation of the manuscript.

* Email: samhuang@nmr.mgh.harvard.edu

Introduction

Speech perception in everyday acoustic environments is a considerable computational challenge. When several persons speak at the same time, the spectrotemporal overlap of competing signals may hinder the segregation of the competing sound streams to form distinct perceptual objects (*i.e.*, object formation) [1]. Even if the relevant and irrelevant sounds can be perceptually grouped into distinct objects, similarity of these objects can make it difficult for the listener to direct attention to correct object in the auditory scene (*i.e.*, object selection) [1]. This could happen, for example, when one hears conflicting pieces of advice in an emergency situation, and the inherently most salient instead of most relevant object tends to prevail. While the top-down modulations of auditory neurons supporting perceptual object formation (for a review, see [2]) under the control of higher-order frontoparietal areas (for reviews, see [3,4]) have been documented, a paucity of information exists on how the higher-order brain regions work together to support selection of relevant sound objects amongst competing or conflicting sound objects.

The question about how different brain regions work together to select relevant objects while ignoring conflicting stimuli in a multitalker environment falls within the cognitive realm of conflict processing. In the visual domain, conflict processing has been intensively studied using the classic Flanker task [5], in which flanking distractor letters or arrows interfere with judgments about central target letters or target arrow direction, respectively. Much like in a multitalker setting where more salient voices can be assumed to complicate speech-object selection in the auditory domain [1], the more salient/numerous flankers significantly interfere with the selection of the relevant visual object and the motor responses associated with it. In addition to the Flanker task, other widely used conflict tasks include the Stroop color-word task [6], requiring the subject to identify the color of the letters instead of reading the word, and the Simon spatial compatibility task where a conflict arises when subjects need to respond with the hand opposite to the side of screen where a visual target appears [7]. A large body of evidence from human neuroimaging studies, using different tasks (although mainly visual) typically report activations in anterior cingulate cortex (ACC), lateral prefrontal cortices (PFC) (including dorsolateral PFC, DLPFC, and inferior frontal cortex, IFC), anterior insula (AI), and parietal cortices [8–14]. However, given the methodological limitations, such as the poor temporal resolution of the prevailing neuroimaging technique of fMRI, it is not completely clear how these regions work together as a functional network during conflict processing.

In order to disentangle specific processes and mechanisms that underlie attentional control during conflict resolution, it is necessary to use imaging tools with high temporal resolution, such as magnetoencephalography (MEG) and EEG that provide a direct measure of post-synaptic neuronal processes. Findings from event-related potential (ERP) studies using various conflict tasks suggest that the components N200 (also known as N2) [15] and N450 [16] are related to stimulus-level conflict, while the error-related negativity (ERN) component [15] reflects response-level conflict (for a review, see [17]). A limitation of such conventional ERP analyses are that task-modulated non-phase-locked "induced" dynamics of EEG data are not-present trial-averaged responses, and that they do not allow inferences of interregional dynamics during conflict processing [18]. However, accumulating evidence suggests that functional coupling across distant brain areas during attention and cognitive control can be explicitly quantified based on interregional phase locking of neuronal oscillations [19,20], occurring at distinct frequency ranges. It appears that low-frequency (<30 Hz) oscillations at the theta (4–7 Hz), alpha (7–15 Hz), and beta (15–30 Hz) ranges are particularly relevant for longer-range coupling associated with top-down modulation of neurons [21–23]. Evidence from human studies suggests that such coupling may be enhanced in task-relevant networks during auditory attention [24], as well as visually-delivered working memory [25] and conflict-processing tasks [26,27]. It has been also noninvasively shown that, during auditory orienting, interregional interactions at the gamma band are modulated by the phase of theta in humans [28]. As suggested by extracellular measurements in cats [29] and human MEG studies [30], inter-regional phase locking may also increase at the beta band during attention and/or cognitive control tasks.

Previous auditory fMRI studies suggest that ACC is essential for selective attention to task-relevant sound features [31,32] and auditory feedback monitoring [33]. It is specifically activated when the subject is asked to pay attention selectively to one of two dichotically presented phonemes and ignore a simultaneously presented competing stimulus [34]. However, only a small number of auditory behavioral [35,36] and neuroimaging [32,34] studies on perceptual conflicts have been conducted in the auditory domain, especially at the early stage of object identification and selection, that is, the stimulus conflict. Here, we therefore tested the hypothesis that ACC may also support selective listening in complex auditory settings such as multitalker environments. To achieve this goal, we used non-invasive estimates of neuronal oscillations [24,37,38] to investigate the ACC and DLPFC oscillatory phase locking patterns predicting fast and efficient conflict processing using a modified auditory flanker interference task, in which participants were required to identify a spoken "A" or "O" from acoustically similar or distinct flankers. Source localization of neuronal oscillations was facilitated by using anatomical MRI constraints to limit the potential solutions to the cortical gray matter [39,40], where non-invasively measurable MEG and EEG activities are generated [41], and by combining the complementary information provided by simultaneously measured MEG and EEG [42]. A priori regions of interest (ROIs) including the caudal ACC (cACC) and DLPFC in each hemisphere were first defined based on the Desikan-Killiany atlas [43]. The cACC seed roughly corresponded to the anterior mid-cingulate cortex area that has also been termed "dorsal ACC" in previous conflict processing studies [44]. Seed-based oscillatory phase locking estimates between these ROIs and all cortical locations were then calculated using the debiased weighted phase lag index (wPLI), to test the specific hypothesis that conflict processing is associated with increased cortico-cortical low-frequency phase locking between ACC and lateral prefrontal regions.

Materials and Methods

Participants

The study protocol was approved by the Partners Human Research Committee, the Institutional Review Board (IRB) of the Massachusetts General Hospital. Potential subjects were first screened with a phone interview to ensure that they had normal hearing and had not been exposed regularly to environments with excessively loud noise. Twelve right-handed college-level educated adults with normal hearing and no neurological disorders, psychiatric conditions, or learning disabilities, gave written informed consent prior to testing.

Task and stimuli

During MEG/EEG acquisitions, subjects ($N = 12$, age 20–33 years, 6 females) were presented with an auditory spatial-phonetic flanker interference task modified based on previous psychoacoustic studies [35] (**Figure 1**). Each sound trial, presented at a randomly varying inter-trial onset interval of 2.95–3.05 s, included two 400 ms "flankers" simulated horizontally from 45° to the right and left using generic head-related transfer functions [45], and a 400 ms target sound coming from straight ahead that started 300 ms after the flankers. The delay was introduced to the target, as very few subjects were able to discriminate the target from simultaneous flankers. The setting was thus analogous to certain previous visuospatial flanker studies [46,47], with the additional delay being also justified because of the serial nature of phonetic sound-object processing [48]. The flankers and targets consisted of a voice sounding out the American English letters "A" or "O", obtained from the Psychology Experiment Building Language (PEBL) Sound Archive version 0.1. The pitch of the flankers was digitally manipulated to be 3.1 semitones lower or higher than the target, such that the listener always heard three sounds coming from three different directions at three different pitches. Equiprobably, the subject heard either a congruent set of voices ("A_{Left}-A_{Middle}-$A_{\mathbf{Right}}$" or "O_{Left}-O_{Middle}-O_{Right}") or an incongruent/conflicting set of voices ("A_{Left}-O_{Middle}-A_{Right}" or "O_{Left}-A_{Middle}-O_{Right}"). In all trials, subjects were instructed to ignore the flanking distractors and pay attention only to the middle target by pressing a button with the index finger of one hand if the target was "A" and with the index finger of the opposite hand if the target was "O". The hand/target letter order was switched after each of two 16-minute runs (324 trials per run), in an counterbalanced order across the subjects. Subjects' responses were recorded together with the MEG/EEG raw data and reaction time (RT) was measured from the moment of the target appearance to the moment of button pressing. Two subjects were excluded from the final MEG/EEG analyses because they could not perform the tasks.

Data acquisition

We recorded 306-channel MEG (Elekta-Neuromag, Helsinki, Finland) and 74-channel EEG data simultaneously in a magnetically shielded room (sampling rate 1 kHz, passband 0.03–330 Hz). The average reference was utilized for all analyses of

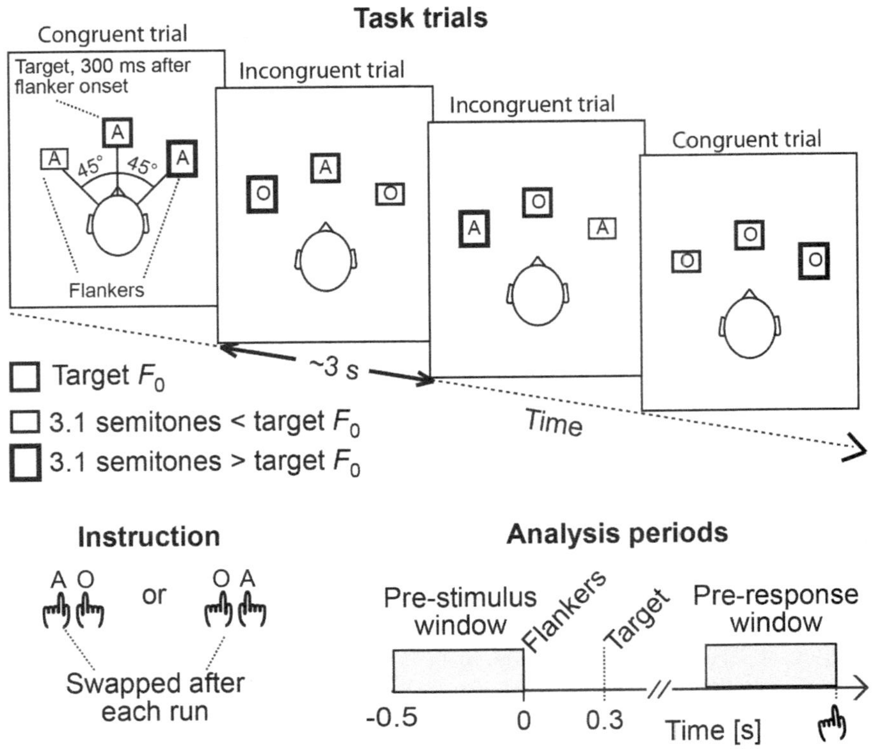

Figure 1. Task design and oscillatory analysis periods. *Task trials*: Subjects were instructed to pay attention to the target sounds and ignore flanking distractor sounds, which were phonetically either congruent (50%) or conflicting (50%) with the target. The flankers arrived 45° to the right and left of the target, at a 3.1 semitones lower or higher pitch than the target. *Instruction*: In a counterbalanced order across runs/subjects, subjects were asked to press a button either with the left index finger to "A" and with the right index finger to "O", or vice versa. *Analysis periods*: To determine oscillatory power and phase locking patterns that predict efficient conflict processing, the analyses were concentrated on the time periods that preceded each stimulus trial ("Pre-stimulus window") and each behavioral response ("Pre-response window").

EEG data. The position of the head relative to the MEG sensor array was monitored continuously using four head position indicator (HPI) coils attached to the scalp. Electrooculogram (EOG) was also recorded to monitor eye artifacts. T1-weighted structural MRIs were obtained for combining anatomical and functional data using a multi-echo MPRAGE pulse sequence (TR = 2510 ms; 4 echoes with TEs = 1.64 ms, 3.5 ms, 5.36 ms, 7.22 ms; 176 sagittal slices with $1 \times 1 \times 1$ mm^3 voxels, 256×256 mm^2 matrix; flip angle = 7°). Multi-echo FLASH data were obtained with 5° and 30° flip angles (TR = 20 ms, TE = 1.89+2n ms [n = 0–7], 256×256 mm^2 matrix, 1.33-mm slice thickness) for reconstruction of head boundary-element models (BEM).

Data analysis

Neuronal bases of auditory conflict processing were studied using a cortically constrained MEG/EEG MNE approach [24,38]. The MNE method reconstructs the intracranial sources of activity by identifying the distribution of dipoles with minimum total power that accounts for the magnetic field distribution recorded over the scalp. The cortically constrained approach takes into account the shape of the cortex and thus provides a better spatial resolution than an MNE only confined to the intracranial volume [39,40]. Our overall workflow consists of (i) preprocessing of the MEG/EEG data (removal of artifacts and estimation of noise covariance matrix), (ii) preprocessing of the anatomical MRI data (reconstruction of the cortical surface to set up individual MEG/EEG source space, and the reconstruction of the scalp, outer skull, and inner skull surfaces), (iii) alignment of the MEG and MRI coordinate frames and computing forward solutions, and (iv) computing the MNE inverse operator for source estimates.

External MEG noise was suppressed and subject movements, estimated continuously at 200-ms intervals, were compensated for using the signal-space separation method [49] (Maxfilter, Elekta-Neuromag, Helsinki, Finland). The MEG/EEG data were down-sampled (333 samples/s, passband 0.5–110 Hz). Epochs coinciding with over 150 µV EOG, 100 µV EEG, 2 pT/cm MEG gradiometer, or 4 pT MEG magnetometer peak-to-peak signals were excluded from further analyses.

For building the cortically constrained source space, we used FreeSurfer 5.3 [50] (http://surfer.nmr.mgh.harvard.edu/) to determine the shapes of the surfaces separating the scalp, skull, and brain compartments, and to build the triangular cortical surface mesh from T1-weighted anatomical 3D-volume MRI data by exploiting the gray-white matter boundary generated by the software. The FreeSurfer software was used due to the following advantages [50–52]: first, in addition to folded surfaces, it also computes inflated and flattened representations of the cortex, and can thus expose the parts of the cortex embedded in the sulci. Further, it provides an automated parcellation of the cortex that can be used in inquiring source waveforms in specific ROI. Finally, an additional benefit of the surface-based analysis is that cortical surfaces can be aligned across individuals for the computation of group statistics using a morphing procedure in a spherical coordinate system [50] and several recent studies have shown that the method has the highest stability in gray matter volume estimate compared to two other volume-based methods [53], and better alignments of cortical landmarks than volume-based registrations [54]. To achieve sufficient anatomical detail for the visualization of the folded cortical mantle, the triangular tessellations of each hemisphere contain roughly 100,000 potential vertices, spaced at ~1 mm. For inverse computations, the dense triangulations were decimated to ~1,000 vertices per hemisphere for computational efficiency.

To calculate MRI-guided depth-weighted ℓ_2 MNE [55], the information from structural segmentation of the individual MRIs and the MEG sensor and EEG electrode locations were used to compute the forward solutions for all putative source locations in the cortex using a three-compartment BEM [55].

The covariance matrix and the forward solution computed in the previous procedures were used to obtain a distributed cortically constrained minimum-norm inverse operator that relates the sensor measurements to dipole current estimates in the source space. The individual forward solutions for current dipoles placed at these vertices comprised the columns of the gain matrix (**A**). A noise covariance matrix (**C**) was estimated from the raw MEG/EEG data during a 20–200-ms pre-stimulus baseline. These two matrices, along with the source covariance matrix (**R**), were used to calculate the MNE inverse operator $\mathbf{W} = \mathbf{RA}^T (\mathbf{ARA}^T + \mathbf{C})^{-1}$, which is applied to the sensor-level data to yield the source time courses.

To investigate seed-based cortico-cortical phase locking patterns, the entire MEG/EEG raw data time series at each time point were multiplied by the inverse operator **W** and noise normalized to yield the estimated source activity as a function of time across the entire cortex [40]. In addition, the frontal seed regions, including cACC and DLPFC, were selected from each hemisphere using the Freesurfer anatomical atlas [43]. The DLPFC was, specifically, defined based on the "rostral middle-frontal cortex" label [43], which encompasses the junction of Brodmann's areas 9, 10, and 46 [56]. An average raw data time course was then calculated within these seed regions, with the waveform signs of sources aligned on the basis of surface-normal orientations to avoid phase cancellations.

Accepted MEG/EEG trial epochs were analyzed using the MNE and MNE-Python [57], and FieldTrip tools (http://www.ru.nl/fcdonders/fieldtrip). To investigate the phase locking between the cACC and DLPFC seed regions and all cortical locations, a FFT with Hanning window was applied on (**a**) the raw data epochs in each vertex of the right and left hemisphere and (**b**) on the corresponding trials of the pooled raw time courses of the right and left seed regions, separately for the 500-ms periods preceding each sound triplet and each behavioral response. Our presumption was that long-range inter-regional phase locking patterns would occur in theta and alpha, and lower beta ranges. Therefore, the FFT was applied at 2-Hz intervals at 6–20 Hz at the 500-ms windows and a Hanning taper. The 500-ms window length was selected on the basis of the RT data, such that the analysis window would not overlap with the target sound onset. We then calculated the phase locking between the seeds and each vertex the left and right hemisphere using the debiased wPLI. In addition to controlling for the sample-size bias, the debiased wPLI provides an index of nonzero phase lags across the regions/locations of interest that helps avoid spurious inflation of synchronization indices due to EEG and MEG point spread and crosstalk [58]. The resulting seed-based debiased wPLI estimates, mapped across all cortical locations in each subject, were then normalized to the Freesurfer standard brain representation for surface-based group statistical analyses [59].

In addition to the main analysis concentrating on the seed-based phase locking, we also estimated the power of neuronal oscillations across the available band during 500-ms pre-stimulus and pre-response periods, using a FFT with a Hanning taper at 2-Hz intervals between 4 and 30 Hz and an adaptive time-window of 3 cycles. At 30–110 Hz, 3-Hz frequency smoothing was used, resulting in three orthogonal Slepian tapers being applied to the 500-ms time window [60]. Analogous to [38], the available frequency band was divided to consecutive one-octave wide sub ranges, which corresponded to theta (4–7.5 Hz), alpha (7.5–15 Hz), beta (15–30 Hz), lower gamma (30–60 Hz), and higher gamma (60–110 Hz) bands (*i.e.*, the highest band was less than one octave).

Statistical analysis

RT and hit rate (HR) differences were analyzed using t-tests. The HR distributions were cubically and the RT distributions logarithmically transformed to render them approximately Gaussian [61], as confirmed by using the Jarque-Bera test. To test our specific hypotheses, we examined correlations between behavioral performance (RT to incongruent normalized by the RT to congruent trials) *vs.* cortical phase locking and power changes during periods preceding stimulus presentation and during the 500-ms period preceding the behavioral responses. For the pre-stimulus analyses, we calculated the correlations between the baseline preceding the incongruent trials and the normalized RT conflict effect. For the pre-response analyses, a 2×2 factorial design was utilized to control for the effects of responding hand (right *vs.* left) and task type (incongruent *vs.* congruent). To control for multiple comparisons, the resulting statistical estimates were tested against an empirical null distribution of maximum cluster size across 10,000 iterations with a vertex-wise threshold of $P<0.05$ and cluster-forming threshold of $P<0.05$ (Bonferroni corrected by the number of hemispheres), yielding clusters corrected for multiple comparisons across the surface.

Results

The behavioral analyses showed a significant conflict effect, demonstrating that the task was functioning as anticipated. RTs to the incongruent trials were significantly longer than those to the congruent trials ($t_9 = 7.5$, $p<0.001$; mean ± SD $RT_{Congruent} = 569 \pm 116$ ms; mean ± SD $RT_{Incongruent} = 637 \pm 118$ ms), and HRs were significantly lower to the incongruent than congruent trials ($t_9 = -3.2$, $p = 0.01$; mean ± SD $HR_{Congruent} = 98 \pm 2\%$; mean ± SD $HR_{Incongruent} = 95 \pm 4\%$).

Seed-based phase locking patterns correlating with behavioral conflict processing

Our main purpose was to examine cortico-cortical functional connectivity patterns that predict efficient behavioral performance during the modified auditory flanker task. This analysis concentrated on two distinct time periods, preceding the stimulus trials and preceding each behavioral response that followed the stimuli. **Figure 2** shows estimates of "sustained" baseline connectivity patterns, which predicted fast and efficient conflict processing, i.e., reduced RT lags, in the subsequent stimulus trials. Significant correlations ($p<0.05$, cluster-based Monte Carlo simulation test) between reduced RT lags and increased phase locking patterns (debiased wPLI) were observed at the theta range (6 Hz) between the right cACC and right lateral frontal regions, including FEF. Reduced conflict-induced RT lags also correlated with increased theta/alpha connectivity between cACC and medial frontal cortex regions bilaterally at 6 Hz, and between the right cACC and left medial/superior frontal cortex at 8 Hz. Note that in this case the connectivity patterns are unlikely to be explained by biases caused

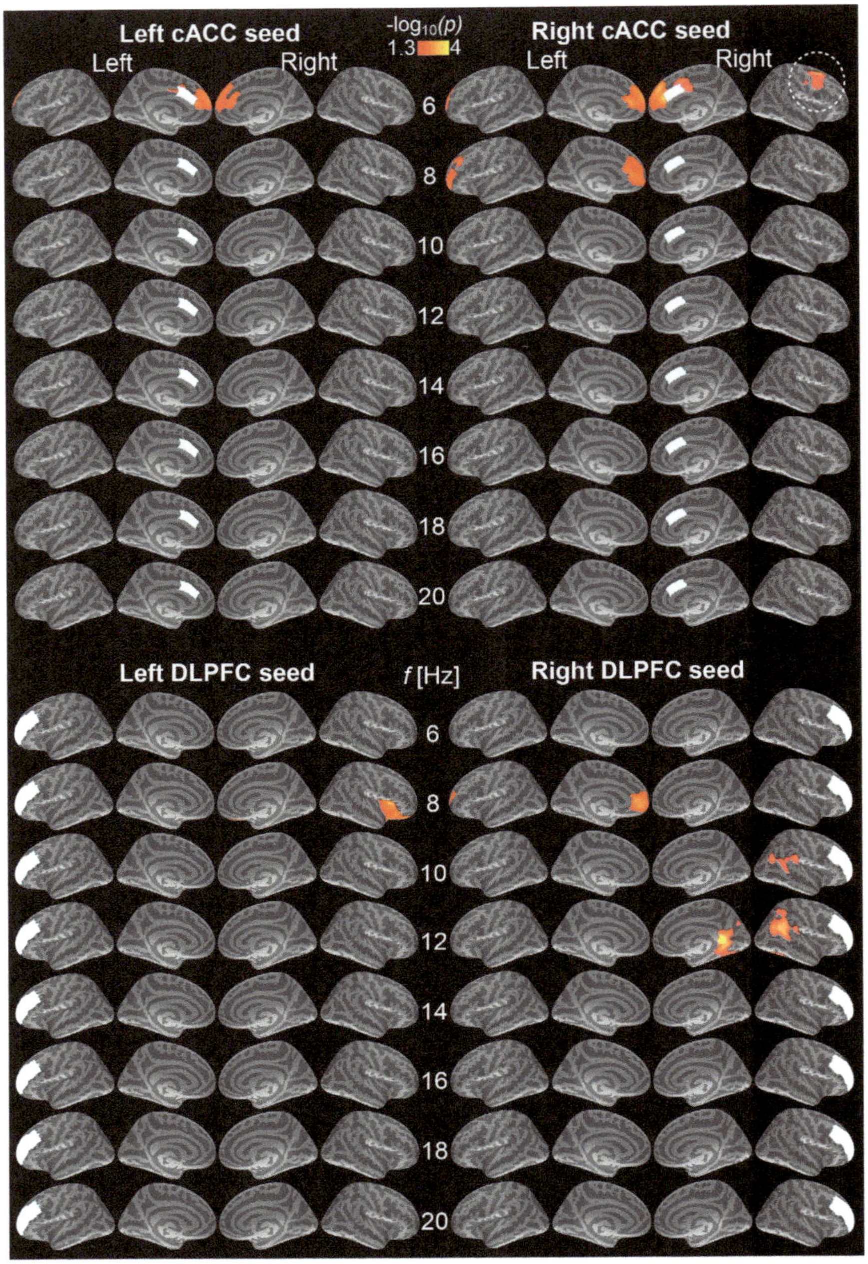

Figure 2. Baseline correlations between conflict-induced RT lags and cortical phase locking to the caudal anterior cingulate (cACC) and dorsolateral prefrontal cortex (DPLPC) seeds during 500-ms periods preceding conflicting trials. All significant findings reflect correlations between reduced RT lags and increased seed-based phase locking patterns ($p<0.05$, cluster-based Monte Carlo simulation test). (Top) Left and right cACC seed data. Interestingly, at 6 Hz (i.e., theta), faster RTs after conflicting sounds correlated with increased connectivity between the right cACC and right lateral prefrontal areas (encircled), and between bihemispheric cACC seeds and adjacent medial frontal cortex locations. (Bottom) Left and right DLPFC seed data. Faster RTs after incongruent trials were strongly correlated with increased alpha phase locking between the right DLPFC and right retrosplenial (12 Hz) and inferior parietal/TPJ regions (10–12 Hz), as well as at 8 Hz, between the left DLPFC and right anterior insula and between right DLPFC and left anteromedial frontal cortex. The results reflect $-\log_{10}(p)$ of the initial *t*-statistics, masked to the locations where the cluster-based Monte Carlo simulation test was significant ($p<0.05$).

by the anatomical adjacency, i.e., EEG/MEG point spread and cross talk, because the debiased wPLI index emphasizes synchronization patterns with nonzero phase lags [58].

During the pre-stimulus baseline period, the strongest behavioral correlations involving the DLPFC seed connectivity patterns were observed at the alpha range (10–12 Hz): Reduced RT lags associated with incongruent trials correlated with increased phase locking between the right DLPFC and right inferior parietal/temporoparietal junction (TPJ), as well as the right retrosplenial cortices. In addition, analogous behavioral correlations were observed with increased 8-Hz phase locking between the left DLPFC and right anterior insula as well as with phase locking between the right DLPFC and left anterior medial frontal cortex. **Table 1** shows the details of the cluster statistics reflecting correlations between the conflict-induced RT lags and the phase

Table 1. Correlations between RT lags caused by conflict and seed-based phase locking patterns during the pre-stimulus baseline period.

Target hemisphere	Seed	f [Hz]	Max value	Size (mm²)	x_{MNI}	y_{MNI}	z_{MNI}	Cluster-wise *P*	Anatomical coverage
Left									
	Left cACC								
		6	−2.2	3922	−8	58	17	0.0022	Superior frontal
	Right cACC								
		6	−2.4	4118	−5	38	8	0.0017	Medial frontal
		8	−2.2	6661	−6	35	8	0.0001	Medial frontal
	Right DLPFC								
		8	−2.4	3347	−7	42	2	0.0116	Medial frontal
Right									
	Left cACC								
		6	−2.0	3149	9	41	35	0.0111	Superior frontal
	Right cACC								
		6	−3.0	4605	6	33	18	0.0001	Medial frontal
		6	−2.3	3126	27	8	47	0.0112	Lateral prefrontal
	Left DLPFC								
		8	−2.5	3657	26	12	−17	0.0047	Anterior insula, IFC, orbitofrontal
	Right DLPFC								
		10	−1.9	2930	47	−35	28	0.0155	TPJ/inferior parietal
		12	−3.7	4975	14	−48	3	0.0001	Retrosplenial/precuneus
		12	−2.8	5534	44	−54	23	0.0001	IPS, TPJ/inferior parietal

Monte Carlo simulation results of the data in **Fig. 2** are demonstrated. The maximum values of initial GLM reflect $-\log10(p)\times \mathrm{sign}(t)$.

locking differences after incongruent vs. congruent stimuli, as measured from the 500-ms periods preceding each stimulus.

Figure 3 shows the results reflecting efficient conflict processing, during the post-stimulus/pre-response period, as estimated from a full factorial model estimating the correlations between the RT lags to incongruent vs. congruent trials and phase locking differences after incongruent vs. congruent stimuli. Most importantly, consistent with the hypothesis that efficient conflict processing depends on cingulofrontal connectivity, we found that reduced conflict-induced RT lags correlated with increased 8-Hz alpha phase locking between the bilateral cACC seeds and right lateral prefrontal regions. In the right lateral prefrontal cortex, these behavioral correlation patterns encompassed the likely location of right FEF, associated with the dorsal attention network, and the right DLPFC. In addition, behavioral correlations emerged with increased phase locking between the following regions: the left cACC and right medial parietal cortex at 12 Hz, left DLPFC and left superior/medial pre- and post-central regions at 8 Hz, and right DLPFC seed and right superior frontal gyrus regions at 18 Hz.

Figure 4 highlights the effects, concentrating on the theta/alpha phase locking between the cACC seeds and right lateral frontal cortices before (at 6 Hz) and after the occurrence of the conflicting information (at 8 Hz), which predict efficient/fast conflict processing performance. In addition to the significant behavioral correlations, the data in **Figure 4** also show that when the contribution of behavioral performance has been removed from the model, during the post-stimulus/pre-response period of the main contrast, a significant ($p<0.05$, cluster-based Monte Carlo simulation test) decrease of debiased wPLI between the cACC and right lateral frontal regions is observed after the incongruent vs. congruent trials. This leaves room for an interpretation that the occurrence of a conflicting information has a tendency to disrupt an existing phase locking pattern between the cACC and lateral frontal cortex, rather than eliciting a new functional connectivity pattern, and that the resolution of a conflict depends on the restoration of the sustained functional coupling between the medial and lateral frontal regions. **Table 2** shows the cluster statistics of correlations between conflict-induced RT lags and connectivity patterns emerging during the 500-ms periods preceding each behavioral response.

Cortical power mapping patterns correlating with behavioral conflict resolution

Finally, we also correlated behavioral measures with cortical power mapping results during the same time periods that were examined in the functional connectivity analyses. These analyses revealed a significant correlation between increased left lateral prefrontal cortex high-gamma power (60–110 Hz) during the pre-stimulus baseline period and reduced conflict-induced RT lags (**Figure 5**). No significant correlations emerged in the other frequency bands during the baseline period, or in any frequency band during the period preceding the behavioral responses.

Discussion

We studied seed-based oscillatory phase locking patterns associated with conflict processing during an auditory flanker interference task. Consistent with our hypothesis, the results demonstrate that efficient conflict resolution during sound object selection, as measured with reduced conflict-induced RT lags, is predicted by theta/alpha phase coupling between the cACC and right lateral frontal cortex regions intersecting FEF and DLPFC. Notably, the correlation patterns observed were not fully consistent with a hypothesis that cACC is a region only transiently recruited to detect conflicting coactivations of information processing streams. On the contrary, our statistical model showed that, when the variability of behavioral performance was regressed out, the occurrence of conflict actually disrupts the sustained connectivity between the cACC and lateral frontal regions. Our results, thus, seem to suggest that the cACC is involved in networks that bias processing of task-relevant sound information in situations requiring sustained engagement of control mechanisms.

It is generally agreed that cognitive control utilizes a network of brain regions including DLPFC, ACC, and posterior parietal regions [62]. Further, an emerging view is that discrete areas process information in a coordinated manner rather than as distinct modules [63]. Coordinated activity between neurons in different networks and brain regions may be mediated by spike synchrony with local field potential (LFP) oscillations [64] as well as synchrony of LFP oscillations, which provide windows of time when the effectiveness of a proximal spike on a distal neuron's postsynaptic potential is enhanced [20,63,65]. Our finding of the cACC phase-locked with the FEF and portions of DLPFC in theta/alpha band during conflict resolution is in line with this proposal, and further demonstrates a functional correlation of cognitive control processes and oscillatory theta-band activity between the ACC, the FEF, and the DLPFC.

Our results that the ability to allocate attention to relevant sound objects and disregard those with conflicting information correlates with cACC connectivity with lateral frontal cortices are consistent with previous studies that link cACC with conflict processing [66–68], error-related reinforcement learning [69], selection of goal-directed actions [70], and allocation of attentional resources [71,72]. Although most previous studies consider vision, there is an abundance of evidence that ACC also plays a role in auditory attention and cognitive control [12,31–33]. For example, there is evidence [73] that conflict-related EEG activations, which presumably originate in ACC [74], correlate with the degree of ambiguity of choice-tasks trials that do not involve actual conflicts. This suggests that the underlying circuits might also contribute to disambiguation of complex stimulus scenes. Further, conflict-related mid frontal theta oscillations have been previously identified in a number of EEG studies [27,75]. By exploiting the temporal and spatial resolution of combined MEG/EEG methods and anatomical MRI, our findings provide convincing evidence regarding the source of the mid frontal theta, as well as its involvement in early stage of perceptual processing before the response selection. Importantly, our findings extend previous literature and show that the functional network involving cACC, FEF, and DLPFC, not only monitors instantaneous occurrences of conflicts, but also exerts sustained attentional control needed for the selection of relevant sound objects in complex auditory environments.

During the post-stimulus/pre-response period, most significant correlations with cACC theta/alpha phase locking patterns emerged in the right FEF. Accumulating evidence suggests that the right FEF is a key part of the dorsal attention network (DAN) that governs voluntary deployment of spatial attention to task-relevant locations (for a review, see [76]), and this area could also be associated with auditory spatial attention [77]. Recent neurophysiological studies in non-human primates further suggest that FEF initiates top-down signals that helps bias saliency maps in posterior parietal cortices (e.g., in the monkey homologue of human intraparietal sulcus, IPS) that prioritize stimuli occurring in task relevant locations [78]. One might therefore conclude that cACC provides top-down feedback that, analogously to its proposed role during visual attention [79], helps the network

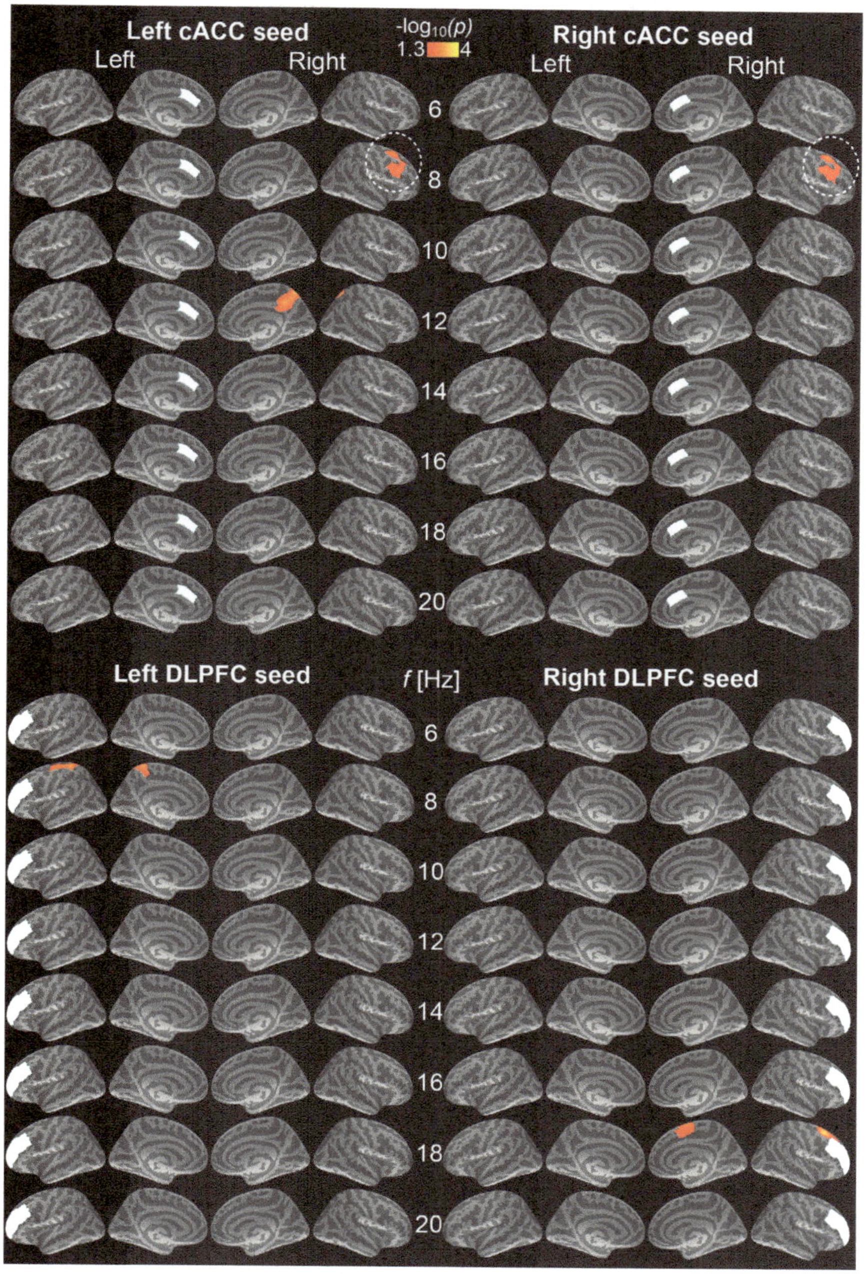

Figure 3. Correlations between conflict-induced RT lags and phase locking to the caudal anterior cingulate (cACC) and dorsolateral prefrontal cortex (DPLPC) seeds during 500-ms periods preceding incongruent trials. All statistically significant findings reflect correlations between reduced RT lags and increased seed-based phase locking after incongruent vs. congruent trials ($p<0.05$, cluster-based Monte Carlo simulation test). (Top) Left and right cACC seed data. Most interestingly, at 8 Hz, reduced conflict-induced RT lags correlated with increased connectivity between the bilateral cACC and right lateral prefrontal areas encompassing FEF and posterior aspects of DLPFC (encircled). At 12 Hz, reduced conflict-induced RT lags also correlate with increased phase locking between the left cACC and right medial parietal cortex. (Bottom) Left and right DLPFC seed data. Reduced conflict-induced RT lags correlated with increased 8-Hz alpha phase locking between the left DLPFC and left postcentral/precentral regions, as well as increased 18-Hz beta phase locking between the right DLPFC and right superior frontal/pre-supplementary motor area (pre-SMA) regions. The results reflect $-\log_{10}(p)$ of the initlal t-statistics, masked to the locations where the cluster-based Monte Carlo simulation test was significant ($p<0.05$).

involving FEF and IPS boost attention toward sound objects originating from the task-relevant spatial direction (here, straight ahead) and suppress those from task-irrelevant directions (here, 45° right/left) during auditory attention. Notably, it has been long speculated that altered connectivity of cingulate regions with FEF and parietal cortices underlies impaired selective attention in schizophrenia, reflected by the patients' inability to distinguish relevant vs. irrelevant objects in their perceptual field [80].

In addition to FEF, we also found the cACC phase-locked with the posterior aspects of right DLPFC at the theta/alpha bands. This finding is consistent with the known bidirectional anatomical connections between ACC and DLPFC [81], and with observations that these two areas work in concert to enhance top-down

Table 2. Correlations between the RT lag caused by conflict and seed-based phase locking differences between periods preceding behavioral responses to incongruent vs. congruent sounds.

Target hemisphere	Seed	f [Hz]	Max value	Size (mm^2)	x_{MNI}	y_{MNI}	z_{MNI}	Cluster-wise P	Anatomical coverage
Left									
	Left DLPFC								
		8	−2.4	3659	−28	−35	58	0.0038	SMA, postcentral
Right									
	Left cACC								
		8	−1.9	3325	29	13	46	0.0095	Lateral PFC, FEF
		12	−2.6	2983	5	−63	55	0.0130	Precuneus
	Right cACC								
		8	−2.1	3740	29	13	46	0.0018	Lateral PFC, FEF
	Right DLPFC								
		18	−2.7	3531	28	14	44	0.0068	Lateral PFC, FEF

Monte Carlo simulation results of the data in **Fig. 3** are demonstrated. The maximum values of initial GLM reflect $-\log10(p)\times\text{sign}(t)$.

control [82]. Our findings are also in line with a proposition that theta oscillations are the electrophysiological mechanism underlying these interactions [83]. For example, a recent animal study reported extensive interactions between ACC and lateral frontal cortices at the theta range [84]. An open question, however, is how the functions of ACC vs. DLPFC are orchestrated during attentional control in the face of interferences and conflicts. The "conflict monitoring" hypothesis [85] suggests a system where ACC monitors and detects conflicts caused by distracting stimuli, and signals them to DLPFC that exerts the ultimate control [86]. The present results are not fully consistent with this notion, as the significant correlation between efficient behavioral conflict resolution and cACC–DLPFC/FEF connectivity was also observable during the pre-stimulus period, that is, before the conflict had even occurred. The presence of effects during the baseline period resembles recent observations in monkey neurophysiological studies [87]. Moreover, when the between-subject behavioral variability was covaried out from our statistical models concerning the post-stimulus/pre-response period, it appeared that the occurrence of a conflict results in a transient decrease in cACC–DLPFC/FEF phase locking. Overall, the results would seem to be most consistent with the notion that cACC and DLPFC work together in a more sustained fashion to suppress distraction and boost attention to relevant stimuli.

However, it is important to note that the present MEG/EEG source estimates are likely less anatomically specific than those achievable with fMRI, not to mention invasive recordings. That is, there is fMRI evidence that the different subregions of ACC may be differentially recruited during conflict processing and distraction suppression. Specifically, a recent study [88] suggested that whereas dorsal aspects of ACC, which overlap with the present cACC seed regions, are associated with biasing attention toward relevant stimuli, the more rostral ACC areas were associated only with conflict detection.

Another interesting finding of the current study is the link between pre-stimulus alpha and performance. Specifically, during the pre-stimulus baseline period, it was found that increased alpha phase locking between the left DLPFC and right AI, as well as between the right DLPFC vs. left anterior MFC and right inferior parietal/TPJ, correlated with fast and efficient behavioral conflict. Although alpha power increases have been often linked to cortical "idling", there is accumulating evidence that inter-regional phase locking at this frequency range mediates top-down effects of attention. Evidence supporting this notion has been shown in animal studies suggesting that interregional alpha and beta synchronization in areas roughly corresponding to primate DLPFC and ACC that generated top-down attentional signals [63], as well as in animal and human studies reporting increases of alpha coherence in visual cortices [29,89] and strengthening of alpha phase synchrony between occipital visual cortex and parietal [90] or PFC [91] regions by attention.

At the beta frequency range, we found that auditory-behavioral conflict resolution correlated with increased phase locking between the right DLPFC and the right pre-SMA. The pre-SMA has anatomical connections with the DLPFC [92,93], and these regions have been implicated in the internally generated aspects of action planning, such as choice and intention. Numerous studies have documented beta oscillations associated with movement behavior and response inhibition, but beta power has also been implicated in broader cognitive processes (for a review, see [94]). In fact, it has been proposed that inter-areal coherence, at the beta frequency range, may have an essential role in cognitive functions including selective attention, working memory, object recognition, perception or sensory-motor integration, due to the prominent

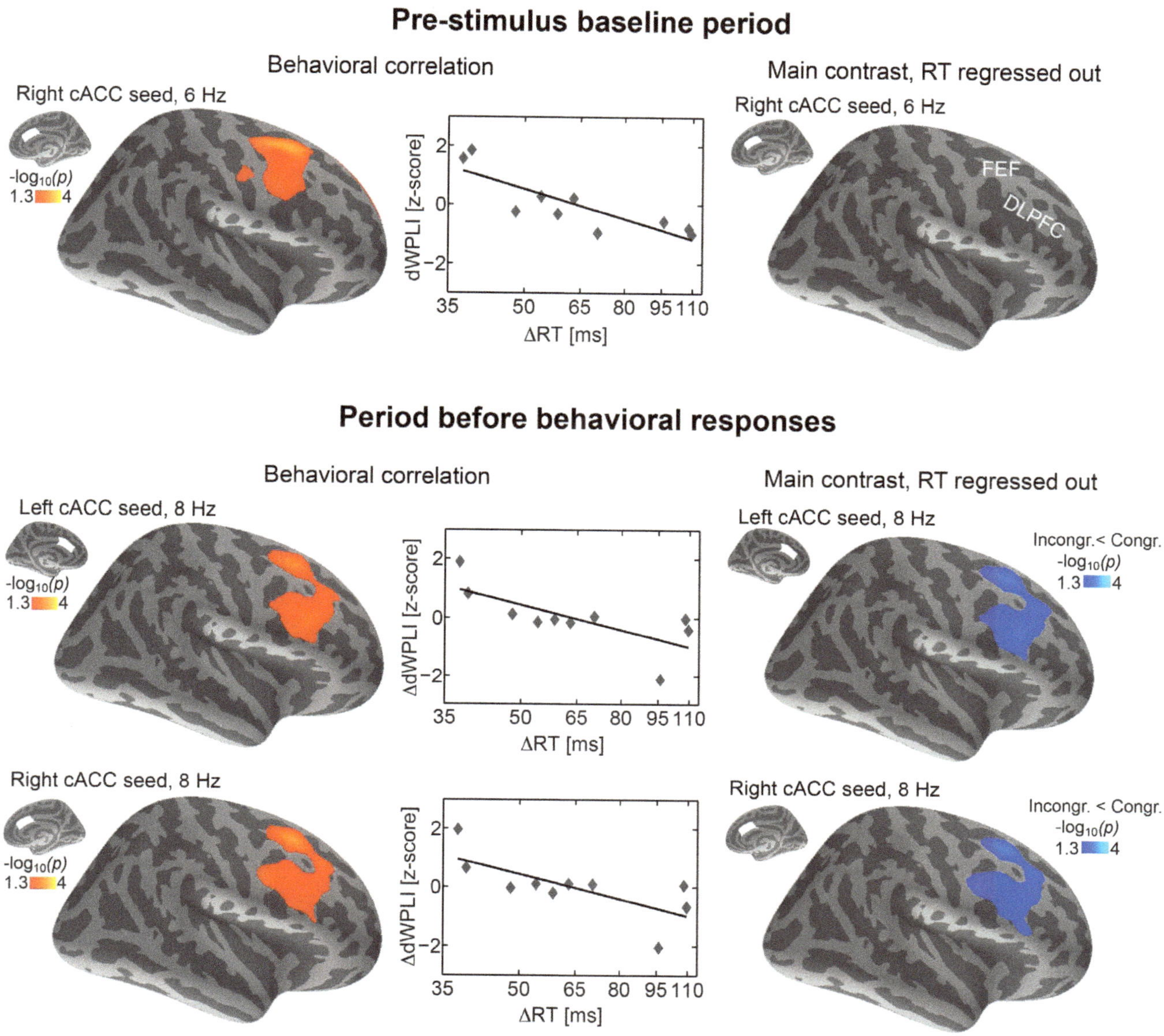

Figure 4. Behavioral conflict resolution and theta/alpha connectivity patters between medial and lateral frontal cortices. (**Top**) The results during the baseline periods. The connectivity between cACC and lateral frontal cortex, specifically FEF, at 6 Hz predicted faster conflict processing, possibly associated with sustained allocation of attention that is necessary for efficient conflict monitoring and resolution during selective listening. The scatter diagram shows the ΔRT (natural logarithmic scale) plotted against lateral frontal cluster average debiased weighted phase lag index (wPLI), with a best-fitting linear trend, depicting the correlation between fast conflict resolution and cACC-lateral frontal theta phase locking. (**Bottom**) Analyses during the 500-ms period preceding each behavioral response are shown. Stronger connectivity between the bilateral cACC and right lateral frontal cortices (FEF, DLPFC) at 8 Hz predicted fast conflict resolution performance, i.e., reduced ΔRT between incongruent and congruent trials. When the effect of behavioral variability was covaried out, the main contrast showed a significant decrease of post-conflict connectivity between the approximately same regions. The scatter diagrams show the ΔRT (natural logarithmic scale) plotted against the lateral frontal debiased wPLI cluster averages for the cACC seed, with the best-fitting linear trend.

role of beta-band oscillations in top-down projections [94]. Interestingly, there is evidence from modeling studies showing that synchronization can tolerate longer synaptic delays for beta than gamma oscillation [23,95], suggesting that long-distance oscillatory synchronization may be more robustly realized at beta frequencies. Our data confirms and extends pervious findings of pre-SMA's involvement in conflict situations [96] and demonstrates that synchronized beta-band oscillations may be the underlying neural mechanism supporting inter-regional communication during conflict processing. Future studies are needed to discern whether its exact role is related to resolving competition between motor plans during response selection, or to conflict-related information processing *per se*.

Our finding that the subjects' ability to resolve conflicts between competing auditory inputs correlated with alpha-band phase locking between the right DLPFC and the retrospenial/precuneus cortex during the baseline period is consistent with recent resting state studies in monkeys and humans demonstrating functional connectivity between the DLPFC and the retrospenial/precuneus regions [97]. It has been proposed that the retrospenial cortex might be the neural substrate between the interaction between the DLPFC and hippocampus [98], and that it plays an essential role

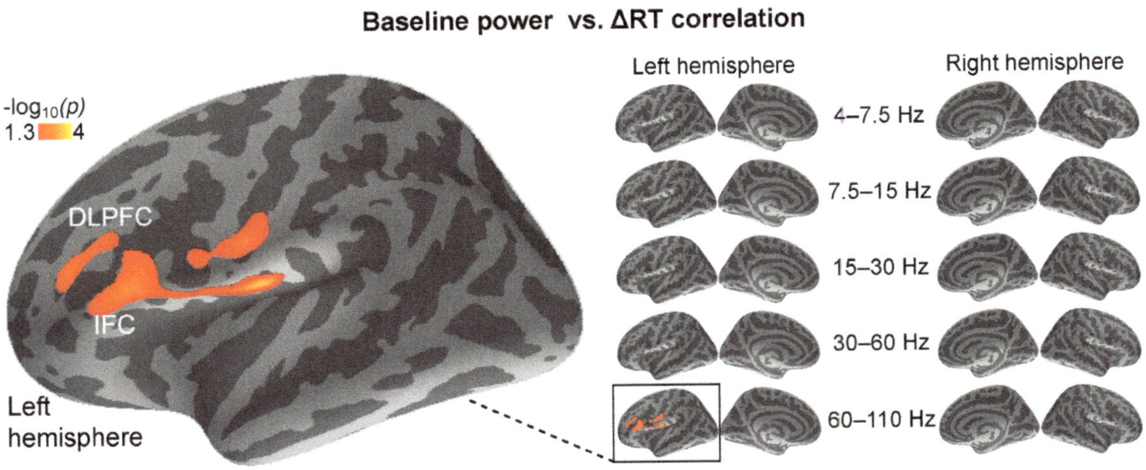

Figure 5. Correlation analyses between the power of pre-stimulus baseline oscillations and behavioral performance. Efficient behavioral conflict processing, as reflected by shorter conflict-induced RT lags, correlated with increased oscillatory power at the higher (60–110 Hz) gamma band during the pre-stimulus period ($p<0.05$, cluster-based Monte Carlo simulation test). The significant correlation were concentrated in the left lateral and inferior frontal cortices, consistent with previous fMRI studies suggesting their role in speech-sound related auditory attention tasks [102]. No significant correlations were observed in the other frequency bands, in the other brain regions, or during the periods immediately before the behavioral responses. The figure shows the significance of initial GLM, masked to the locations that survived the post-hoc correction based on the cluster-based Monte Carlo simulation test.

in cognitive context processing [for a review, see 99]. For example, in an fMRI/MEG study investigating neural synchronization in the contextual processing, activations associated with stronger contextual association were found in retrospenial, parahippocampal and occipital cortices. Importantly, greater phase locking at beta band between these regions were also observed. Taken together, we speculate that the increased phase locking between the right DLPFC and the retrospenial/precuneus cortex observed in the current study might reflect enhanced contextual processing originates in the DLPFC in the face of increasing conflicts/ interferences.

Notably, there was a significant correlation between efficient behavioral conflict resolution and increased oscillatory power at the higher (60–110 Hz) gamma band, which concentrated in the left inferior frontal cortex (IFC) during the pre-stimulus period. Previous fMRI studies have shown that IFC are associated with proactive interference [100,101] and may play an important role in speech-related auditory attention tasks [102]. Further, several neurophysiological studies have also observed sustained gamma oscillations in left IFC associated with phonological processing [103] and maintaining auditory patterns in short-term memory [104]. Our results suggest that IFC gamma oscillations may be essential in maintaining relevant auditory objects during selective attention tasks, and support the concept that attention can rely on gamma-band synchronization that helps integrate neural activities related to a specific sensory object into a stable, salient and coherent representation [19]. More generally, this result is consistent with previous findings associating sustained prefrontal gamma-power increases with successful auditory attention performance [38].

Finally, it is noteworthy that the degree of conflict in each individual trial is essentially modulated by what happened during the preceding trials. The conflict monitoring theories [105] suggest that such a "conflict adaptation' occurs because the preceding conflicts trigger stronger top-down control, which improves performance on subsequent trials of similar context. An alternative theory, however, suggested that these effects are related to a priming effect through episodic memory [106]. Although the exact mechanisms may still be debatable, the trial structure is nevertheless a factor that could affect responses and brain activations at the level of individual trials. Relevantly to the current study, previous fMRI studies have shown that the DLPFC activity gets stronger with an increasing predictability and decreasing experience of conflict, that is, when the probability of conflicts increases [9] or an increasing number of incongruent trials occur in a row during visual flanker task studies, respectively [11,107,108]. Future studies with runs having different probabilities of conflict could help elucidate how such a factor may affect cortico-cortical phase locking between cACC and DLPFC.

Conclusions

Our results demonstrate the importance of sustained connectivity, observed as theta/alpha phase locking between ACC and lateral frontal cortices including the right FEF and DLPFC, for efficient auditory conflict processing, and suggest brain regions of control and attention networks may communicate through synchronous oscillations to manage auditory scenes with multiple overlapping signals. The broader functional relevance of this observation is supported by recent results that pre-stimulus preparatory cACC–FEF alpha coherence is reduced in subjects with autism spectrum disorders during antisaccade tasks [109]. In the context of previous theories, the present results are most consistent with a prediction that ACC may play a role in "regulatory" networks that suppress distractions and boost attention to relevant objects in multisource acoustic environments. The cortical power estimates suggest that gamma-band activity in the left IFC plays a role in selective attention to speech-sound objects.

Acknowledgments

We thank Nao Suzuki, and Drs. Wei-Tang Chang and John W. Belliveau for their advice and support.

Author Contributions

Conceived and designed the experiments: JA. Performed the experiments: JA SH SR. Analyzed the data: JA. Contributed reagents/materials/analysis tools: MH. Contributed to the writing of the manuscript: SH JA MH.

References

1. Shinn-Cunningham BG (2008) Object-based auditory and visual attention. Trends Cogn Sci 12: 182–186.
2. Jääskeläinen IP, Ahveninen J (2014) Auditory-cortex short-term plasticity induced by selective attention. Neural Plast 2014: 216731.
3. Larson E, Lee AK (2013) The cortical dynamics underlying effective switching of auditory spatial attention. Neuroimage 64: 365–370.
4. Alain C, Arnott SR (2000) Selectively attending to auditory objects. Front Biosci 5: D202–212.
5. Eriksen B, Eriksen C (1974) Effects of noise letters upon identification of a target letter in a nonsearch task. Percept Psychophys 16: 143–149.
6. Stroop JR (1935) Studies of interference in serial verbal reactions. Journal of Experimental Psychology 12: 643–662.
7. Simon JR, Rudell AP (1967) Auditory S-R compatibility: the effect of an irrelevant cue on information processing. J Appl Psychol 51: 300–304.
8. Luks TL, Simpson GV, Dale CL, Hough MG (2007) Preparatory allocation of attention and adjustments in conflict processing. Neuroimage 35: 949–958.
9. Casey BJ, Thomas KM, Welsh TF, Badgaiyan RD, Eccard CH, et al. (2000) Dissociation of response conflict, attentional selection, and expectancy with functional magnetic resonance imaging. Proc Natl Acad Sci U S A 97: 8728–8733.
10. MacDonald AW 3rd, Cohen JD, Stenger VA, Carter CS (2000) Dissociating the role of the dorsolateral prefrontal and anterior cingulate cortex in cognitive control. Science 288: 1835–1838.
11. Kerns JG, Cohen JD, MacDonald AW 3rd, Cho RY, Stenger VA, et al. (2004) Anterior cingulate conflict monitoring and adjustments in control. Science 303: 1023–1026.
12. Roberts KL, Hall DA (2008) Examining a Supramodal Network for Conflict Processing: A Systematic Review and Novel Functional Magnetic Resonance Imaging Data for Related Visual and Auditory Stroop Tasks. Journal of Cognitive Neuroscience 20: 1063–1078.
13. Liu X, Banich MT, Jacobson BL, Tanabe JL (2004) Common and distinct neural substrates of attentional control in an integrated Simon and spatial Stroop task as assessed by event-related fMRI. Neuroimage 22: 1097–1106.
14. Fan J, Flombaum JI, McCandliss BD, Thomas KM, Posner MI (2003) Cognitive and brain consequences of conflict. Neuroimage 18: 42–57.
15. Folstein JR, Van Petten C (2008) Influence of cognitive control and mismatch on the N2 component of the ERP: a review. Psychophysiology 45: 152–170.
16. Szucs D, Soltesz F (2012) Functional definition of the N450 event-related brain potential marker of conflict processing: a numerical stroop study. BMC Neurosci 13: 35.
17. Larson MJ, Clayson PE, Clawson A (2014) Making sense of all the conflict: A theoretical review and critique of conflict-related ERPs. International Journal of Psychophysiology 93: 283–297.
18. Cohen MX (2014) Advantages and Limitations of Time- and Time-Frequnecy-Domain Analysis. Analyzing Neural Time Series Data: Theory and Practice. Cambridge, MA: MIT. 15–29.
19. Jensen O, Kaiser J, Lachaux JP (2007) Human gamma-frequency oscillations associated with attention and memory. Trends Neurosci 30: 317–324.
20. Womelsdorf T, Fries P (2007) The role of neuronal synchronization in selective attention. Curr Opin Neurobiol 17: 154–160.
21. Engel AK, Fries P, Singer W (2001) Dynamic predictions: oscillations and synchrony in top-down processing. Nat Rev Neurosci 2: 704–716.
22. von Stein A, Sarnthein J (2000) Different frequencies for different scales of cortical integration: from local gamma to long range alpha/theta synchronization. International Journal of Psychophysiology 38: 301–313.
23. Kopell N, Ermentrout GB, Whittington MA, Traub RD (2000) Gamma rhythms and beta rhythms have different synchronization properties. Proc Natl Acad Sci U S A 97: 1867–1872.
24. Huang S, Chang WT, Belliveau JW, Hamalainen M, Ahveninen J (2014) Lateralized parietotemporal oscillatory phase synchronization during auditory selective attention. Neuroimage 86: 461–469.
25. Schack B, Klimesch W, Sauseng P (2005) Phase synchronization between theta and upper alpha oscillations in a working memory task. Int J Psychophysiol 57: 105–114.
26. Moore RA, Gale A, Morris PH, Forrester D (2006) Theta phase locking across the neocortex reflects cortico-hippocampal recursive communication during goal conflict resolution. Int J Psychophysiol 60: 260–273.
27. Nigbur R, Cohen MX, Ridderinkhof KR, Stürmer B (2011) Theta Dynamics Reveal Domain-specific Control over Stimulus and Response Conflict. Journal of Cognitive Neuroscience 24: 1264–1274.
28. Doesburg SM, Green JJ, McDonald JJ, Ward LM (2012) Theta modulation of inter-regional gamma synchronization during auditory attention control. Brain Res 1431: 77–85.
29. von Stein A, Chiang C, König P (2000) Top-down processing mediated by interareal synchronization. Proc Natl Acad Sci U S A 97: 14748–14753.
30. Gross J, Schmitz F, Schnitzler I, Kessler K, Shapiro K, et al. (2004) Modulation of long-range neural synchrony reflects temporal limitations of visual attention in humans. Proc Natl Acad Sci U S A 101: 13050–13055.
31. Benedict RH, Shucard DW, Santa Maria MP, Shucard JL, Abara JP, et al. (2002) Covert auditory attention generates activation in the rostral/dorsal anterior cingulate cortex. J Cogn Neurosci 14: 637–645.
32. Haupt S, Axmacher N, Cohen MX, Elger CE, Fell J (2009) Activation of the caudal anterior cingulate cortex due to task-related interference in an auditory Stroop paradigm. Hum Brain Mapp 30: 3043–3056.
33. Christoffels IK, Formisano E, Schiller NO (2007) Neural correlates of verbal feedback processing: An fMRI study employing overt speech. Hum Brain Mapp 28: 868–879.
34. Westerhausen R, Moosmann M, Alho K, Belsby SO, Hamalainen H, et al. (2010) Identification of attention and cognitive control networks in a parametric auditory fMRI study. Neuropsychologia 48: 2075–2081.
35. Chan JS, Merrifield K, Spence C (2005) Auditory spatial attention assessed in a flanker interference task. Acta Acust United Ac 91: 554–563.
36. Espinoza-Varas B, Jang H (2011) Selective attention to pitch amid conflicting auditory information: context-coding and filtering strategies. Psychol Res 75: 159–178.
37. Ahveninen J, Jääskeläinen IP, Belliveau JW, Hämäläinen M, Lin FH, et al. (2012) Dissociable influences of auditory object vs. spatial attention on visual system oscillatory activity. PLoS ONE 7: e38511.
38. Ahveninen J, Huang S, Belliveau JW, Chang WT, Hamalainen M (2013) Dynamic oscillatory processes governing cued orienting and allocation of auditory attention. J Cogn Neurosci 25: 1926–1943.
39. Dale AM, Sereno MI (1993) Improved Localizadon of Cortical Activity by Combining EEG and MEG with MRI Cortical Surface Reconstruction: A Linear Approach. Journal of Cognitive Neuroscience 5: 162–176.
40. Hämäläinen MS, Lin FS, Mosher JC (2010) Anatomically and Functionally Constrained Minimum-Norm Estimates. In: Hansen O, Kringelbach M., and Salmelin, R., editor. MEG: An Introduction to Methods. New York, NY: Oxford University Press. 186–215.
41. Buzsaki G, Anastassiou CA, Koch C (2012) The origin of extracellular fields and currents–EEG, ECoG, LFP and spikes. Nat Rev Neurosci 13: 407–420.
42. Sharon D, Hämäläinen MS, Tootell RB, Halgren E, Belliveau JW (2007) The advantage of combining MEG and EEG: comparison to fMRI in focally stimulated visual cortex. Neuroimage 36: 1225–1235.
43. Desikan R, Segonne F, Fischl B, Quinn B, Dickerson B, et al. (2006) An automated labeling system for subdividing the human cerebral cortex on MRI scans into gyral based regions of interest. Neuroimage 31: 968–980.
44. Shenhav A, Botvinick MM, Cohen JD (2013) The expected value of control: an integrative theory of anterior cingulate cortex function. Neuron 79: 217–240.
45. Algazi VR, Duda RO, Thompson M, Avendano C (2001) The CIPIC HRTF database; 2001 October 21–24; Mohonk Mountain House, New Paltz, NY. 99–102.
46. Kopp B, Rist F, Mattler U (1996) N200 in the flanker task as a neurobehavioral tool for investigating executive control. Psychophysiology 33: 282–294.
47. Machado L, Guiney H, Struthers P (2013) Identity-based inhibitory processing during focused attention. Q J Exp Psychol (Hove) 66: 138–159.
48. DeWitt I, Rauschecker JP (2012) Phoneme and word recognition in the auditory ventral stream. Proc Natl Acad Sci U S A 109: E505–514.
49. Taulu S, Simola J, Kajola M (2005) Applications of the Signal Space Separation Method. IEEE Trans Signal Proc 53: 3359–3372.
50. Fischl B, Sereno MI, Dale AM (1999) Cortical surface-based analysis. II: Inflation, flattening, and a surface-based coordinate system. Neuroimage 9: 195–207.
51. Fischl B, Liu A, Dale AM (2001) Automated manifold surgery: constructing geometrically accurate and topologically correct models of the human cerebral cortex. IEEE Trans Med Imaging 20: 70–80.
52. Fischl B, Salat DH, van der Kouwe AJ, Makris N, Segonne F, et al. (2004) Sequence-independent segmentation of magnetic resonance images. Neuroimage 23 Suppl 1: S69–84.
53. Klauschen F, Goldman A, Barra V, Meyer-Lindenberg A, Lundervold A (2009) Evaluation of automated brain MR image segmentation and volumetry methods. Hum Brain Mapp 30: 1310–1327.
54. Ghosh SS, Kakunoori S, Augustinack J, Nieto-Castanon A, Kovelman I, et al. (2010) Evaluating the validity of volume-based and surface-based brain image registration for developmental cognitive neuroscience studies in children 4 to 11 years of age. Neuroimage 53: 85–93.
55. Hämäläinen M, Hari R, Ilmoniemi R, Knuutila J, Lounasmaa O (1993) Magnetoencephalography - theory, instrumentation, and applications to noninvasive studies of the working human brain. Rev Mod Phys 65: 413–497.
56. Yendiki A, Greve DN, Wallace S, Vangel M, Bockholt J, et al. (2010) Multi-site characterization of an fMRI working memory paradigm: reliability of activation indices. Neuroimage 53: 119–131.

57. Gramfort A, Luessi M, Larson E, Engemann DA, Strohmeier D, et al. (2013) MNE software for processing MEG and EEG data. Neuroimage.
58. Vinck M, Oostenveld R, van Wingerden M, Battaglia F, Pennartz CM (2011) An improved index of phase-synchronization for electrophysiological data in the presence of volume-conduction, noise and sample-size bias. Neuroimage 55: 1548–1565.
59. Fischl B, Sereno MI, Tootell RB, Dale AM (1999) High-resolution intersubject averaging and a coordinate system for the cortical surface. Hum Brain Mapp 8: 272–284.
60. Percival DB, Walden AT (1993) Spectral analysis for physical applications: multitaper and conventional univariate techniques. Cambridge, UK: Cambridge University Press.
61. Bland JM, Altman DG (1996) Transforming data. BMJ 312: 770.
62. Lesh TA, Westphal AJ, Niendam TA, Yoon JH, Minzenberg MJ, et al. (2013) Proactive and reactive cognitive control and dorsolateral prefrontal cortex dysfunction in first episode schizophrenia. NeuroImage: Clinical 2: 590–599.
63. Totah NKB, Jackson ME, Moghaddam B (2012) Preparatory Attention Relies on Dynamic Interactions between Prelimbic Cortex and Anterior Cingulate Cortex. Cerebral Cortex.
64. Varela F, Lachaux JP, Rodriguez E, Martinerie J (2001) The brainweb: phase synchronization and large-scale integration. Nat Rev Neurosci 2: 229–239.
65. Buzsaki G, Draguhn A (2004) Neuronal oscillations in cortical networks. Science 304: 1926–1929.
66. Braver TS, Barch DM, Gray JR, Molfese DL, Snyder A (2001) Anterior cingulate cortex and response conflict: effects of frequency, inhibition and errors. Cereb Cortex 11: 825–836.
67. Botvinick MM, Cohen JD, Carter CS (2004) Conflict monitoring and anterior cingulate cortex: an update. Trends Cogn Sci 8: 539–546.
68. Carter CS, Braver TS, Barch DM, Botvinick MM, Noll D, et al. (1998) Anterior cingulate cortex, error detection, and the online monitoring of performance. Science 280: 747–749.
69. Holroyd CB, Coles MG (2002) The neural basis of human error processing: reinforcement learning, dopamine, and the error-related negativity. Psychol Rev 109: 679–709.
70. Rushworth MF, Walton ME, Kennerley SW, Bannerman DM (2004) Action sets and decisions in the medial frontal cortex. Trends Cogn Sci 8: 410–417.
71. Fan J, McCandliss BD, Fossella J, Flombaum JI, Posner MI (2005) The activation of attentional networks. Neuroimage 26: 471–479.
72. Sauseng P, Hoppe J, Klimesch W, Gerloff C, Hummel FC (2007) Dissociation of sustained attention from central executive functions: local activity and interregional connectivity in the theta range. Eur J Neurosci 25: 587–593.
73. Szmalec A, Verbruggen F, Vandierendonck A, De Baene W, Verguts T, et al. (2008) Stimulus ambiguity elicits response conflict. Neurosci Lett 435: 158–162.
74. van Veen V, Carter CS (2002) The anterior cingulate as a conflict monitor: fMRI and ERP studies. Physiol Behav 77: 477–482.
75. Cohen MX, Donner TH (2013) Midfrontal conflict-related theta-band power reflects neural oscillations that predict behavior. Journal of Neurophysiology 110: 2752–2763.
76. Corbetta M, Shulman GL (2002) Control of goal-directed and stimulus-driven attention in the brain. Nat Rev Neurosci 3: 201–215.
77. Huang S, Belliveau JW, Tengshe C, Ahveninen J (2012) Brain networks of novelty-driven involuntary and cued voluntary auditory attention shifting. PLoS One 7: e44062.
78. Miller EK, Buschman TJ (2013) Cortical circuits for the control of attention. Curr Opin Neurobiol 23: 216–222.
79. Weissman DH, Gopalakrishnan A, Hazlett CJ, Woldorff MG (2005) Dorsal anterior cingulate cortex resolves conflict from distracting stimuli by boosting attention toward relevant events. Cereb Cortex 15: 229–237.
80. Benes FM, Cunningham GC, Berretta S, Gisabella B (2009) Course and pattern of cingulate pathology in schizophrenia. In: Vogt BA, editor. Cingulate Neurobiology and Disease Oxford University Press. 679–705.
81. Barbas H (2000) Connections underlying the synthesis of cognition, memory, and emotion in primate prefrontal cortices. Brain Research Bulletin 52: 319–330.
82. Badre D, Wagner AD (2004) Selection, Integration, and Conflict Monitoring: Assessing the Nature and Generality of Prefrontal Cognitive Control Mechanisms. Neuron 41: 473–487.
83. van Driel J, Ridderinkhof KR, Cohen MX (2012) Not All Errors Are Alike: Theta and Alpha EEG Dynamics Relate to Differences in Error-Processing Dynamics. The Journal of Neuroscience 32: 16795–16806.
84. Womelsdorf T, Johnston K, Vinck M, Everling S (2010) Theta-activity in anterior cingulate cortex predicts task rules and their adjustments following errors. Proceedings of the National Academy of Sciences 107: 5248–5253.
85. Cohen JD, Botvinick M, Carter CS (2000) Anterior cingulate and prefrontal cortex: who's in control? Nat Neurosci 3: 421–423.
86. Biehl S, Ehlis AC, Muller L, Niklaus A, Pauli P, et al. (2013) The impact of task relevance and degree of distraction on stimulus processing. BMC Neuroscience 14: 107.
87. Johnston K, Levin HM, Koval MJ, Everling S (2007) Top-down control-signal dynamics in anterior cingulate and prefrontal cortex neurons following task switching. Neuron 53: 453–462.
88. Orr JM, Weissman DH (2009) Anterior Cingulate Cortex Makes 2 Contributions to Minimizing Distraction. Cerebral Cortex 19: 703–711.
89. Fries P, Womelsdorf T, Oostenveld R, Desimone R (2008) The Effects of Visual Stimulation and Selective Visual Attention on Rhythmic Neuronal Synchronization in Macaque Area V4. The Journal of Neuroscience 28: 4823–4835.
90. Doesburg SM, Green JJ, McDonald JJ, Ward LM (2009) From local inhibition to long-range integration: a functional dissociation of alpha-band synchronization across cortical scales in visuospatial attention. Brain Res 1303: 97–110.
91. Palva S, Palva JM (2007) New vistas for ± frequency band oscillations. Trends in neurosciences 30: 150–158.
92. Luppino G, Matelli M, Camarda R, Rizzolatti G (1993) Corticocortical connections of area F3 (SMA-proper) and area F6 (pre-SMA) in the macaque monkey. The Journal of Comparative Neurology 338: 114–140.
93. Johansen-Berg H, Behrens TEJ, Robson MD, Drobnjak I, Rushworth MFS, et al. (2004) Changes in connectivity profiles define functionally distinct regions in human medial frontal cortex. Proc Natl Acad Sci U S A 101: 13335–13340.
94. Wang XJ (2010) Neurophysiological and Computational Principles of Cortical Rhythms in Cognition. Physiological Reviews 90: 1195–1268.
95. Bibbig A, Traub RD, Whittington MA (2002) Long-Range Synchronization of γ and β Oscillations and the Plasticity of Excitatory and Inhibitory Synapses: A Network Model. Journal of Neurophysiology 88: 1634–1654.
96. Soutschek A, Taylor PC, Muller HJ, Schubert T (2013) Dissociable networks control conflict during perception and response selection: a transcranial magnetic stimulation Study. J Neurosci 33: 5647–5654.
97. Petrides M, Pandya DN (1984) Projections to the frontal cortex from the posterior parietal region in the rhesus monkey. J Comp Neurol 228: 105–116.
98. Morris R, Pandya DN, Petrides M (1999) Fiber system linking the mid-dorsolateral frontal cortex with the retrosplenial/presubicular region in the rhesus monkey. J Comp Neurol 407: 183–192.
99. Bar M (2004) Visual objects in context. Nat Rev Neurosci 5: 617–629.
100. Jonides J, Smith EE, Marshuetz C, Koeppe RA, Reuter-Lorenz PA (1998) Inhibition in verbal working memory revealed by brain activation. Proc Natl Acad Sci U S A 95: 8410–8413.
101. Badre D, Poldrack RA, Pare-Blagoev EJ, Insler RZ, Wagner AD (2005) Dissociable controlled retrieval and generalized selection mechanisms in ventrolateral prefrontal cortex. Neuron 47: 907–918.
102. Yoncheva YN, Zevin JD, Maurer U, McCandliss BD (2010) Auditory selective attention to speech modulates activity in the visual word form area. Cereb Cortex 20: 622–632.
103. Mainy N, Kahane P, Minotti L, Hoffmann D, Bertrand O, et al. (2007) Neural correlates of consolidation in working memory. Hum Brain Mapp 28: 183–193.
104. Kaiser J, Ripper B, Birbaumer N, Lutzenberger W (2003) Dynamics of gamma-band activity in human magnetoencephalogram during auditory pattern working memory. Neuroimage 20: 816–827.
105. Botvinick MM, Braver TS, Barch DM, Carter CS, Cohen JD (2001) Conflict monitoring and cognitive control. Psychol Rev 108: 624–652.
106. Mayr U, Awh E, Laurey P (2003) Conflict adaptation effects in the absence of executive control. Nat Neurosci 6: 450–452.
107. Botvinick M, Nystrom LE, Fissell K, Carter CS, Cohen JD (1999) Conflict monitoring versus selection-for-action in anterior cingulate cortex. Nature 402: 179–181.
108. Durston S, Davidson MC, Thomas KM, Worden MS, Tottenham N, et al. (2003) Parametric manipulation of conflict and response competition using rapid mixed-trial event-related fMRI. Neuroimage 20: 2135–2141.
109. Kenet T, Orekhova EV, Bharadwaj H, Shetty NR, Israeli E, et al. (2012) Disconnectivity of the cortical ocular motor control network in autism spectrum disorders. Neuroimage 61: 1226–1234.

3

High-Resolution Mechanical Imaging of Glioblastoma by Multifrequency Magnetic Resonance Elastography

Kaspar-Josche Streitberger[1]◑, Martin Reiss-Zimmermann[2]◑, Florian Baptist Freimann[3], Simon Bayerl[4], Jing Guo[1], Felix Arlt[5], Jens Wuerfel[6,7], Jürgen Braun[8], Karl-Titus Hoffmann[2], Ingolf Sack[1]*

1 Department of Radiology, Charité - Universitätsmedizin Berlin, Berlin, Germany, **2** Department of Neuroradiology, Universitätsmedizin Leipzig, Leipzig, Germany, **3** Department of Neurosurgery, Universitätsmedizin Göttingen, Göttingen, Germany, **4** Department of Neurosurgery, Charité - Universitätsmedizin Berlin, Berlin, Germany, **5** Department of Neurosurgery, Universitätsmedizin Leipzig, Leipzig, Germany, **6** Institute of Neuroradiology, Universitätsmedizin Göttingen, Göttingen, Germany, **7** NeuroCure, Charité - Universitätsmedizin Berlin, Berlin, Germany, **8** Institute of Medical Informatics, Charité - Universitätsmedizin Berlin, Berlin, Germany

Abstract

Objective: To generate high-resolution maps of the viscoelastic properties of human brain parenchyma for presurgical quantitative assessment in glioblastoma (GB).

Methods: Twenty-two GB patients underwent routine presurgical work-up supplemented by additional multifrequency magnetic resonance elastography. Two three-dimensional viscoelastic parameter maps, magnitude $|G^*|$, and phase angle φ of the complex shear modulus were reconstructed by inversion of full wave field data in 2-mm isotropic resolution at seven harmonic drive frequencies ranging from 30 to 60 Hz.

Results: Mechanical brain maps confirmed that GB are composed of stiff and soft compartments, resulting in high intratumor heterogeneity. GB could be easily differentiated from healthy reference tissue by their reduced viscous behavior quantified by φ (0.37±0.08 vs. 0.58±0.07). $|G^*|$, which in solids more relates to the material's stiffness, was significantly reduced in GB with a mean value of 1.32±0.26 kPa compared to 1.54±0.27 kPa in healthy tissue (P = 0.001). However, some GB (5 of 22) showed increased stiffness.

Conclusion: GB are generally less viscous and softer than healthy brain parenchyma. Unrelated to the morphology-based contrast of standard magnetic resonance imaging, elastography provides an entirely new neuroradiological marker and contrast related to the biomechanical properties of tumors.

Editor: Wang Zhan, University of Maryland, College Park, United States of America

Funding: IS received a grant of the German Research Foundation (DFG Sa901/10). The funders had no role in study design, data collection and analysis, decision to publish, or preparation of the manuscript.

Competing Interests: The authors have declared that no competing interests exist.

* Email: ingolf.sack@charite.de

◑ These authors contributed equally to this work.

Introduction

Despite recent advances in operative and postoperative treatment, glioblastoma (GB) still remains one of the most malicious and aggressive and malignant forms of cancer [1,2]. It accounts for >50% of all primary neuroepithelial tumors and approximately 20% of all brain tumors [3]. In developed countries, the incidence of GB is 3.5 per 100,000 population per year [4,5,6]. The term GB was first introduced in 1926 by Percival Bailey and Harvey Cushing and refers to the cellular origin from glioblasts and the histological heterogeneity of this brain tumor [7]. The classification of the World Health Organization (WHO) ranks GB as a grade IV tumor due to its histological characteristics with aggressive and infiltrative growth and overall poor prognosis [8]. Despite aggressive surgical resection, radiotherapy, and chemotherapy the prognosis for patients newly diagnosed with GB remains poor with a 2-year survival rate of only 13–26% and a mean survival time of 12–15 months [2].

Neuroradiological assessment of GB and differentiation from solitary intracranial metastases or lymphomas is challenging due to the tumor's heterogeneous composition resulting from the presence of cysts, necrosis, and hemorrhage [9,10]. As a consequence, diagnostic biopsy remains inevitable for a definitive diagnosis despite possible complications [11]. Advanced magnetic resonance imaging (MRI) methods such as diffusion tensor imaging provide structural information related to water mobility in white matter tracts but cannot reveal the consistency and mechanical constitution of biological tissue[12,13]. Targeting the mechanical properties of GB potentially provides information about the tumor's structural heterogeneity as well as its perifocal tissue infiltration which is of relevance for diagnosis, therapy planning and treatment monitoring.

Today, the viscoelastic properties of the brain can be assessed noninvasively by magnetic resonance elastography (MRE) [14]. Combining time-harmonic vibrations in the low audible range with motion-sensitive MRI, cerebral MRE [15,16,17] has proven sensitive to mechanostructural changes in the human brain associated with aging [18,19] and diseases [20,21,22,23,24,25]. Recent results in mouse models suggest that cerebral MRE is sensitive to demyelination, inflammation, and extracellular matrix alterations [26,27,28] and may thus provide new information about structural changes of cerebral tissue in brain tumors. Indeed, initial findings in different intracranial tumor entities [29] including meningeomas [30,31] indicate the feasibility of MRE for the presurgical assessment of neuronal tumor consistency.

However, previous studies were limited by low spatial resolution of the mechanical parameter maps achievable by MRE at a single harmonic drive frequency. Recent advances in fast image acquisition schemes [32,33] and wave field reconstruction methods [34,35,36,37] enabled us to acquire 3D wave fields at multiple vibration frequencies, generating cerebral MRE maps with a spatial resolution comparable to that of normal MRI [38,39].

In this study we applied multifrequency MRE (MMRE) for in vivo high resolution mechanical imaging of GB tissue including perifocal brain parenchyma as a surrogate for infiltrative tumor growth, and distant tumor edema in comparison to tumor and reference tissue. The lack of clearly delineable solid-type tissue within many tumors led us to further specify regions with homogeneous appearance in standard T2- and contrast-enhanced T1-weighted MR images.

By these regions, we address for the first time whether high-resolution multifrequency MRE can measure the heterogeneity of GB tissue mechanics which is likely linked to the well known microstructural heterogeneity of GB including neovascularisation and central hemorrhage. Despite the fact that any spatial averaging over-simplifies the tumor's intrinsic heterogeneity, we will tabulate mechanical property values of GB as a starting point for quantification, diagnostic assessment and therapy planning of GB by MRE.

Methods

Twenty-two patients with histologically proven GB (mean age 64.5±15.1 years; 10 women) were included in this study. Each patient underwent clinical MRI and MRE prior to further diagnostic (e.g., biopsy) or therapeutic procedures. In addition to MRE, a clinical protocol including T1-, T2-, and proton-density-weighted sequences was applied before and after administration of gadolinium-based contrast agent for further evaluation of the lesion. Imaging slices for MRE were positioned in transverse orientation according to tumor site.

The study was approved by the ethics committee of the Charité - Universitätsmedizin Berlin (EA1/261/12). All patients gave informed written consent prior to MRE.

MMRE

A custom-designed nonmagnetic driver based on piezoelectric ceramics [33] was mounted at the end of the patient table. The vibrations were transmitted by a carbon fiber rod connected to a custom-designed head cradle located inside the head coil. Eleven of the experiments were performed on a 1.5T MRI scanner (Magnetom Sonata; Siemens Erlangen, Germany), the remaining eleven experiments were carried out on a 3T MRI scanner (Trio; Siemens Erlangen, Germany) using a 4-channel (1.5T) and a 12-channel (3T) head coil. The imaging sequence parameters for both systems are listed below. After acquisition of a localizer and a 3D T1-weighted sequence for anatomical reference, a single-shot spin-echo echo-planar imaging sequence with trapezoidal flow-compensated motion-encoding gradients (MEG), consecutively applied along all three axes of the scanner coordinate system, was used for rapid motion field acquisition [40]. A custom-made head cradle was used to generate mechanical shear waves inside the brain by inducing a gentle nodding motion of the head. To allow the mechanical waves to propagate into the tissue, the vibration was initiated through a trigger pulse by the scanner at least 100 ms before the start of the MEG. The vibration frequencies (f) used in this experiment were 30, 35, 40, 45, 50, 55, and 60 Hz. The trigger pulse was delayed in consecutive time-resolved scans by increments of $1/(8*f)$, yielding 8 dynamics of a wave cycle. For 10 (1.5T) and 15 (3T) adjacent slices of $2\times2\times2$ mm^3 resolution, 7 frequencies, 8 wave dynamics, and 3 MEG directions were applied. Further imaging parameters were: repetition time (TR) 2400 ms (1.5T) and 3000 ms (3T); echo time (TE) 99 ms (1.5T) and 71ms (3T); field of view (FoV) 192×176 mm^2 (1.5T) and 250×188 mm^2 (3T); matrix size 88×96 (1.5T) and 128×64 (3T); no parallel imaging at 1.5T, GRAPPA factor of 2 at 3T; MEG frequencies (number of MEG periods): 25 (1), 26 (1), 30 (1), 50 (2), 50 (2), 50 (2), 54 (2) Hz corresponding to 30, 35, 40, 45 ,50, 55, 60 Hz vibration frequency, respectively (note: MEG frequency and period number were chosen to accomplish the highest encoding efficiency according to the principle of fractional motion encoding [41] and given by equation 4e in [40]); MEG amplitude 30 mT/m (1.5T) and 35 mT/m (3T); ~1 min scan time for each frequency, resulting in a total acquisition time of ~7 min for a full multislice MMRE examination.

Data Postprocessing

Wave image postprocessing followed the strategy outlined in [42]. In brief: First, the complex MR images were smoothed using a 2D Gaussian filter with a kernel of 5 pixel edge length and sigma = 0.65 for noise reduction. Subsequent gradient-based unwrapping was performed as described by [43]. First-order in-plane derivatives along the image coordinate axes x_k ($k = 1,2$) (x_1 is the phase-encoding direction and x_2 the read-out direction) of the spin phase φ_j ($j = 1,2,3$) were calculated by:

$$u_{j,k} = \frac{\partial u_j}{\partial x_k} = -i\xi\cdot\exp(-i\phi_j)\cdot\frac{\partial}{\partial x_k}\exp(i\phi_j) \qquad (1)$$

Factor ξ scales the spin phase ϕ_j to the physical displacement component u_j (in meters) according to [40]. After Fourier transformation in time, equation (1) yields six complex-valued strain images $u^*_{j,k}(\omega_l)$ at angular drive frequency ω_l, resulting in a total of 42 images at each slice invoked by the reconstruction algorithm. These images were further smoothed by a 2D Butterworth lowpass filter with a threshold of 100 m^{-1}. Low wave numbers as resulted by compression waves were considered sufficiently suppressed by the derivative operators. Other than in previous work [33,38,39], we abandoned curl components for wave inversion since interslice phase artifacts, as addressed by [44], impair the derivative operator in the x_3 direction. Instead of three curl components for each frequency, six independent strain wave images were obtained using eq.(1). All six images were used for stabilizing the wave inversion as described in the following. This strategy is further outlined in [42].

We applied multifrequency dual elasto visco (MDEV) inversion [33,38,39]. This algorithm provides two independent mechanical constants, $|G^*|$ and φ, corresponding to the magnitude and phase of the complex shear modulus G*. $|G^*|$ provides an indication of the softness or firmness of the tissue while φ provides an indication of the viscous, i.e. dissipative, tissue properties. Of note, both parameters are model-free and provide just another representation of the storage and loss modulus usually parameterized in MRE. It is well known that the loss and storage modulus of brain tissue display dispersion within the examined frequency range [18]. In MDEV inversion-based MRE, we sacrifice the information provided by frequency-resolved complex shear moduli for generating spatially highly resolved maps of $|G^*|$ and φ [33]. As a result, $|G^*|$ and φ refer to the amplitude and phase angle of the oscillatory response to a harmonic stress, respectively. The effective harmonic frequency of $|G^*|$ and φ is given by the mean of all vibration frequencies weighted by the wave amplitudes they produced.

Accounting for complex-valued shear strain images $u^*_{j,k}(\omega_l)$ and making the usual assumptions in MRE such as homogeneity, linear viscoelasticity, and isotropy, we obtain the following inversion equations:

$$|G^*| = \rho \frac{\sum_{j=1}^{3}\sum_{k=1}^{2}\sum_{l=1}^{7}\omega_l^2|u^*_{j,k}(\omega_l)|}{\sum_{j=1}^{3}\sum_{k=1}^{2}\sum_{l=1}^{7}|\Delta u^*_{j,k}(\omega_l)|} \tag{2a}$$

$$\phi = \arccos\left(-\frac{\sum_{j=1}^{3}\sum_{k=1}^{2}\sum_{l=1}^{7}\left[\Delta u'_{j,k}(\omega_l)u'_{j,k}(\omega_l)+\Delta u''_{j,k}(\omega_l)u''_{j,k}(\omega_l)\right]}{\sum_{j=1}^{3}\sum_{k=1}^{2}\sum_{l=1}^{7}|\Delta u^*_{j,k}(\omega_l)||u^*_{j,k}(\omega_l)|}\right) \tag{2b}$$

Given that $u^*_{j,k}$ represents in-plane strain components and Δ denotes the 2D-Laplacian, our inversion is entirely 2D-based. By these equations we implemented the method proposed in [39] where data and data derivatives are projected onto the ones vector instead of derivative vector as done in classical least squares solutions of the wave equation [45]. The ones-vector model refers to the almost trivial regression of repeated measurements by computing the observational average (see eqs. 2.81 and 2.82 in [46]).

Morphological Tumor Assessment

MRI-based tumor morphology was classified and graded using T2-weighted (T2w) images as well as contrast-enhanced T1-weighted (T1w) images. These images were used to assess tumor morphology including e.g. the presence of cysts, homogenous appearing tumor portion, and necrosis. The tumor volume was calculated using the OsiriX-Imaging software (Geneva, Switzerland) and the MiaLite plugin (SPIE medical imaging 2011, Lake Buena Vista, Florida, USA) by defining contrast enhancing tissue on T1-weighted images. Assessment of tumor morphology and tumor size was performed by experienced neuroradiologists (M.R.-Z., K.-T.H.). Regions of interest (ROI) were manually selected on the basis of image contrast in the MRE magnitude images for the tumor, the edema, and healthy tissue (normal appearing white matter) in a corresponding contralateral region as demonstrated in Figure 1. The selection was done by one observer experienced in neurological MRI and MRE (K.-J.S.) and further confirmed or revised by two experienced neuroradiologists (M.R.-Z., J.W.). Standard deviations of $|G^*|$ and φ were calculated for the tumor ROI to indicate the heterogeneity of the tumor's viscoelastic properties. Additionally, we selected a region of apparently high homogeneity within the tumor region based on morphological MRI (HAM –homogeneous appearing matter) to further compartmentalize the tumor and therewith to address the intra-tumor heterogeneity. In order to study the effect of uncertainties in tumor margins, invasion of surrounding tissue, and partial volume effects, a perifocal ROI was automatically defined by dilatation of the tumor ROI by three pixels minus the tumor region, yielding a small ring around the tumor as illustrated in Figure 1. All regions were single objects delineated in multiple slices. Similarly, tumor volume determination was based on three dimensions, i.e., area analysis was performed on consecutive sections in adjacent slices.

Statistical Analysis

The results are tabulated as arithmetic mean ± standard deviation. The regional differences between tumor, homogenous appearing matter, perifocal region, edema, and corresponding healthy tissue in $|G^*|$ and φ were analyzed by two-tailed paired Student's t-test and Wilcoxon signed-rank test. The Gaussian distribution of the data was tested using the Lilliefors test and the Shaprio-Wilk test. Possible correlations between age and the viscoelastic properties of our regions of interest as well as between tumor volume and viscoelastic properties of the tumor were tested using linear and rank correlation. A P-value <0.05 was considered statistically significant. All calculations were performed using the MATLAB Statistics Toolbox (MathWorks, Natick, Massachusetts, USA).

Results

The results regarding tumor morphology are summarized in Table 1. Figure 2 presents two cases with stiff and soft spatially averaged properties within the tumor ROI (On average, patient #15 [upper row] has an approximately 33% stiffer tumor compared to surrounding tissue. Vice versa, patient #14 has approximately 33% reduced tumor stiffness [bottom row]). In the

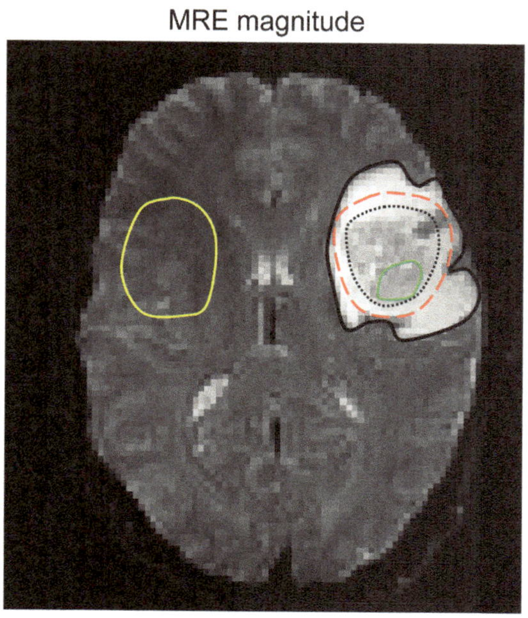

Figure 1. Example illustrating how the regions of interest (ROI) are defined one slice of the MRE magnitude image of patient #10: healthy tissue (yellow), tumor (black dotted line), perifocal margin (red dashed line), and edema (black solid line). The green line demarcates the region chosen for homogeneous appearing matter (HAM).

Table 1. Patient data, morphological classification on the basis of conventional MRI, size, and location of all tumors included in this study.

Pat. #	Sex	Age yrs.	Tumor size mm^3	Morphology	Morph. staging	Location	Hemisphere	MRI field strength in T
1	m	55	5.9	mostly homogenous appearing tumor	1	parietal	left	3
2	m	61	83.0	mostly homogenous appearing tumor, few cysts	1	temporal	left	3
3	m	75	10.0	homogenous appearing tumor with central necrosis	1	parietal	left	3
4	f	60	22.6	large central necrosis with haemorrhage	3	parieto-occipital	left	3
5	m	42	37.8	mostly homogenous tumor with cysts	1	temporo-occipital	right	3
6	m	79	67.9	mostly homogenous tumor	1	corpus callosum	bilateral	3
7	f	86	17.9	many small cysts, no hemorrhage	2	frontal	right	3
8	m	80	46.5	large central hemorrhage	3	frontal	right	3
9	f	72	39.0	homogenous appearing tumor with small cystic fraction	2	parietal+ventricle	right	3
10	f	54	14.0	indistinct tumor edge with necrotic fraction, only a few cysts and homogenous portion	3	fronto-temporal	left	1.5
11	f	53	9.7	mostly homogenous appearing tumor with central necrosis, no cysts, no hemorrhage	1	parieto-occipital	left	1.5
12	f	65	30.8	diffuse tumor with few homogenous appearing fractions	3	parietal	left	1.5
13	m	76	16.8	mostly homogenous tumor with discrete central necrosis, no cysts	1	occipital, CC	right	1.5
14	f	72	22.1	cystic tumor, no hemorrhage	2	frontal	bilateral (l>r)	1.5
15	m	61	31.6	tumor with central necrosis and hemorrhage, only small homogenous appearing portion	3	temporal	right	1.5
16	f	61	25.1	mostly homogenous appearing tumor, few cysts, discrete haemorrhage	1	occipital	right	1.5
17	m	18	99.8	mostly cystic, homogenous appering tumor rostrally, discrete haemorrhage	2	frontal	right	1.5
18	m	59	140	mostly cystic, no hemorrhage	2	temporo-parietal	links	1.5
19	m	75	20.2	mostly homogenous appearing tumor, few cysts	1	fronto-temporal	links	1.5

upper row, an extended edematous region is visible. Both types of GB present compartments of soft properties with distinct dissipative behavior. While the soft GB compartment in patient #15 has low φ values, the soft GB region in #14 presents with higher dissipative properties, indicating necrotic liquefaction (yellow arrows). The heterogeneity of mechanical tissue properties is further reflected by group-averaged values given for GB, HAM, perifocal region, edema, and contralateral healthy reference tissue in Table 2. Intrinsic tumor heterogeneity is indicated by the standard deviation values for $|G^*|$ and φ within the tumor regions.

The mean $|G^*|$ value for all tumors was 1.32±0.26 kPa ranging, from 0.85 kPa (softest tumor) to 1.83 kPa (stiffest tumor). On average, healthy tissue was significantly stiffer than GB with a mean value of 1.54±0.27 kPa and a range of 0.99–2.08 kPa ($P = 0.001$); however, in a group of 5 tumors, higher $|G^*|$ values compared to reference tissue were observed ($P = 0.015$).

Mean φ was 0.37±0.08 for the tumor tissue and 0.58±0.07 for the corresponding healthy tissue. Interestingly, this reduction in φ was seen in all tumors ($P = 2.9\times10^{-10}$) regardless of their $|G^*|$ values, which suggests less dissipative (viscous) GB properties compared to healthy tissue.

Within the tumor, homogenous appearing matter showed a higher $|G^*|$ compared to full GB regions ($P = 0.012$) without different appearance to healthy tissue ($P = 0.228$), suggesting that HAM consists of less affected tissue than the remaining GB. Nevertheless, φ_{HAM} was still lower than $\varphi_{\mathrm{healthy}}$ ($P = 0.00013$) without significant difference to φ_{tumor} ($P = 0.40$). This high sensitivity of φ to GB is further represented by the normalized ratios $\varphi_{\mathrm{tumor}}/\varphi_{\mathrm{healthy}}$ which are below 1 in all patients indicating the viability of φ as diagnostic biomarker.

Figure 3 shows $|G^*|$ and φ values of all tumors normalized by healthy tissue parameters ($|G^*|_{\mathrm{GB}}/|G^*|_{\mathrm{ref}}$ and $\varphi_{\mathrm{GB}}/\varphi_{\mathrm{ref}}$). This figure illustrates the softer tissue properties in the majority of GB and less dissipative (more elastic) properties in all tumors studied.

Additionally, lines of standard deviations are shown for the two tumors displayed in figure 2 (patients #14 und #15) in order to indicate the heterogeneity of values encountered within tumor regions. Intriguingly, standard deviations of $|G^*|_{\mathrm{GB}}/|G^*|_{\mathrm{ref}}$ do not overlap in both cases, which corroborates the visual appearance of their distinct mechanical tumor properties in Figure 2.

No correlation between tumor size and $|G^*|$ or phase angle φ was seen with correlation coefficients of $R = -0.391$ ($P = 0.072$) and $R = 0.101$ ($P = 0.655$), respectively. A correlation between the viscoelastic tissue parameters ($|G^*|$, φ) and morphological tumor staging (Table 1) was also not seen ($R = -0.235$, $P = 0.292$ and $R = -0.063$, $P = 0.781$ respectively).

$|G^*|$ in the perifocal region was not significantly different to $|G^*|$ in GB ($P = 0.306$), whereas φ showed a significant increase in the perifocal region ($P = 0.01$). The significant correlation between $|G^*|$ of tumor and perifocal region ($R = 0.571$, $P = 0.0055$) indicates the extension of the tumor's viscoelastic properties into surrounding tissue.

In 16 of 22 GB included in this study, perifocal edema was visible in T2w MRI and could be outlined for MRE parameter analysis. On average, edema tissue was significantly stiffer than GB ($P = 0.004$), whereas φ was not significantly altered between tumor and edema ($P = 0.99$). No correlation between $|G^*|$ of tumor and edema was observed ($R = 0.34$, $P = 0.197$).

Lower values for $|G^*|_{\mathrm{healthy}}$ at 1.5T (1.36±0.21 kPa) than at 3T field strength (1.71±0.22 kPa, $P = 0.001$) were observed, while none of the other parameters given in Table 2 was significantly different between 3T and 1.5T. Specifically, three of the five cases

Table 1. Cont.

Pat. #	Sex	Age yrs.	Tumor size mm³	Morphology	Morph. staging	Location	Hemisphere	MRI field strength in T
20	m	62	17.8	mostly homogenous appearing tumor, few cysts	1	temporal	rechts	1.5
21	f	75	7.7	cystic tumor with central necrosis	3	parietal	left	3
22	f	78	33.2	cystic tumor with central necrosis	3	frontal	right	3

Morphological staging was performed according to the predominant tissue type of homogenous appearing mass (= 1), cysts (= 2), and necrosis/hemorrhage(= 3).
CC = corpus callosum.

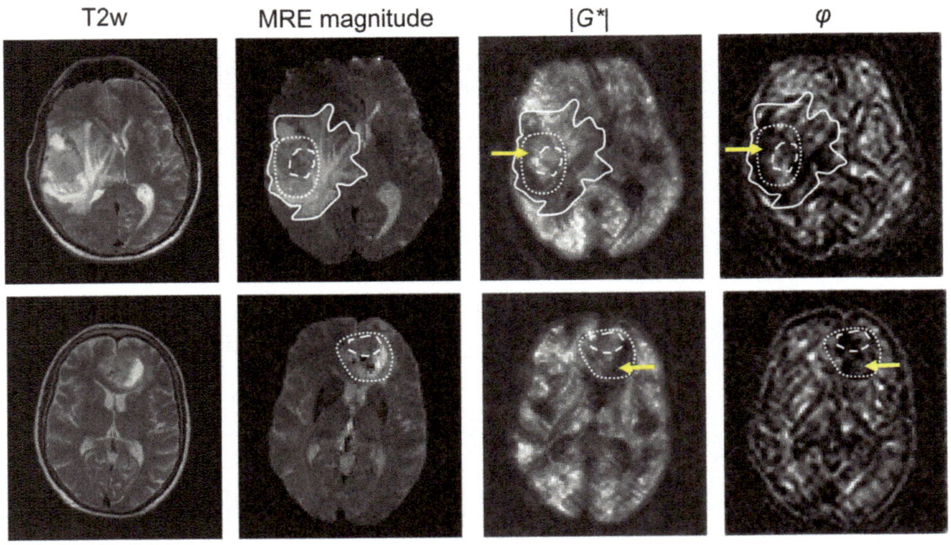

Figure 2. Anatomical T2-weighted images (T2w), MRE magnitude images, and 3DMMRE parameter maps (|G*| and φ) of 2 GB patients (upper row: patient #15, bottom row: patient #14, corresponding to the tables). The selected regions of tumor (dotted lines) and edema (solid line in #15) were used for the parameter evaluation as given in Table 2. The region of HAM is indicated by the dashed line. The yellow arrows indicate compartments of soft tissue properties (low |G*|) but different dissipative behavior (φ) in both tumors. |G*| was scaled from 0 to 3 kPa, φ was scaled from 0 to 2.5 rad.

with a higher $|G^*|_{tumor}$ than $|G^*|_{healthy}$ were measured at 1.5T, which corroborates the independence of MRE parameters from MRI field strength [47].

Discussion

Noninvasive characterization of GB remains a challenge in the present clinical routine. Conventional MRI provides only little information about tissue structure and intraparenchymal tissue connectivity. GB may include cystic, solid, and necrotic fractions as well as diffuse tumor infiltrations of the surrounding tissue; each fraction may alter the mechanical tissue properties measured by MRE.

This manuscript presents the first analysis of viscoelastic constants of intracranial tumors obtained with high spatial resolution MDEV inversion MMRE. To eliminate artifacts resulting from ill-posed inverse problems related to time-harmonic wave patterns and improve MRE parameter maps, we included multifrequency information in the solution of the inverse problem of time-harmonic elastography. The mechanical parameters elucidated in this study are well known in material science and provide full information on the complex shear modulus of human brain tissue. While $|G^*|$ relates to our haptic distinction between stiff and soft materials, φ represents the dispersion of the complex modulus, which is dictated by the topology of the underlying cellular network [48]. A highly elastic material such as agarose gel has a low φ value and is thus regarded as less dissipative than biological soft tissues composed of dense and irregular viscoelastic networks including energy-absorbing motile chains. This example illustrates the importance of considering both elastic and viscous terms for characterizing the mechanical properties of a material: agarose gel and biological tissue can have the same elasticity while their distinct viscous behavior may be appreciated by manual palpation.

$|G^*|$ and φ are not correlated with each other, and the two parameters convey different and independent mechanical information. In our study, this fact is illustrated by Figure 2, φ was clearly different in GB and healthy brain tissue, while $|G^*|$ was lower in only 17 of the 22 tumors. The uniform reduction in the dissipative GB properties may suggest a causal relationship between homeostatic tumor pressure and malignant growth as recently proposed [49] and may in the future be used as a neuroradiological marker of tumor malignancy similar to recent findings in liver tumors [50].

The heterogeneity of $|G^*|$ deserves further investigations in GB animal models. Since neither a correlation between $|G^*|$ and tumor size was observed (geometry bias) nor system-specific reasons may account for the higher stiffness in five of our patients (three were investigated at 1.5 T and two at 3 T) we expect that $|G^*|$ bears potentially valuable information for the characterization of GB. The large variability in morphological tumor assessment scores resulting from the fact that GB may be solid masses or contain cystic and necrotic fractions reflects the potential source of heterogeneity in $|G^*|$. The fact that $|G^*|$ is not correlated to the morphological score underlines the novelty of information measured by MRE.

Although encouraging, our study has some limitations: since we conducted a pilot study, we investigated the feasibility of high-resolution MMRE in a relatively small group of patients. Future studies should include more patients and compare the findings in different tumor entities. Furthermore, no other mechanical tests could be performed to provide reference values since MRE is unique for the in vivo assessment of tumor consistency. The subjective haptic impression of surgeons in our departments varied widely, preventing us from using their scores as a gold standard of tumor consistency. Future studies in animal models can tackle this issue by using indentation tests or other microelastography methods. Finally, we cannot draw any conclusions regarding the cause of variability and the sensitivity of $|G^*|$ to diagnostically relevant tissue changes. This information has to be gathered by MRE in animal models and in a higher number of patients including post-treatment follow-up.

In summary, using multislice MMRE in combination with MDEV inversion enabled us to characterize intracranial tumors

Table 2. $|G^*|$ and φ values of the selected regions of interest (ROIs) as well as the parameter ratios of tumor ROI to healthy tissue ROI (normal appearing white matter) of the 22 patients included in the study.

Pat. #	$\lvert G^*\rvert_{tumor}$ kPa	$\lvert G^*\rvert_{HAM}$ kPa	$\lvert G^*\rvert_{healthy}$ kPa	$\lvert G^*\rvert_{perifocal}$ kPa	$\lvert G^*\rvert_{edema}$ kPa	φ_{tumor} rad	φ_{HAM} rad	$\varphi_{healthy}$ rad	$\varphi_{perifocal}$ rad	φ_{edema} rad	$\lvert G^*\rvert_{tumor}/\lvert G^*\rvert_{healthy}$	$\varphi_{tumor}/\varphi_{healthy}$
1	1.83 (0.308)	1.75	1.70	1.91	2.12	0.51 (0.32)	0.31	0.66	0.52	0.43	1.08	0.78
2	1.24 (0.471)	1.23	1.54	1.03	1.15	0.38 (0.28)	0.28	0.58	0.47	0.39	0.80	0.66
3	1.35 (0.431)	1.31	1.24	1.29	1.77	0.30 (0.24)	0.47	0.47	0.31	0.39	1.09	0.64
4	1.32 (0.724)	1.02	1.87	1.46	2.19	0.45 (0.31)	0.26	0.50	0.45	0.47	0.71	0.90
5	1.29 (0.541)	1.61	1.74	1.42	1.66	0.38 (0.29)	0.39	0.60	0.44	0.33	0.74	0.63
6	1.52 (0.464)	1.84	1.65	1.38	1.53	0.48 (0.25)	0.44	0.68	0.46	0.30	0.92	0.71
7	1.55 (0.446)	2.07	1.73	2.03	no edema	0.46 (0.23)	0.73	0.57	0.53	no edema	0.90	0.81
8	0.97 (0.420)	1.04	1.66	1.41	1.90	0.34 (0.28)	0.61	0.58	0.43	0.51	0.59	0.59
9	1.47 (0.539)	1.89	1.68	1.33	1.27	0.44 (0.25)	0.42	0.60	0.43	0.28	0.88	0.73
10	1.57 (0.320)	1.50	1.37	1.73	1.83	0.26 (0.15)	0.27	0.57	0.36	0.36	1.15	0.45
11	1.39 (0.548)	1.18	1.51	1.12	1.83	0.39 (0.25)	0.26	0.63	0.38	0.53	0.92	0.61
12	0.85 (0.358)	0.99	1.11	1.27	no edema	0.35 (0.23)	0.47	0.41	0.42	no edema	0.76	0.85
13	1.34 (0.359)	1.19	1.63	1.88	1.55	0.17 (0.15)	0.56	0.58	0.32	0.29	0.82	0.29
14	1.01 (0.323)	1.26	1.53	1.33	no edema	0.36 (0.23)	0.3	0.58	0.52	no edema	0.66	0.63
15	1.32 (0.395)	1.51	0.99	1.09	1.23	0.43 (0.24)	0.67	0.59	0.31	0.38	1.34	0.73
16	1.08 (0.261)	1.24	1.26	1.13	1.22	0.34 (0.21)	0.38	0.50	0.29	0.25	0.86	0.67
17	0.95 (0.349)	1.06	1.32	0.89	no edema	0.39 (0.27)	0.2	0.73	0.30	no edema	0.72	0.54
18	1.14 (0.415)	1.33	1.27	1.34	1.39	0.37 (0.19)	0.46	0.56	0.55	0.33	0.9	0.66
19	1.79 (0.287)	1.95	1.69	1.45	no edema	0.37 (0.25)	0.32	0.61	0.47	no edema	1.06	0.61
20	1.22 (0.154)	1.25	1.35	1.04	no edema	0.43 (0.21)	0.35	0.55	0.59	no edema	0.91	0.79
21	1.43 (0.299)	1.86	2.08	1.39	1.82	0.36 (0.2)	0.41	0.55	0.42	0.35	0.69	0.65
22	1.49 (0.321)	1.86	1.91	1.44	1.53	0.34 (0.2)	0.37	0.61	0.44	0.35	0.77	0.55
Mean	1.32	1.45	1.54	1.38	1.63	0.37	0.41	0.58	0.43	0.37	0.88	0.66
SD	0.26	0.34	0.27	0.29	0.32	0.08	0.14	0.07	0.09	0.08	0.19	0.15

The standard deviations of $|G^*|$ and φ within the tumor indicating the tumor heterogeneity are given in the brackets.
tumor: region of GB, HAM: region of homogeneous appearing matter, healthy: region of normal appearing white matter, perifocal: ring of tissue obtained by dilatation of the tumor region, edema: region of edematous tissue.

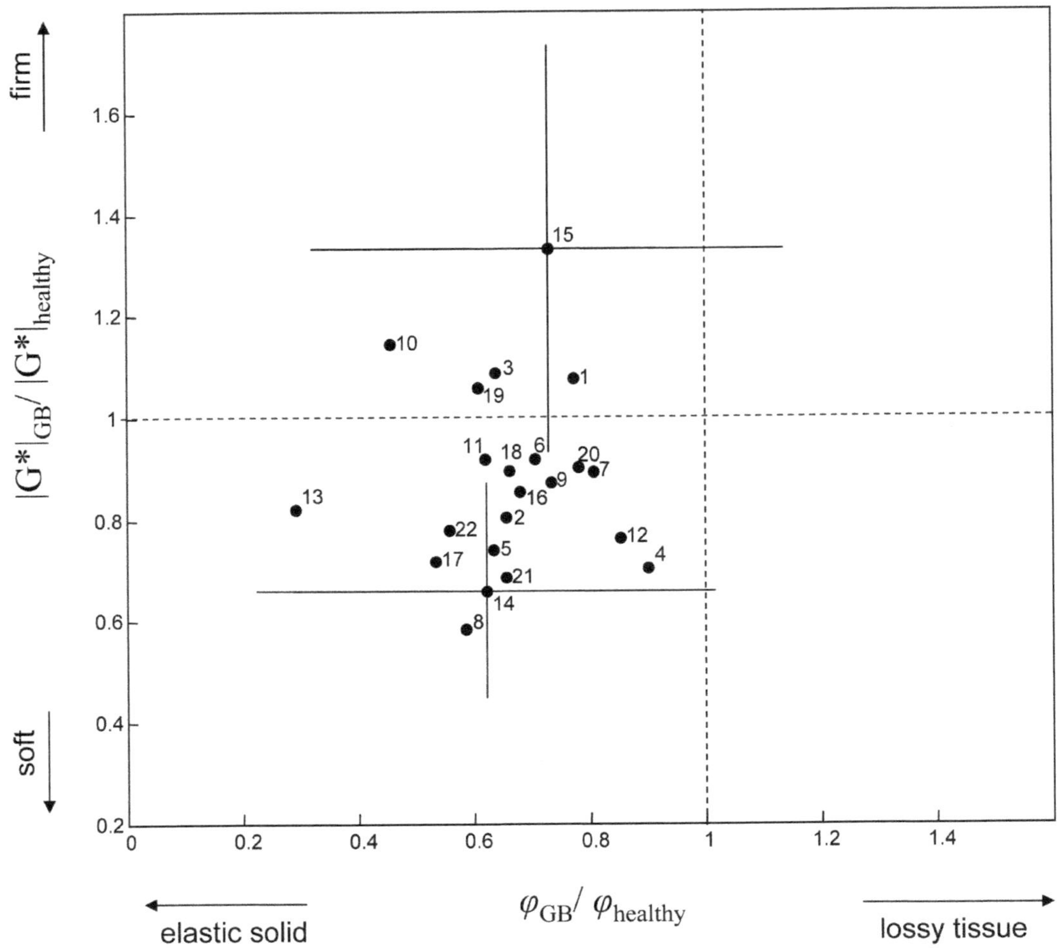

Figure 3. Viscoelastic properties of GB based on the parameter ratios of |G*| and φ between tumor and healthy reference tissue (ref). Numbers correspond to the list of tumors in tables 1 and 2. For illustration purposes, standard deviations (SD) indicating intratumoral heterogeneity are shown for the two tumors presented in figure 2 (solid lines in 14, and 15). All SD values are given in table 2.

by high-resolution mechanical parameter maps of the human brain. In our cohort of 22 GB patients, the mechanical tissue parameter $|G^*|$ indicated that GB are generally softer than healthy tissue, although we noted a large heterogeneity of values. A second mechanical parameter, φ, which is related to the dissipative behavior of tissue, was significantly reduced in all cases. High-resolution MRE may provide an early imaging marker sensitive to pathological changes of mechanical networks in brain tissue. Its diagnostic value, in particular concerning post-treatment follow-up, has to be verified by future studies.

Acknowledgments

We thank all of the patients for their participation in this study.

Author Contributions

Conceived and designed the experiments: KJS JB KTH IS. Performed the experiments: KJS MRZ JG. Analyzed the data: KJS IS JG JW. Contributed reagents/materials/analysis tools: FA SB FBF. Wrote the paper: IS.

References

1. Furnari FB, Fenton T, Bachoo RM, Mukasa A, Stommel JM, et al. (2007) Malignant astrocytic glioma: genetics, biology, and paths to treatment. Genes Dev 21: 2683–2710.
2. Stupp R, Mason WP, van den Bent MJ, Weller M, Fisher B, et al. (2005) Radiotherapy plus concomitant and adjuvant temozolomide for glioblastoma. N Engl J Med 352: 987–996.
3. CBTRUS Central Brain Tumor Registry of the United States: CBTRUS Statistical Report: Primary Brain and Central Nervous System Tumors Diagnosed in the United States in 2004–22008.
4. Davis FG, Kupelian V, Freels S, McCarthy B, Surawicz T (2001) Prevalence estimates for primary brain tumors in the United States by behavior and major histology groups. Neuro Oncol 3: 152–158.
5. Dolecek TA, Propp JM, Stroup NE, Kruchko C (2012) CBTRUS statistical report: primary brain and central nervous system tumors diagnosed in the United States in 2005–2009. Neuro Oncol 14 Suppl 5: v1–49.
6. Porter KR, McCarthy BJ, Freels S, Kim Y, Davis FG (2010) Prevalence estimates for primary brain tumors in the United States by age, gender, behavior, and histology. Neuro Oncol 12: 520–527.
7. Bailey P, Cushing H (1926) A classification of the tumors of the glioma group on a histogenic basis with a correlated study of prognosis. Philadelphia: J B Lippincott Co.
8. Louis DN, Ohgaki H, Wiestler OD, Cavenee WK, Burger PC, et al. (2007) The 2007 WHO classification of tumours of the central nervous system. Acta Neuropathol 114: 97–109.
9. Toh CH, Wei KC, Ng SH, Wan YL, Lin CP, et al. (2011) Differentiation of brain abscesses from necrotic glioblastomas and cystic metastatic brain tumors with diffusion tensor imaging. AJNR Am J Neuroradiol 32: 1646–1651.
10. Buhring U, Herrlinger U, Krings T, Thiex R, Weller M, et al. (2001) MRI features of primary central nervous system lymphomas at presentation. Neurology 57: 393–396.

11. Bernstein M, Parrent AG (1994) Complications of CT-guided stereotactic biopsy of intra-axial brain lesions. J Neurosurg 81: 165–168.
12. Romano A, Scheel M, Hirsch S, Braun J, Sack I (2012) In vivo waveguide elastography of white matter tracts in the human brain. Magn Reson Med 68: 1410–1422.
13. Johnson CL, McGarry MD, Gharibans AA, Weaver JB, Paulsen KD, et al. (2013) Local mechanical properties of white matter structures in the human brain. Neuroimage 79: 145–152.
14. Muthupillai R, Ehman RL (1996) Magnetic resonance elastography. Nature Med 2: 601–603.
15. Kruse SA, Rose GH, Glaser KJ, Manduca A, Felmlee JP, et al. (2008) Magnetic resonance elastography of the brain. Neuroimage 39: 231–237.
16. Sack I, Beierbach B, Hamhaber U, Klatt D, Braun J (2008) Non-invasive measurement of brain viscoelasticity using magnetic resonance elastography. NMR Biomed 21: 265–271.
17. Green MA, Bilston LE, Sinkus R (2008) In vivo brain viscoelastic properties measured by magnetic resonance elastography. NMR Biomed 21: 755–764.
18. Sack I, Beierbach B, Wuerfel J, Klatt D, Hamhaber U, et al. (2009) The impact of aging and gender on brain viscoelasticity. Neuroimage 46: 652–657.
19. Sack I, Streitberger KJ, Krefting D, Paul F, Braun J (2011) The influence of physiological aging and atrophy on brain viscoelastic properties in humans. PlosOne 6: e23451.
20. Streitberger KJ, Wiener E, Hoffmann J, Freimann FB, Klatt D, et al. (2011) In vivo viscoelastic properties of the brain in normal pressure hydrocephalus. NMR Biomed 24: 385–392.
21. Freimann FB, Streitberger KJ, Klatt D, Lin K, McLaughlin J, et al. (2012) Alteration of brain viscoelasticity after shunt treatment in normal pressure hydrocephalus. Neuroradiology 54: 189–196.
22. Wuerfel J, Paul F, Beierbach B, Hamhaber U, Klatt D, et al. (2010) MR-elastography reveals degradation of tissue integrity in multiple sclerosis. Neuroimage 49: 2520–2525.
23. Murphy MC, Huston J 3rd, Jack CR Jr, Glaser KJ, Manduca A, et al. (2011) Decreased brain stiffness in Alzheimer's disease determined by magnetic resonance elastography. J Magn Reson Imaging 34: 494–498.
24. Streitberger KJ, Sack I, Krefting D, Pfuller C, Braun J, et al. (2012) Brain viscoelasticity alteration in chronic-progressive multiple sclerosis. PLoS One 7: e29888.
25. Lipp A, Trbojevic R, Paul F, Fehlner A, Hirsch S, et al. (2013) Cerebral magnetic resonance elastography in supranuclear palsy and idiopathic Parkinson's disease. NeuroImage: Clinical 3: 381–387.
26. Schregel K, Wuerfel E, Garteiser P, Gemeinhardt I, Prozorovski T, et al. (2012) Demyelination reduces brain parenchymal stiffness quantified in vivo by magnetic resonance elastography. Proc Natl Acad Sci U S A 109: 6650–6655.
27. Riek K, Millward JM, Hamann I, Mueller S, Pfueller CF, et al. (2012) Magnetic resonance elastography reveals altered brain viscoelasticity in experimental autoimmune encephalomyelitis. NeuroImage: Clinical 1: 81–90.
28. Freimann FB, Muller S, Streitberger KJ, Guo J, Rot S, et al. (2013) MR elastography in a murine stroke model reveals correlation of macroscopic viscoelastic properties of the brain with neuronal density. NMR Biomed 26: 1534–1539.
29. Simon M, Guo J, Papazoglou S, Scholand-Engler H, Erdmann C, et al. (2013) Non-invasive characterization of intracranial tumors by MR-Elastography. The New Journal of Physics 15: 085024.
30. Murphy MC, Huston J 3rd, Glaser KJ, Manduca A, Meyer FB, et al. (2013) Preoperative assessment of meningioma stiffness using magnetic resonance elastography. J Neurosurg 118: 643–648.
31. Xu L, Lin Y, Han JC, Xi ZN, Shen H, et al. (2007) Magnetic resonance elastography of brain tumors: preliminary results. Acta Radiol 48: 327–330.
32. Johnson CL, McGarry MD, Van Houten EE, Weaver JB, Paulsen KD, et al. (2012) Magnetic resonance elastography of the brain using multishot spiral readouts with self-navigated motion correction. Magn Reson Med doi: 10.1002/mrm.24473. [Epub ahead of print].
33. Hirsch S, Guo J, Reiter R, Papazoglou S, Kroencke T, et al. (2013) MR Elastography of the Liver and the Spleen Using a Piezoelectric Driver, Single-Shot Wave-Field Acquisition, and Multifrequency Dual Parameter Reconstruction. Magn Reson Med 71: 267–277.
34. Papazoglou S, Hirsch S, Braun J, Sack I (2012) Multifrequency inversion in magnetic resonance elastography. Phys Med Biol 57: 2329–2346.
35. Baghani A, Salcudean S, Honarvar M, Sahebjavaher RS, Rohling R, et al. (2011) Travelling wave expansion: a model fitting approach to the inverse problem of elasticity reconstruction. IEEE Trans Med Imaging 30: 1555–1565.
36. Barnhill E, Kennedy P, Hammer S, van Beek EJ, Brown C, et al. (2013) Statistical mapping of the effect of knee extension on thigh muscle viscoelastic properties using magnetic resonance elastography. Physiol Meas 34: 1675–1698.
37. Murphy MC, Huston J 3rd, Jack CR Jr, Glaser K, Senjem ML, et al. (2013) Measuring the Characteristic Topography of Brain Stiffness with Magnetic Resonance Elastography. PLoS One 8: e81668.
38. Guo J, Hirsch S, Fehlner A, Papazoglou S, Scheel M, et al. (2013) Towards an elastographic atlas of brain anatomy. PLoS One 8: e71807.
39. Braun J, Guo J, Lützkendorf R, Stadler J, Papazoglou S, et al. (2014) High-resolution mechanical imaging of the human brain by three-dimensional multifrequency magnetic resonance elastography at 7T. Neuroimage 90: 308–314.
40. Hirsch S, Klatt D, Freimann F, Scheel M, Braun J, et al. (2012) In vivo measurement of volumetric strain in the human brain induced by arterial pulsation and harmonic waves. Magn Reson Med doi: 10.1002/mrm.24499. [Epub ahead of print].
41. Rump J, Klatt D, Braun J, Warmuth C, Sack I (2007) Fractional encoding of harmonic motions in MR elastography. Magn Reson Med 57: 388–395.
42. Jiang X, Asbach P, Streitberger K-J, Thomas A, Braun J, et al. (2014) In vivo high resolution magnetic resonance elastography of the uterine corpus and cervix. European Radiology in print: DOI: 10.1007/s00330-00014-03305-00338.
43. Papazoglou S, Xu C, Hamhaber U, Siebert E, Bohner G, et al. (2009) Scatter-based magnetic resonance elastography. Phys Med Biol 54: 2229–2241.
44. Murphy MC, Huston J 3rd, Glaser K, Manduca A, Felmlee J, et al. (2012) Phase Correction for Interslice Discontinuities in Multislice EPI MR Elastography. In: ISMRM IPotsAMo, editor; Montreal. pp. 3426.
45. Oliphant TE, Manduca A, Ehman RL, Greenleaf JF (2001) Complex-valued stiffness reconstruction for magnetic resonance elastography by algebraic inversion of the differential equation. Magn Reson Med 45: 299–310.
46. Aster RC, Borchers B, Thurber CH (2013) Parameter Estimation and Inverse Problems. Amsterdam: Elsevier.
47. Hamhaber U, Klatt D, Papazoglou S, Hollmann M, Stadler J, et al. (2010) In vivo magnetic resonance elastography of human brain at 7 T and 1.5 T. J Magn Reson Imaging 32: 577–583.
48. Sack I, Joehrens K, Wuerfel E, Braun J (2013) Structure sensitive elastography: on the viscoelastic powerlaw behavior of in vivo human tissue in health and disease. Soft Matter 9: 5672–5680.
49. Basan M, Risler T, Joanny JF, Sastre-Garau X, Prost J (2009) Homeostatic competition drives tumor growth and metastasis nucleation. Hfsp J 3: 265–272.
50. Garteiser P, Doblas S, Daire JL, Wagner M, Leitao H, et al. (2012) MR elastography of liver tumours: value of viscoelastic properties for tumour characterisation. Eur Radiol 22: 2169–2177.

4

Hippocampal and Left Subcallosal Anterior Cingulate Atrophy in Psychotic Depression

Kelly Rowe Bijanki*, Brendan Hodis, Michael C. Brumm, Emily L. Harlynn, Laurie M. McCormick

Department of Psychiatry, University of Iowa Roy J. and Lucille A. Carver College of Medicine, Iowa City, Iowa, United States of America

Abstract

Background: Psychotic depression is arguably the most diagnostically stable subtype of major depressive disorder, and an attractive target of study in a famously heterogeneous mental illness. Previous imaging studies have identified abnormal volumes of the hippocampus, amygdala, and subcallosal region of the anterior cingulate cortex (scACC) in psychotic depression, though studies have not yet examined the role of family history of depression in these relationships.

Methods: 20 participants with psychotic depression preparing to undergo electroconvulsive therapy and 20 healthy comparison participants (13 women and 7 men in each group) underwent structural brain imaging in a 1.5 T MRI scanner. 15 of the psychotic depression group had a first-degree relative with diagnosed affective disorders, while the healthy control group had no first-degree relatives with affective disorders. Depression severity was assessed with the Hamilton Depression Rating Scale and duration of illness was assessed in all patients. Automated neural nets were used to isolate the hippocampi and amygdalae in each scan, and an established manual method was used to parcellate the anterior cingulate cortex into dorsal, rostral, subcallosal, and subgenual regions. The volumes of these regions were compared between groups. Effects of laterality and family history of affective disorders were examined as well.

Results: Patients with psychotic depression had significantly smaller left scACC and bilateral hippocampal volumes, while no group differences in other anterior cingulate cortex subregions or amygdala volumes were present. Hippocampal atrophy was found in all patients with psychotic depression, but reduced left scACC volume was found only in the patients with a family history of depression.

Conclusions: Patients with psychotic depression showed significant reduction in hippocampal volume bilaterally, perhaps due to high cortisol states associated with this illness. Reduced left scACC volume may be a vulnerability factor related to family history of depression.

Editor: Kewei Chen, Banner Alzheimer's Institute, United States of America

Funding: Funding for this study was provided by a Collaborative Interdisciplinary Project Grant from the University of Iowa College of Medicine (LM) (http://obermann.uiowa.edu/programs/interdisciplinary-research-grants) and a Nellie Ball Trust Foundation Grant (LM) (https://research.uiowa.edu/grantbulletin/show.php/25137). The funders had no role in study design, data collection and analysis, decision to publish, or preparation of the manuscript.

Competing Interests: The authors have declared that no competing interests exist.

* Email: kelly-rowe@uiowa.edu

Introduction

Depression is the highest contributor to disease burden in middle- and high-income countries [1], and among all of its subtypes, psychotic depression is the most severe variant [2,3]. Psychotic depression represents a mood disorder distinct from non-psychotic major depression based on differences in symptomatology, disease course, treatment response, cognitive dysfunction, and biological features [4]. Approximately 20% of people with major depression are thought to experience psychosis, though this number rises to 50–60% in groups of patients with treatment-refractory major depression [5]. Patients with psychotic depression can be sensitively (84%) and specifically (99%) discerned from their non-psychotically depressed counterparts on the basis of their endorsements of unusual thought content, an item on the Brief Psychiatric Rating Scale [6,7]. Patients with psychotic depression are reported to show greater cognitive deficits, have previous episodes with psychosis, longer duration of episodes, and a greater likelihood of recurrence [7]. In addition, they show greater hypothalamo-pituitary-adrenal axis activation and have higher cortisol levels than their non-psychotically depressed counterparts [8]. Psychotic depression has been advanced as the most diagnostically stable presentation of major depressive disorder [9]; in one study, 92.3% of patients with psychotic depression experienced previous and/or subsequent psychotic episodes [10]. From a research perspective, this diagnostic stability makes patients with psychotic depression an ideal group to study. Kronmuller and colleagues have elegantly articulated the importance of reducing variability in chronicity and severity of depressive illness for the purposes of research [11].

Reports of volumetric brain abnormalities in major depressive disorder have been mixed, likely owing to the heterogeneity of depressive symptoms and etiologies, as well as demographic differences among samples. Many studies report abnormalities of the hippocampus, amygdala, ventral anterior cingulate and prefrontal cortex in depressive illness [12–14]. Overall, it appears that there are significant effects of illness chronicity on hippocampus and amygdala atrophy in major depressive disorder, where longer illness duration correlates with more severe tissue loss [13,15,16]. One previous study [4] has examined hippocampus and amygdala volumes in three groups: psychotic major depression, non-psychotic major depression, and healthy controls. Results indicated that patients with psychotic depression had significant amygdala atrophy compared with the other two groups, and there were no significant group differences in hippocampal volumes. In contrast, a more recent study [50] examined virtually identical participant groups and found no significant differences between psychotic and non-psychotic major depressive disorder patients in amygdala or hippocampus volumes. However, they did observe that patients with major depression (regardless of the presence of psychosis) tended to have larger amygdala volumes than controls.

In recent years, research on depression has turned toward the ventral anterior cingulate cortex and the two sub-regions that comprise it; the subcallosal and subgenual regions (scACC and sgACC respectively). Decreased activity has been noted in these areas in response to antidepressant medication, placebo treatment, and electroconvulsive therapy (ECT). Increased activity in these regions is noted in treatment non-responders, the currently depressed and transiently sad people compared to healthy controls [17]. One recent study [50] examined group-wise differences in the volume of this brain region in patients with psychotic depression as compared with non-psychotic major depression and healthy controls, reporting no significant differences between depression groups, but significant atrophy in the left subgenual region compared with controls.

An important terminological shift must be acknowledged in the literature on the ventral anterior cingulate. Early research on the anatomy and function of the area used the term "subgenual" to define the entirety of the ventral anterior cingulate cortex underlying the genu of the corpus callosum. In recent years, the term "subgenual" has been revised to include only a small volume of the posterior ventral ACC, also frequently termed "Brodmann Area 25" (Figure 1, yellow region). The anterior section of the ventral ACC, or ventral Brodmann Area 24 has since been termed "subcallosal" (Figure 1, green region). For example, decreased activity has been shown in the "subgenual cingulate" (identical to the subcallosal + subgenual cingulate as defined in the current study) in patients with familial unipolar major depressive disorder and that this decrease in activity corresponded with a 48% reduction in volume of the structure [18].

In the current study we aimed to examine the neural correlates of psychotic depression using structural MRI volumetric techniques. Based on findings reported across the depression literature, we defined six regions of interest for the current study: the hippocampus, the amygdala, and four parcellations of the anterior cingulate cortex (dorsal, rostral, subcallosal, and subgenual). Two previous reports from our lab [19,20] have suggested the left subcallosal cingulate and the hippocampus as major mediators of treatment response in ECT for psychotic depression. We anticipated seeing group differences in volumes in these regions, especially on the left side. In contrast with the previous study by Vassilopoulou and colleagues, we also aimed to examine the role of family history of affective disorders in any observed volumetric abnormality of these structures. Furthermore, the current study expands on previous findings [4] by including measures of the anterior cingulate cortex and by examining patients whose depression may have been more homogeneous (in that all participants in the current study experienced very severe psychotic depression and were being treated with ECT at the time of neuroimaging). The current study additionally expands on the findings of Drevets et al. [18] by examining patients with psychotic depression and including measures of medial temporal lobe structures.

Methods

Participants

The current study included 20 participants with psychotic unipolar major depression (here termed "psychotic depression") and 20 age- and sex-matched healthy comparison participants (see Table 1 for demographics). Healthy comparisons were recruited from the community through newspaper advertisements and were screened using an abbreviated version of the Comprehensive Assessment of Symptoms and History. Comparison participants were excluded if they had current or past major medical, neurological, or psychiatric illnesses, or if they had a family history of schizophrenia or affective disorders.

The participants in the psychotic depression group took part in a larger study that reported neuroimaging findings before and after ECT [19,20]. All participants met DSM-IV criteria for major depression with psychotic features and completed an MRI scan prior to or early in treatment with ECT (scans gathered after an average of 3.5 ECT doses). Eighteen participants (90%) underwent inpatient hospitalization at the University of Iowa Hospitals and Clinics and were referred for ECT by their psychiatrist on clinical grounds; the other two participants (10%) had been referred for ECT treatment on an outpatient basis. Data on the duration of depressive episode, as well as family histories of affective disorders and information on medication usage (Table 1) were taken from interviews conducted by trained psychiatrists during the course of treatment and documented in the participants' medical records. Participants had a range of current episode duration: 55% had been depressed for less than 6 months; 20% had been depressed for between 6 and 12 months; 5% had been depressed for between 12 and 24 months; 20% had been depressed for greater than 24 months at the time of data collection. Participants were rated as having a family history of affective disorder if there was unequivocal documentation of a first-degree relative (i.e. parent, sibling, or child) with diagnosed depression, bipolar disorder and/or suicide attempt based upon review of their medical records. Medications were assessed an average of 8 days prior to MRI scan and excluded "pro re nata" medications given for acute care of psychotic depression during hospitalization.

All participants in the psychotic depression group had a pre-ECT score of at least 30 on the 28-item Hamilton Depression Rating Scale (indicating severe depression) and had at least one psychotic symptom. Participants were excluded if they had a diagnosis of bipolar disorder or schizophrenia, met criteria for alcohol or illicit drug abuse or dependence within the past three months, or had been treated with a previous course of ECT within the past three months. After complete description of the study to the participants, written informed consent was obtained. This study was approved by The University of Iowa Institutional Review Board (200402013).

Measures

All participants in the psychotic depression group completed clinical interviews using the Scales for the Assessment of Negative and Positive Symptoms (SANS/SAPS) [21,22]. Scores from the

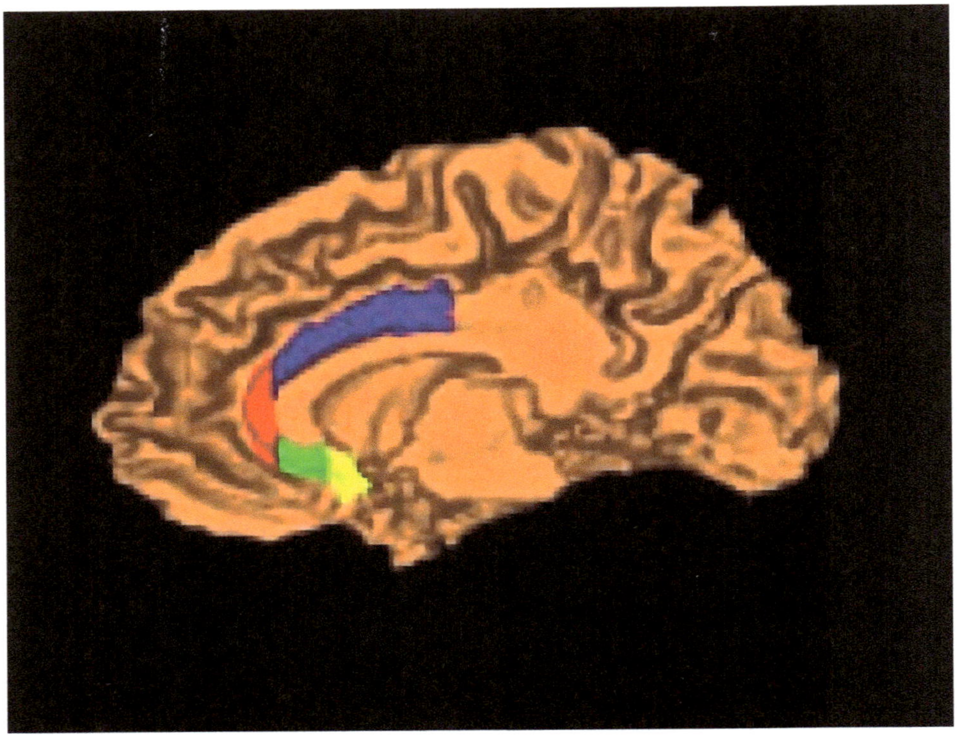

Figure 1. Parcellations of the anterior cingulate cortex. Dorsal anterior cingulate cortex (ACC) shown in blue, rostral ACC in red, subcallosal ACC in green, subgenual ACC in yellow. Figure reprinted with permission from John Wiley and Sons, from McCormick et al., (2008), license number 3103240766914.

SANS/SAPS were divided into three dimensions: (1) psychoticism (scale 0–10), based on global ratings of delusions and hallucinations; (2) disorganization (scale 0–15), based on global ratings of bizarre (disorganized) behavior, positive formal thought disorder, and inappropriate affect; and (3) negative symptoms (scale 0–25), based on global ratings of alogia, anhedonia-asociality, avolition-apathy, affective flattening, and attention. The most common psychotic symptom in the current sample was delusional guilt.

In addition, all psychotic depression participants completed the 28-item Hamilton Depression Rating Scale (HAM-D) [23], as well as the Hamilton Anxiety Rating Scale (HAM-A) [24]. Both are clinician-administered instruments that assess symptoms and

Table 1. Demographic Comparison between Psychotic Depression and Healthy Control groups.

	Psychotic Depression Mean (SD) [n = 20]	HC Mean (SD) [n = 20]	DF	Statistic	*p*-value
Age	46.0 (9.5)	45.4 (9.9)	38	$t = -0.201$	$p = 0.841$
Education	13.3 (2.8)	14.5 (1.6)	38	$t = 1.737$	$p = 0.090$
Sex	65% F (13 f: 7 m)	65% F (13 f: 7 m)	1	$X^2 = 0.000$	$p > 0.999$
HAM-D	38.5 (5.4)	–	–	–	–
HAM-A	28.8 (7.9)	–	–	–	–
Family History of Affective Disorders	75%	–	–	–	–
Medication Use					
Antidepressant	95%	–	–	–	–
Anxiolytic	25%	–	–	–	–
Antipsychotic	40%	–	–	–	–
Lithium	5%	–	–	–	–

Note: Age and education reported in years. HAM-D = Hamilton Depression Rating Scale, HAM-A = Hamilton Anxiety Rating Scale, HC = healthy control, DF = degrees of freedom, SD = standard deviation. Family history of affective disorders included evidence of depression, bipolar disorder, or suicide attempt in a first degree relative. Data on family histories of affective disorders and medication usage were taken from interviews conducted by trained psychiatrists during the course of treatment and documented in the participants' medical records. Medications were assessed an average of 8 days prior to MRI scan and excluded "pro re nata" medications given for acute care of psychotic depression during hospitalization.

severity of a patient's depressive and anxious symptoms, with higher scores indicating increasing severity of symptoms. Scores above 30 on the HAM-D and HAM-A are generally taken to indicate "very severe" anxiety and depression.

Neuroimaging

Multimodal magnetic resonance imaging (MRI) scans were obtained using either a 1.5-T GE Signa scanner (10 psychotic depression participants and 20 healthy controls; GE Medical Systems, Milwaukee, WI) or on a 1.5-T Siemens Avanto scanner (10 psychotic depression participants; Erlangen, Germany). The sequences collected included a standard T1-weighted three-dimensional spoiled gradient recall acquisition (TE = 5 ms; TR = 24 ms; flip angle = 30°−50°; two excitations; FOV = 26 cm; matrix = 256×256; slice thickness = 1.5–1.7 mm). Two-dimensional T2 sequences were also acquired (TE = 24–98 ms; TR = 3000–9500 ms; flip angle = 90°−180°; one excitation; FOV = 26 cm; matrix = 256×256; slice thickness = 3.0 mm). All scans were visually assessed for quality and for motion artifacts.

Automated processing of the structural images was performed using BRAINS2 (Brain Research: Analysis of Images, Networks, and Systems) software [25], which includes automated AC-PC alignment, image alignment, image intensity standardization, tissue classification, and brain extraction. Then, automated neural nets were used to parcellate the hippocampi and amygdalae bilaterally [26,27]. These neural nets were then reviewed by human raters following procedures as outlined by [28] and, when necessary, hand-corrected following procedures as outlined by [29].

The hand-tracing methods for parcellating the ACC (Figure 1) have been described at length elsewhere [30], and the previous methods were strictly followed for the identification of the dorsal, rostral, and subgenual ACC. For the current study, the previous parcellation method for the subcallosal ACC was modified slightly; the subcallosal region includes only the continuation of the rostral cingulate gyrus as it wraps around the genu of the corpus callosum, rather than additionally including paracingulate gyrus. The anterior boundary of the subcallosal ACC is defined by the anteriormost slice where the forceps major of the corpus callosum is no longer connected through the genu on the coronal view. The posterior boundary is placed one slice anterior to where the putamen first is visible within the basal ganglia. The superior boundary is formed by the ventral continuation of the callosal sulcus. The inferior boundary of this region is defined by the termination of the primary cingulate sulcus (whether or not a secondary sulcus is evident) [31].

Twenty-one psychotic depression participants and 20 HC participants received structural neuroimaging scans. One psychotic depression participant was excluded from the study due to profound damage from a traumatic brain injury. Two other psychotic depression participants' scans failed the amygdala and hippocampus neural net application and were excluded from those analyses, though their ACC regions were parcellated satisfactorily. One HC participant's scan failed the amygdala ANN but his or her data were usable for hippocampal and ACC measures. Therefore, the following samples were available for analysis: amygdala (18 psychotic depression, 19 HC), hippocampus (18 psychotic depression, 20 HC), ACC subregions (20 psychotic depression, 20 HC). Of the two psychotic depression participants whose amygdala and hippocampus neural nets failed, one had a positive family history of affective disorders.

Statistical Analyses

All data underlying the current manuscript are presented as Supplementary Files (Dataset S1, Dataset S2, Variable Definitions S1), including raw numerical data and variable descriptions. Statistical analyses used the standard alpha level of .05 for statistical significance and used two-tailed tests. Demographic data were examined to demonstrate that there were no significant differences between the experimental and control groups, using independent samples t-tests (age, education) and chi-squared tests (sex) (Table 1). For methodological reasons, half of the psychotic depression group received their neuroimaging scans on a different scanner (Siemens) than the rest of the participants (GE). For this reason, we used a multivariate general linear model to confirm that there were no effects of scanner on the imaging measures used in the study.

Next, independent samples t-tests were used to examine the volumetric differences in the regions of interest (hippocampus, amygdala, dorsal ACC, rostral ACC, subcallosal ACC, subgenual ACC, and total intracranial volume) between the experimental and control groups. The hippocampus test precluded an assumption of equal variances, so the degrees of freedom for that test were adjusted accordingly. After the initial hypothesis testing, these group-wise comparisons were re-calculated using a multivariate model adjusting for total intracranial volume (indicated with asterisks in Table 2). Finally, the results of these comparisons were further adjusted for the false discovery rate [32], and results remaining significant after that adjustment are indicated with pluses (Table 2).

A more detailed examination of laterality effects in the hippocampus and subcallosal ACC was conducted using independent samples t-tests and repeating the statistical adjustments for total intracranial volume and false discovery rate. Finally, we examined the psychotic depression group to see if there was an effect of family history of affective disorders on hippocampal and subcallosal ACC volumes, again using independent samples t-tests.

Results

There were no significant differences between participants with psychotic depression and healthy comparisons in terms of sample size, age, education, or sex (see Table 1). Patients with psychotic depression additionally completed the Hamilton Depression and Anxiety Rating Scales (HAM-D and HAM-A) (Table 1), as well as Scales for the Assessment of Negative and Positive Symptoms of Schizophrenia (SANS: mean = 12.9, SD = 3.4; SAPS-Psychoticism: mean = 3.3, SD = 1.8; SAPS-Disorganization: mean = 0.5, SD = 0.8). The psychotic depression group was further characterized in terms of family history of affective disorders, where fifteen of the twenty participants with psychotic depression had a family history of a first-degree relative with an affective disorder. There were no differences between psychotic depression patients with and without family histories in terms of baseline HAM-D score ($t = -.065$, $DF = 19$, $p = .949$). Psychotic depression patients had an average duration of current episode of less than six months (55%), and the majority used antidepressant medications (Table 1). Because of the possibility of confounding due to the use of two different scanners in the neuroimaging acquisition, we used a multivariate general linear model to confirm that there were no effects of scanner on the imaging measures used in the study. This analysis confirmed that there was a non-significant effect of scanner on the brain regions examined in the current study (Pillai's Trace = 0.315, $F = .880$, $p = .577$).

Group-wise comparisons examined regional brain volumetric differences between psychotic depression and HC participants in

Table 2. Comparison of psychotic depression group with healthy controls on brain volumetrics.

	Psychotic Depression Mean (SD)	HC Mean (SD)	DF	Statistic	*p*-value
Total ICV	1345.74 (170.18)	1388.78 (160.59)	38	t = 0.823	*p* = 0.416
Hippocampus[a]	4.12 (0.37)	4.58 (0.52)	34.33	t = 3.166	*p* = 0.003*+
Amygdala[b]	2.18 (0.30)	2.28 (0.36)	36	t = 0.948	*p* = 0.349
Subcallosal ACC	0.71 (0.23)	0.93 (0.22)	38	t = 3.036	*p* = 0.004*+
Subgenual ACC	1.02 (0.28)	1.04 (0.29)	38	t = −0.196	*p* = 0.845
Dorsal ACC	7.39 (1.26)	7.00 (0.88)	38	t = −1.139	*p* = 0.262
Rostral ACC	4.32 (1.66)	4.20 (1.04)	38	t = −0.263	*p* = 0.794

Note: Raw means and standard deviations presented (reported in cubic centimeters).
*comparisons that remain significant after adjustment for total ICV.
+comparisons that remain significant after adjustment for false discovery rate.
[a]sample included 18 psychotic depression and 20 HC participants with no significant differences between groups on demographic variables (age *p* = 0.772, education *p* = 0.114, sex *p* = 0.804).
[b]sample included 19 psychotic depression and 19 HC participants. Hippocampal t-test adjusted because of violation of the assumption of equal variances.
ICV = intracranial volume, reported in cubic centimeters. ACC = anterior cingulate cortex.

raw volumes of the hippocampus, amygdala, dorsal ACC, rostral ACC, subcallosal ACC, and subgenual ACC. These analyses showed that the only significant differences between groups were in the hippocampus and the subcallosal ACC (see Table 2). These comparisons were calculated twice; once uncorrected, and once controlled for total intracranial volume and adjusted for false discovery rate.

Laterality effects were then assessed. While both sides of the hippocampus were found to be significantly smaller in psychotic depression participants than healthy comparisons, the reduction in subcallosal ACC volume was driven primarily by left-sided atrophy (Table 3). Hippocampal volume in the psychotic depression group averaged 10.1% smaller than healthy controls, while the left subcallosal ACC was 31.4% smaller than controls. Furthermore, it was found that within the psychotic depression group, those with a positive family history of affective disorders (15 of the 20 participants) had significant atrophy of the left subcallosal ACC ($t = 3.809$, $df = 24.590$, $p = .001$) when compared with healthy controls, while the five without family history showed normal volume of the structure ($t = .497$, $df = 23$, $p = .624$). On average, psychotic depression patients with a family history of affective disorders had left scACC volumes 38.5% smaller than healthy controls. By comparison, there was no effect of family history of affective disorder on the finding of hippocampal atrophy ($t = .531$, $df = 16$, $p = .603$). Both subgroups of depressed patients had significantly smaller hippocampal volumes than healthy comparison subjects (positive family history: $t = 2.350$, $df = 10.888$, $p = .039$; negative family history: $t = 2.972$, $df = 32$, $p = .006$).

Discussion

Participants with psychotic depression were compared with healthy controls on measures of the hippocampus, amygdala, dorsal ACC, rostral ACC, subcallosal ACC, and subgenual ACC. As hypothesized, this study demonstrates a pattern of significantly smaller bilateral hippocampus and left-sided subcallosal cingulate volumes in patients with psychotic depression when compared to age-matched healthy control participants. Left subcallosal ACC atrophy was highly significant only in the group of psychotic depression subjects with a family history of affective disorders, while hippocampal atrophy was found bilaterally and was not dependent on whether there was a family history of affective disorders.

Left scACC atrophy in patients with depression who also have a family history of affective disorders is consistent with three previous studies, all of which examined the undifferentiated "subgenual" region, which included what are now termed the subcallosal and subgenual subregions [18,33,34]. The current finding is consistent with that of [18], which reported a 48% reduction in left "subgenual" cingulate volume in a group of patients with familial unipolar depression compared with healthy controls. The second study [33] showed a 20% reduction in left "subgenual" cingulate volumes in patients with affective disorders compared with healthy controls, and a 24% reduction in patients with familial affective disorders compared to patients with non-familial affective disorders. The third study [34] further showed that women with MDD had significantly smaller left "subgenual" ACC volumes than controls, with no reduction on the right. Another study has shown a 23.8% reduction in the volume of the subgenual cingulate bilaterally in familial major depressive disorder [35]. Histological analysis showed that this volume reduction was related to decreased numbers of glia in the region while the number of neurons remained unchanged [35]. It is unclear why only the left sided atrophy of the subcallosal cingulate cortex appears to be driven by genetics in the current sample, in that it was only observed in those psychotic depression patients with a family history of affective disorders. However, one previous study [50] in patients with psychotic depression reported a similar finding, and similarly constrained to the left subgenual cingulate.

Several previous studies have identified the presence of bilateral hippocampal atrophy in MDD patients, which was supported by the findings of the current study [12,13,15,16]. We did not confirm the previous finding from Keller et al. [4], who reported amygdala atrophy rather than hippocampal atrophy specifically in psychotic depression. This discrepancy could be related to the use in the current study of a new, automated method for measuring amygdala and hippocampus volumes, rather than the manual method used in the previous study, which was originally developed for use in a pediatric population [36]. The current study also used a 1.5 T MRI (3T in Keller et al.), as well as older (mean age 45 in the current study; 36 in Keller et al.), and more depressed participants (mean HAM-D = 38 current study; mean HAM-D = 30 in Keller et al.).

Table 3. Laterality effects on hippocampus and subcallosal ACC volumes in psychotic depression compared to age-matched healthy comparisons.

	Psychotic Depression Mean (SD) [n = 20]	HC Mean (SD) [n = 20]	DF	Statistic	*p*-value
Left Hippocampus[a]	2.05 (0.181)	2.30 (0.276)	33.08	t = 3.303	$p = 0.002$ *+
Right Hippocampus[a]	2.07 (0.214)	2.28 (0.262)	36	t = 2.797	$p = 0.008$ *+
Left subcallosal ACC	0.289 (0.087)	0.421 (0.174)	38	t = 3.035	$p = 0.004$ *+
Right subcallosal ACC	0.425 (0.213)	0.507 (0.143)	33.25	t = 1.420	$p = 0.165$

Note: Raw means and standard deviations presented (reported in cubic centimeters).
*comparisons that remain significant after adjustment for total ICV.
+comparisons that remain significant after adjustment for false discovery rate.
[a]sample included 18 participants with psychotic depression and 20 HC participants with no significant differences between groups on demographic variables (age $p = 0.772$, education $p = 0.114$, sex $p = 0.804$). Left hippocampal and right subcallosal ACC t-tests adjusted because of violation of the assumption of equal variances.
ICV = intracranial volume, reported in cubic centimeters. ACC = subcallosal anterior cingulate cortex.

The exact neurobiological underpinnings of depression and psychotic depression remain to be completely elucidated, though there are hints at the mechanisms, one of which is related to glucocorticoid toxicity of the hippocampus following prolonged exposure to the stress hormone cortisol. Intense stress, such as that experienced during severe depression, can cause reduced expression of brain-derived neurotrophic factor (BDNF) in the hippocampus and elevated expression of cortisol, leading to decreased hippocampal neurogenesis and overall atrophy of the structure [37,38]. Patients with psychotic depression may be especially vulnerable to decreased hippocampal neurogenesis and overall atrophy because they (more so than their non-psychotic depressed counterparts) experience elevated cortisol expression [4,39] ECT, and to a lesser extent antidepressant medications, have been shown to promote synaptogenesis and neurogenesis in the hippocampus [40–42]. Psychotic depression is highly responsive to ECT treatment, with a 95% response rate [43] and the mechanism of this response may be linked to increased neurogenesis in the hippocampus [42]. It is possible that in psychotic depression, ECT is the most effective treatment because it most strongly promotes neurogenesis in the hippocampus, perhaps even to such an extent that it can overcome the stress-induced atrophy of the structure.

The ACC and the hippocampus are connected through the limbic system and may function as pacemakers for theta oscillations in the brain [44–46]. Previous studies have shown that theta activity in the ACC could predict treatment response to antidepressants, and that ECT could change theta activity in the scACC in depressed patients [47,19]. The scACC is also the primary brain target for deep brain stimulation (DBS) for treatment-resistant depression in a large multi-site study [48]. Resolution of depressive symptoms with DBS of the scACC has also been associated with changes in theta activity and pre-treatment theta activity may even predict response to DBS [49].

The current study included a sample of patients with psychotic depression that was so severe and treatment resistant to necessitate treatment with ECT. The current study was limited by a relatively small sample, a lower-powered MR scanner, and included only cross-sectional data. In order to remedy the limitations of the current study, future studies with this population should include both pre- and post-ECT MRI with a higher resolution 3T scanner and with diffusion weighted imaging to allow tractography studies to specifically look at hippocampal-ACC connections. It will also be important to further assess whether these findings are specific to psychotic depression or high cortisol states, and whether they exist in other subtypes of MDD severe enough to require ECT. However, the current study has shown for the first time that the volume of the hippocampus is significantly smaller in patients with psychotic depression than in controls, and that there are significant effects of family history on atrophy of the scACC specifically. These findings may provide further insight into the pathophysiology of psychotic depression, and highlight the importance of consideration of family history and brain structural changes over the course of the illness.

Supporting Information

Dataset S1 All data underlying the current manuscript are presented here in comma-separated variable format for easy access.

Dataset S2 All data underlying the current manuscript are presented here in IBM SPSS software file format with variable definitions and other descriptive information embedded.

Variable Definitions S1 Definitions for each variable heading in Dataset S1 and Dataset S2.

Acknowledgments

The authors thank the participants of the current study for the time and energy they contributed to the project. Without their support, this study would never have been possible.

Author Contributions

Conceived and designed the experiments: LM MB. Performed the experiments: LM MB. Analyzed the data: KB BH MB EH LM. Contributed reagents/materials/analysis tools: BH KB. Contributed to the writing of the manuscript: KB BH MB EH LM.

References

1. WHO (2008) The global burden of disease: 2004 update. Geneva: World Health Organization.
2. Lykouras E, Malliaras D, Christodoulou GN, Papakostas Y, Voulgari A, et al. (1986) Delusional depression: phenomenology and response to treatment: a prospective study. Acta Psychiatr Scand 73: 324–329.

3. Rothschild AJ, Benes F, Hebben N, Woods B, Luciana M, et al. (1989) Relationships between brain CT scan findings and cortisol in psychotic and nonpsychotic depressed patients. Biol Psychiatry 26: 565–575.
4. Keller J, Shen L, Gomez RG, Garrett A, Solvason HB, et al. (2008) Hippocampal and amygdalar volumes in psychotic and nonpsychotic unipolar depression. Am J Psychiatry 165: 872–880.
5. Dubovsky SL (1991) What we don't know about psychotic depression. Biol Psychiatry 30: 533–536.
6. Overall JE, Gorham DE (1961) The brief psychiatric rating scale. Psychol Rep. 10; 799–812.
7. Keller J, Schatzberg AF, Maj M (2007) Current issues in the classification of psychotic major depression. Schizophr Bull 33: 877–885.
8. Hill SK, Keshavan MS, Thase ME, Sweeney JA (2004) Neuropsychological dysfunction in antipsychotic-naïve first-episode unipolar psychotic depression. Am J Psychiatry 161: 996–1003.
9. Charney DS, Nelson JC (1981) Delusional and nondelusional unipolar depression: further evidence for distinct subtypes. Am J Psychiatry 138: 328–333.
10. Helms PM, Smith RE (1983) Recurrent psychotic depression: Evidence of diagnostic stability. J Affect Disord. 5: 51–54.
11. Kronmuller KT, Schroder J, Kohler S, Gotz B, Victor D, et al. (2009) Hippocampal volume in first episode and recurrent depression. Psychiatry Res. 174: 62–66.
12. Videbech P, Ravnkilde B (2004) Hippocampal volume and depression: a meta-analysis of MRI studies. Am J Psychiatry 161: 1957–1966.
13. Campbell S, MacQueen G (2006) An update on regional brain volume differences associated with mood disorders. Curr Opin Psychiatry 19: 25–33.
14. Drevets WC, Price JL, Furey ML (2008) Brain structural and functional abnormalities in mood disorders: implications for neurocircuitry models of depression. Brain Struct Funct 213: 93–118.
15. MacQueen GM, Campbell S, McEwen BS, Macdonald K, Amano S, et al. (2003) Course of illness, hippocampal function, and hippocampal volume in major depression. Proc Natl Acad Sci U S A 100: 1387–1392.
16. Sheline YI, Sanghavi M, Mintun MA, Gado MH (1999) Depression duration but not age predicts hippocampal volume loss in medically healthy women with recurrent major depression. J Neurosci. 19: 5034–5043.
17. Mayberg HS (2009) Targeted electrode-based modulation of neural circuits for depression. J Clin Invest. 119: 717–725.
18. Drevets WC, Price JL, Simpson JR, Todd RD, Reich T, et al. (1997) Subgenual prefrontal cortex abnormalities in mood disorders. Nature. 386: 824–827.
19. McCormick LM, Boles Ponto LL, Pierson RK, Pierson RK, Johnson HJ, et al. (2007) Metabolic correlates of antidepressant and antipsychotic response in patients with psychotic depression undergoing electroconvulsive therapy. J ECT 23: 265–273.
20. McCormick LM, Yamada T, Yeh M, Brumm MC, Thatcher RW (2009) Antipsychotic effect of electroconvulsive therapy is related to normalization of subgenual cingulate theta activity in psychotic depression. J Psychiatr Res 43: 553–560.
21. Andreasen NC (1984) Scale for the assessment of positive symptoms. Iowa City: University of Iowa.
22. Andreasen NC (1982) Negative symptoms in schizophrenia: definition and reliability. Arch Gen Psychiatry 39: 784–788.
23. Hamilton M (1960) A rating scale for depression. J Neurol Neurosurg Psychiatry. 23: 56–63.
24. Hamilton M (1959) The assessment of anxiety states by rating. Br J Med Psychol. 32: 50–55.
25. Magnotta VA, Harris G, Andreasen NC, O'Leary DS, Yuh WTC, et al. (2002) Structural MR image processing using the BRAINS2 toolbox. Comput Med Imaging Graph. 26: 251–264.
26. Powell HWR, Richardson MP, Symms MR, Boulby PA, Thompson PJ, et al. (2008) Preoperative fMRI predicts memory decline following anterior temporal lobe resection. J Neurol Neurosurg Psychiatry 79: 686–693.
27. Schumann CM, Hamstra J, Goodlin-Jones BL, Lotspeich LJ, Kwon H, et al. (2004) The amygdala is enlarged in children but not adolescents with autism; the hippocampus is enlarged at all ages. Neurobiol Disease 24: 6392–6401.
28. Aylward EH, Liu D, Nopoulos PC, Ross CA, Pierson RK, et al. (2012) Striatal volume contributes to the prediction of onset of Huntington disease in incident cases. Biol Psychiatry 71: 822–828.
29. Pantel J, O'Leary DS, Cretsinger K, Bockhold HJ, Keefe H, et al. (2000) A new method for the in vivo volumetric measurement of the human hippocampus with high neuroanatomical accuracy. Hippocampus 10: 752–758.
30. McCormick LM, Ziebell S, Nopoulos P, Cassell M, Andreasen NC, et al. (2006) Anterior cingulate cortex: an MRI-based parcellation method. Neuroimage 32: 1167–1175.
31. Coryell W, Nopoulos P, Drevets W, Wilson T, Andreasen NC (2005) Subgenual prefrontal cortex volumes in major depressive disorder and schizophrenia: Diagnostic specificity and prognostic implications. Am J Psychiatry 162: 1706–1712.
32. Benjamini Y, Hochberg Y (1995) Controlling the false discovery rate: a practical and powerful approach to multiple testing. J R Stat Soc Series B Stat Methodol 57: 289–300.
33. Hirayasu Y, Shenton ME, Salisbury DF, Kwon JS, Wible CG, et al. (1999) Subgenual cingulate cortex volume in first-episode psychosis. Am J Psychiatry 156: 1091–1093.
34. Botterton KN, Raichle ME, Drevets WC, Heath AC, Todd RD (2002) Volumetric reduction in left subgenual prefrontal cortex in early onset depression. Biol Psychiatry 51: 342–344.
35. Ongur D, Drevets WC, Price JL (1998) Glial reduction in the subgenual prefrontal cortex in mood disorders. Proc Natl Acad Sci U S A 95: 13290–13295.
36. Kates WR, Abrams MT, Kaufmann WE, Breiter SN, Reiss AL (1997) Reliability and validity of MRI measurement of the amygdala and hippocampus in children with fragile X syndrome. Psychiatry Res 75: 31–48.
37. Nestler EJ, Barrot M, DiLeone RJ, Eisch AJ, Gold SJ, et al. (2002) Neurobiology of Depression. Neuron 34: 13–25.
38. Sheline YI (2003) Neuroimaging studies of mood disorder effects on the brain. Biol Psychiatry 54: 338–352.
39. Hill SC, Keshavan MS, Thase ME, Sweeney JA (2004) Neuropsychological dysfunction in antipsychotic-naïve first-episode unipolar psychotic depression. Am J Psychiatry 161: 996–1003.
40. Malberg JE, Eisch AJ, Nestler EJ, Duman RS (2000) Chronic antidepressant treatment increases neurogenesis in adult rat hippocampus. J Neurosci. 20: 9104–9110.
41. Scott BW, Wojtowicz TJ, McIntyre Burnham W (2000) Neurogenesis in the dentate gyrus of the rat following electroconvulsive shock seizures. Exp Neurol 165: 231–236.
42. Nordanskog P, Dahlstrand U, Larsson MR, Larsson EM, Knutsson L, et al. (2010) Increase in hippocampal volume after electroconvulsive therapy in patients with depression: a volumetric magnetic resonance imaging study. J ECT 26, 62–67.
43. Petrides G, Fink M, Husain MM (2001) ECT remission rates in psychotic versus nonpsychotic depressed patients: a report from CORE. J ECT. 17: 244–253.
44. Buzsaki G (2002) Theta oscillations in the hippocampus. Neuron, 33: 325–340.
45. Ishii R, Shinosaki K, Inouye T (1999) Medial prefrontal cortex generates frontal midline theta rhythm. Neuroreport, 10: 675–679.
46. Asada H, Fukuda Y, Tsunoda S, Yamaguchi M, Tonoike M (1999) Frontal midline theta rhythms reflect alternative activation of prefrontal cortex and anterior cingulate cortex in humans. Neurosci Lett, 274: 29–32.
47. Pizzagalli DA (2011) Frontocingulate dysfunction in depression: toward biomarkers of treatment response. Neuropsychopharmacology Rev. 36: 183–206.
48. Lozano AM, Giacobbe P, Hamani C, Rizvi SJ, Kennedy SH, et al. (2012) A multicenter pilot study of subcallosal cingulate area deep brain stimulation for treatment-resistant depression. J Neurosurg 116(2): 315–322.
49. Broadway JM, Holtzheimer PE, Hilimire MR (2012) Frontal theta cordance predicts 6-month antidepressant response to subcallosal cingulate deep brain stimulation for treatment-resistant depression: a pilot study. Neuropsychopharmacology. 37: 1764–1772.
50. Vassilopoulou K, Papathanasiou M, Michopoulos I, Boufidou F, Oulis P, et al. (2013) A magnetic resonance imaging study of hippocampal, amygdala and subgenual prefrontal cortex volumes in major depression subtypes: melancholic versus psychotic depression. J Affect Disord. 146: 197–204.

5

Optimal Brain MRI Protocol for New Neurological Complaint

William A. Mehan Jr., R. Gilberto González*, Bradley R. Buchbinder, John W. Chen, William A. Copen, Rajiv Gupta, Joshua A. Hirsch, George J. Hunter, Scott Hunter, Jason M. Johnson, Hillary R. Kelly, Mykol Larvie, Michael H. Lev, Stuart R. Pomerantz, Otto Rapalino, Sandra Rincon, Javier M. Romero, Pamela W. Schaefer, Vinil Shah

Neuroradiology Division, Massachusetts General Hospital, Harvard Medical School, Boston, Massachusetts, United States of America

Abstract

Background/Purpose: Patients with neurologic complaints are imaged with MRI protocols that may include many pulse sequences. It has not been documented which sequences are essential. We assessed the diagnostic accuracy of a limited number of sequences in patients with new neurologic complaints.

Methods: 996 consecutive brain MRI studies from patients with new neurological complaints were divided into 2 groups. In group 1, reviewers used a 3-sequence set that included sagittal T1-weighted, axial T2-weighted fluid-attenuated inversion recovery, and axial diffusion-weighted images. Subsequently, another group of studies were reviewed using axial susceptibility-weighted images in addition to the 3 sequences. The reference standard was the study's official report. Discrepancies between the limited sequence review and the reference standard including Level I findings (that may require immediate change in patient management) were identified.

Results: There were 84 major findings in 497 studies in group 1 with 21 not identified in the limited sequence evaluations: 12 enhancing lesions and 3 vascular abnormalities identified on MR angiography. The 3-sequence set did not reveal microhemorrhagic foci in 15 of 19 studies. There were 117 major findings in 499 studies in group 2 with 19 not identified on the 4-sequence set: 17 enhancing lesions and 2 vascular lesions identified on angiography. All 87 Level I findings were identified using limited sequence (56 acute infarcts, 16 hemorrhages, and 15 mass lesions).

Conclusion: A 4-pulse sequence brain MRI study is sufficient to evaluate patients with a new neurological complaint except when contrast or angiography is indicated.

Editor: Jan Kassubek, University of Ulm, Germany

Funding: The authors have no support or funding to report.

Competing Interests: The authors have declared that no competing interests exist.

* Email: rggonzalez@mgh.harvard.edu

Introduction

Diagnostic medical imaging is one of the major driving forces behind rising healthcare expenditures. Between 2000 and 2006, Medicare spending on imaging services more than doubled, increasing to $14 billion[1]. The volume of brain MR studies performed may continue to rise in the future due to the expansion of health care insurance under the Patient Protection and Affordable Care Act (PPACA) and as a result of an aging population. At our institution, patients with various neurologic complaints are often imaged with MRI protocols that may involve a large number of pulse sequences, resulting in long scan times. There have been major advances in MRI hardware and software technology since the days of the first nuclear magnetic resonance (NMR) images in 1974. These advancements have provided us with an array of available MR sequences to choose from for our neuroimaging protocols. Long scan times related to multiple sequence acquisitions likely result in patient inconvenience and discomfort. It is unclear whether the multiple MR sequences performed are necessary and which of the sequences add value to the interpretation of the study. Optimizing the number of sequences in a routine screening brain MR protocol could improve efficiency as well as increase patient compliance and satisfaction by reducing scan time. Our goal was to investigate the diagnostic accuracy of brain MRI protocols containing a limited number of basic sequences in the evaluation of patients with new neurologic complaints.

Methods

Patient Selection

This retrospective study was approved by the Partners Human Research Committee, our hospital's Institutional Review Board

Table 1. Patient Demographics and MRI Findings Group 1.

Parameter	Group 1 (n = 497)	Group 2 (n = 499)
Age (years)	**mean 54.3 (range 0.5–98)**	**mean 51.3 (range 0.5–93)**
Male:Female (%)	**43:57**	**38:62**
Significant MRI Findings	84	117 (23.4%)
Acute/subacute infarction	39 (46.4%)	67 (57.3%)
Intracranial hemorrhages	9 (10.7%)	7 (6.0%)
Posterior reversible encephalopathy syndrome (PRES)	2 (2.4%)	4 (3.4%)
Vascular lesions*	4 (4.8%)	4 (3.4%)
Cavernous malformations	4 (4.8%)	1(0.9%)
Active demyelinating lesions	3 (3.6%)	2(1.7%)
Hydrocephalus	1 (1.2%)	3 (2.6%)
Metastases	5 (6.0%)	9 (7.7%)
Meningiomas or schwannomas	8 (9.5%)	7 (6.0%)
Mass lesions**	4 (4.8%)	11 (9.4%)
Infectious/Inflammatory lesions	3 (3.6%)	2(1.7%)
Cortical dysplasia	2 (2.4%)	0
Major discrepancies	21	19 (16.2%)
Enhancing lesions***	12 (57.1%)	17 (89.5%)
Punctate acute/subacute infarcts	4 (19.0%)	0
Cortical dysplasias	2(9.5%)	0
Vascular lesions	3 (14.3%)	2 (10.5%)
Microhemorrhage discrepancies		
Microhemorrhages	Group 1 (n = 19)	Group 2 (n = 28)
Discrepancies	15 (77.8%)	0

* Venous sinus thrombosis, ICA dissection, arterial thrombus, absent vertebrobasilar flow voids, MCA branch thrombosis
** Cerebellar mass, brainstem mass, optic nerve sheath mass, thalamic masses, lobar masses, pituitary/sellar masses, corpus callosal mass, clival mass, colloid cysts
***Included probable metastases, probable primary tumors, inflammatory/demyelinating lesions, and indeterminate punctate enhancing foci

(IRB). Consent was not obtained and patient records/information was anonymized and de-identified prior to analysis.

We performed a retrospective study of consecutive brain MR examinations performed at our institution, a major urban academic medical center, between February 20, 2010 and April 21, 2010. Studies included patients of all ages who underwent brain MR imaging for the evaluation of new neurologic complaints for which there was no established diagnosis stated on the radiology requisition. We included studies referred from the emergency department, inpatient and outpatient settings. Both intravenous contrast- enhanced and unenhanced studies were included as were studies that contained MR angiogram (MRA) and MR venogram (MRV) sequences. Image review commenced in June 2012, at least 24 months after the examinations were performed. Exclusion criteria were MR studies performed for follow-up evaluation of pre-existing neurological conditions (e.g. serial neuro-oncology studies) and specialized MR protocols (e.g. pituitary, orbits, brainstem and internal auditory canal studies).

All MRI examinations were performed on either 1.5T (Tesla) or 3T MR systems (GE Healthcare Clinical Systems, Wauwatosa, WI, USA; Siemens Medical Solutions, Erlangen, Germany). A total of 9 MRI scanners were used during the period that was reviewed. Eight scanners had field strengths of 1.5T. Six were manufactured by General Electric; 3 were located within the hospital and 3 were located at free standing imaging centers. Two 1.5T MRI scanners were manufactured by Siemens and were located within the hospital. Additionally, a single Siemens 3T scanner was located within the hospital. All MR images in the study were reviewed on a PACS system (Agfa Impax 5.3, Agfa Healthcare, Mortsel, Belgium).

Study Interpretation

The total number of consecutive MRI studies was partitioned into two separate data sets (group 1, MR studies from February 20, 2010 through March 23, 2010; group 2, MR studies from March 24, 2010 through April 21, 2010).

The group 1 neuroradiologists reviewed a three-sequence abbreviated image set composed of sagittal T1-weighted images, axial T2-weighted FLAIR images, and images derived from a single diffusion-weighted imaging sequence, which included images with and without diffusion gradients, as well as derived apparent diffusion coefficient maps. The neuroradiologists interpreted those three MRI sequences while blinded to both the additional MRI sequences that were acquired, and to the official radiologic report. For each case, a group 1 neuroradiologist formulated an impression based on the three limited sequences and then subsequently compared it to the unblinded impression in the reference official radiologic report. For any discrepancy between the two interpretations, the neuroradiologist was instructed to revisit the limited MR sequences and determine

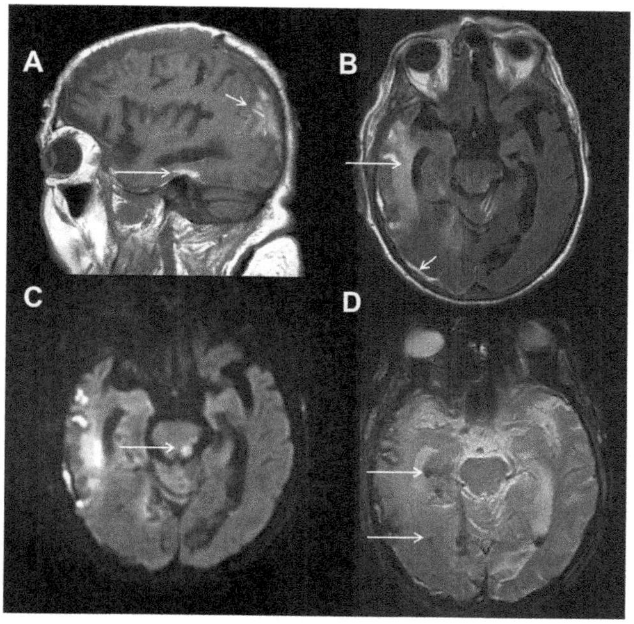

Figure 1. Intracranial hemorrhages and diffuse axonal injury. 83 year old female status post fall. Sagittal T1-weighted image (A) shows hyperintense signal involving the lateral right temporal lobe consistent with cortical contusion and subacute blood products (white arrow). Axial T2-weighted FLAIR image (B) depicts edema in the right temporal lobe from traumatic contusion (long white arrow) and a subdural hemorrhage overlying the lateral right temporal and occipital lobes (short white arrow). Axial diffusion weighted trace image (C) shows a focus of restricted diffusion within the left dorsolateral midbrain compatible with non-hemorrhagic diffuse axonal injury (white arrow). Axial gradient recalled echo image (D) shows a punctate focus of susceptibility effect within the right temporal lobe compatible with hemorrhagic diffuse axonal injury (white arrow).

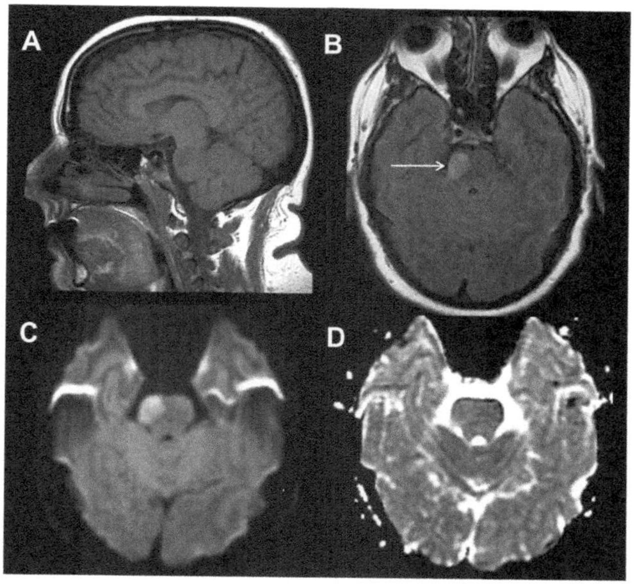

Figure 2. Brainstem mass lesion. 38 year old female with transient left sided weakness. Sagittal T1-weighted image (A) shows a subtle hypointense lesion within the pons. Axial T2-weighted FLAIR image (B) demonstrates a hyperintense, expansile mass-like lesion within the right mid pons (white arrow). Axial diffusion weighted trace (C) and apparent diffusion coefficient images (D) reveal slightly increased diffusivity within the lesion compatible with a demyelinating lesion, neoplasm, or subacute infarction.

whether, in retrospect, the discrepant findings could have been made on the limited sequences, but were missed due to perceptual error.

The second phase of the study involved a different set of staff neuroradiologists with experience ranging from 2 to 20 years. The group 2 neuroradiologists reviewed a four-sequence abbreviated image set composed of the three basic sequences that were reviewed by the group 1 neuroradiologists, with the addition of an axial magnetic susceptibility sensitive sequence (either T2* gradient recalled echo (GRE), or susceptibility weighted imaging (SWI), including susceptibility weighted angiography (SWAN)). The neuroradiologists interpreted those four MRI sequences while blinded to both the additional MRI sequences that were acquired, and to the official radiologic report. For each case, a group 2 neuroradiologist formulated an impression based on the four limited sequences and then subsequently compared it to the unblinded impression in the official radiologic report, (the reference standard). For any discrepancy between the two interpretations, the neuroradiologist revisited the limited MR sequences and determined whether, in retrospect, the discrepant findings could have been appreciated on the limited sequences, but were missed due to perceptual error.

The limited sequence interpretations by the neuroradiologists in groups 1 and 2 were performed on the same PACS workstations as the original interpretations, and they are located in the same interpretation areas as in the original clinical interpretation. The only history that was permitted to the new study reviewer was the limited one provided with the original request for imaging. The neuroradiologists in groups 1 and 2 were allowed to review previous MRI studies when available, but only the limited MRI sequences on the prior study could be reviewed when formulating an impression. Readers in both groups were not permitted to review post-contrast, MRA, or MRV images, if these were acquired.

In order to eliminate recall bias, the assignment of MRI cases to each neuroradiologist was reviewed. If any case had been previously reviewed by the neuroradiologist to which the case was assigned, then the case was reassigned to an additional neuroradiologist (RGG) who reviewed the case with the same instructions.

We designated findings and discrepancies as major if they were likely to have a significant impact on patient management. Level 1 findings were designated as those requiring immediate communication at our institution: acute infarction, intracranial hemorrhage and unexpected mass lesion. The following imaging findings were also designated as major: subacute infarctions; posterior reversible encephalopathy syndrome (PRES); vascular malformations; malformations of cortical development (including focal cortical dysplasia); hydrocephalus; parenchymal lesions suspicious for infection, inflammatory disease, primary or secondary CNS neoplasm; and other mass lesions. Abnormalities of the major intracranial flow voids including arterial dissection, venous sinus thrombosis and intra-arterial thrombus were also considered major abnormalities. Acute/subacute infarctions required observation of decreased diffusivity in DWI sequences. Microhemorrhages (punctate parenchymal foci of susceptibility effect) were

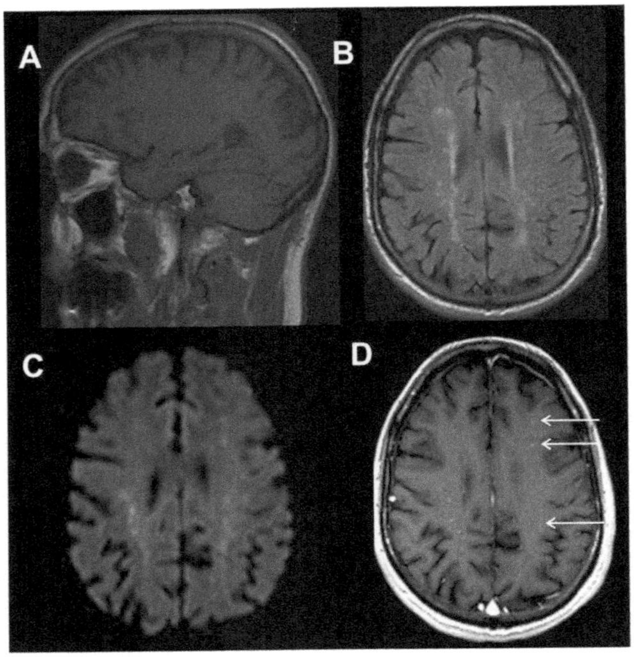

Figure 3. Foci of enhancement in a 57 year old male with ataxia. Sagittal T1-weighted image (A) shows no definite abnormality. Axial T2-weighted FLAIR image (B) demonstrates multiple punctate hyperintense foci involving the deep and periventricular white matter of the bilateral cerebral hemispheres with corresponding restricted diffusion on the axial diffusion weighted trace (C) image. Axial T1-weighted post contrast image (D) reveals numerous punctate foci of enhancement corresponding to the deep and periventricular white matter lesions (white arrows). In this patient, the differential diagnosis included intravascular lymphoma, granulomatous disease, neurosarcoidosis, and vasculitis.

considered potentially important findings. Other typically incidental findings were designated as non-major.

Statistical Analysis

A descriptive analysis of the data from groups 1 and 2 was performed.

Results

Out of a total of ~3750 brain MRI studies, 998 brain MRI studies met our eligibility criteria. The first 497 studies were placed in group 1, and the remaining 499 in group 2.

In group 1, 84 major findings were identified (16.9% of studies, Table 1). All 41 level 1 findings (28 acute infarcts, 9 hemorrhages, and 4 mass lesions) were identified on the limited sequences. Examples of cases with accurately interpreted major findings included traumatic brain injury with multi-compartment intracranial hemorrhages (Figure 1) and neoplasms (Figure 2). Of these 84 major findings, there were 21 discrepancies between the interpretation based on the abbreviated MRI protocol, and the official interpretation from the radiologic report, yielding an error rate of 25.0%.

The most common discrepant major findings were enhancing intracranial lesions (12 cases) (Figure 3). There were 4 small acute or subacute infarctions that were missed by two of the group 1 readers. All of these abnormalities were identified on the diffusion MR sequences when the readers re-examined these studies. Thus,

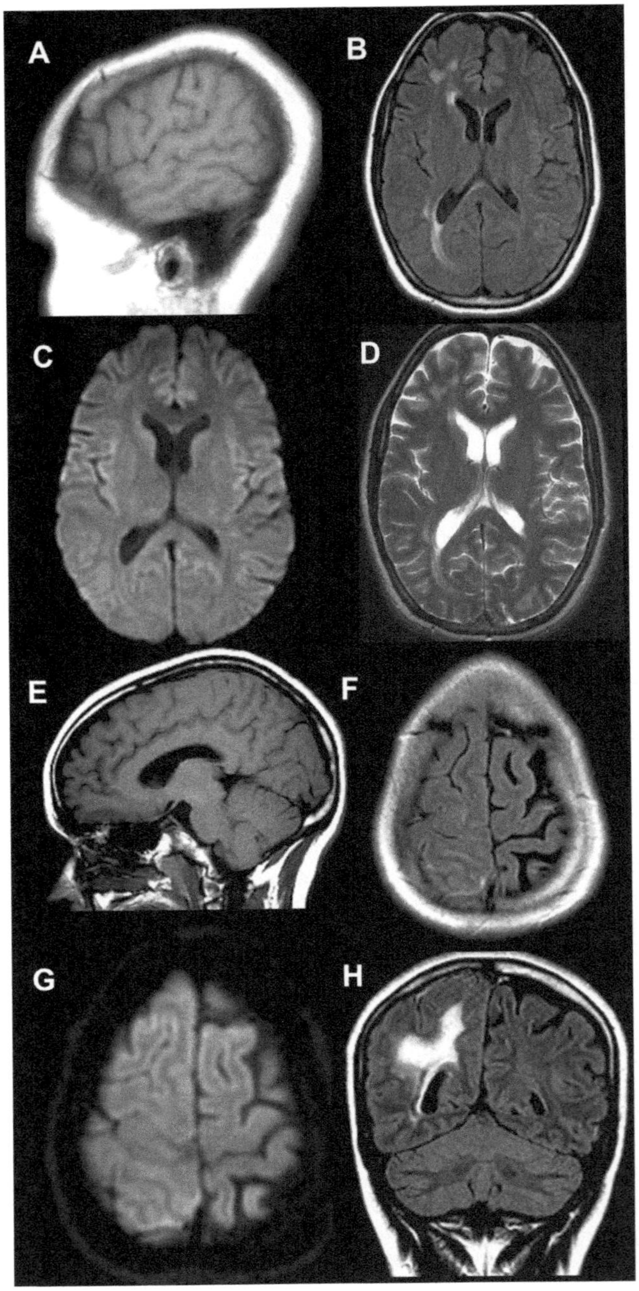

Figure 4. 22 year old female with right frontal hemispheric dysplasia. Sagittal T1-weighted image (A) shows no definite abnormality. Axial FLAIR image (B) demonstrates subtle enlargement of the right hemisphere with focal areas of signal hyperintensity within the subcortical white matter of the right frontal and parietal lobes but without corresponding restricted diffusion on the axial diffusion weighted trace (C) image. Additionally noted is ipsilateral ventricular enlargement. Pachygyria was also demonstrated within the right frontal and parietal lobes, better demonstrated on more superior axial FLAIR images. Axial T2-weighted image (D) also demonstrates these findings. Sagittal T1-weighted image (E) shows no definite abnormality. Axial FLAIR image (F) demonstrates asymmetric cortical thickening, gyral enlargement within the right frontal and parietal lobes without restricted diffusion on the axial diffusion weighted trace (G) image, consistent with pachygyria. Coronal FLAIR image (H) reveals asymmetric cortical thickening, abnormal sulcation and white matter signal hyperintensity in the right parietal lobe. The group 1 reader described the right frontal lobe signal abnormality, but did not diagnose the full extent of the hemispheric abnormality. These findings are more apparent on the coronal FLAIR sequence, not available to the reader.

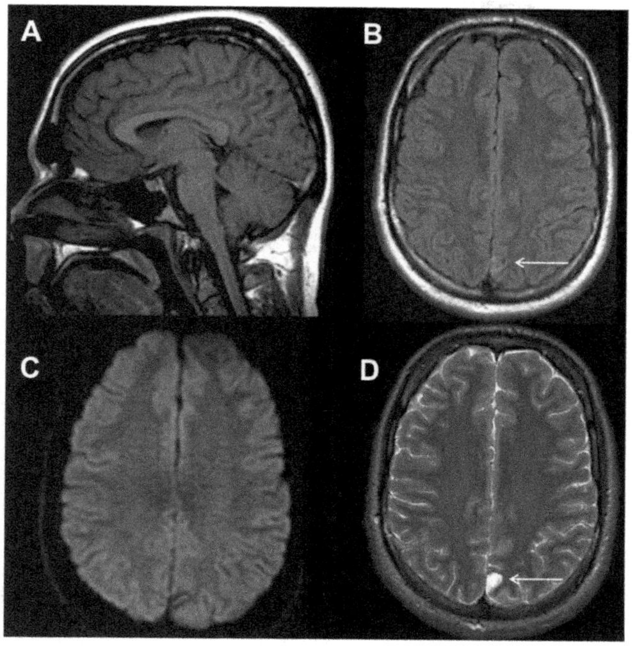

Figure 5. Cortical dysplasia versus dysembryoplastic neuroepithelial tumor in an 18 year old male with seizures. Sagittal T1-weighted image (A) shows no definite abnormality. Axial T2-weighted FLAIR image (B) demonstrates a subtle focal area of signal hyperintensity within the cortex and subcortical white matter of the left parafalcine parietal lobe(white arrow) with no corresponding restricted diffusion on the axial diffusion weighted trace (C) image. Axial T2-weighted image (D) again demonstrates the hyperintense lesion within the cortex and subcortical white matter of the left parafalcine parietal lobe (white arrow), which is compatible with cortical dysplasia or dysembryoplastic neuroepithelial tumor. This finding is subtle and was not seen prospectively when using the limited sequences. However, the lesion can be seen on the FLAIR images in retrospect. Furthermore, for seizure patients, additional sequences, including isotropic multiplanar sequences, could be added that would help in identifying subtle abnormalities.

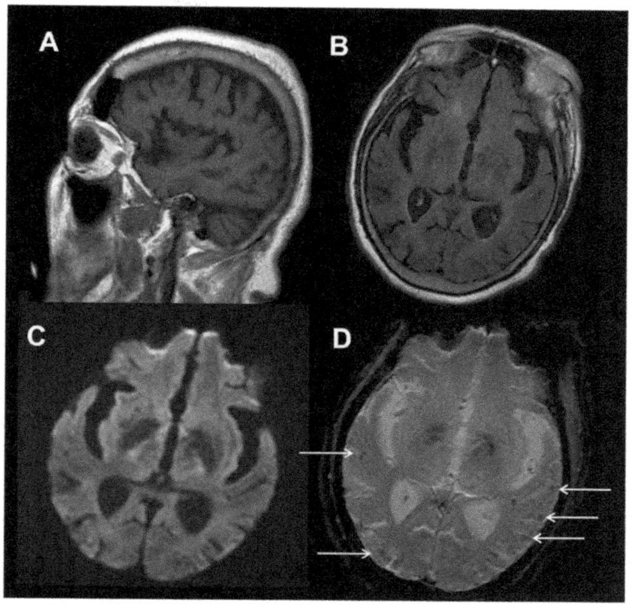

Figure 6. Cerebral amyloid angiopathy in a 78 year old female with altered mental status. Sagittal T1-weighted image (A) shows age appropriate parenchymal volume loss. Axial FLAIR image (B) demonstrates a small number of nonspecific hyperintense foci that are not unusual in a patient of this age. The axial diffusion weighted image (C) demonstrates no evidence of acute ischemia. Sequences A-C (group 1 sequences) show no definite abnormality that would explain the patient's symptoms. Axial gradient recalled echo image (D) reveals multiple punctate foci of susceptibility effect (white arrows) involving peripheral grey-white matter junctions, consistent with chronic micro-hemorrhages, which was not identified by the group 1 reader. This sequence alone (in addition to the other 3 sequences) provides the information needed to make the diagnosis of cerebral amyloid angiopathy.

these discrepancies were due to perceptual error. The diagnosis of cortical dysplasia was not made in 2 studies by group 1 readers. Abnormalities on the limited sequences were identified (Figure 4), but the diagnosis was not suggested. In the other case, a small non-enhancing lesion was only observed upon repeat review of the study (Figures 5).

There were 3 vascular abnormalities that were not identified on the abbreviated sequences; 2 cases of middle cerebral artery branch (MCA) thrombus in patients with concurrent acute infarctions and a case of transverse sinus thrombosis. The cases of MCA branch occlusion were not visualized on the 3-sequence series, although the acute infarctions in the MCA distribution were identified. The group 1 reader who did not identify the venous thrombosis reported that they would not have seen this lesion without an MR venogram.

In group 1, there were 19 cases that had evidence of probable microhemorrhage (3.8%). Out of these 19 cases, 15 were not identified by group 1 readers on the abbreviated MR sequences (77.8%) (Figure 6).

In the group 2 evaluation, there were 117 major findings in the 499 MR studies (23.4%, Table 2). Examples of cases with accurately detected major findings included early infarctions (Figures 7, 8, and 9) and neoplasms (Figure 10). Of these, 19 major findings were not identified on the abbreviated 4-sequence MRI series resulting in an error rate of 16.2%. Enhancing parenchymal lesions were the most commonly missed major findings (17 cases). The other major discrepancies were vascular lesions; one case of ICA dissection (Figure 11) and one case of vertebrobasilar arterial occlusion (Figure 12). In both of these cases, the readers reported that the absence of the flow voids was not identifiable without the aid of a non-inversion recovery T2-weighted sequence or MR angiogram (Figures 11D-F and 12E-G). There were 28 cases with probable microhemorrhages in the group 2 data set. All of these were identified by the group 2 readers.

Discussion

Since the introduction of MRI for the clinical evaluation of brain pathology, a large number of pulse sequences have been developed, and those with the highest clinical value have been extensively evaluated. However, there is little documented research on the optimal set of MRI sequences for the evaluation of patients with specific clinical presentations. In this evaluation of MRI used in patients with a new neurological complaint, we found that a limited-sequence imaging protocol can identify nearly all significant brain abnormalities with the major exceptions of small,

Table 2. Patient Demographics and MRI Findings Group 2.

Parameter	Group 2 (n=499)
Age (years)	**mean 51.3 (range 0.5–93)**
Male:Female (%)	**38:62**
Significant MRI Findings	117
Acute/subacute infarction	67 (57.3%)
Intracranial hemorrhages	7 (6.0%)
Posterior reversible encephalopathy syndrome (PRES)	4 (3.4%)
Vascular lesions*	4 (3.4%)
Cavernous malformations	1(0.9%)
Active demyelinating lesions	2(1.7%)
Hydrocephalus	3 (2.6%)
Metastases	9 (7.7%)
Meningiomas or schwannomas	7 (6.0%)
Mass lesions**	11 (9.4%)
Infectious/Inflammatory lesions	2(1.7%)
Cortical dysplasia	0
Major discrepancies	19
Enhancing lesions***	17 (89.5%)
Punctate acute/subacute infarcts	0
Cortical dysplasias	0
Vascular lesions	2 (10.5%)
Microhemorrhage discrepancies	
Microhemorrhages	Group 2 (n=28)
Discrepancies	0

* Venous sinus thrombosis, ICA dissection, arterial thrombus, absent vertebrobasilar flow voids, MCA branch thrombosis
** Cerebellar mass, brainstem mass, optic nerve sheath mass, thalamic masses, lobar masses, pituitary/sellar masses, corpus callosal mass, clival mass, colloid cysts
***Included probable metastases, probable primary tumors, inflammatory/demyelinating lesions, and indeterminate punctate enhancing foci

contrast-enhancing lesions and vascular lesions that are revealed by MR angiography. The 4-sequence protocol was superior to the 3-sequence protocol due to improved detection of probable microhemorrhages, and we conclude that it is sufficiently robust for the routine evaluation of patients who have new neurological symptoms and do not have a clear clinical indication for the use of contrast (e.g. history of a primary non-CNS malignancy or suspicion of demyelinating/inflammatory disorders) or direct evaluation of the cerebral vasculature (e.g. vascular risk factors with high suspicion for acute ischemia).

The T2-weighted FLAIR sequence has been shown to be the single most sensitive sequence for the detection of brain pathology [1–16]. Saleh et al. demonstrated in 1026 consecutive outpatient MRI studies that this sequence alone had positive and negative predictive values of 96.1% and 98.4%, respectively, for lesions detectable by a complete MRI protocol that included contrast enhancement [17]. The data presented here are fully consistent with this work. However, the T2-weighted FLAIR sequence is not sensitive in detecting small enhancing lesions, small structural lesions, early ischemia, and microhemorrhages, and it cannot be relied upon as the only sequence. The use of diffusion MRI and susceptibility sequences are excellent supplemental sequences for the detection of the latter two types of abnormalities.

Cerebral microhemorrhages are a common finding, but have indeterminate prognostic and therapeutic significance [18]. Using the 3-sequence protocol, 78% of cases with probable cerebral microhemorrhages were undetected by readers viewing the T1, T2-weighted FLAIR and diffusion sequences. This is similar to prior reports [19,20]. All probable microhemorrhages were correctly identified by readers who were able to view an axial susceptibility sequence as part of the 4 sequence protocol. This finding is consistent with the known superiority of susceptibility-weighted sequences in identifying small foci of susceptibility effect [18–23].

The use of the 3-sequence protocol resulted in lack of detection of 25% of major abnormalities, with over half of these being enhancing lesions. An improved detection rate was manifest with the 4-sequence protocol, with a lack of detection of 16% of major findings, but 90% of these were enhancing lesions. Enhancing lesions included meningiomas, active inflammatory/demyelinating lesions, metastases and probable primary brain tumors, as well as indeterminate punctate areas of parenchymal enhancement. Our findings suggest that intravenous gadolinium-based contrast should be administered in patients with a history of malignancy or suspected demyelinating/inflammatory disorders.

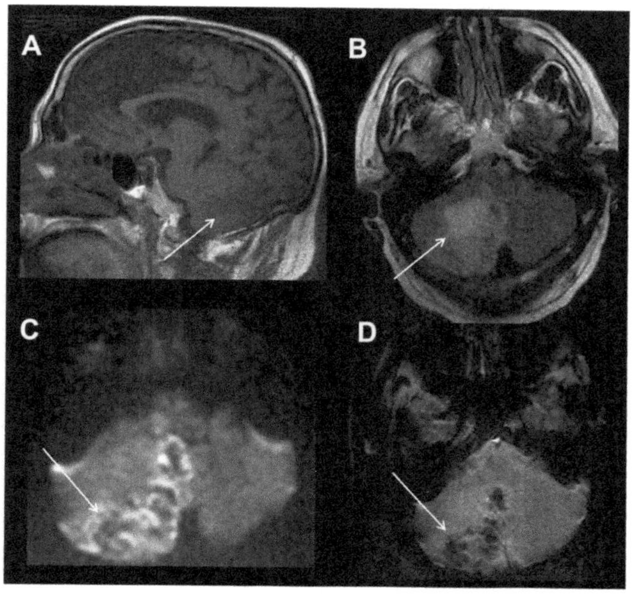

Figure 7. Hemorrhagic acute cerebellar infarction in a 79 year old male with a focal neurological deficit. Sagittal T1-weighted image (A) shows hypointense signal within the right inferior cerebellar hemisphere (white arrow). Axial T2-weighted FLAIR image (B) demonstrates geographic hyperintense signal and mass effect within the right inferior cerebellar hemisphere (white arrow). Axial diffusion weighted trace image (C) shows restricted diffusion in the right cerebellar hemisphere compatible with infarction (white arrow) as well as areas of hypointensity reflecting hemorrhage. Axial gradient recalled echo image shows susceptibility effect within the right cerebellar hemisphere, which is consistent with hemorrhage (white arrow).

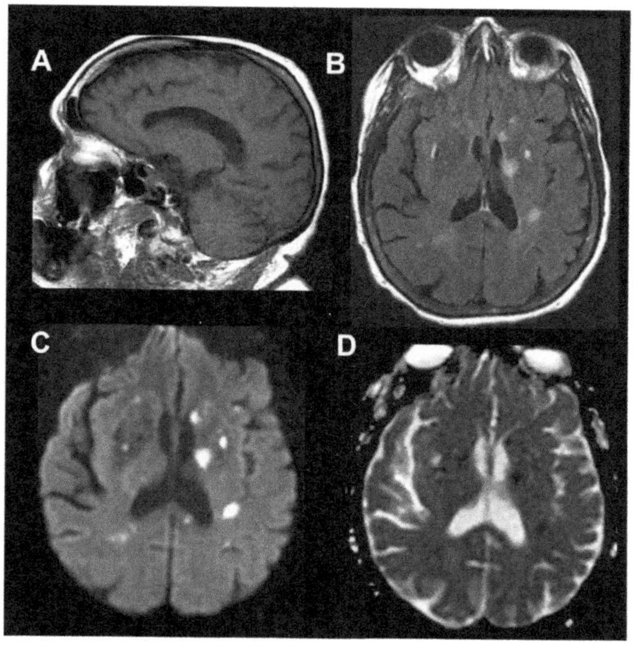

Figure 8. Acute infarctions in a 77 year old female with altered mental status. A 77-year-old woman underwent MRI examination because of altered mental status. Her complete examination included 12 pulse sequences, but all significant abnormalities are apparent in images derived from the three pulse sequences that comprised the abbreviated examination described in phase 1 of this study. A sagittal T1-weighted image (A) reveals no apparent abnormality. Axial T2-weighted FLAIR images (B) demonstrate multiple small hyperintense lesions in deep gray matter and white matter structures. The lesions are markedly hyperintense in diffusion-weighted images (C) and apparent diffusion coefficient maps derived from the DWI sequence (D) show restricted diffusion within the lesions, confirming that they are ischemic infarcts.

Several significant vascular lesions were not identified on the 3- or 4-sequence protocols, even upon revisiting the study, but were identified on MRA or MRV. Two of the missed vascular abnormalities in group 1 were occlusions in MCA branches. In cases where arterial dissection, vascular thrombosis or occlusion is clinically suspected, a vascular imaging sequence such as an MRA or MRV may add considerable value (Figures 11D-F and 12E-G).

One case of cortical dysplasia in group 1 was not initially identified, but the dysplasia was discernible in retrospect (Figure 5). The finding is subtle but visible on FLAIR images, and more obvious on T2 images. In these patients with a history of seizures, additional sequences could be added to the protocol for diagnostic imaging, including the use of high resolution, isotropic multiplanar sequences that would aid in identifying the structural abnormalities that may often be subtle.

The limited 4-sequence MRI protocol should increase efficiency and reduce scan length. The amount of time saved using the 4-sequence protocol is difficult to precisely calculate due to the variable pre-scan preparation times; however, we estimate that the time saved ranges from 5 to 25 minutes per study compared to our standard protocols. Further efficiencies in study acquisition may be possible through optimization of the limited sequence parameters. Also, substantial time savings in the interpretation of the 4-sequence MRI studies are expected since there will be fewer images per study for the neuroradiologist to review.

The 4-sequence MRI protocol will only be efficient and of value if the limited sequences allow the neuroradiologist to make a correct diagnosis with a limited rate of patient recall for additional sequences. The data in our study suggest that the patient recall rate will be very low and on the order of "misses" using the standard protocol.

A proper review of the patient's history should allow the neuroradiologist to tailor the MRI sequences to be performed for any given indication. The limited 4-sequence MRI screening protocol is only appropriate for the patient with new neurological complaints without an existing diagnosis. For example, a patient with known metastatic cancer will receive a contrast-enhanced MRI study. For patients undergoing the limited screening protocol, unexpected findings may be detected that warrant work-up with additional MR sequences. In these cases, we envision a hybrid solution. A large number of cases are monitored in 'real-time' by the neuroradiologist, which allows for immediate tailoring of the examination based on the findings on the limited sequences. Current technology even permits the neuroradiologist to remotely monitor cases and tailor them off-site. However, there will be some cases that cannot be monitored and such patients may require additional sequences to be performed at another time.

This study has several limitations. It has a retrospective design, although effort was made to minimize bias by analyzing consecutive cases. Despite our diligent attempt to minimize bias, results should be interpreted with caution as they have not yet been validated in a prospective fashion or using active clinical

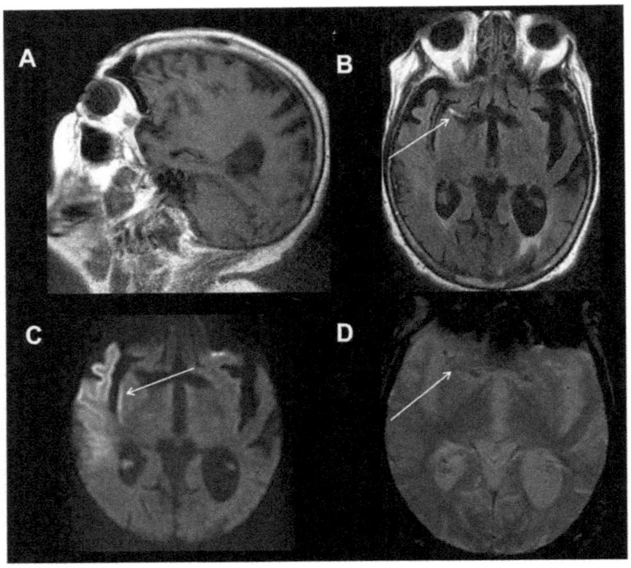

Figure 9. Acute stroke in a 78 year old female with altered mental status. Sagittal T1-weighted image of the right temporal lobe/insula (A) is normal. Axial T2-weighted FLAIR image (B) shows hyperintense signal within the M1 segment of the right middle cerebral artery (MCA), suggesting slow flow or clot (white arrow). Axial diffusion weighted image (DWI) (C) shows restricted diffusion within the right temporal lobe and insula, diagnostic of acute stroke to this region (white arrow). Axial gradient recalled echo (GRE) susceptibility image (D) shows subtle linear susceptibility effect within the right MCA, consistent with recent passage of embolic material (white arrow).

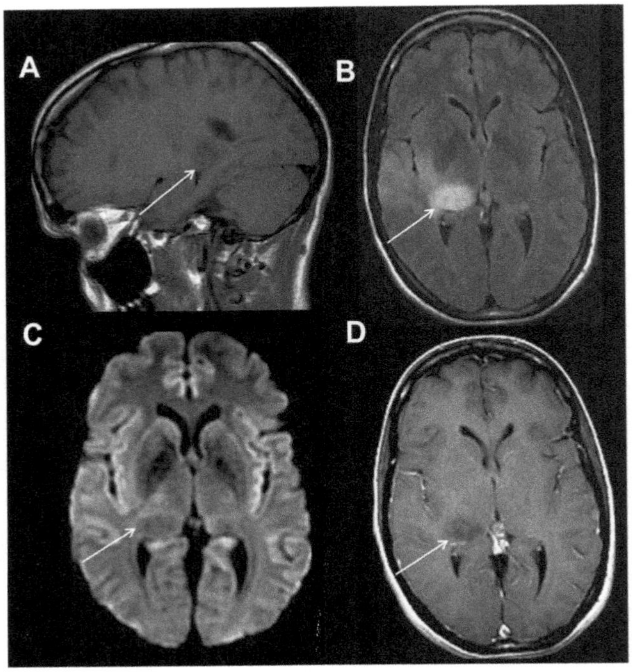

Figure 10. Right thalamic neoplasm identified in a 48 year old female with seizures. Limited pre-contrast set of imaging sequences are sufficient to clearly identify an expansile lesion within the pulvinar of the right thalamus; a finding requiring immediate communication for action (Level I) (white arrows). It is hypointense on sagittal T1-weighted image (A) and has associated hyperintensity on axial T2-weighted FLAIR extending into the adjacent insular-opercular region (B). Even within the confines of the limited set of sequences, neoplastic differential considerations are still able to be favored over acute ischemia as no evidence of restricted diffusion is seen on diffusion-weighted imaging (DWI) sequences; specifically low signal on DWI trace images (C) and elevated diffusivity on Apparent-Diffusion-Coefficient images (not shown). Post-contrast imaging, not initially available to the readers within the limited set of review sequences, demonstrated no abnormal enhancement (D).

cases. A prospective study is currently being designed to confirm the findings described here. An additional limitation is that the impressions from each original MRI interpretation were used as the reference standard. There may have been findings on brain MRI that were mentioned only in the body of a report and not in the impression. This most notably occurred in patients with probable microhemorrhages. Another limitation is that the original MRI interpretations were performed in the true clinical setting where the neuroradiologist may have been interrupted or distracted by phone calls, teaching and consultations, which is different than the clinical research conditions under which the group 1 and 2 neuroradiologists reviewed the cases. However, the group 1 and 2 neuroradiologsists interpreted their cases using the same PACS workstations in the same clinical work areas as those of the original interpretations and, therefore, were subject to similar disturbances and distractions. In addition, for the original clinical interpretations, the readers also had access to the full medical record that is readily accessible at the workstation, as well as the ability to contact the referring the physician for further information. Thus the reading of the limited sequences was more restricted than the original reading, thus providing an added measure of assurance on the validity of the results. The heterogeneity of our institutions MRI scanners, which had different manufacturers and field strengths, may be considered as another limitation. Bearing that in mind, the national installed base of clinical magnets has far greater heterogeneity than our institutions and one might argue that these studies cannot reflect the diversity of clinical practice. Additionally, this paper describes an effort to limit the number of sequences required for routine performance and is not making any comment with respect to interpretation times. Finally, the readers were primarily experienced neuroradiologists, which is not necessarily true for all those interpreting brain MRIs. We have not attempted to validate error rates utilizing this protocol amongst general radiologists or other specialists.

Conclusions

A four-sequence MRI protocol that includes sagittal T1 weighted images, axial T2-weighted FLAIR images, axial diffusion-weighted images, and T2*-weighted images reliably detects nearly all non-enhancing brain MRI findings in patients without a known history of a neurologic disease undergoing evaluation for a new neurologic complaint. If a patient has persistent unexplained symptoms, an additional MRI study including post-contrast and high-resolution imaging should reveal abnormalities characterized by blood brain barrier breakdown or small structural lesions. Clinical information suggesting a vascular lesion should be evaluated using an angiographic or venographic sequence.

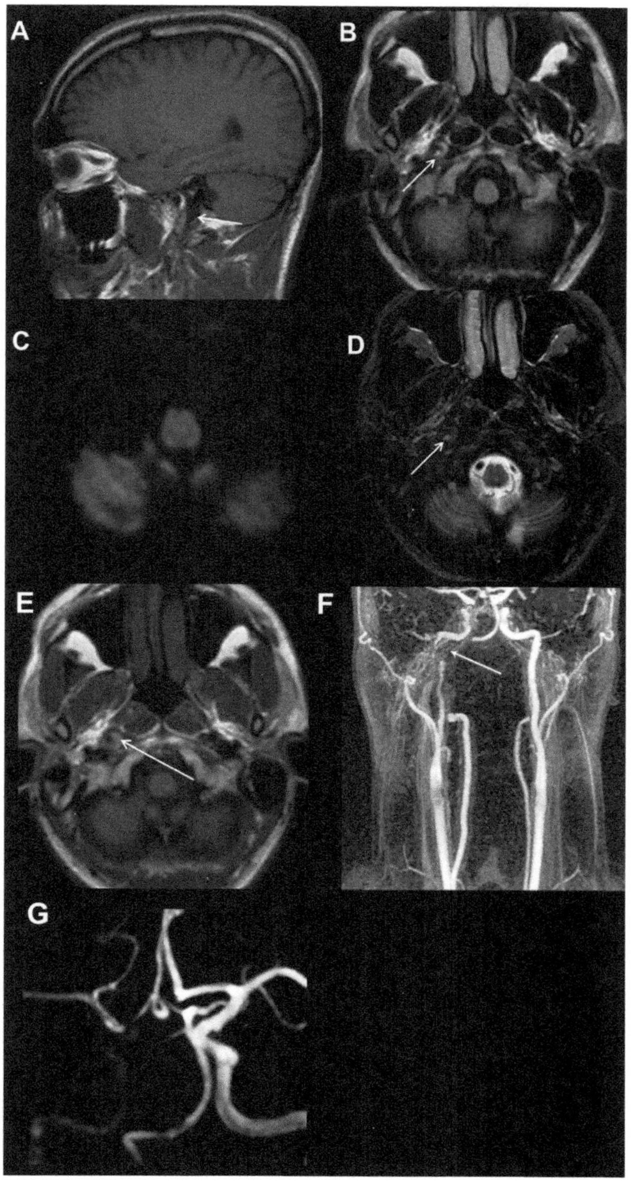

Figure 11. Internal carotid artery dissection in a 41 year old male with headache. The dissection was not identified on the limited 3 sequence review. Sagittal T1-weighted image (A) shows narrowing of the distal cervical portion of the right internal carotid artery with T1 hyperintense intramural hematoma (white arrow). Axial FLAIR image (B) demonstrates loss of the normal right internal carotid artery flow void (white arrow), which is more conspicuous on the axial T2-weighted image (D). Axial diffusion weighted trace image (C) shows no restricted diffusion in the region of the right internal carotid artery. Axial pre-contrast T1-weighted image (E) demonstrates an eccentric T1 hyperintense intramural hematoma (white arrow) in the distal cervical right internal carotid artery. MR angiography maximum intensity projection images reveal irregular critical narrowing (white arrow) of the distal cervical right ICA (F) and asymmetrical flow-related signal in the right intracranial ICA (G).

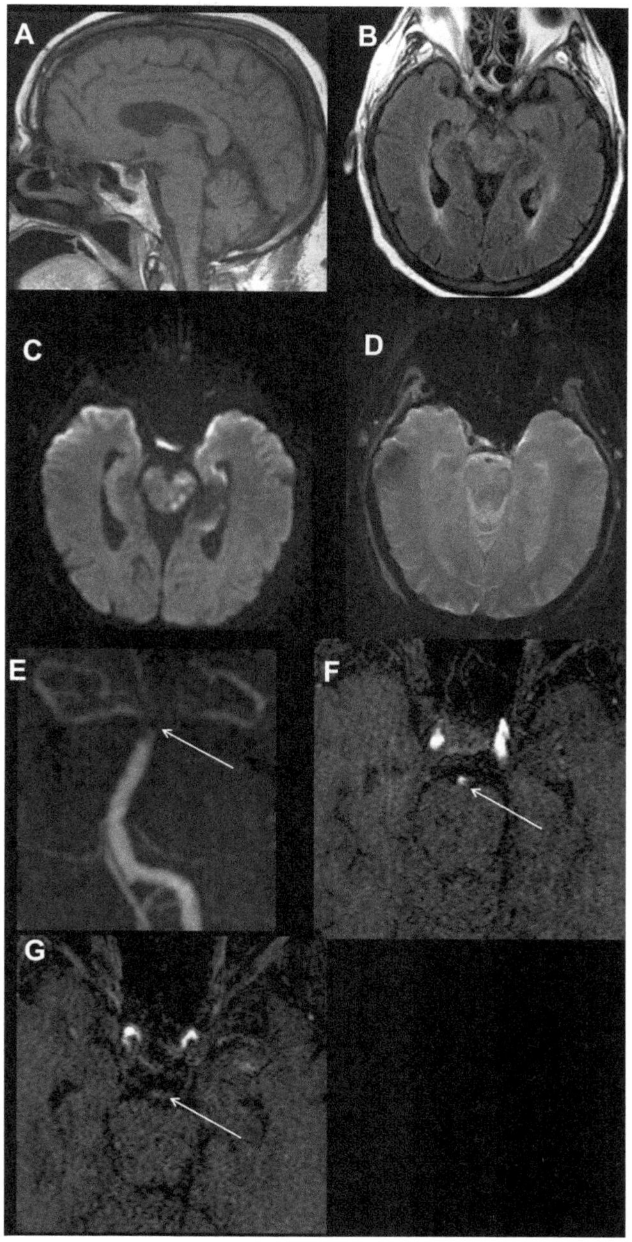

Figure 12. 72-year-old female with altered mental status and ischemic stroke. On the 4-sequence MRI protocol (A-D), the axial FLAIR image (B) demonstrates multifocal ill-defined areas of signal hyperintensity within the midbrain with corresponding restricted diffusion on the axial diffusion weighted trace image (C), consistent with infarctions. Additional foci of infarction were seen in the left occipital lobe, left mesial temporal lobe, both thalami and the cerebellum (images not shown). No definite abnormality is seen on the sagittal T1-weighted image (A) or axial T2* image (D). MR angiography was also requested. MRA maximum intensity projection image (E) reveals thrombus with the distal basilar (white arrow) and proximal posterior cerebral arteries, which is confirmed on the axial source MR angiography images (F, G) (white arrow). Even in retrospect, this finding was not apparent on any of the sequences included in the 4-sequence MRI protocol. MRA imaging adds significant value in cases with clinical suspicion for vascular occlusion or thrombosis.

Author Contributions

Conceived and designed the experiments: WAM RGG. Performed the experiments: WAM RGG BRB JWC WAC RG JAH GJH SH JMJ HRK ML MHL SRP OR SR JMR PWS VS. Analyzed the data: WAM RGG BRB JWC WAC RG JAH GJH SH JMJ HRK ML MHL SRP OR SR JMR PWS VS. Wrote the paper: WAM RGG BRB JWC WAC RG JAH GJH SH JMJ HRK ML MHL SRP OR SR JMR PWS VS.

References

1. Hashemi RH, Bradley WG Jr, Chen DY, Jordan JE, Queralt JA, et al. (1995) Suspected multiple sclerosis: MR imaging with a thin-section fast FLAIR pulse sequence. Radiology 196: 505–510.
2. Brant-Zawadzki M, Atkinson D, Detrick M, Bradley WG, Scidmore G (1996) Fluid-attenuated inversion recovery (FLAIR) for assessment of cerebral infarction. Initial clinical experience in 50 patients. Stroke 27: 1187–1191.
3. Ashikaga R, Araki Y, Ishida O (1997) MRI of head injury using FLAIR. Neuroradiology 39: 239–242.
4. Noguchi K, Ogawa T, Seto H, Inugami A, Hadeishi H, et al. (1997) Subacute and chronic subarachnoid hemorrhage: diagnosis with fluid-attenuated inversion-recovery MR imaging. Radiology 203: 257–262.
5. Thurnher MM, Thurnher SA, Fleischmann D, Steuer A, Rieger A, et al. (1997) Comparison of T2-weighted and fluid-attenuated inversion-recovery fast spin-echo MR sequences in intracerebral AIDS-associated disease. AJNR Am J - Neuroradiol 18: 1601–1609.
6. Demaerel P, Bosmans H, Caerts B, Herpels V, Vercruysse J, et al. (1998) Fast FLAIR MRI in childhood white-matter abnormalities. Neuroradiology 40: 355–358.
7. Maubon AJ, Pothin A, Ferru JM, Berger VM, Daures JP, et al. (1998) Unselected brain 0.5-T MR imaging: comparison of lesion detection and characterization with three T2-weighted sequences. Radiology 208: 671–678.
8. Aprile I, Iaiza F, Lavaroni A, Budai R, Dolso P, et al. (1999) Analysis of cystic intracranial lesions performed with fluid-attenuated inversion recovery MR imaging. AJNR Am J Neuroradiol 20: 1259–1267.
9. Bakshi R, Kamran S, Kinkel PR, Bates VE, Mechtler LL, et al. (1999) Fluid-attenuated inversion-recovery MR imaging in acute and subacute cerebral intraventricular hemorrhage. AJNR Am J Neuroradiol 20: 629–636.
10. Meiners LC, van Gils AD, De Kort G, Van Der Graaf Y, Jansen GH, et al. (1999) Fast fluid-attenuated inversion recovery (FLAIR) compared with T2-weighted spin-echo in the magnetic resonance diagnosis of mesial temporal sclerosis. Invest Radiol 34: 134–142.
11. Palmer S, Bradley WG, Chen DY, Patel S (1999) Subcallosal striations: early findings of multiple sclerosis on sagittal, thin-section, fast FLAIR MR images. Radiology 210: 149–153.
12. Taillibert S, Oppenheim C, Baulac M, Dormont D, Marsault C, et al. (1999) Yield of fluid-attenuated inversion recovery in drug-resistant focal epilepsy with noninformative conventional magnetic resonance imaging. Eur Neurol 41: 64–72.
13. Casey SO, Sampaio RC, Michel E, Truwit CL (2000) Posterior reversible encephalopathy syndrome: utility of fluid-attenuated inversion recovery MR imaging in the detection of cortical and subcortical lesions. AJNR Am J Neuroradiol 21: 1199–1206.
14. Essig M, Wenz F, Schoenberg SO, Debus J, Knopp MV, et al. (2000) Arteriovenous malformations: assessment of gliotic and ischemic changes with fluid-attenuated inversion-recovery MRI. Invest Radiol 35: 689–694.
15. Herskovits EH, Itoh R, Melhem ER (2001) Accuracy for detection of simulated lesions: comparison of fluid-attenuated inversion-recovery, proton density–weighted, and T2-weighted synthetic brain MR imaging. AJR Am J Roentgenol 176: 1313–1318.
16. Maeda M, Yamamoto T, Daimon S, Sakuma H, Takeda K (2001) Arterial hyperintensity on fast fluid-attenuated inversion recovery images: a subtle finding for hyperacute stroke undetected by diffusion-weighted MR imaging. AJNR Am J Neuroradiol 22: 632–636.
17. Saleh A, Wenserski F, Cohnen M, Furst G, Godehardt E, et al. (2004) Exclusion of brain lesions: is MR contrast medium required after a negative fluid-attenuated inversion recovery sequence? Br J Radiol 77: 183–188.
18. Koennecke HC (2006) Cerebral microbleeds on MRI: prevalence, associations, and potential clinical implications. Neurology 66: 165–171.
19. Lin DD, Filippi CG, Steever AB, Zimmerman RD (2001) Detection of intracranial hemorrhage: comparison between gradient-echo images and b(0) images obtained from diffusion-weighted echo-planar sequences. AJNR Am J Neuroradiol 22: 1275–1281.
20. Lam WW, So NM, Wong KS, Rainer T (2003) B0 images obtained from diffusion-weighted echo planar sequences for the detection of intracerebral bleeds. J Neuroimaging 13: 99–105.
21. Atlas SW, Mark AS, Grossman RI, Gomori JM (1988) Intracranial hemorrhage: gradient-echo MR imaging at 1.5 T. Comparison with spin-echo imaging and clinical applications. Radiology 168: 803–807.
22. Chan S, Kartha K, Yoon SS, Desmond DW, Hilal SK (1996) Multifocal hypointense cerebral lesions on gradient-echo MR are associated with chronic hypertension. AJNR Am J Neuroradiol 17: 1821–1827.
23. Tsushima Y, Aoki J, Endo K (2003) Brain microhemorrhages detected on T2*-weighted gradient-echo MR images. AJNR Am J Neuroradiol 24: 88–96.

6

Atlas-Based Quantification of Cardiac Remodeling Due to Myocardial Infarction

Xingyu Zhang[1], Brett R. Cowan[1], David A. Bluemke[2], J. Paul Finn[3], Carissa G. Fonseca[3], Alan H. Kadish[4], Daniel C. Lee[4], Joao A. C. Lima[5], Avan Suinesiaputra[1], Alistair A. Young[1], Pau Medrano-Gracia[1]*

1 Department of Anatomy with Radiology, University of Auckland, Auckland, New Zealand, **2** National Institute of Biomedical Imaging and Bioengineering, Bethesda, Maryland, United States of America, **3** Department of Radiology, University of California Los Angeles, Los Angeles, California, United States of America, **4** Feinberg Cardiovascular Research Institute, Northwestern University Feinberg School of Medicine, Chicago, Illinois, United States of America, **5** The Donald W. Reynolds Cardiovascular Clinical Research Center, The Johns Hopkins University, Baltimore, Maryland, United States of America

Abstract

Myocardial infarction leads to changes in the geometry (remodeling) of the left ventricle (LV) of the heart. The degree and type of remodeling provides important diagnostic information for the therapeutic management of ischemic heart disease. In this paper, we present a novel analysis framework for characterizing remodeling after myocardial infarction, using LV shape descriptors derived from atlas-based shape models. Cardiac magnetic resonance images from 300 patients with myocardial infarction and 1991 asymptomatic volunteers were obtained from the Cardiac Atlas Project. Finite element models were customized to the spatio-temporal shape and function of each case using guide-point modeling. Principal component analysis was applied to the shape models to derive modes of shape variation across all cases. A logistic regression analysis was performed to determine the modes of shape variation most associated with myocardial infarction. Goodness of fit results obtained from end-diastolic and end-systolic shapes were compared against the traditional clinical indices of remodeling: end-diastolic volume, end-systolic volume and LV mass. The combination of end-diastolic and end-systolic shape parameter analysis achieved the lowest deviance, Akaike information criterion and Bayesian information criterion, and the highest area under the receiver operating characteristic curve. Therefore, our framework quantitatively characterized remodeling features associated with myocardial infarction, better than current measures. These features enable quantification of the amount of remodeling, the progression of disease over time, and the effect of treatments designed to reverse remodeling effects.

Editor: Wolfgang Rudolf Bauer, University Hospital of Würzburg, Germany

Funding: This project was supported by award numbers R01HL087773 and R01HL121754 from the National Heart, Lung, and Blood Institute. The content is solely the responsibility of the authors and does not necessarily represent the official views of the National Heart, Lung, and Blood Institute or the National Institutes of Health. MESA was supported by contracts N01-HC-95159 through N01-HC-95169 from the NHLBI and by grants UL1-RR-024156 and UL1-RR-025005 from NCRR. DETERMINE was supported by St. Jude Medical, Inc; and the National Heart, Lung and Blood Institute (R01HL91069). A list of participating DETERMINE investigators can be found at http://www.clinicaltrials.gov. David A. Bluemke is supported by the NIH intramural research program. Xingyu Zhang would like to gratefully acknowledge financial support from the China Scholarship Council. The funders had no role in study design, data collection and analysis, decision to publish, or preparation of the manuscript.

Competing Interests: Daniel C. Lee received research funding from St. Jude Medical, Inc. All other authors have no competing interests.

* Email: p.medrano@auckland.ac.nz

Introduction

A computational atlas of image-derived shapes refers to an alignment of maps that relate individual anatomical geometry and function to the distribution of biological variations across a population, which can be described at different scales from genotype to phenotype [1]. Atlas-based analyses of patients and healthy volunteers have recently been explored in several different medical areas. For that purpose, large imaging databases, which enable the construction of probabilistic shape atlases for specific organs or diseases, have been established. Atlas-based analysis of brain anatomy and pathology is well advanced (e.g. [2]), including analysis of occipitalization in children [3], and MRI-based probabilistic atlases of neuroanatomy [4]. In the heart, atlas-based analysis has recently shown the potential to reveal new measures of geometry and function [1]. For example, atlas-based methods have been used to quantify subtle differences in heart shape between individuals born prematurely compared with full term age

Table 1. Demographics for the MESA and DETERMINE datasets (mean±std).

	Units	DETERMINE	MESA
Sex (Female/Male) ‡		60/238	1034/975
Age†	years	62.76±10.80	61.47±10.15
Height‡	cm	173.91±9.80	165.97±9.99
Weight†	kg	79.91±28.00	76.75±16.50
Systolic BP	mmHg	127.50±20.14	126.00±22.00
Diastolic BP‡	mmHg	73.86±11.34	71.49±10.33
EDV‡	ml	196.32±52.94	125.45±31.17
ESV‡	ml	118.60±48.86	47.48±18.74
MASS‡	g	168.55±41.19	126.24±36.03

†$p<0.05$; ‡$p<0.01$.
For continuous variables, p values report a Wilcoxon signed-rank test of the null hypothesis. For categorical variables the p-value reports a χ^2 test of the null hypothesis.

matched controls [5]. In patients with cardiovascular disease, certain changes in heart shape over time, known as remodeling, are indicative of worse prognostic outcome [6]. After myocardial infarction, remodeling associated with an increase in heart size is a predictor of mortality, and remodeling associated with sphericalization of heart shape is linked with decreased survival [7]. However, standard clinical indices used to describe remodeling are typically simple measures of mass and volume, such as end-diastolic (ED) volume (largest volume), end-systolic (ES) volume (smallest volume) or left ventricular mass. These ignore much of the available shape information. We hypothesized that atlas-based analysis of patients with myocardial infarction would enable better quantification of remodeling features associated with myocardial infarction.

The Cardiac Atlas Project (CAP, http://www.cardiacatlas.org) is a world-wide web-accessible resource, comprising a population atlas of asymptomatic and pathological hearts [8]. The CAP facilitates large-scale data sharing of cardiac imaging studies and their corresponding derived analyses that describe the cardiac shape, structure and function across various population groups. The data has been contributed from several studies, including Defibrillators to Reduce Risk by Magnetic Resonance Imaging Evaluation (DETERMINE) [9], comprising patients with myocardial infarction, and the Multi Ethnic Study of Atherosclerosis (MESA) [10], comprising asymptomatic volunteers. We used cases from both studies to examine the principal components of shape variation between the two cohorts, and thereby characterize shape changes associated with myocardial infarction.

Cardiovascular magnetic resonance (CMR) imaging is a non-invasive modality, which provides detailed, quantitative data of the heart structure and function. Compared to other imaging modalities, CMR does not use ionizing radiation, and is not

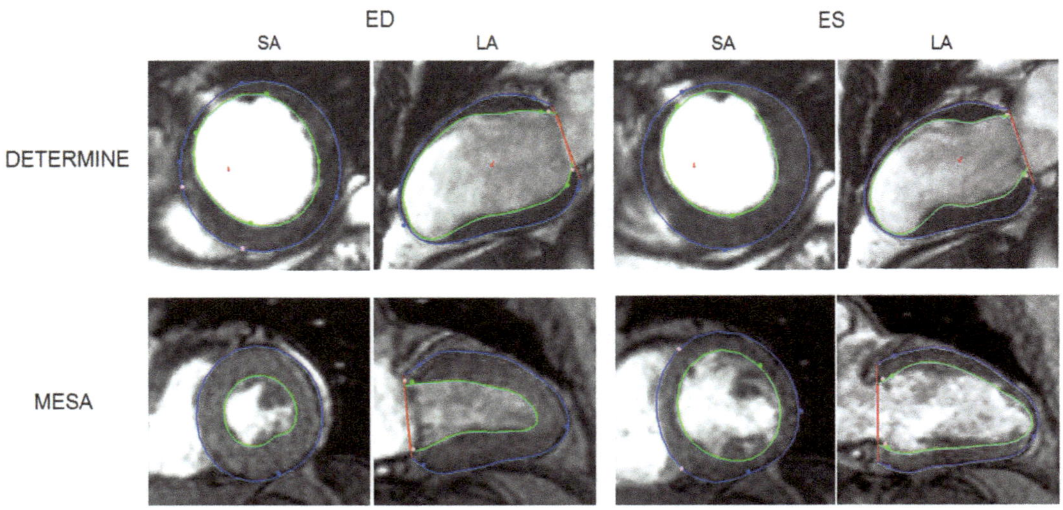

Figure 1. Image and shape differences for volunteers imaged from DETERMINE (top), and MESA (bottom), for the same short-axis (SA), long-axis (LA) planes at end diastole (ED) and end systole (ES). Green and blue contours and markers show the model's endocardial and epicardial boundaries and guide points, respectively. Light color markers denote fiducial landmarks (right ventricular free wall insertion points, mitral valve hinge points) used to define the location of the model shape parameters in consistent positions relative to the anatomy of the heart.

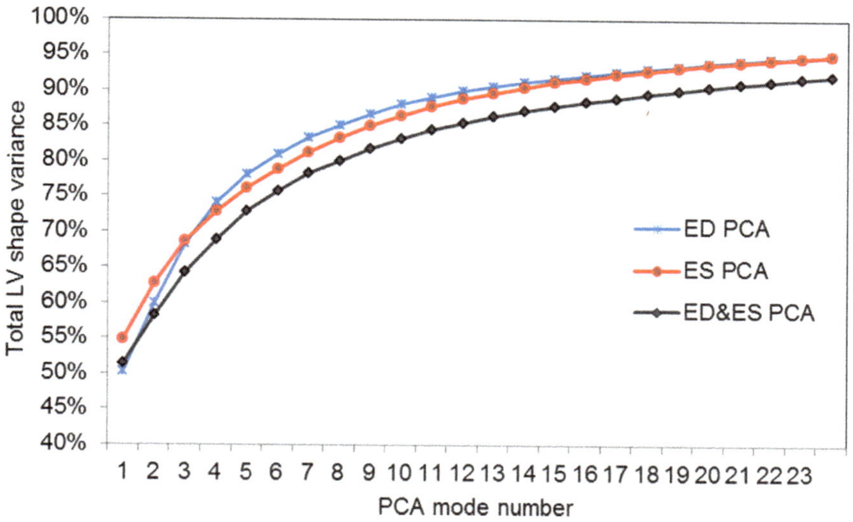

Figure 2. Scree plot of PCA analysis at ED and ES.

dependent on restricted views of the heart. As a result, many large research studies are using CMR to collect phenotypic data on cardiac disease. Model-based image analyses were developed in the last decades from the availability of large-scale data set of CMR images. This has led to the growing number of statistical analysis applications for cardiac shape and motion [1]. One particular shape representation is a finite element model, which provides an efficient and accurate representation of complex geometries [11]. This method has been shown to provide a compact and powerful representation of shape and function of the LV, and has been validated against ex-vivo LV mass, against manually-drawn contours in patients with regional wall motion abnormalities, and against cardiac output flow in healthy subjects [12,13]. However, the statistical analysis of shape parameters has previously been limited by the lack of substantial sample size and/or bias between acquisition protocols.

In this study, we applied principal component analysis (PCA) to characterize the cardiac shape features in a large number of CMR cases. PCA is a widely used dimensionality reduction technique, which has been applied to heart shape analysis [14], motion analysis [15], 3D segmentation [16], and population analysis [17] [18]. After extracting shape features using PCA, we applied a logistic regression to analyze the differences between myocardial infarction patients and asymptomatic volunteers. We also compared the performance (goodness of fit) of the model with standard clinical indices, including LV mass and volume. We found that the shape indices derived from the principal components of the shape variation characterized remodeling better than standard LV mass and volume indices.

Data and Methods

2.1 CMR Data

CMR datasets of 300 patients with myocardial infarction from DETERMINE and 1991 asymptomatic volunteers from MESA were obtained from the CAP database for inclusion in this study. These represented a random sample of the MESA baseline and DETERMINE CMR examinations contributed to CAP with local Institutional Review Board approval. This retrospective study was approved by the Health and Disability Ethics Committees of the New Zealand Government, under reference MEC/08/04/052. Informed participant consent compatible with sharing of de-identified data was obtained in writing in all cases. Imaging studies and derived analyses were de-identified, prior to analysis, in a HIPAA compliant manner [US Health Insurance Portability and Accountability Act of 1996 (HIPAA; Pub.L. 104–191, 110 Stat. 1936, enacted August 21, 1996)], annotated using standard ontological schema, stored in a web-accessible picture archiving and communication system database, and analyzed using atlas-based techniques [8]. The asymptomatic cases were regarded as the control group since, at the time of recruitment, they did not present any clinical symptoms of cardiovascular disease [19]. Table 1 shows the cohort characteristics. Patients were taller and heavier than the asymptomatic group, with larger LV mass, end-diastolic volume (EDV), end-systolic volume (ESV), and blood pressures. They were also more likely to be male. The CMR imaging protocol was different between the two cohorts: the DETERMINE protocol used steady state free precession (SSFP) imaging with 10–12 short axis slices and two long axis slices typically with 6 mm thickness, 4 mm gap, field of view 360–400 mm, 256×192 matrix, flip angle 60°, echo time 1.41 ms, repetition time 2.8 ms, with 20–40 frames per slice (temporal resolution <50 ms) and pixel size from 1.4 to 2.5 mm/pixel depending on patient size. The MESA protocol used fast gradient-recalled echo (GRE) imaging with 10–12 short axis slices and one (four chamber) long axis slice with typical parameters 6 mm thickness, 4 mm gap, field of view 360–400 mm, 256×160 matrix, flip angle 20°, echo time 3–5 ms, repetition time 8–10 ms with 20–30 frames per slice (temporal resolution <50 ms) and pixel size from 1.4 to 2.5 mm/pixel depending on patient size.

2.2 Finite Element Modeling

For the MESA cohort, short-axis hand-drawn contours on the inner and outer surfaces of the left ventricle were available from the MESA MRI core laboratory. These contours were fitted by the finite element model by linear least squares as described previously [20]. For the DETERMINE cohort, expert observers performed the analysis using guide-point modeling [13] to interactively customize a time-varying 3D cardiac finite element model of the

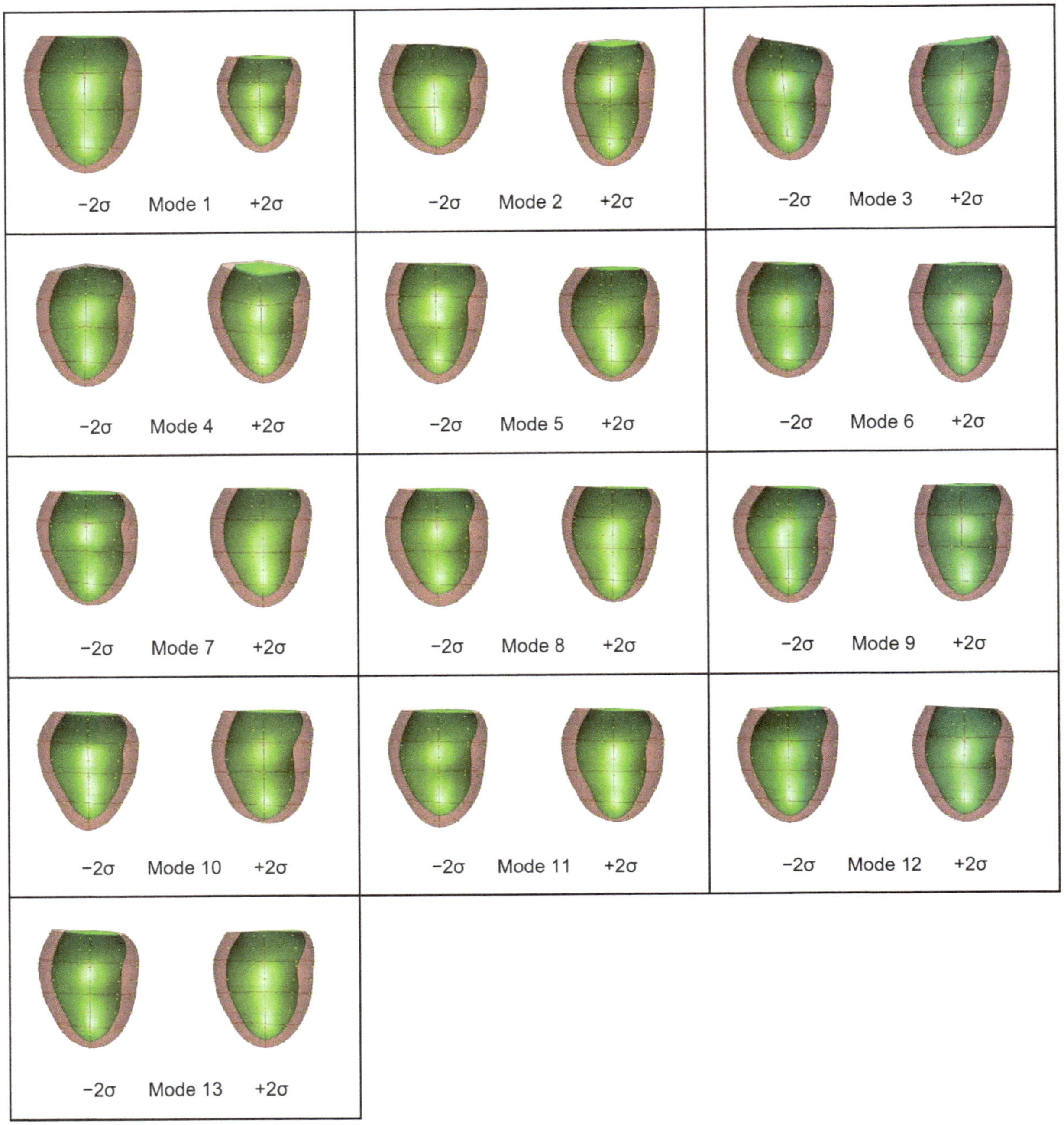

Figure 3. PCA first 13 modes using shape vectors at ED.

LV to MR images (Figure 1) using custom software (CIM version 6.0, University of Auckland, New Zealand). LV mass and volume at ED and ES were subsequently calculated from the fitted cardiac LV shape models. The model comprised 16 bicubic finite elements with C^1 continuity, (see [12,13] for details). Briefly, the model was interactively fitted by least-squares optimization to guide points provided by the analyst, as well as computer-generated points calculated from the image using an edge detection algorithm. Automatic feature tracking was used to track points throughout the cardiac cycle using non-rigid registration in both short and long axis images [12]. The model was registered to each case using fiducial landmarks defined at the hinge points of the mitral valve and the insertions of the right ventricular free wall into the interventricular septum. This method has been previously validated against autopsy LV mass, in patients against manually drawn contours and in healthy volunteers against flow-derived measurements of cardiac output [13]. The finite element coordinates were used to provide the atlas coordinates of the LV: each point was assumed to be in approximately the same anatomical location in every heart [21].

2.3 Alignment

For statistical analysis, the shape models were evenly sampled at sufficient resolution to capture all the shape features available. The

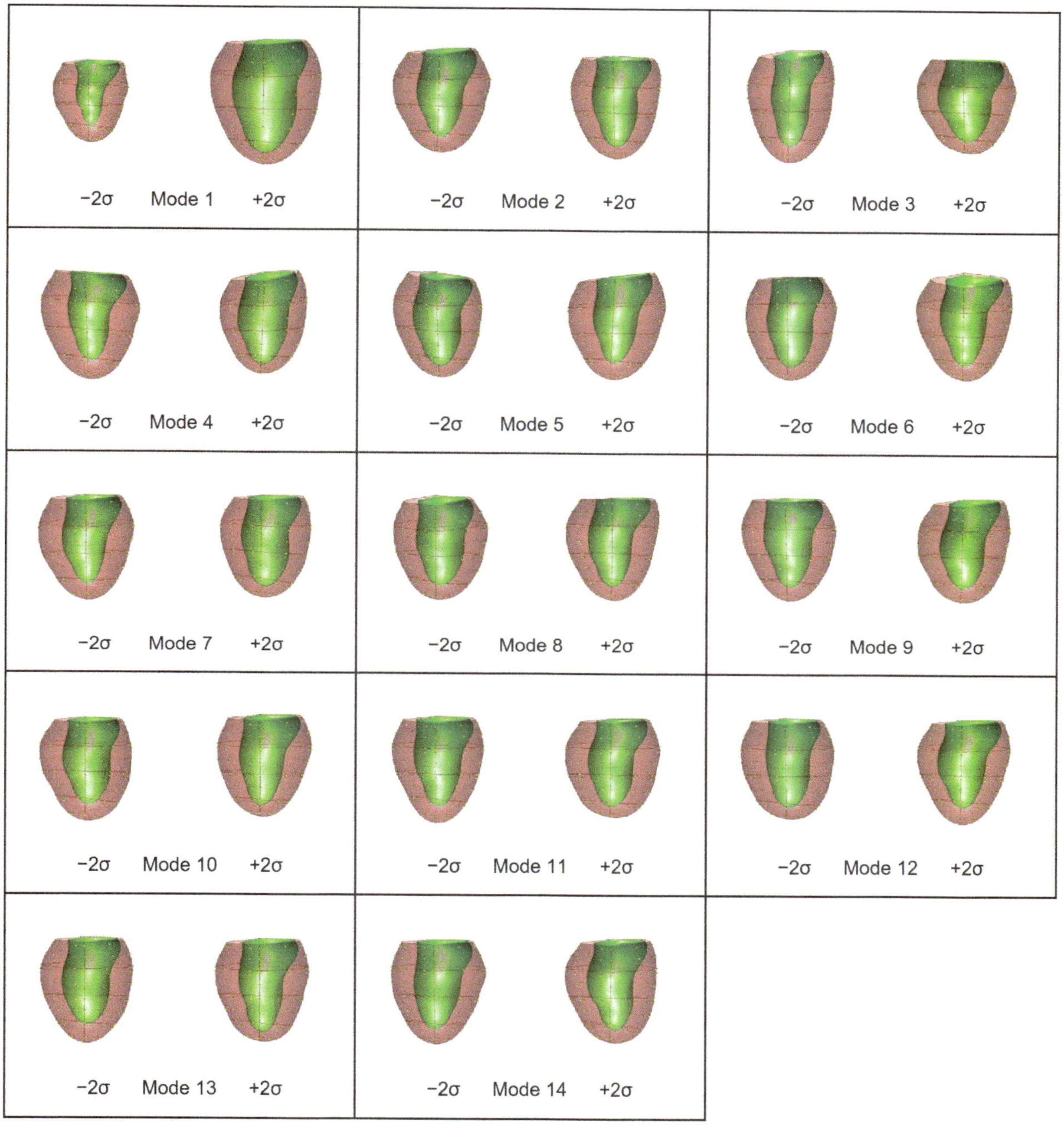

Figure 4. PCA first 14 modes using only shape vectors at ES.

surface sampling process resulted in 2738 Cartesian (xi,yi,zi) points. A Procrustes alignment method [22] was applied to the sampled point data to determine similarity transformations between shapes: i.e. isotropic scale, translation and rotation. This algorithm finds the optimal scale, rotation matrix and translation vector, which minimizes the overall distance between two sets of points with respect to the Euclidean norm. All LV models from the DETERMINE and MESA datasets were aligned using translation and rotation to their mean shape whenever required. Scale variations were not removed since heart size is a clinical indicator of disease.

2.4 Correction of Acquisition Bias

As outlined in Section 2.1, the MESA cohort was acquired using a different imaging protocol (GRE) to the DETERMINE cohort (SSFP). It is known that these two protocols result in small differences in the placement of inner and outer surfaces of the heart. SSFP typically gives rise to larger estimates of left ventricle (LV) cavity volume and smaller estimates of LV mass than GRE. The shape bias has been shown to be regionally variable, and can be effectively removed using a maximum likelihood correction algorithm [23]. Briefly, a transformation between GRE models and SSFP models was learned using data from 40 asymptomatic individuals who were scanned using both protocols. The optimal

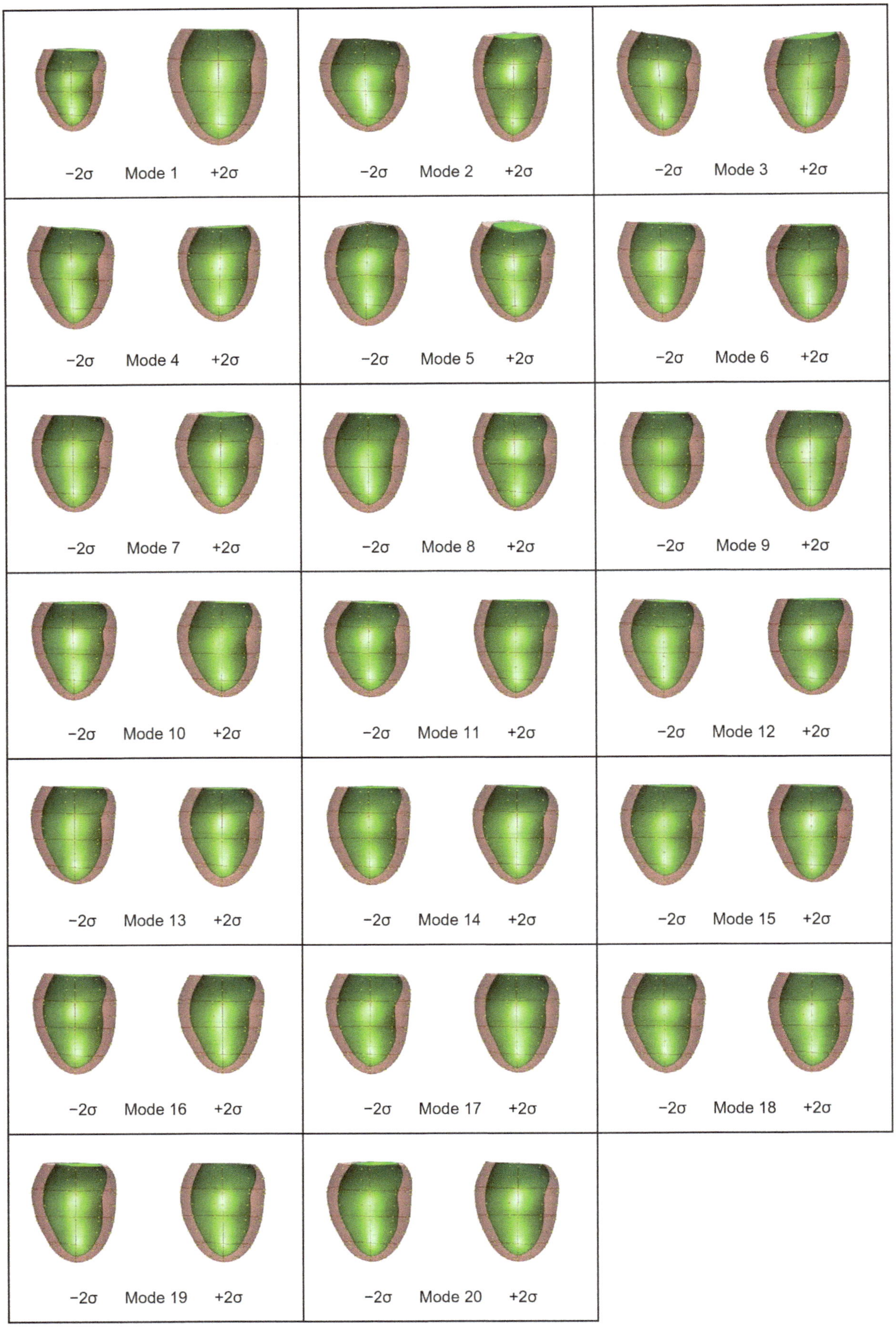

Figure 5. First 20 modes at ED using PCA of a combination of ED and ES.

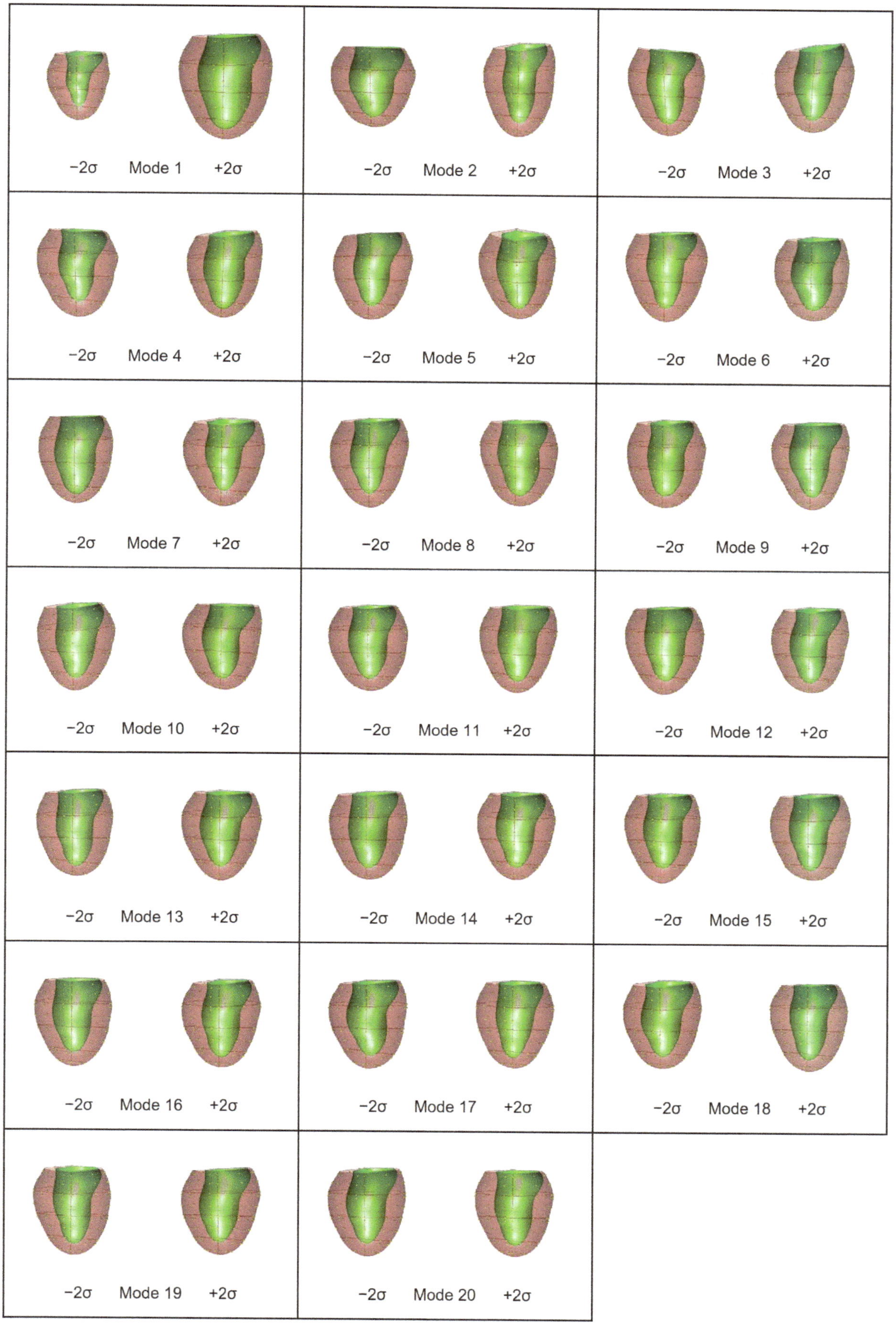

Figure 6. First 20 modes at ES using PCA of a combination of ED and ES.

Table 2. Logistic regression analysis of the baseline model.

Parameter	Coefficient	Standard Error	Standardized coefficient	Odds Ratio(OR)	OR 95% Confidence Interval	
Intercept*	−18.8662	1.9036				
Age‡	0.0233	0.0085	0.1308	1.0240	1.0070	1.0410
Sex	0.4107	0.2263	0.1132	1.5080	0.9680	2.3500
Height*	0.0943	0.0111	0.5316	1.0990	1.0750	1.1230
Weight*	−0.0216	0.0046	−0.2148	0.9790	0.9700	0.9880
SBP	0.0045	0.0053	0.0536	1.0040	0.9940	1.0150
DBP	0.0002	0.0105	0.0010	1.0000	0.9800	1.0210

‡$p<0.01$ * $p<0.0001$.

transformation was found using maximum likelihood methods and was validated previously [23]. All MESA shape models were then transformed using this method, with the transformed shapes then being directly comparable to SSFP models.

2.5 Principal component analysis and Logistic regression classification

Principal component analysis [24] is currently one of the most widely used dimension reduction procedures. Using orthogonal transformations, PCA projects the data onto a linear space of maximum-variation directions, known as *modes*. After the projection, the number of modes retained is typically well below the number of original variables, yet still retains a high percentage of the overall variability in the original set. The first mode accounts for as much of the variability in the data as possible, and each succeeding mode in turn has the highest residual variance possible under the linear orthogonality constraint. The coordinates (x, y, z) of the surface sampling points were concatenated into a shape vector. Shape vectors from all cases were formed into a matrix. The eigenvectors of the covariance matrix formed the principal component modes, and their corresponding eigenvalues indicate the proportion of the total variation explained by each mode. Selecting the number of PCA modes to retain in subsequent analysis is contingent on the application. In this paper, enough

Table 3. Logistic regression analysis of the modes at ES.

Parameter	Coefficient	Standard Error	Standardized coefficient	Odds Ratio(OR)	OR 95% Confidence Interval	
Intercept*	−16.8281	4.1446				
Age‡	0.0467	0.0178	0.2629	1.0480	1.0120	1.0850
Sex	−0.4471	0.4698	−0.1232	0.6400	0.2550	1.6060
Height†	0.0506	0.0245	0.2851	1.0520	1.0020	1.1040
Weight‡	−0.0306	0.0086	−0.3048	0.9700	0.9540	0.9860
SBP‡	0.0310	0.0114	0.3732	1.0320	1.0090	1.0550
DBP	−0.0239	0.0206	−0.1378	0.9760	0.9380	1.0170
mode1*	0.0214	0.0018	1.8503	1.0220	1.0180	1.0250
mode2*	0.0209	0.0030	0.7308	1.0210	1.0150	1.0270
mode3*	0.0111	0.0026	0.3281	1.0110	1.0060	1.0160
mode4*	0.0463	0.0049	1.1490	1.0470	1.0370	1.0580
mode5	−0.0011	0.0039	−0.0250	0.9990	0.9910	1.0060
mode6‡	−0.0126	0.0044	−0.2509	0.9870	0.9790	0.9960
mode7*	0.0264	0.0043	0.4954	1.0270	1.0180	1.0350
mode8	0.0085	0.0046	0.1508	1.0090	0.9990	1.0180
mode9*	−0.0245	0.0052	−0.3856	0.9760	0.9660	0.9860
mode10*	0.0260	0.0063	0.3877	1.0260	1.0140	1.0390
mode11	0.0054	0.0067	0.0736	1.0050	0.9920	1.0190
mode12‡	−0.0242	0.0064	−0.3150	0.9760	0.9640	0.9890
mode13	−0.0022	0.0072	−0.0248	0.9980	0.9840	1.0120
mode14*	0.0386	0.0077	0.4035	1.0390	1.0240	1.0550

†$p<0.05$; ‡$p<0.01$; * $p<0.0001$.

Table 4. Logistic regression analysis of the modes at ED.

Parameter	Coefficient	Standard Error	Standardized coefficient	Odds Ratio(OR)	OR 95% Confidence Interval	
Intercept	−6.5146	3.5722				
Age*	0.0508	0.0153	0.2859	1.0520	1.0210	1.0840
Sex	−0.4259	0.4037	−0.1174	0.6530	0.2960	1.4410
Height	0.0119	0.0212	0.0674	1.0120	0.9710	1.0550
Weight*	−0.0385	0.0078	−0.3826	0.9620	0.9480	0.9770
SBP	−0.0078	0.0093	−0.0936	0.9920	0.9740	1.0110
DBP	−0.0002	0.0174	−0.0010	1.0000	0.9660	1.0340
mode1*	−0.0212	0.0017	−1.6175	0.9790	0.9760	0.9820
mode2*	−0.0201	0.0024	−0.6924	0.9800	0.9750	0.9850
mode3*	0.0112	0.0025	0.3573	1.0110	1.0060	1.0160
mode4	0.0019	0.0028	0.0497	1.0020	0.9960	1.0070
mode5*	−0.0186	0.0037	−0.4163	0.9820	0.9750	0.9890
mode6*	−0.0557	0.0056	−1.0397	0.9460	0.9360	0.9560
mode7	−0.0061	0.0049	−0.1010	0.9940	0.9840	1.0030
mode8*	0.0528	0.0067	0.7886	1.0540	1.0400	1.0680
mode9‡	−0.0142	0.0045	−0.1954	0.9860	0.9770	0.9950
mode10	0.0112	0.0069	0.1442	1.0110	0.9980	1.0250
mode11*	0.0875	0.0102	0.9628	1.0910	1.0700	1.1140
mode12	0.0006	0.0071	0.0062	1.0010	0.9870	1.0150
mode13	0.0105	0.0074	0.0929	1.0110	0.9960	1.0250

†p<0.05; ‡p<0.01; * p<0.0001.

modes were retained to explain 90% of the total variance. Three PCA cases were considered, the first using only shape vectors at ED, the second using shape vectors at ES, and the third using a combination of ED and ES (ED&ES). The ED&ES PCA was formed by concatenating the shape vectors from ED and ES into a single shape vector.

After PCA, a logistic regression model [25] was used to identify which modes were most associated with the differences between myocardial infarct patients and asymptomatic patients. The weights of the PCA components (up to 90% of the total variability) were used as predictors for classification. In statistics, logistic regression is a type of probabilistic, statistical classification model, which is used to predict a binary response from continuous, binary, or canonical variables. MESA cases (non-patients) were assigned a zero label whereas DETERMINE cases (patients) were assigned a one label. These values were used to obtain the coefficients in the regression models. Thus, the following equation can be used to calculate the probability that a new case belongs to the patient class [26]:

$$P=\frac{1}{1+\exp[-(\beta_0+\sum\beta_iX_i)]}$$

where P is the probability of the a certain case belonging to the myocardial infarction set, X_i are the values of the predictors, which in our case represent the PCA modes, β_i are the coefficient terms of X_i, and β_0 is the intercept. The β terms were found by maximum likelihood estimation. After the coefficients have been estimated, the goodness-of-fit of the resulting model can be examined to determine how well the regression model distinguishes between non-patients and patients. Three common statistics used to quantify the goodness-of-fit of the model are deviance, Akaike information criterion (AIC) and Bayesian information criterion (BIC) [27,28]:

$$Deviance=-2\log(L)$$
$$AIC=-2\log(L)+2k$$
$$BIC=-2\log(L)+2k*\log(n)$$

where the L represents the log-likelihood of the model (i.e. the value that is maximized by computing the maximum likelihood value for the βi parameters), k is the number of estimated parameters and n is the sample size. In all three measures, a lower number is indicative of a better model. In addition to these three measures, we also evaluated the area under the curve (AUC) of the receiver operating characteristic curves, since this is also an overall measure of goodness of fit (better models having values closer to 1.0).

Results

PCA was performed on the shape models at ED and ES as well as their combination (ED&ES). A scree plot [29] is given in Fig. 2 showing the cumulative variance explained by each mode. The shape variation described by each mode is shown in Fig. 3 for ED, Fig. 4 for ES, and Fig. 5 and Fig. 6 for ED&ES. Although most of the modes do not correspond with traditional shape measures, the first three modes in each case can be understood in terms of commonly used clinical measures of remodeling. Mode 1 explained 50% of the total variance at ED and 55% at ES. In both cases the first mode was primarily associated with the size of

Table 5. Logistic regression analysis of the modes combined ED and ES.

Parameter	Coefficient	Standard Error	Standardized coefficient	Odds Ratio(OR)	OR 95% Confidence Interval	
Intercept	−15.9741	4.7246				
Age	0.0384	0.0214	0.2157	1.0390	0.9960	1.0840
Sex	−0.2512	0.5221	−0.0692	0.7780	0.2800	2.1640
Height	0.0530	0.0285	0.2991	1.0540	0.9970	1.1150
Weight*	−0.0371	0.0097	−0.3694	0.9640	0.9450	0.9820
SBP	0.0195	0.0137	0.2345	1.0200	0.9930	1.0470
DBP	−0.0145	0.0246	−0.0834	0.9860	0.9390	1.0340
mode1*	0.0160	0.0015	1.8174	1.0160	1.0130	1.0190
mode2*	−0.0122	0.0021	−0.5272	0.9880	0.9840	0.9920
mode3	−0.0024	0.0025	−0.0971	0.9980	0.9930	1.0020
mode4*	0.0438	0.0046	1.5528	1.0450	1.0350	1.0540
modes5†	0.0068	0.0029	0.2227	1.0070	1.0010	1.0130
mode6	0.0012	0.0037	0.0329	1.0010	0.9940	1.0080
mode7†	−0.0314	0.0045	−0.8131	0.9690	0.9610	0.9780
mode8†	0.0089	0.0043	0.1963	1.0090	1.0000	1.0180
mode9	−0.0023	0.0045	−0.0479	0.9980	0.9890	1.0060
mode10	0.0096	0.0050	0.1906	1.0100	1.0000	1.0200
mode11	−0.0006	0.0051	−0.0115	0.9990	0.9890	1.0090
mode12‡	−0.0217	0.0056	−0.3548	0.9790	0.9680	0.9890
mode13*	−0.0263	0.0067	−0.4121	0.9740	0.9610	0.9870
mode14*	0.0264	0.0065	0.3784	1.0270	1.0140	1.0400
mode15*	0.0293	0.0086	0.4079	1.0300	1.0130	1.0470
mode16‡	0.0195	0.0071	0.2479	1.0200	1.0060	1.0340
mode17	0.0092	0.0070	0.1122	1.0090	0.9960	1.0230
mode18	0.0076	0.0073	0.0935	1.0080	0.9930	1.0220
mode19	−0.0126	0.0082	−0.1451	0.9870	0.9720	1.0030
mode20	0.0033	0.0080	0.0371	1.0030	0.9880	1.0190

†$p<0.05$; ‡$p<0.01$; * $p<0.0001$.

the LV. Mode 2 explained 10% of the total variance at ED and was primarily associated with the sphericity of the left ventricle. The third mode of ED was associated with mitral valve orientation. At ES the second mode accounting for 8% of the variance was associated with wall thickening. The third mode at ES was associated with sphericity. We retained 90% of the cumulative variance, which resulted in 13 modes at ED, 14 modes at ES and 20 modes for the ED&ES combination.

Five logistic regression models were studied using all available data. The coefficients (β), standard error, associated p-values, standardized coefficients and odds ratios (OR) were calculated for each model. A p-value of 0.05 or lower was considered significant. The first model included age, sex, height, weight, systolic blood pressure and diastolic blood pressure (Table 1). This was considered the baseline model (Table 2). The second model included the baseline model variables plus 14 ES PCA modes (ES PCA, Table 3). The third model consisted of the baseline variables plus 13 ED PCA modes (ED PCA, Table 4). The fourth model consisted of the baseline variables plus the modes obtained from the ED&ES combination of the ED and ES shape parameters (ED&ES PCA, Table 5). The fifth model included the baseline variables plus the ED volume (EDV), the ES volume (ESV) and the LV mass (MASSVOL, Table 6). The baseline model showed that the age, height and weight were statistically significant predictors of disease (Table 2). These were also significant in the baseline plus ES PCA model (Table 3), along with most of the PCA modes (except modes 5, 8, 11 and 13). The baseline plus ED modes (Table 4) also showed that most PCA modes were significantly associated with disease (except modes 4, 7, 10, 12 and 13). The baseline plus mass and volume model showed that EDV, ESV and MASS were all associated with disease (Table 6).

The standardized coefficients show which modes have greater effect on the probability that the case is a patient. Mode 1 and mode 4 have greater effect in the classification model at ES. Mode 1, mode 6 and mode 2 have greater effect in the classification model at ED. EDV, ESV and MASS are highly related with the disease, according to Table 6. The Odds ratios were relative measures of the effects of the shape indicators between the myocardial infarction patients and the normal people. Some shape indicators (OR>1), for instance, the mode 1 and mode 4 in the ES model (Table 3) and ED&ES model (Table 5) show higher odds of myocardial infarction than others. Some shape indicators (OR<1) show lower odds of the disease, for example, mode 1 and mode 6 in the ED model (Table 4). There are several modes whose OR is not significant as their confidence intervals overlap the null value (OR = 1).

Table 6. Logistic regression analysis of the modes for LV volume and Mass.

Parameter	Coefficient	Standard Error	p value	Standardized coefficient	Odds Ratio(OR)	OR 95% Confidence Interval	
Intercept	−14.6045	2.9025	<.0001				
Age	0.0246	0.0128	0.0538	0.1384	1.0250	1.0000	1.0510
Sex	−0.2043	0.3522	0.5619	−0.0563	0.8150	0.4090	1.6260
Height‡	0.0650	0.0176	0.0002	0.3664	1.0670	1.0310	1.1040
Weight*	−0.0321	0.0068	<.0001	−0.3197	0.9680	0.9560	0.9810
SBP	0.0126	0.0080	0.1136	0.1515	1.0130	0.9970	1.0290
DBP	−0.0138	0.0158	0.3826	−0.0792	0.9860	0.9560	1.0170
EDV‡	−0.0245	0.0070	0.0005	−0.5374	0.9760	0.9630	0.9890
ESV*	0.1175	0.0099	<.0001	2.0280	1.1250	1.1030	1.1470
MASS‡	−0.0185	0.0048	0.0001	−0.3894	0.9820	0.9730	0.9910

†$p<0.05$; ‡$p<0.01$; * $p<0.0001$.

The goodness of fit was compared between the five models with the indices of Deviance, AIC, BIC and AUC of each model, which are listed in Table 7. Overall, all the PCA mode models as well as the mass-volume model showed good performance. The ED&ES PCA model achieved the best performance in terms of Deviance, AIC, SC, and AUC values, followed closely by the ES PCA model and the ED PCA model. All PCA models better characterized patients from non-patients than traditional mass and volume measures. The ROC curves are shown in Fig. 7.

Discussion

We have proposed an atlas-based disease analysis framework by means of shape parameters from LV finite element models with a large number of subjects. The framework consisted of three steps: (1) fitting a finite element model to the LV MR images, (2) principal component analysis of the aligned shape parameters, and (3) quantification of the association with disease using logistic regression. We hypothesized that patients with myocardial infarction have significant shape differences with respect to the normal population, due to cardiac remodeling. The results supported this hypothesis, with most modes significantly associated with disease. The PCA analysis also performed better than traditional indices of remodeling (mass and volume). This method can therefore be used as a clinical tool for the characterization of the patterns of change associated with remodeling. These methods can also be used to track individual patients over time, by quantifying the degree to which their shape modes conform to the remodeling spectrum. Patients who are moving toward the adverse side of the spectrum may benefit from more aggressive treatment regimes. Conversely, the reverse remodeling associated with treatment can also be quantified. Although in this study we applied the method to patients with myocardial infarction, this framework is generalizable to any disease group.

Note that we did not attempt to correct for colinearity between EDV, ESV and Mass in the MASSVOL model, or between SBP and DPB in the baseline model. EDV and ESV were strongly correlated (Pearson coefficient $\rho = 0.911$, $p<0.05$), as were ESV and Mass (Pearson coefficient $\rho = 0.664$, $p<0.05$), which would affect these coefficient estimates and odds ratios in the model. However, all three were input together in the MASSVOL baseline model to show the combined goodness-of-fit of traditional indicators, in order to assess the improvement given by the PCA modes. SBP, DBP (Pearson coefficient $\rho = 0.604$, $p<0.05$) and other baseline variables were included in all the regression models to control for any differences between the patient and asymptomatic groups (Table 1).

The finite-element method is a powerful representation of the LV model, which also provides traditional indicators such as volume and mass. This method has been used to characterize cardiac motion [30,31] and deformation in a variety of disease groups [32]. Extensions to the right ventricle and atria have also been proposed [33,34]. In this study, we have limited the application of these models to the description of shape; however, these models also have the capability of simulating the excitation, contraction and relaxation of cardiac mechanics [35].

PCA clusters the variability of the finite element models into orthogonal modes that can be interpreted from a global shape point of view. In [5], PCA was used to determine the shape differences between people born pre-term and people born full-term. PCA has the disadvantage that the modes are in general difficult to interpret from a clinical perspective. However, in the present study the first three modes were associated with well understood clinical indicators such as size or sphericity.

Table 7. Comparison of the five logistic models.

	Deviance	AIC	BIC	AUC
Baseline Model	1254.44	1268.44	1308.34	0.7404
MASSVOL Model	602.641	622.641	679.644	0.9530
ED PCA Model	411.088	451.088	565.094	0.9810
ES PCA Model	319.881	361.881	481.587	0.9883
ED&ES PCA Model	260.753	314.753	468.661	0.9905

Interestingly, both size and sphericity are associated with adverse outcomes after myocardial infarction [7,36,37]. In the current study, the ED_ES PCA regression model performed the best with an AUC of 0.9905. Adding ESV, EDV and MASS into this model did not improve this performance greatly (results not shown), indicating that the discriminatory information included in these mass and volume measures are already captured in the ED&ES PCA model. Adding stroke volume or ejection fraction to the MASSVOL model also did not improve the results greatly, since these are very dependent on the ESV and EDV already in the model.

Although heart size is known to be dependent on patient body habitus, we did not correct the shape vectors for height or weight, as done clinically using indexing methods. This was because the baseline model already included height and weight, so all PCA logistic regression analyses were automatically corrected for height and weight.

Further work is needed in several areas. Although PCA is one of the most common dimensionality reduction techniques, other techniques may be more appropriate, such as independent component analysis [18]. Secondly, logistic regression classification method is only one of many methods which can be used for the characterization of disease. For example, in [38] a three-dimensional cortical gray matter density map was established and validated using sparse multinomial logistic regression in the classification of schizophrenia. In [39], a maximum a posteriori classifier was used to distinguish brain tissue types. Expectation-maximization (EM) [40] and k-Nearest-Neighbor [41] classification have been successfully applied to evaluate brain tumors from MRI. Neural networks and support vector machines have been used to identify brain structures with MRI [42] and to predict wall motion scores [43]. Evaluation and comparison of these methods for the evaluation of cardiac disease should be performed. Thirdly, the transformation from GRE to SSFP models was learned using 40 normal volunteers. While [23] showed that this was sufficient to robustly characterize the transformation, more cases would provide a greater variation of heart shape and might improve the transformation parameters.

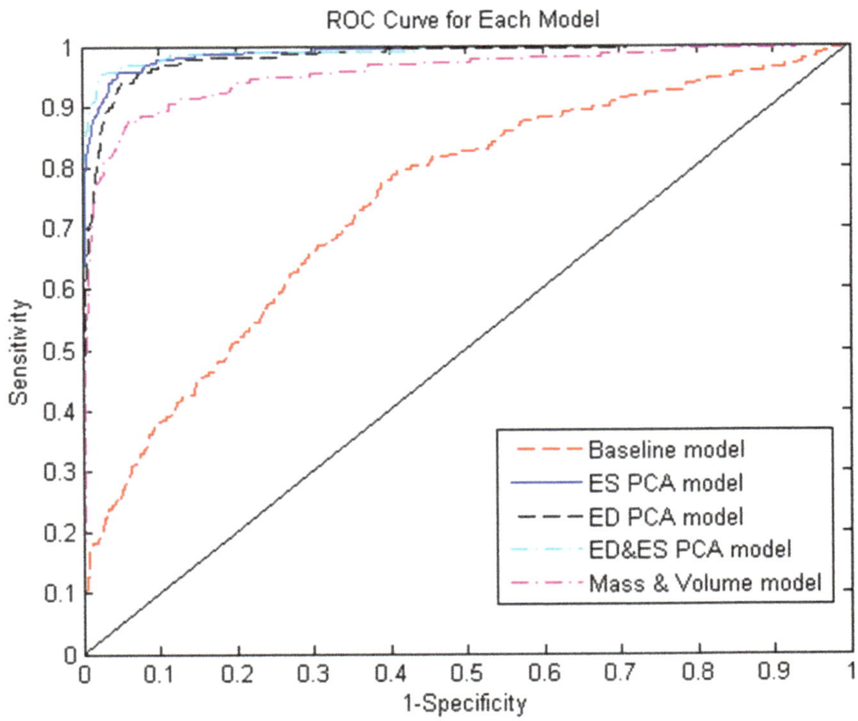

Figure 7. ROC curve for the logistic regression classification for each model.

Author Contributions

Conceived and designed the experiments: XZ BRC AS AAY PMG. Performed the experiments: XZ AS PMG. Analyzed the data: XZ BRC DAB JPF CGF AHK DCL JACL AS AAY PMG. Contributed reagents/materials/analysis tools: XZ BRC DAB JPF CGF AHK DCL JACL AS AAY PMG. Wrote the paper: XZ BRC DAB JPF CGF AHK DCL JACL AS AAY PMG.

References

1. Young AA, Frangi AF (2009) Computational cardiac atlases: from patient to population and back. Experimental Physiology 94: 578–596.
2. Thompson PM, Woods RP, Mega MS, Toga AW (2000) Mathematical/computational challenges in creating deformable and probabilistic atlases of the human brain. Human brain mapping 9: 81–92.
3. Gholve PA, Hosalkar HS, Ricchetti ET, Pollock AN, Dormans JP, et al. (2007) Occipitalization of the Atlas in ChildrenMorphologic Classification, Associations, and Clinical Relevance. The Journal of Bone & Joint Surgery 89: 571–578.
4. Evans AC, Kamber M, Collins DL, MacDonald D (1994) An MRI-based probabilistic atlas of neuroanatomy. Magnetic resonance scanning and epilepsy: Springer. pp. 263–274.
5. Lewandowski AJ, Augustine D, Lamata P, Davis EF, Lazdam M, et al. (2013) Preterm Heart in Adult Life Cardiovascular Magnetic Resonance Reveals Distinct Differences in Left Ventricular Mass, Geometry, and Function. Circulation 127: 197–206.
6. Sutton MGSJ, Sharpe N (2000) Left ventricular remodeling after myocardial infarction pathophysiology and therapy. Circulation 101: 2981–2988.
7. Wong SP, French JK, Lydon A-M, Manda SOM, Gao W, et al. (2004) Relation of left ventricular sphericity to 10-year survival after acute myocardial infarction. The American journal of cardiology 94: 1270–1275.
8. Fonseca CG, Backhaus M, Bluemke DA, Britten RD, Do Chung J, et al. (2011) The Cardiac Atlas Project—an imaging database for computational modeling and statistical atlases of the heart. Bioinformatics 27: 2288–2295.
9. Kadish AH, Bello D, Finn J, Bonow RO, Schaechter A, et al. (2009) Rationale and design for the defibrillators to reduce risk by magnetic resonance imaging evaluation (DETERMINE) trial. Journal of cardiovascular electrophysiology 20: 982–987.
10. Bild DE, Bluemke DA, Burke GL, Detrano R, Roux AVD, et al. (2002) Multi-ethnic study of atherosclerosis: objectives and design. American Journal of Epidemiology 156: 871–881.
11. Frangi AF, Niessen WJ, Viergever MA (2001) Three-dimensional modeling for functional analysis of cardiac images, a review. Medical Imaging, IEEE Transactions on 20: 2–5.
12. Li B, Liu Y, Occleshaw CJ, Cowan BR, Young AA (2010) In-line automated tracking for ventricular function with magnetic resonance imaging. JACC: Cardiovascular Imaging 3: 860–866.
13. Young AA, Cowan BR, Thrupp SF, Hedley WJ, Dell'Italia LJ (2000) Left Ventricular Mass and Volume: Fast Calculation with Guide-Point Modeling on MR Images 1. Radiology 216: 597–602.
14. Luo H, O'Donnell T (2001) A 3D statistical shape model for the left ventricle of the heart; Springer. pp. 1300–1301.
15. Augenstein KF, Young AA (2002) Finite element modeling for three-dimensional motion reconstruction and analysis. Measurement of Cardiac Deformations from MRI: Physical and Mathematical Models: Springer. pp. 37–58.
16. Zhu Y, Papademetris X, Sinusas AJ, Duncan JS (2008) Bidirectional segmentation of three-dimensional cardiac MR images using a subject-specific dynamical model. Medical Image Computing and Computer-Assisted Intervention–MICCAI 2008: Springer. pp. 450–457.
17. Medrano-Gracia P, Cowan BR, Bluemke DA, Finn JP, Lima JAC, et al. (2013) Large Scale Left Ventricular Shape Atlas Using Automated Model Fitting to Contours. In: Ourselin S, Rueckert D, Smith N, editors. Lecture Notes in Computer Science; London. Springer. pp. 433–441.
18. Medrano-Gracia P, Cowan B, Finn JP, Fonseca C, Kadish A, et al. (2010) The Cardiac Atlas Project: Preliminary Description of Heart Shape in Patients with Myocardial Infarction. In: Camara O, Pop M, Rhode K, Sermesant M, Smith N et al., editors. Statistical Atlases and Computational Models of the Heart: Springer Berlin Heidelberg. pp. 46–53.
19. Bild DE, Bluemke DA, Burke GL, Detrano R, Diez Roux AV, et al. (2002) Multi-ethnic study of atherosclerosis: objectives and design. Am J Epidemiol 156: 871–881.
20. Medrano-Gracia P, Cowan B, Bluemke D, Finn JP, Lima JC, et al. (2013) Large Scale Left Ventricular Shape Atlas Using Automated Model Fitting to Contours. In: Ourselin S, Rueckert D, Smith N, editors. Functional Imaging and Modeling of the Heart: Springer Berlin Heidelberg. pp. 433–441.
21. Young AA, Crossman DJ, Ruygrok PN, Cannell MB (2011) Mapping system for coregistration of cardiac MRI and ex vivo tissue sampling. Journal of Magnetic Resonance Imaging 34: 1065–1071.
22. Goodall C (1991) Procrustes methods in the statistical analysis of shape. Journal of the Royal Statistical Society Series B (Methodological): 285–339.
23. Medrano-Gracia P, Cowan BR, Bluemke DA, Finn JP, Kadish AH, et al. (2013) Atlas-based analysis of cardiac shape and function: correction of regional shape bias due to imaging protocol for population studies. Journal of Cardiovascular Magnetic Resonance 15: 80.
24. Jolliffe I (2005) Principal component analysis: Wiley Online Library.
25. Hosmer DW, Lemeshow S, Sturdivant RX (2013) Introduction to the Logistic Regression Model. Applied Logistic Regression: John Wiley & Sons, Inc. pp. 1–33.
26. Press SJ, Wilson S (1978) Choosing between logistic regression and discriminant analysis. Journal of the American Statistical Association 73: 699–705.
27. Johnson JB, Omland KS (2004) Model selection in ecology and evolution. Trends in Ecology & Evolution 19: 101–108.
28. Liu Y (2007) On goodness-of-fit of logistic regression model: ProQuest.
29. Zhu M, Ghodsi A (2006) Automatic dimensionality selection from the scree plot via the use of profile likelihood. Computational Statistics & Data Analysis 51: 918–930.
30. Remme E, Young AA, Augenstein KF, Cowan B, Hunter PJ (2004) Extraction and quantification of left ventricular deformation modes. Biomedical Engineering, IEEE Transactions on 51: 1923–1931.
31. Medrano-Gracia P, Cowan BR, Bluemke DA, Finn JP, Kadish AH, et al. (2014) Continuous Spatio-temporal Atlases of the Asymptomatic and Infarcted Hearts. Statistical Atlases and Computational Models of the Heart Imaging and Modelling Challenges: Springer. pp. 143–151.
32. Young AA, Prince JL (2013) Cardiovascular Magnetic Resonance: Deeper Insights Through Bioengineering. Annual review of biomedical engineering 15: 433–461.
33. Gonzales MJ, Sturgeon G, Krishnamurthy A, Hake J, Jonas R, et al. (2013) A three-dimensional finite element model of human atrial anatomy: New methods for cubic Hermite meshes with extraordinary vertices. Medical image analysis 17: 525–537.
34. Zhang Y, Liang X, Ma J, Jing Y, Gonzales MJ, et al. (2012) An atlas-based geometry pipeline for cardiac Hermite model construction and diffusion tensor reorientation. Medical image analysis 16: 1130–1141.
35. Nash MP, Hunter PJ (2000) Computational mechanics of the heart. Journal of elasticity and the physical science of solids 61: 113–141.
36. White HD, Norris RM, Brown MA, Brandt PW, Whitlock RM, et al. (1987) Left ventricular end-systolic volume as the major determinant of survival after recovery from myocardial infarction. Circulation 76: 44–51.
37. Mannaerts HFJ, van der Heide JA, Kamp O, Stoel MG, Twisk J, et al. (2004) Early identification of left ventricular remodelling after myocardial infarction, assessed by transthoracic 3D echocardiography. European heart journal 25: 680–687.
38. Sun D, van Erp TGM, Thompson PM, Bearden CE, Daley M, et al. (2009) Elucidating a magnetic resonance imaging-based neuroanatomic biomarker for psychosis: classification analysis using probabilistic brain atlas and machine learning algorithms. Biological psychiatry 66: 1055–1060.
39. Bourouis S, Hamrouni K, Betrouni N (2008) Automatic MRI brain segmentation with combined atlas-based classification and level-set approach. Image Analysis and Recognition: Springer. pp. 770–778.
40. Prastawa M, Bullitt E, Moon N, Van Leemput K, Gerig G (2003) Automatic brain tumor segmentation by subject specific modification of atlas priors1. Academic Radiology 10: 1341–1348.
41. Vrooman HA, Cocosco CA, Stokking R, Ikram MA, Vernooij MW, et al. (2006) kNN-based multi-spectral MRI brain tissue classification: manual training versus automated atlas-based training; International Society for Optics and Photonics. pp. 61443L-61443L-61449.
42. Akselrod-Ballin A, Galun M, Gomori MJ, Basri R, Brandt A (2006) Atlas guided identification of brain structures by combining 3D segmentation and SVM classification. Medical Image Computing and Computer-Assisted Intervention–MICCAI 2006: Springer. pp. 209–216.
43. Medrano-Gracia P, Suinesiaputra A, Cowan B, Bluemke D, Frangi A, et al. (2013) An atlas for cardiac MRI regional wall motion and infarct scoring. Statistical Atlases and Computational Models of the Heart Imaging and Modelling Challenges: Springer. pp. 188–197.

7

The Functional Connectivity Landscape of the Human Brain

Bratislav Mišić[1*◔], Zainab Fatima[1], Mary K. Askren[2¶], Martin Buschkuehl[3¶], Nathan Churchill[1¶], Bernadine Cimprich[4¶], Patricia J. Deldin[5¶], Susanne Jaeggi[5¶], Misook Jung[6¶], Michele Korostil[1¶], Ethan Kross[5¶], Katherine M. Krpan[7¶], Scott Peltier[5¶], Patricia A. Reuter-Lorenz[5¶], Stephen C. Strother[1¶], John Jonides[5], Anthony R. McIntosh[1], Marc G. Berman[7,8*◔]

1 Rotman Research Institute, Baycrest Centre, Toronto, Ontario, Canada, **2** Department of Radiology, University of Washington, Seattle, Washington, United States of America, **3** MIND Research Institute, Irvine, California, United States of America, **4** School of Nursing, University of Michigan, Ann Arbor, Michigan, United States of America, **5** Department of Psychology, University of Michigan, Ann Arbor, Michigan, United States of America, **6** Department of Psychology, Chungnam University, Daejeon, South Korea, **7** Department of Psychology, University of South Carolina, Columbia, South Carolina, United States of America, **8** Department of Psychology, University of Chicago, Chicago, Illinois, United States of America

Abstract

Functional brain networks emerge and dissipate over a primarily static anatomical foundation. The dynamic basis of these networks is inter-regional communication involving local and distal regions. It is assumed that inter-regional distances play a pivotal role in modulating network dynamics. Using three different neuroimaging modalities, 6 datasets were evaluated to determine whether experimental manipulations asymmetrically affect functional relationships based on the distance between brain regions in human participants. Contrary to previous assumptions, here we show that short- and long-range connections are equally likely to strengthen or weaken in response to task demands. Additionally, connections between homotopic areas are the most stable and less likely to change compared to any other type of connection. Our results point to a functional connectivity landscape characterized by fluid transitions between local specialization and global integration. This ability to mediate functional properties irrespective of spatial distance may engender a diverse repertoire of cognitive processes when faced with a dynamic environment.

Editor: Xi-Nian Zuo, Institute of Psychology, Chinese Academy of Sciences, China

Funding: This work was supported by 1) Tom and Kitty Stoner Foundation (TKF) Grant to MGB, 2) National Institutes of Mental Health (NIMH) Grant MH 60655 to JJ, and 3) National Institutes of Health (NIH) grant NIH-NINR-R01-NRO10939 to BC. The funders had no role in study design, data collection and analysis, decision to publish, or preparation of the manuscript.

Competing Interests: The authors have declared that no competing interests exist.

* Email: bermanm@uchicago.edu (MGB); bmisic@research.baycrest.org (BM)

◔ These authors contributed equally to this work.

¶ These authors also contributed equally to this work and are noted in alphabetical order.

Introduction

Functional brain networks are continually evolving on top of an anatomical skeleton to engender perception, thought and action. Patterns of functional connectivity may change either spontaneously [1–3], in response to task demands [4–7] or in response to disease or pharmacological interventions [8–10]. It is unclear, however, whether these various sources of connectivity change can be characterized in a principled way to predict brain states.

One hypothesis is that short-range functional connections are more stable than long-range connections. The laminar, cytoarchitectonic and columnar organization of the neocortex suggests that proximal areas may participate in similar functions [11]. As a result, short-range functional connections may be relatively stable and less likely to be affected by changes in task demands. Conversely, long-range functional connections between distal brain areas with dissimilar functions may be less stable and more likely to change due to task. Therefore, changes in tasks and psychological conditions may elicit relatively large changes in functional connectivity between distal areas and relatively small changes between proximal areas.

An alternative hypothesis is that task-dependent changes in functional connectivity do not depend on the distance between areas. Complex network theory suggests that, for optimal information processing, functional networks must simultaneously enable local segregation and global integration, thereby allowing for the interplay between specialization and integration of function [12–14]. To strike an adaptive balance between integration and segregation, task-dependent reconfiguration of functional networks would require flexible functional connectivity that is not biased by the distance between areas. According to this hypothesis, changes in brain states will be associated with equally stable short- and long-range functional connections.

Here we investigated whether the stability of a functional connection between two brain regions is affected by the length (distance spanned) of that connection. We define stability as a change in functional connectivity across two or more tasks or psychological conditions. We used the Euclidean distance between two regions as a proxy for the length of their functional connection. We analyzed data from four functional magnetic resonance imaging (fMRI) datasets, one magnetoencephalography (MEG) dataset and one positron emission tomography (PET) dataset. The data that we analyzed varied in task conditions, populations, preprocessing parameters, and acquisition parameters and yet even with all of this heterogeneity we demonstrate two key results across all studies. 1) Within a single condition, functional connectivity depends on spatial distance, i.e., short-range functional connections are stronger than long-range connections [a common finding [15]]. 2) Critically, the spatial distance between two regions does not affect the stability of their functional connectivity. Between conditions, changes in functional connectivity do not depend on connection length. Thus, both short- and long-range functional connections are equally likely to change and are equally stable.

While distance is not predictive of stability, whether a connection is between homotopic areas does predict stability. Namely, connections between homotopic areas do not change and therefore are the most stable connections. Importantly, we draw these conclusions based on data from a wide-range of tasks, populations, scanning environments, parcellation schemes, and preprocessing parameters indicating that our results are robust to these idiosyncrasies. These results suggest a simple yet fundamental characteristic of brain network dynamics; that changes in task result in alterations to the entire landscape of functional connections, independent of their lengths.

Results

Dataset Summaries and Rationale for Inclusion

Here we summarize the datasets that we used for our analyses. The interested reader can find all of the details for each individual study under the specific dataset sub-headings in the Materials and Methods section. However, these details are not necessary to understand our results and analyses. This section, and the next section, "Partial Least-Squares (PLS) Analysis Parameters," are the only methods' sections that are required to understand the results and analyses.

Methodological details regarding participants, tasks, and processing parameters for the six datasets used in this analysis are shown in Table 1. Two fMRI datasets contained data from clinically depressed patients and breast cancer patients to examine if *our results were robust for different clinical populations*. The third and fourth fMRI datasets involved healthy adults performing a learning task where participants learned to associate pseudo-words to pictures, and a crossmodal (auditory-visual) attentional cuing task to examine if *our results were robust for on-task performance vs. resting-states*. The MEG dataset was also acquired using healthy adults participating in a visual learning paradigm. The PET data were derived from a study on memory recall in young and old adults. The MEG and PET datasets were included to examine if *our results were robust for different imaging modalities*. In the paragraphs below we describe these studies.

In the depression dataset [16], healthy individuals and individuals diagnosed with major depression had their resting-state connectivity assessed and this resting-state connectivity was compared to a condition where participants were induced to ruminate about two negative, self-generated, autobiographical memories. There was also a resting-state scan after this rumination phase to examine recovery after induced rumination. ***Here changes in connectivity were assessed for changes between rest and induced rumination.***

In the breast cancer dataset, women with breast cancer and healthy-aged matched controls had their brain connectivity assessed during resting-state epochs. Of the patients with breast cancer, half received chemotherapy treatment for breast cancer and half received radiation therapy for breast cancer. Connectivity was assessed before and after chemotherapy treatment, radiation therapy and an equivalent period of elapsed time for the healthy aged-matched controls. ***Here connectivity changes were due to treatment (i.e., chemotherapy and radiation therapy) vs. the mere passage of time for age-matched controls.***

In the cross-modal dataset [17] participants responded to visual and auditory targets. A trial was composed of a stimulus (S1), a delay, and a second stimulus (S2). The two main task types were designed by manipulating the content of S1 and S2. For the Cue 1st (C1) tasks, S1 was a cue that signaled a response compatibility rule to a subsequent lateralized target (S2). In Target 1st (C2) tasks, S1 was the lateralized target followed by the cue stimulus (S2). In a compatible trial, a cue instructed participants to press a button on the same side (left or right) as the lateralized target. In an incompatible trial, participant's pressed the button on the opposite side of the lateralized target. Unlike in the depression and breast cancer datasets, ***here connectivity changes were assessed by examining connectivity changes for changes in the task conditions such as trials when one must respond to a visual target preceded by an auditory cue vs. when one must respond to an auditory target preceded by a visual cue.***

In the learning dataset participants heard an auditory presentation of a pseudoword. After the presentation of the pseudoword participants saw a picture presented for 1 second and were told to intuitively decide if the pairing of pseudoword and picture was correct. There were two conditions: "Learning" and "No-Learning." The "Learning" condition involved a higher co-occurrence of "correct" arbitrary object-pseudoword pairings compared to "incorrect" pairings. Participants learned this novel vocabulary of 30 concrete nouns over the course of five consecutive training blocks. Over the course of the five training blocks the ratio of "correct" to "incorrect" pairings increased. The "No-Learning" condition was structured similarly, but used a parallel set of pseudoword-object pairings and lacked a learning principle because each pairing occurred only once. ***Here changes in connectivity were measured as learning progressed.***

In the MEG dataset [18] participants performed two tasks: an active learning task and a choice reaction time task with no learning component. In the learning task, participants linked 2 scene pairs with 2 color pairs (4 associations) through trial-and-error. The general structure of a trial consisted of scene presentation, a delay interval and a color pair, after which the participants had to record their responses. Participants received on-screen, written feedback (correct/wrong) about their response choices. In the control task, participants were instructed in advance about which colors were correct and scenes preceding these colors were shown randomly. ***Here changes in connectivity were assessed for these different task conditions and for a different imaging modality (i.e., MEG).***

In the PET dataset participants encoded and recalled word pairs. Effective connectivity was assessed using Structural Equation Modeling (SEM). ***Here changes in connectivity were assessed for yet another imaging modality (i.e., PET), for differences in memory recall by age (i.e., aging***

Table 1. Details for the neuroimaging studies that were analyzed.

Study	Modality	Groups	Conditions	ROIs	Parcellation Scheme
Depression	fMRI	Depressed (N = 16) Healthy Control (N = 17)	4: Resting 1, Resting 2, Induced Rumination, Resting 3	116	AAL
Breast Cancer	fMRI	Chemotherapy (N = 16) Radiation therapy (N = 16) Healthy Control (N = 16)	2: Pre-treatment, Post-treatment	116	AAL
Learning	fMRI	Healthy Control (N = 12)	6: Learning conditions	152	AAL/MNI hybrid
Crossmodal	fMRI	Healthy Control (N = 16)	4: Autitory-Visual Cue target combinations	229 voxels	Every 100th gray matter voxel
MEG	MEG	Healthy Control (N = 14)	3: Learning Conditions	32 sources	N/A
PET	PET	Healthy Control (N = 12)	2: Memory encoding and Recall	13 ROIs	N/A

Details for the PET study can be found in [31].

effects) and for effective connectivity rather than functional connectivity.

Correlating Functional Connectivity and Euclidean Distance

The parcellation scheme used for each dataset is specified in Table 1. For datasets that were parceled into ROIs, time series were averaged across all voxels in each ROI. Functional connectivity matrices were then created by correlating the mean ROI timeseries with all other mean ROI timeseries separately for each individual participant and for each condition. Sample Fisher-transformed and group averaged functional connectivity matrices are shown separately for each condition (Fig. 1).

The Euclidean distance between ROI centroids was calculated and correlated with functional connectivity. Euclidean distance significantly predicted functional connectivity for each study, for each group and for each condition, such that ROIs that were spatially closer were more likely to be highly correlated (Fig. 2). This result has been found by other researchers [2,15,19] and may be expected given that contiguous brain areas participate in similar functions. In addition, studies find that contiguous brain areas share similar regional homogeneity [20,21], i.e. temporal signatures, which may also indicate similar functionality. This aspect of functional neuroanatomy also results in the well-known spatial autocorrelation of the BOLD signal [22]. In summary, within a condition, Euclidean distance significantly predicts functional connectivity, i.e., connections between more proximal areas are more highly correlated.

Correlating Changes in Functional Connectivity and Euclidean Distance

The results presented in the previous sub-section indicate that, within a condition, Euclidean distance and functional connectivity are negatively correlated, such that proximal areas tend to be more highly correlated with one another compared to more distal areas. In the present section, we show that there is no reliable relationship between Euclidean distance and changes in functional connectivity due to changes in task or group.

For each dataset we extracted participant- and condition-specific functional connectivity matrices and used a partial least-squares (PLS) analysis [23–25] to find connections that showed significant changes in functional connectivity across tasks and/or groups. The latent variables (LVs) from those analyses are shown in Fig. 3. Connection saliences are weights that describe the extent to which a connection expresses a latent variable or contrast, and therefore they express the degree to which a connection changes according to the latent variable pattern. For the depression dataset the greatest changes in functional connectivity occurred for the individuals diagnosed with depression who are more affected by the induced rumination condition compared to rest. These results are described in more depth in [16].

For the Breast Cancer dataset the greatest changes in functional connectivity occurred pre- and post-chemotherapy, followed by pre- and post-radiation therapy. The healthy group does not show reliable changes over an equivalent period of elapsed time (as expected given that they receive no intervention). Related breast cancer results are described in more depth in [26,27].

In the Crossmodal dataset there is a significant interaction for changes in functional connectivity by cue position (1 vs. 2) and target type (visual vs. verbal). The Crossmodal results are described in more depth in [17]. Lastly, in the learning dataset there are significant changes in functional connectivity from the baseline reaction time condition with no learning (L8) compared to the other learning conditions as learning progresses. When comparing the greatest change in conditions, we compared the last learning session to the baseline reaction time task that required no learning.

The specific LV results are not critical for this investigation (please see the aforementioned studies for analyses and results specific to these studies). What is important is that for each study there were functional connections that significantly changed due to experimental manipulation (i.e. across groups and/or conditions). Based on these significant LVs, we can determine whether changes

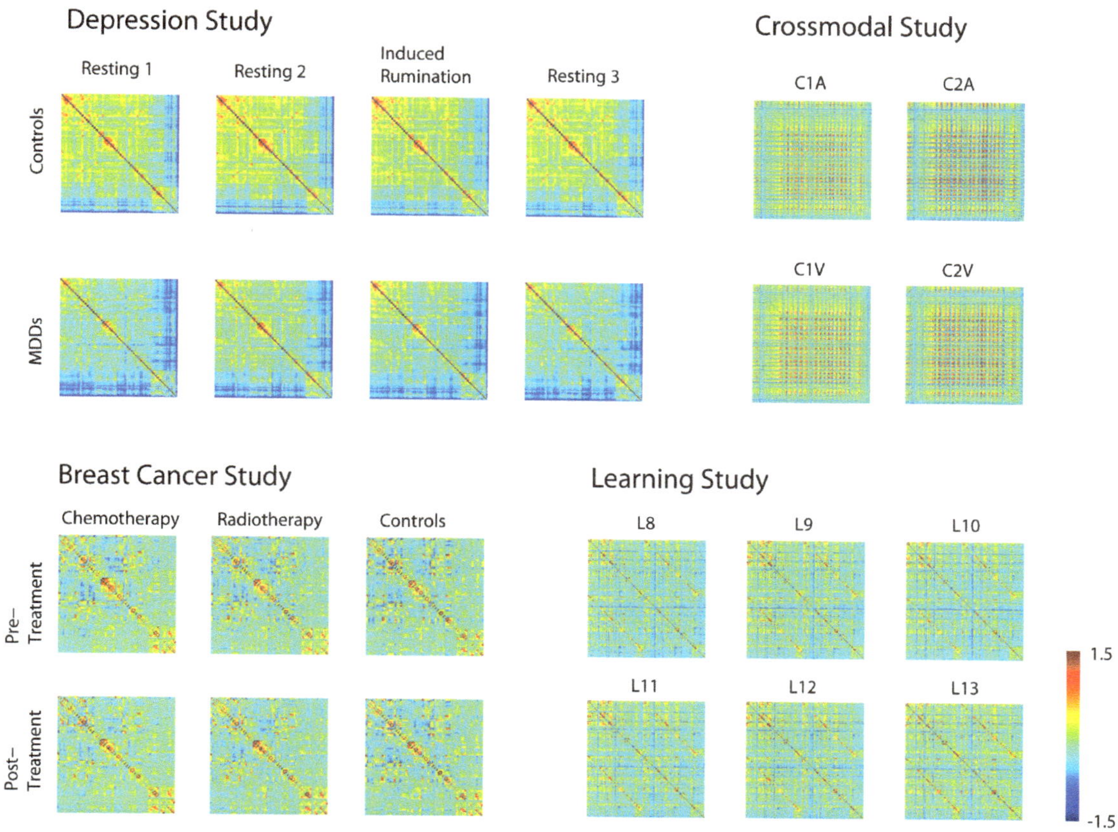

Figure 1. Fisher r-to-z-transformed correlation matrices for all studies exhibiting the correlation between all nodes used to analyze each study. For the PLS analyses, each participant's matrix was used in the analysis.

in functional connectivity are distance-dependent or distance-independent.

To determine whether the lengths of connections predicted connection changes we correlated the saliences of connection changes with Euclidean distance (Fig. 4). The result of that analysis showed no relationship between Euclidean distances and salience values (Fig. 4). These results suggest that all functional connections, independent of the distance between them, are equally likely to change.

We then performed an analysis to examine how differences in correlation values between two conditions in the experiments might change with Euclidean distance. This analysis is much simpler than PLS as we only examine changes in correlation strength between two conditions. Here we selected the two conditions that showed the greatest differences from the PLS analyses and simply subtracted their correlation matrices (e.g., depression dataset: resting 1 vs. induced rumination). When doing so, we again found no relationship between Euclidean distance and changes in functional connectivity between the two conditions (Fig. 5).

It is possible that we observed no systematic relationship between saliences or correlation differences and Euclidean distances because neither saliences nor correlation differences measure the statistical reliability with which a functional connection changes. For instance, saliences are weighted coefficients that represent the magnitude of change. In the PLS framework, the statistical significance of a task effect is assessed at the level of the entire multivariate connectivity profile, but the significance of the task effect on individual functional connections is not tested directly.

To address this problem, we related anatomical distance with the bootstrap ratio associated with each functional connection (Fig. 6). Bootstrap ratios are calculated by taking the ratio of the salience (which reflects the magnitude of a statistical effect) and the bootstrap-estimated standard error of that salience (which reflects the reliability of the salience). Thus, a high-valued bootstrap ratio for a given functional connection indicates both a strong contribution to the latent variable as well as reliability across subjects. Functional connections with large bootstrap ratios show a statistically significant propensity to change due to experimental manipulation. We then correlated the bootstrap ratios with Euclidean distances for each of the four studies, and again found no evidence for a systematic relationship (Fig. 6).

Assessing statistical significance

The results in Figs. 4, 5 and 6 show no obvious relationship between Euclidean distance and changes in functional connectivity, but this is difficult to assess using conventional parametric statistical inference because the data points are dependent. For instance, functional connections are derived from correlation coefficients and are inherently non-independent. Thus, if one possesses knowledge of r(a, b) and r(a, c), it is possible to place limits on the value of r(b, c). As a result, the assumption of independence on which conventional inferential statistics are predicated would be violated, resulting in inflated p-values.

To address this problem, we estimated the p-value for the relationship between distance and change in functional connectivity with respect to a nonparametric null distribution, constructed using independent pairs of distances and correlations, e.g. r(a,

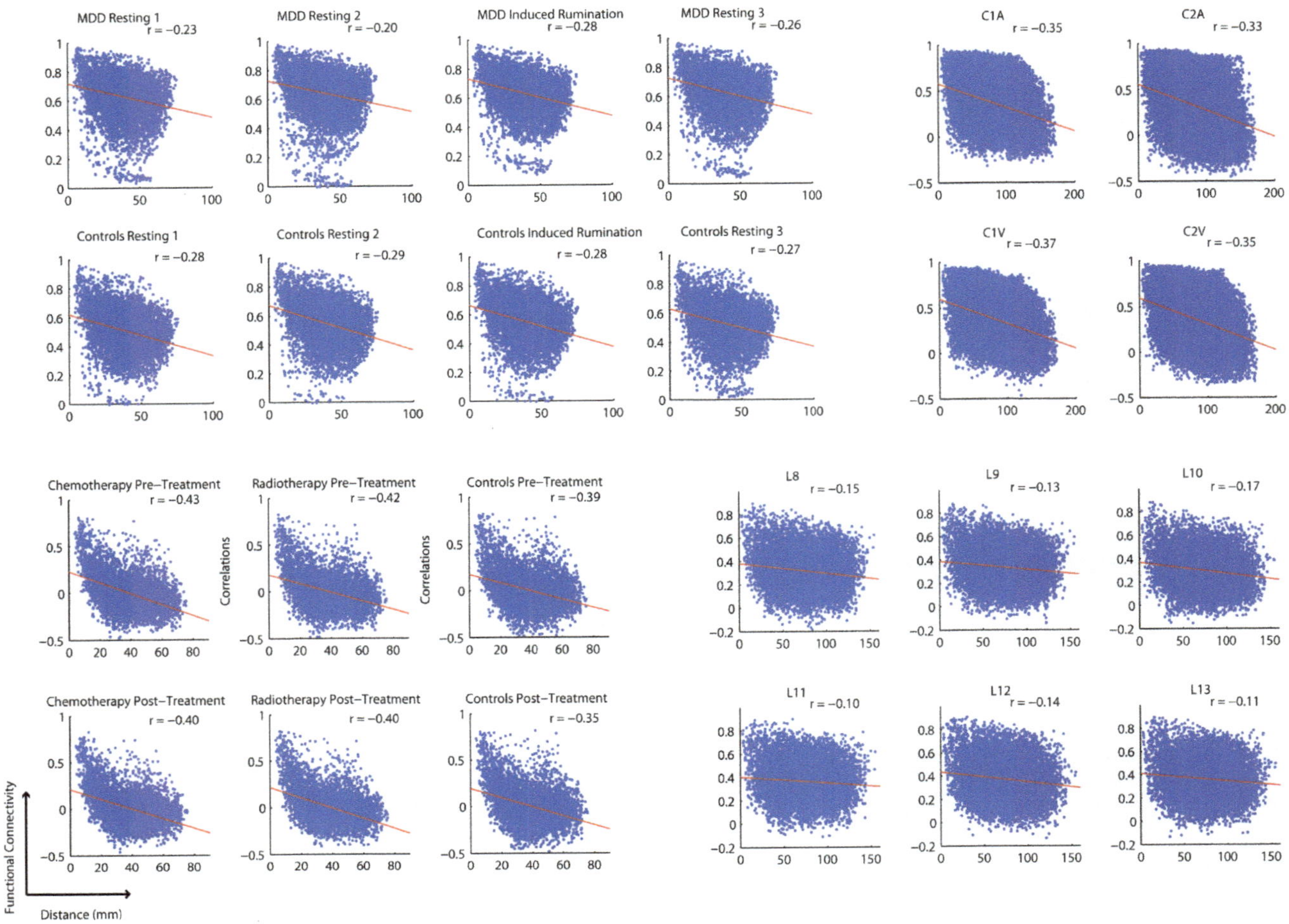

Figure 2. Relationship between the Euclidean distance of parcels and the correlation between parcel timeseries for each fMRI study and for each condition and participant group.

b), r(c, d) and r(e, f) but not r(a, c), etc. For a parcellation with n nodes, there exist floor $(n/2)$ such independent pairs. For a given set of independent pairs, we computed the correlation coefficient between distance and changes in functional connectivity. We then repeated the procedure 1000 times, to construct a sampling distribution of independent correlation coefficients. P-values were calculated as the proportion of independent pairs that were greater than or less than zero. Table 2 displays the mean, standard error and p-value associated with the correlations between salience and anatomical distance, for each of the four studies. The mean correlation values (rho) were low, with small standard errors (SEs). Importantly, one-tailed tests for rho<0 and rho>0 were non-significant, suggesting no evidence of a statistically significant relationship between change in functional connectivity and anatomical distance.

To further illustrate that there is no evidence that these correlations are different from zero, we performed three more analyses. First, to ensure that there were no systematic trends in the dense portions of the plots shown in Fig. 4 and Fig. 5, we re-plotted the changes in correlation data with a 3-dimensional surface plot. As shown in Fig. 7, the areas of the plot with more data points do not show any relationship between changes in correlation and Euclidean Distance.

Second, a principal components analysis (PCA) was conducted as described by [28], to examine possible trends between Euclidean distance and correlation differences in the outlying points. To do so, we performed a PCA on the correlation differences versus Euclidean distances, and for each observation we calculated its displacement from the primary axis of variance. Points that were in the upper or lower 5% in terms of displacement from the primary axis of variance are colored red (Fig. 8). When examining these outlying points, there appears to be no systematic relationship between correlation differences and Euclidean distances.

Third, we were concerned that using the signed value (i.e., positive or negative) of the salience or correlation change could impact the relationship between Euclidean distance and the magnitude of the effect. We calculated the absolute value of the salience and the absolute value of the change in correlation and found that the absolute value of the effects were unrelated to Euclidean distance (Figs. 9 and 10).

In summary, across different groups (healthy, depressed and breast cancer patients) and across different experimental conditions (learning task, crossmodal task, rest) we find the same results. Namely, we consistently find no evidence of a relationship between anatomical distance and changes in functional connectivity. This indicates that across different environmental conditions and groups, the functional connectivity of the whole brain is equally likely to change, independent of the distance between areas.

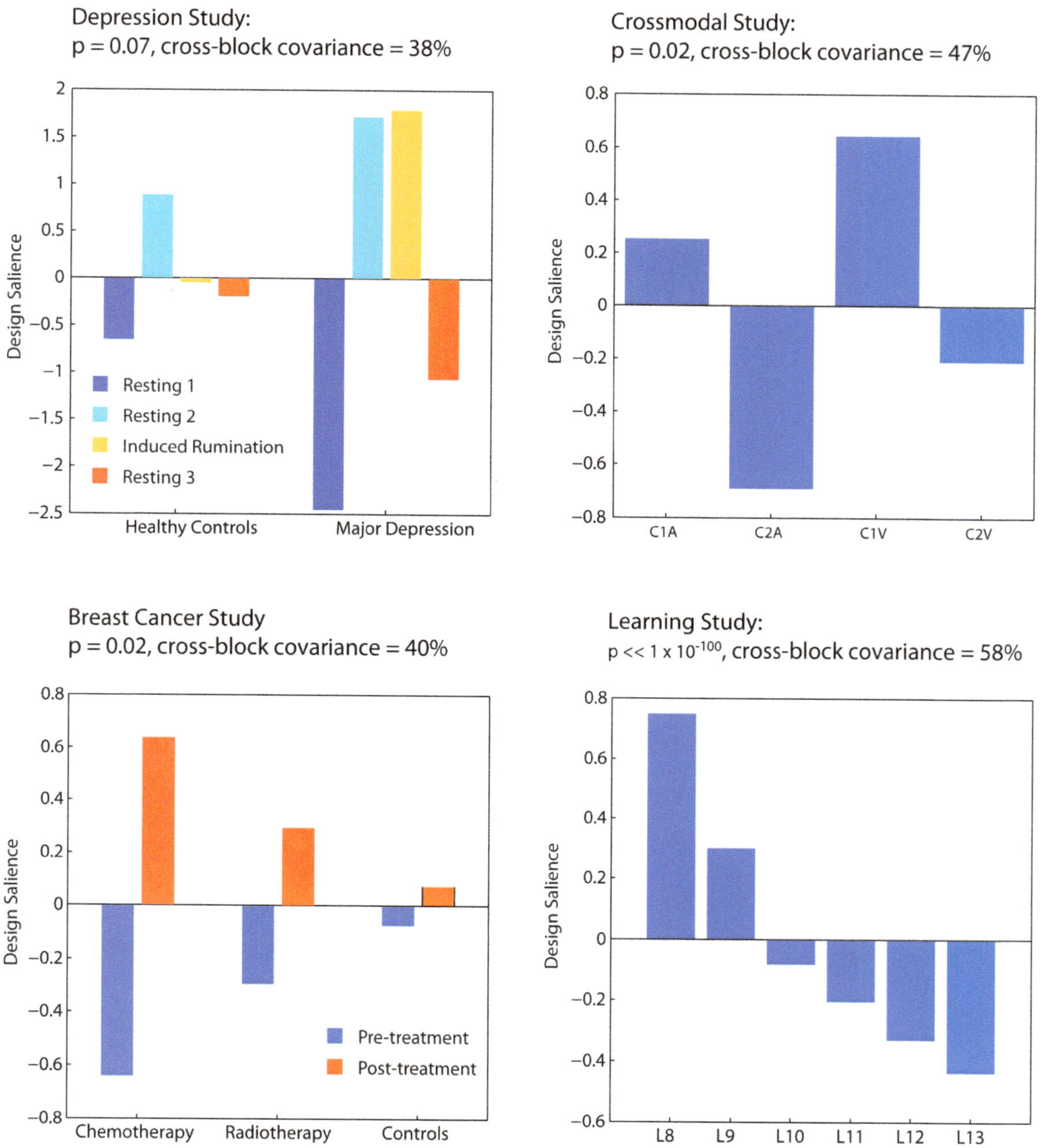

Figure 3. First Latent Variables (LVs) from each of the four fMRI Datasets as uncovered with PLS. The significance of the LVs and the amount of cross-block covariance explained are listed in the titles.

Functional Specialization and Modularity

The previous set of analyses have shown that functional connectivity changes cannot be predicted by the distance of the functional connection across a wide range of populations, tasks, fMRI scanners, preprocessing parameters and parcellation schemes. However, it is possible that the relationship between proximity and functional connectivity change may be influenced by the modular organization of functional networks (Meunier, Lambiotte and Bullmore, 2010). For example, long-distance functional connections may be more likely to change between conditions if they connect regions belonging to different modules, as opposed to the same module.

We applied a community detection algorithm to partition functional brain networks into modules [29,30], allowing us to analyze how functional connections change both within and between modules. Specifically, we used the Louvain algorithm, as implemented in the Brain Connectivity Toolbox (Rubinov & Sporns, 2010). Following 100 runs on each data set, we selected the partition with the highest modularity, Q. We found no evidence of a relationship between functional connectivity changes and Euclidean distance either between or within modules (Fig. 11). In other words, the propensity of a functional connection between two areas to change does not appear to be influenced by the community membership of those areas

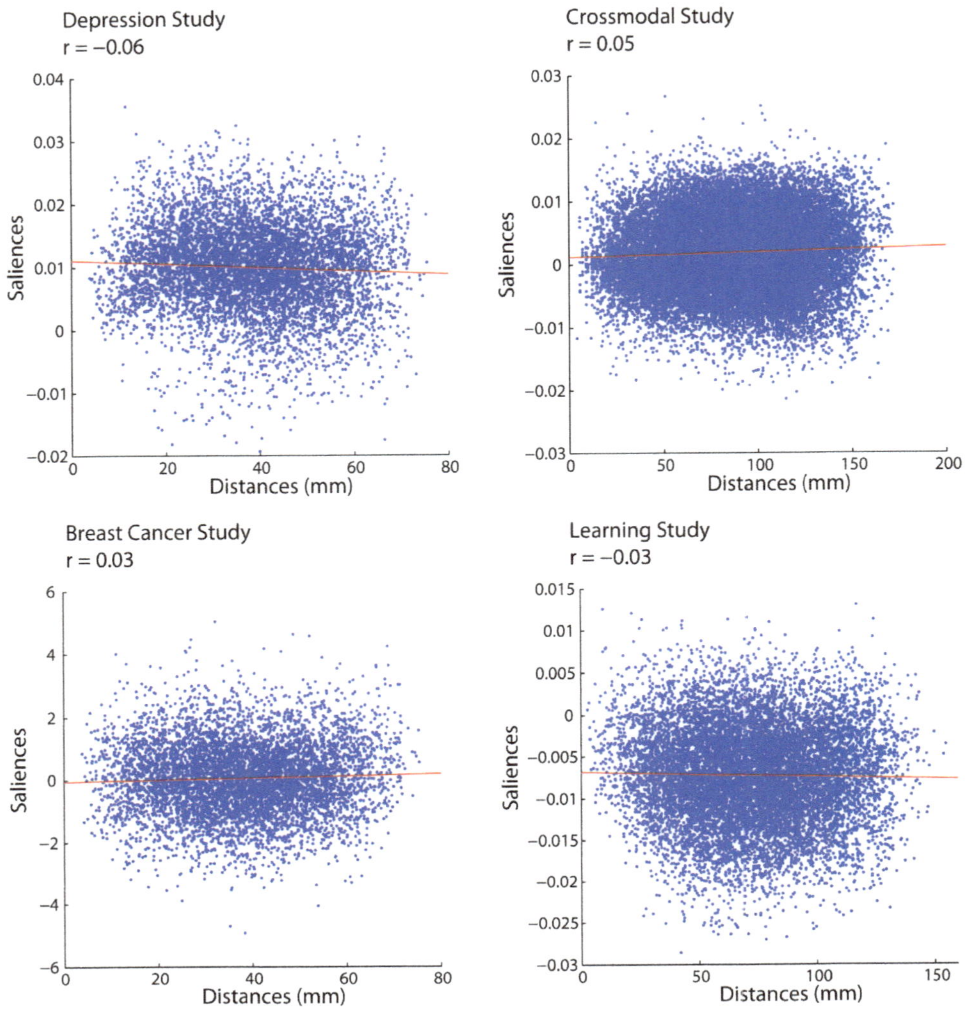

Figure 4. PLS Saliences for the first latent variable in each study plotted against Euclidean distance of each functional connection.

Replication across multiple neuroimaging modalities

Our analyses thus far have focused on a single neuroimaging modality (i.e., fMRI). To examine whether these effects are idiosyncratic to fMRI, we analyzed a MEG dataset [18] and a PET dataset [31] that was published at an earlier time utilizing Structural Equation Modeling (SEM) [32]. In analyzing the MEG dataset, we replicated our previous results and found no relationship between changes in functional connectivity and Euclidean distance (Fig. 12).

We found the same pattern of results for the PET SEM dataset, where significant condition changes in path coefficients were not distance dependent (Fig. 12). It is noteworthy that the path coefficients in SEM represent effective connections, i.e. causal relationships based on known direct anatomical projections. In contrast to functional connections based on zero-order correlations, they are not confounded by potential indirect connections from other areas. This is important because our previous results with functional connectivity could be influenced by other indirect connections. The fact that similar results are observed for SEM suggests that the effects that we report are unlikely to be influenced by indirect connections.

Intra- and inter-hemisphere connections

Finally, we investigated whether spatial proximity had any differential effect on communication within and between hemispheres. For this analysis all functional connections were divided into two classes: intra-or inter-hemispheric. Inter-hemispheric connections were further stratified into those between homotopic and those between non-homotopic brain regions. Fig. 13 shows that even when functional connections are stratified in this way, distance did not predict changes in functional connectivity for either inter- or intra-hemispheric functional connections (Fig. 13A, B).

Interestingly, the relationship between Euclidean distance and change in inter-hemispheric functional connectivity did appear to be affected by whether connections were between homotopic areas. When inter-hemispheric functional connections were further segregated into homotopic and non-homotopic connections, there was still no reliable relationship between changes in functional connectivity and distance (Fig. 13C, D). However, functional connections between homotopic brain areas were associated with smaller change saliences that deviated from zero far less than non-homotopic connections, indicating that they were less likely to change and were more stable than functional connections between non-homotopic areas (Fig. 13D). This is illustrated further in Fig. 13E, which shows the histogram of

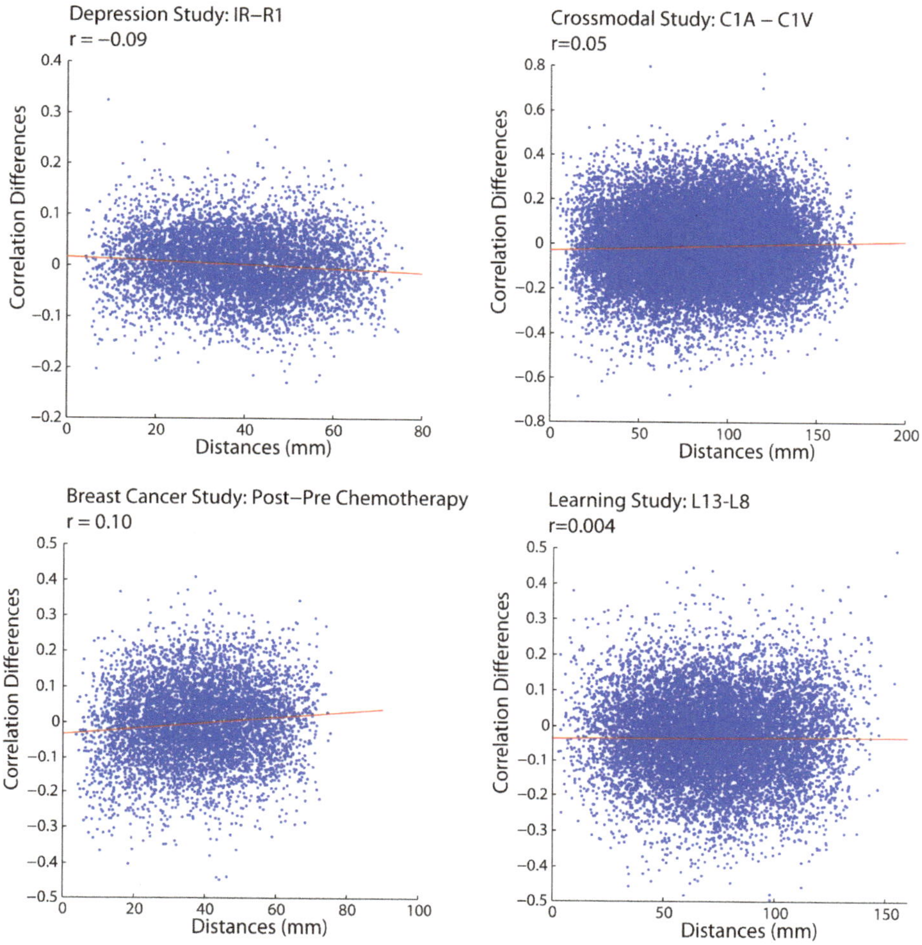

Figure 5. Changes in correlation between conditions of greatest difference in correlation plotted against Euclidean distance.

change saliences for homotopic and non-homotopic functional connections. The homotopic functional connections deviate from zero considerably less than non-homotopic connections.

To statistically assess whether homotopic functional connections were more stable compared to non-homotopic connections, we combined the change saliences for both types of connections and calculated the proportion of each connection type that exceeded the 95% confidence interval of change saliences. We found that, for each study, the proportion of change saliences that exceeded the 95% confidence interval was greater for the non-homotopic connections compared to the homotopic connections. For the Depression, Breast Cancer and Learning studies, these proportions, for the non-homotopic and homotopic connections respectively, were: 5.4% vs. 1.9%, 5.8% vs. 0% and 5% vs. 3.9%. This provides an interesting addition to previous reports, which have shown stronger functional connectivity between homotopic areas compared to functional connectivity between non-homotopic areas [19,33,34].

Discussion

In the present report we investigated whether functional connectivity stability could be predicted by anatomical distance. The goal was to determine whether one of two hypotheses were true: 1) That long-range connections were more likely to change with different manipulations or 2) that all connections, independent of distance, were equally likely to change with different manipulations (i.e., equivalent stability). We implemented a multivariate approach to test these hypotheses, allowing us to simultaneously examine changes in all functional connections in the brain.

We found three important results. First, within a single condition, Euclidean distance significantly predicts functional connectivity; namely, regions that are closer together have stronger functional connectivity and regions further apart have weaker functional connectivity (Fig. 2). We found this result to be robust across different tasks, populations, preprocessing parameters and parcellation schemes. This result is also consistent with previous reports in the literature [2,15,19].

Second, we find that anatomical distance is not a significant predictor of the stability of functional connectivity (Figs. 4–9 & 11), meaning that changes in functional connectivity are not specific to short- or long-range connections; thereby lending support for hypothesis 2. These effects were also robust for a wide range of tasks, populations, preprocessing parameters, parcellation schemes and neuroimaging modalities, suggesting that these effects are not idiosyncratic to particular experimental and analysis parameters.

Third, we find that homotopic functional connections appear to be more stable than any other type of connection. This finding complements previous reports that homotopic functional connections are stronger than other types of functional connections

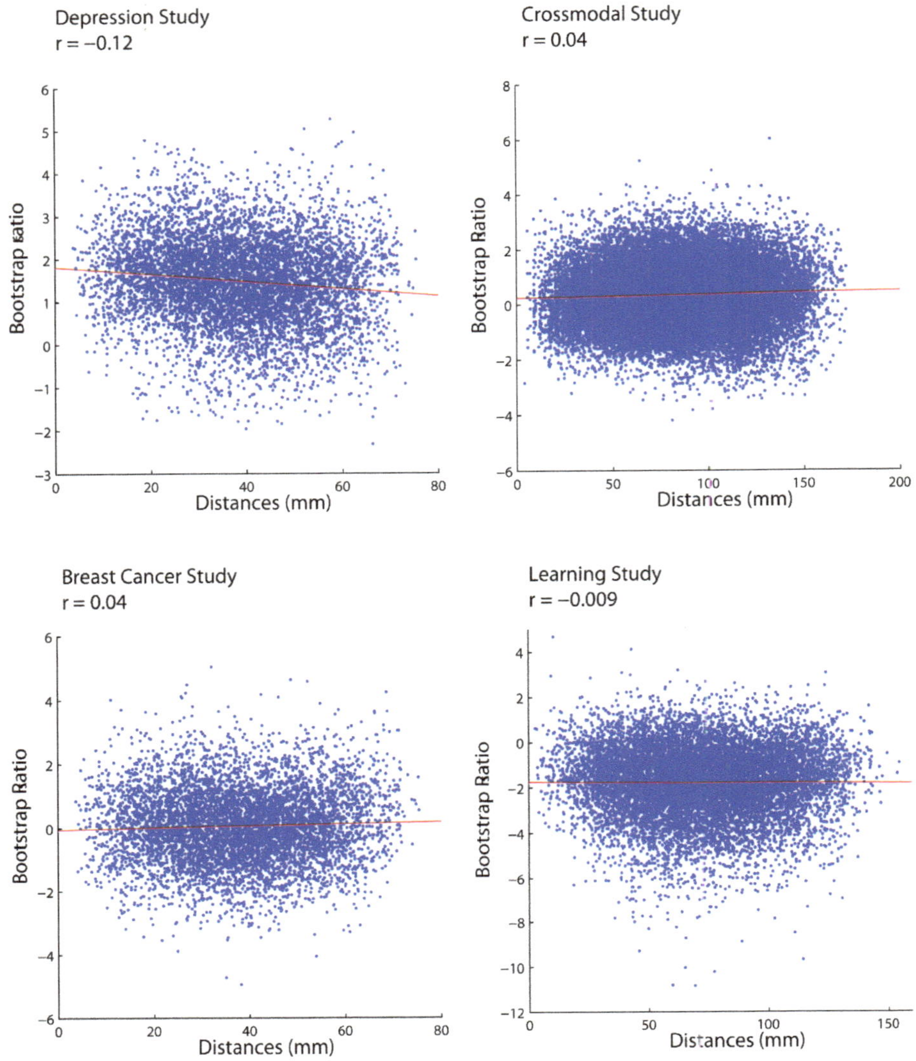

Figure 6. PLS bootstrap ratios for each functional connection are plotted against the Euclidean distance of that connection.

[19,33,34]. We find that functional connections between homotopic brain areas are most stable, and therefore least likely to change.

It is important to consider whether the main result reported here – the weak or non-existent relationship between distance and functional stability – is a "null" result and whether such a finding holds scientific value. Standard inferential statistics do not allow us to rule out such a relationship; rather, they can only indicate that there is no significant evidence to suggest the existence of such a relationship. The present analyses demonstrate that this "null" result is remarkably consistent and robust. First, the independent pairs analysis reported in Table 2 shows that the miniscule correlations between functional connectivity change and anatomically distance are statistically stable, with tight confidence

Table 2. For each study, a sampling distribution of correlations between changes in saliences and Euclidean distances was constructed using only independent pairs of nodes.

fMRI Study	rho	SE	P-value (rho>0)	P-value (rho<0)
Depression	−0.05	0.004	0.34	0.66
Breast Cancer	0.03	0.004	0.57	0.43
Crossmodal	0.05	0.003	0.71	0.29
Learning	−0.03	0.003	0.42	0.58

The table displays the mean correlation (rho) and standard error (SE) from this sampling distribution, as well as P-values associated with one-tailed tests for rho<0 and rho>0.

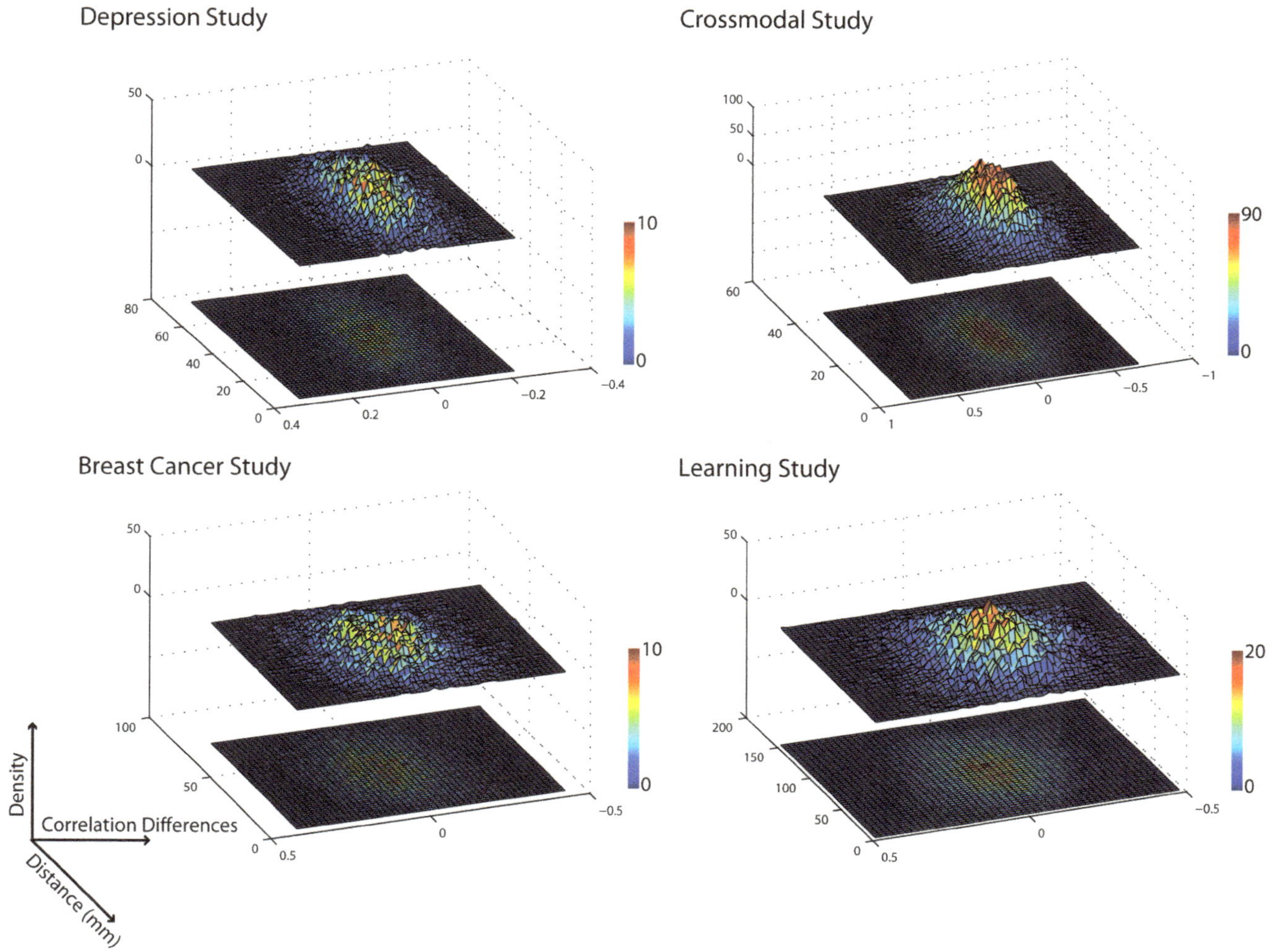

Figure 7. 3-dimensional histogram of correlation differences by Euclidean distance for each study. In the 3-dimensional histogram (top) the number of observations (i.e., density) is represented by color and height. In the 2-dimensional plot (bottom) density is represented by color only.

intervals. Second, the finding is robust and persistent across six different data sets that were deliberately chosen to cover a wide range of populations and brain states. Altogether, the present investigation supports one particular hypothesis: that all functional connections, regardless of their distance, are equally likely to change.

The fact that all functional connections are equally likely to change, regardless of their length, is counterintuitive. Namely, one might expect connections between proximal areas to be more stable given that proximal brain areas tend to be functionally more similar and highly correlated within-condition (Fig. 2). While somewhat counterintuitive, the fact that long- and short-range connections are equally stable may support the balance between local segregation (i.e., the isolation of specialized processing) and global integration (i.e., the combination of different processes) in the brain [12,35]. A functional connectivity landscape in which short-range and long-range connections are equally likely to be strengthened or weakened may facilitate fluid transitions between regional specialization and global integration, thereby allowing the brain to explore a wider range of functional network configurations. This would appear to be a desirable and an adaptive quality, as it would facilitate a more diverse repertoire of cognitive processes.

As mentioned above, one variable that was predictive of functional connectivity change was whether a connection was between homotopic areas. Connections between homotopic areas did not change significantly for changes in task. The source of this stability is likely to be the inter-hemispheric callosal fibers connecting these homotopic regions [19]. This small subset of connections remained relatively stable against a perpetually changing functional connectivity landscape. This stability, combined with increased functional connectivity for those connections [19,33,34], may serve as a grounding principle to maintain steadiness in brain networks in the face of changes in the environment.

Our results show a strong negative relationship between functional connectivity and anatomical distance, but no relationship for changes in functional connectivity and anatomical distance. One may wonder if changes in functional connectivity do not correlate with anatomical distance because of some type of statistical artifact. Namely, within-condition functional connectivity has a robust negative relationship with anatomical distance, and it may be the case that the difference between two such negative trends automatically results in a "flat", non-significant trend as observed in these data. This explanation is highly unlikely because it would imply that the changes in individual data points between two conditions are non-systematic and completely

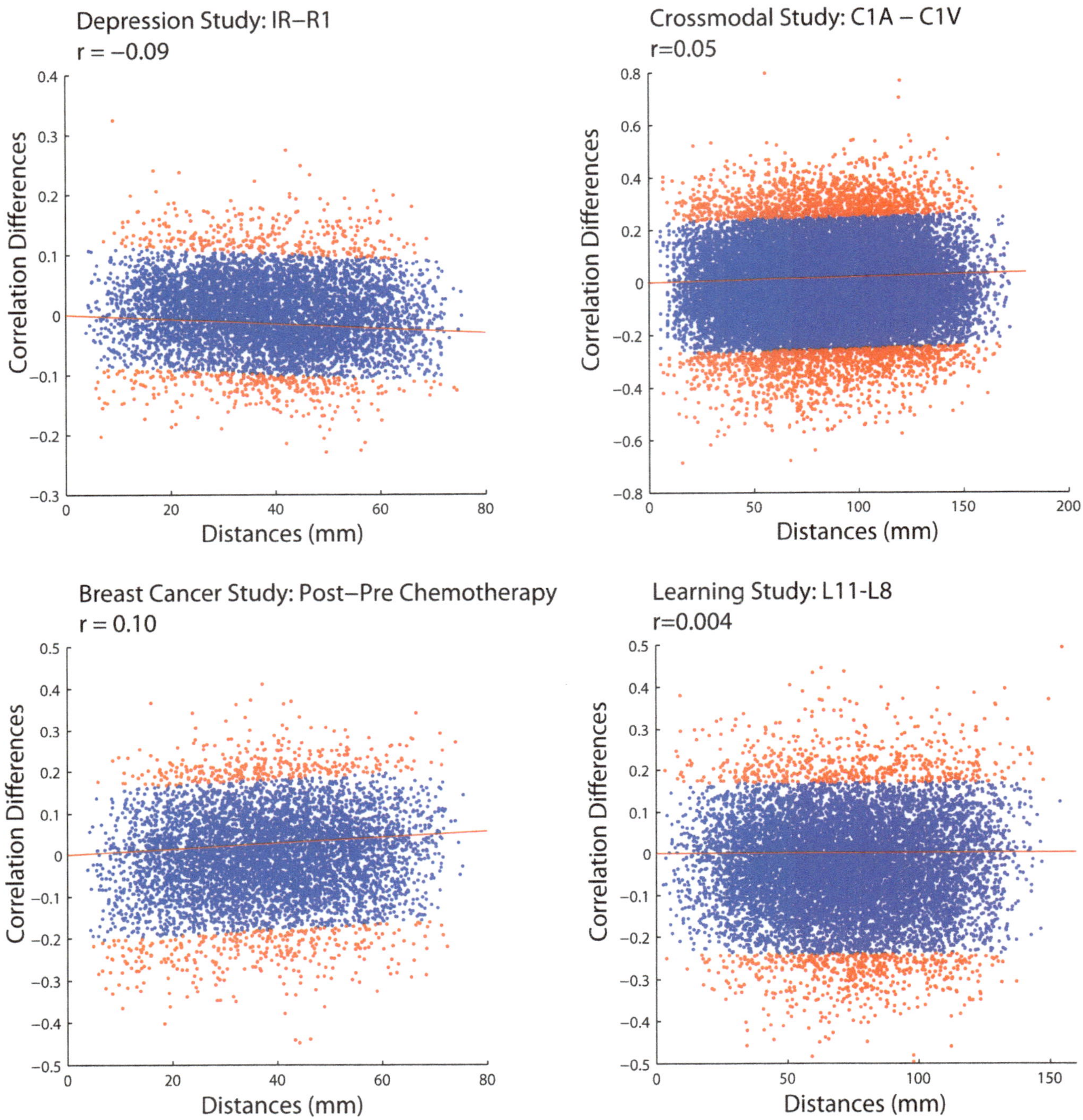

Figure 8. PCA analysis of scatter plots displaying the relationship between correlation differences and Euclidean distance. The PCA analysis was used to determine if outlying points exhibited a different relationship with Euclidean distance than the majority of the points. Points that were in the upper or lower 5% in terms of displacement from the primary axis of variance are colored red and suggest that there is no systematic relationship between correlation differences and Euclidean distances for the outlying points. The red line represents the primary axis of variance.

random, whereas our PLS results show that the changes in functional connectivity between conditions are statistically significant and highly reliable across participants. As such, we consider it unlikely that these results are driven by this type of statistical artifact.

One possible limitation of the present study is that we use Euclidean distance as a proxy for anatomical distance. The former may not be completely representative of the lengths spanned by anatomical projections due to the well-known folding of cortical tissue. Note, however, that we find the relationship between changes in functional connectivity and Euclidean distance to be the same for long and short distances. Additionally, if we look only at relatively long distances that would be unaffected by folding, we still find no relationship between Euclidean distance and changes in functional connectivity.

In conclusion, the present investigation presents the first detailed report that the changes in cognitive state are supported by long-range and short-range functional connections in equal

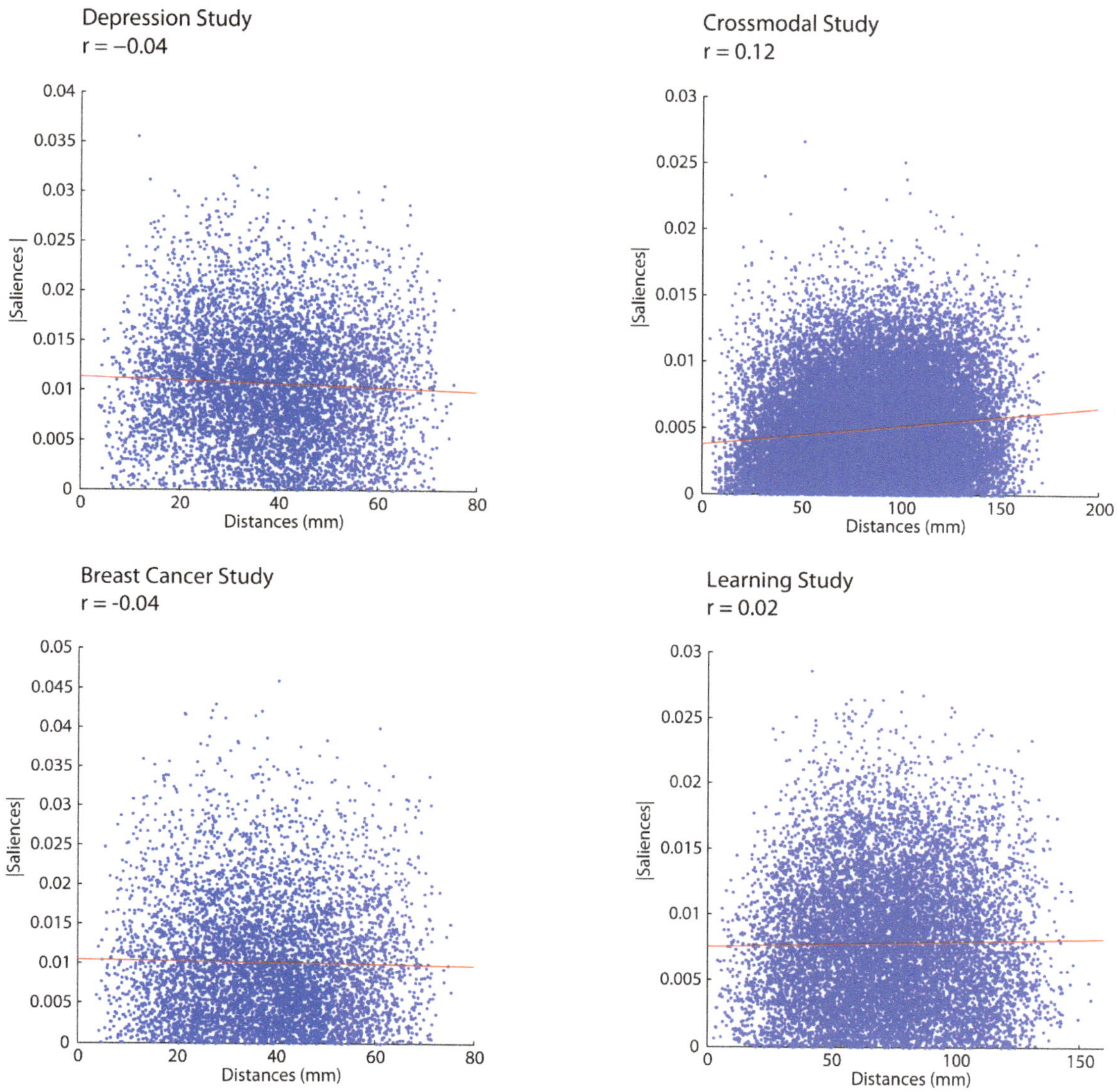

Figure 9. Absolute value of the Saliences for each of the four fMRI studies plotted against Euclidean distance.

measure. At the same time, connections between homotopic areas are among the most stable, which may provide stability in the face of a changing environment. These may be fundamental brain phenomena to strike a balance between local segregation and global integration.

Materials and Methods

Partial least-squares (PLS) Analysis

These analysis parameters are the same as those presented in [16]. Whole-brain fMRI timeseries were parcellated into 116 brain areas based on the AAL template [36] for the depression and breast cancer datasets, and with the template (that aggregated across four atlases) for the Learning dataset. For the Crossmodal dataset every 100th voxel in gray matter was used in the analysis. These timeseries were then correlated together to form a full correlation matrix for all regions correlated with all other regions for each participant and condition.

Partial least-squares (PLS) analysis is a multivariate statistical analysis that is used to relate two sets of variables together. In the case of neuroimaging one set of variables could be brain data (e.g., BOLD signal per voxel per time point) while the other set of variables could be the experimental study design (e.g., groups and experimental conditions). The first step in PLS is to compute the covariance between the two sets of variables (i.e., the "cross-block" covariance). The second step of PLS is to perform a singular value decomposition on the "cross-block" covariance matrix to determine the combination of variables in each set that are optimally related to each other (i.e., that accounts for the greatest proportion of "cross-block" covariance). This combination, termed a latent variable (LV), is comprised of a linear combination (i.e., weighted) of variables from both sets (i.e., brain and experimental sets), as well as a scalar singular value. For the brain set this combination is a spatial-temporal pattern (saliences) and for the design set this combination is a contrast between groups and conditions. The mutually orthogonal LVs are extracted in order of magnitude, i.e. the first LV explains the most "cross-block" covariance, the second LV explains the second most "cross-block" covariance, etc. In the present study the brain data were not activations (i.e., voxels in time), but rather were functional connections between the parcels. This produced 6670 unique connections for the AAL parceled data (i.e., (116*115)/2). As a result, the latent variable represents a

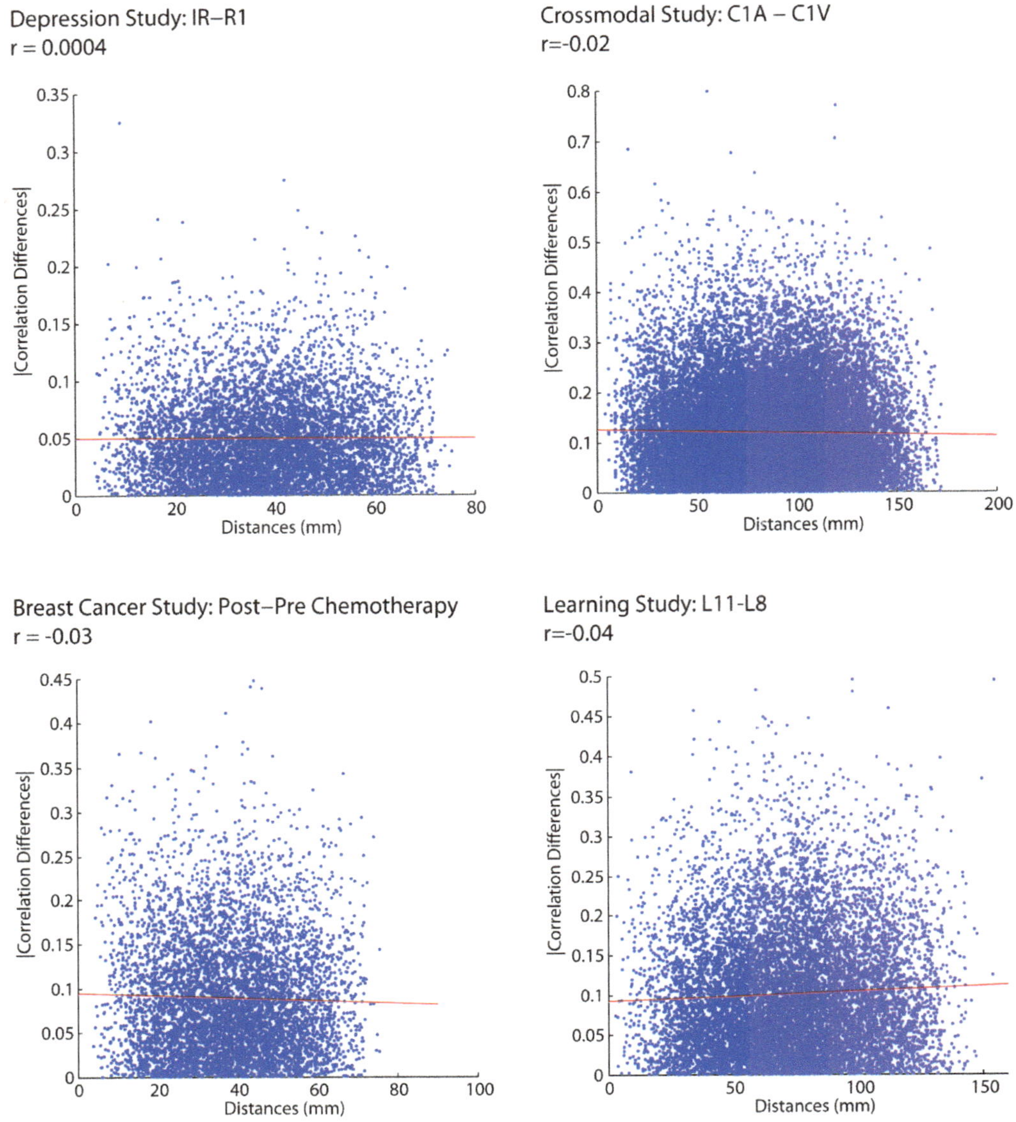

Figure 10. Absolute value of the correlation differences for each of the four fMRI studies plotted against Euclidean distance.

weighted combination of functional connections that optimally relate to our groups and conditions (e.g., for the depression dataset: depressed vs. control for the 4 different experimental conditions).

The significance of each LV is assessed with permutation testing. A set of 500 permuted samples were created by randomly re-ordering participants and condition labels without replacement for the brain set (note: groups and conditions are permuted because PLS is uncovering the interactions between group and condition effects) while the labels for the design set are maintained resulting in 500 new covariance matrices. These covariance matrices embody the null hypothesis and are then each subjected to singular value decomposition as before resulting in a null distribution of singular values. The significance of the original LV is assessed with respect to this null distribution; the p-value is calculated as proportion of permuted singular values that exceed the original singular value.

The reliability with which each functional connection expresses the LV pattern is determined with bootstrapping. A set of 500 bootstrap samples are created by re-sampling participants with replacement within each condition (i.e., preserving condition labels, but not participant labels). Each new covariance matrix is subjected to singular value decomposition as before and the saliences of the bootstrapped dataset are used to build a sampling distribution of the saliences from the original dataset. The purpose of a constructed a bootstrapped sampling distribution is to determine the reliability of each salience; saliences that are highly dependent on which participants are included in the analysis will have wide distributions. A single index of reliability ("bootstrap" ratio) is calculated by taking the ratio of the salience to its bootstrap estimated standard error. A bootstrap ratio for a given functional connection is large when that functional connection has a large and stable salience.

Depression Dataset Details

The methods for this depression dataset are the same as those from [16].

Participants. Sixteen participants diagnosed with clinical depression (mean age = 26.6 std. age = 6.12, 11 female) and

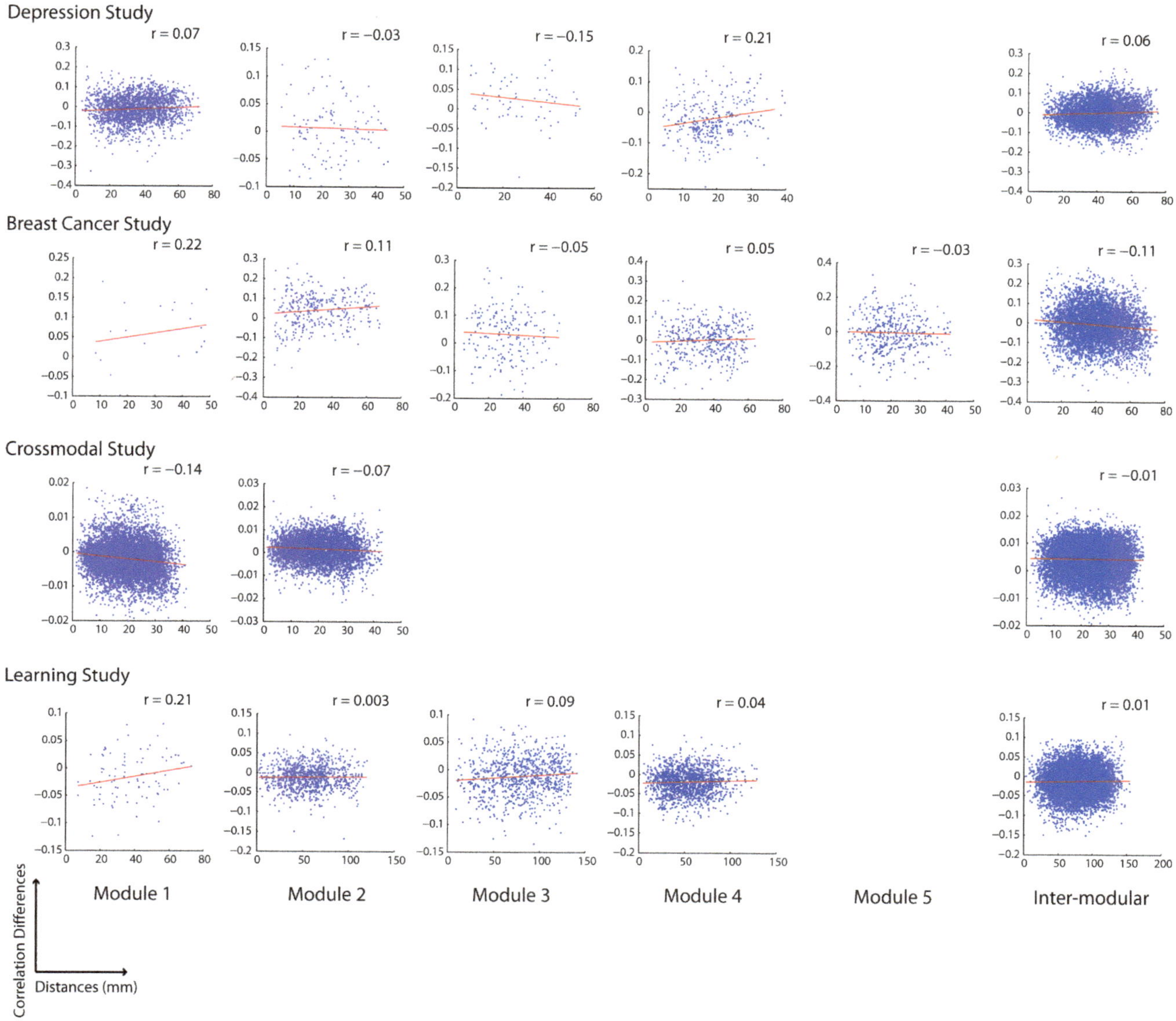

Figure 11. Relationship between Euclidean distance and Salience for functional connections within and between modules.

seventeen non-depressed controls (mean age = 24.4 std. age = 5.83, 13 female) participated in our study. Participants' diagnosis of MDD vs. a non-diagnosis was determined by a trained clinician administering the Structured Clinical Interview Diagnostic (SCID) IV [37]. All participants provided written informed consent in accordance with the Institutional Review Board of the University of Michigan, which approved this study. Participants were compensated $25/hour for their participation.

fMRI Acquisition and Analysis parameters. Images were acquired on a GE Signa 3-Tesla scanner equipped with a standard quadrature head coil. Functional T2* weighted images were acquired using a spiral sequence with 40 contiguous slices with 3.44×3.44×3 mm voxels (repetition time (TR) = 2000 ms; echo time (TE) = 30 ms; flip angle = 90°; field of view (FOV) = 22 cm). A T1-weighted gradient echo anatomical overlay was acquired using the same FOV and slices (TR = 250 ms, TE = 5.7 ms, flip angle = 90°). Additionally, a 124-slice high-resolution T1-weighted anatomical image was collected using spoiled-gradient-recalled acquisition (SPGR) in steady-state imaging (TR = 9 ms, TE = 1.8 ms, flip angle = 15°, FOV = 25–26 cm, slice thickness = 1.2 mm).

Each SPGR anatomical image was corrected for signal inhomogeneity and skull-stripped using FSL's Brain Extraction Tool [38]. These images were then segmented with SPM5 (Wellcome Department of Cognitive Neurology, London) into grey matter, white matter and cerebrospinal fluid and normalization parameters for warping into MNI space were recorded.

Functional images were corrected for differences in slice timing using 4-point sinc-interpolation [39] and were corrected for head movement using MCFLIRT [40]. To reduce noise from spike artifacts, the data were winsorized prior to normalization [41] by exploring time courses for each voxel and finding values that were 3 standard deviations (SDs) away from the mean of that voxel's time course. Spikes that were above 3 SDs from the mean were made equal to the mean +3 SDs and spikes that were 3 SDs below the mean were made equal to the mean −3 SDs. The segmented normalization parameters were then applied to the functional

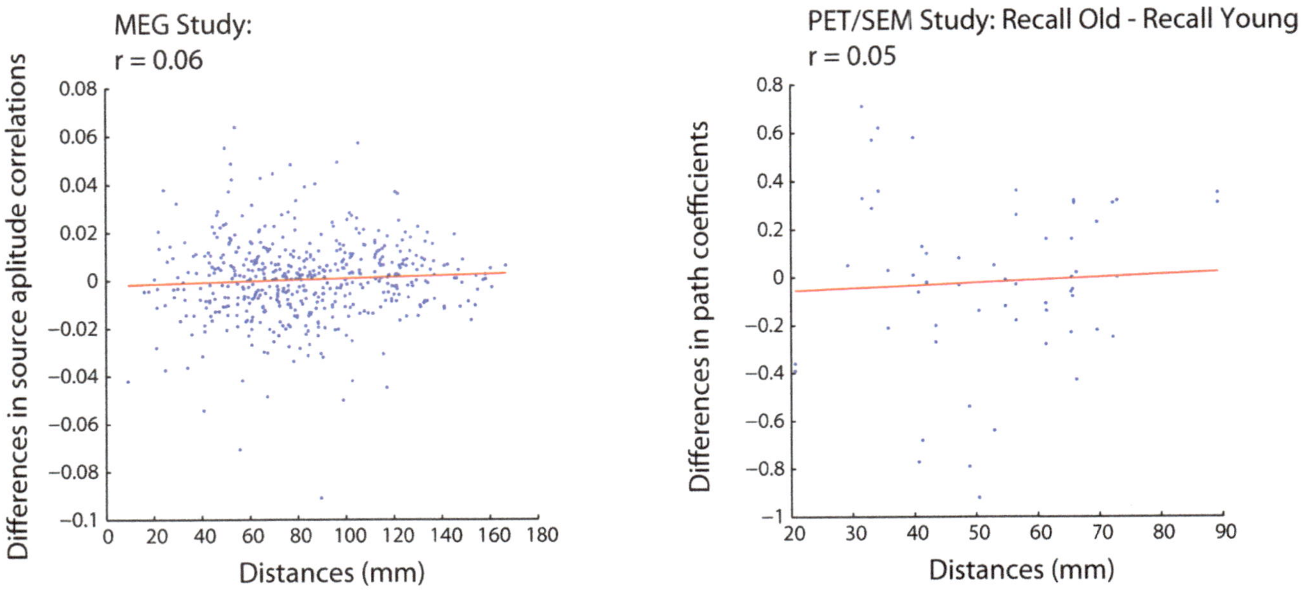

Figure 12. Relationship between changes in coherence and Euclidean distance for the MEG dataset (left) and differences in path coefficients from an SEM analysis of the PET dataset (right).

images maintaining their original 3.44×3.44×3 mm resolution and they were spatially smoothed with a Gaussian kernel of 8 mm.

To correct for physiological artifacts, all of our functional data were corrected using the PHYCAA algorithm. This is an adaptive multivariate model that estimates and removes physiological noise components from fMRI data, without requiring external measures of heartbeat and respiration [42].

Furthermore, 24 motion parameters were calculated, which included the linear, squared, derivative, and squared derivative of the six rigid-body movement parameters [43]. A principal component analysis was performed on these 24 motion parameters and only the first principal component, which accounted for nearly 90% of the motion variance, was covaried out from each voxel's time course to remove any signal that could be attributed to motion (Berman et al., 2013). Lastly, functional images were parceled into 116 different ROIs based on the AAL template [36] for analysis.

Task Parameters. Participants initially performed two resting-state scans back-to-back that were 8 minutes in length. Participants were instructed to look at a fixation cross at the center of the screen and were told not to think about any particular thought (i.e., they could think about whatever they wanted to). After acquiring anatomical images of the brain, participants were then taken out of the scanner and were asked to generate four negative autobiographical memories. In order to facilitate the generation of the memories, we provided four distinct prompts such as "Please recall a specific time when you were rejected by someone you loved or still love" or "Please recall a specific time when you were very embarrassed." Following such a prompt, participants had to indicate whether they were able to think of a prompted event and if they were successful in doing so they were asked to re-live the event for 30 s as well as they could. Next, they had to rate how positively and negatively they felt about that event using a visual-analog scale. Finally, they were asked to describe the event in a few sentences and to create a 2 to 3 word long cue that reminded them of the event.

Following the creation of these events, participants went back into scanner. Now only considering the two most negatively rated events, we simultaneously showed the event description and its cue and instructed participants to pair the two so that they were able to easily recall the memory after seeing the corresponding cue. In a next step, participants were asked to practice recalling the events after seeing the corresponding cue. For this purpose, participants had to press a key as soon as they were able to bring to mind the cued event. The cues were repeated until participants were able to vividly recall the corresponding event in less than 5 s.

Following this practice session, the induction period started. Participants were presented with the cue of one of the two memories that they rated as being most negative. The cue stayed on the screen for 3 min and participants were instructed to re-live that experience as vividly as possible in their imagination and to go back to the time and place of the experience in their imagination and to re-experience it happening to them all over again. After 3 min the cue of the second negatively rated event was presented on the screen. After this negative mood induction, participants again performed another resting-state scan where they fixated on centrally on a fixation cross for 8 minutes.

Breast Cancer Dataset Details

Similar methods with the same participants performing a verbal working memory-task can be found in [26,27].

Participants. Sixteen women (mean age = 49.3, std. = 10.7) with breast cancer that underwent chemotherapy, sixteen women (mean age = 55.0, std. = 8.9) with breast cancer who underwent radiation therapy and sixteen aged-matched non-cancer controls (mean age = 51.4, std. = 7.9) participated in our study. Participants were tested before and after treatment. For the non-cancer controls an equal amount of time separated their two imaging sessions, which was approximately 5 months. All participants provided written informed consent in accordance with the Institutional Review Board of the University of Michigan, which approved this study.

fMRI acquisition parameters. Images were acquired on a GE Signa 3 Tesla scanner equipped with a standard quadrature head coil. Functional T2* weighted images were acquired using a spiral sequence with 25 contiguous slices with 3.75×3.75×5 mm

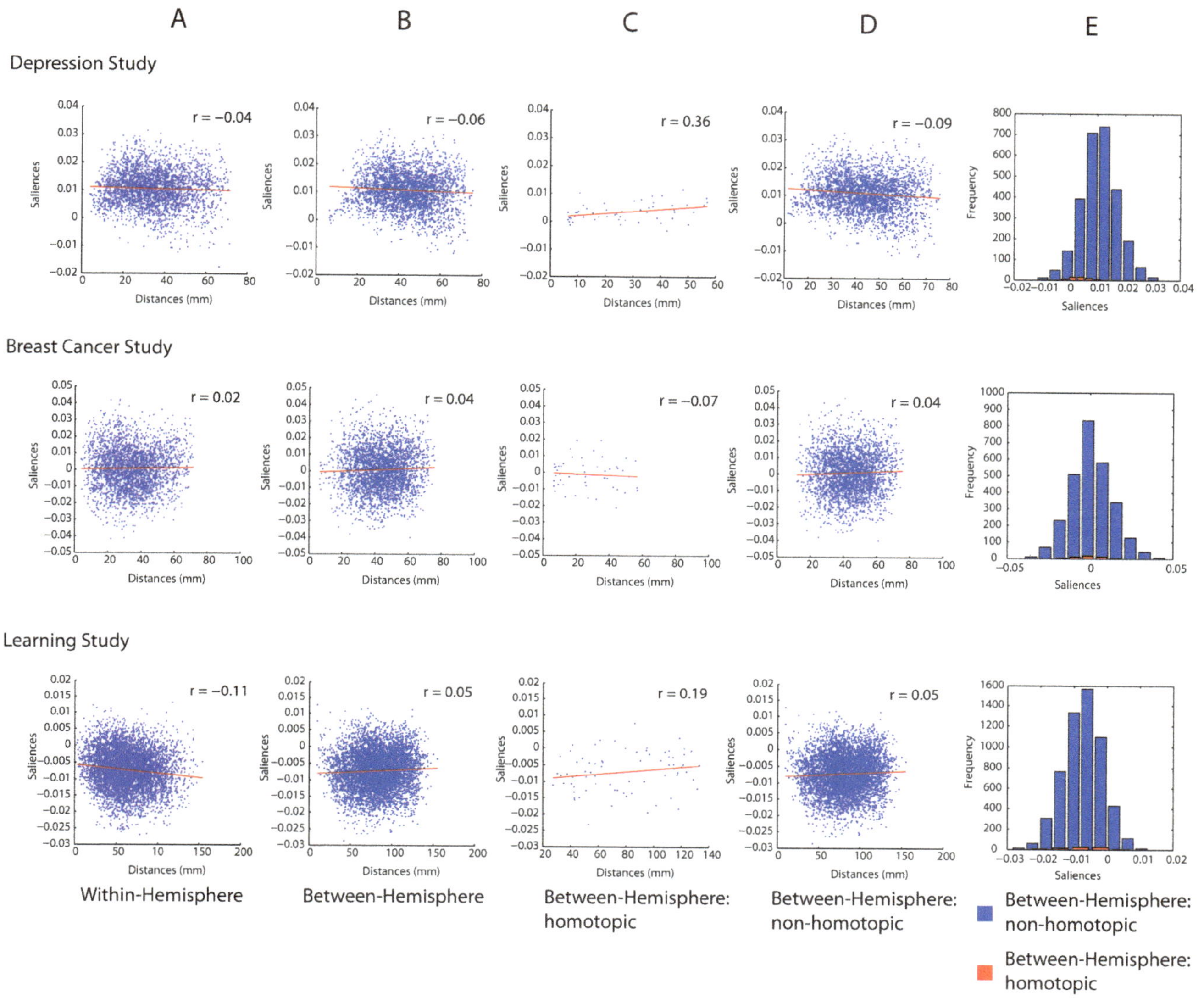

Figure 13. Relationship between changes in functional connectivity for nodes within a hemisphere (A), between hemispheres (B), between homotopic areas (C) and between non-topic areas (D). (E) Histogram showing the changes in functional connectivity for homotopic and non-homotopic areas.

voxels (repetition time (TR) = 1500 ms; echo time (TE) = 30 ms; flip angle = 70°; field of view (FOV) = 24 cm). A T1-weighted gradient echo anatomical overlay was acquired using the same FOV and slices (TR = 225 ms, TE = 5.7 ms, flip angle = 90°). Additionally, a 124-slice high-resolution T1-weighted anatomical image was collected using spoiled-gradient-recalled acquisition (SPGR) in steady-state imaging (TR = 9 ms, TE = 1.8 ms, flip angle = 15°, FOV = 25–26 cm, slice thickness = 1.2 mm).

fMRI Preprocessing Parameters. Each SPGR was corrected for signal in-homogeneity and skull-stripped using FSL's Brain Extraction Tool [38]. These images were then normalized with SPM5 (Wellcome Department of Cognitive Neurology, London); the normalization parameters for warping to the standard MNI template were recorded and applied to the functional images.

Functional images were corrected for differences in slice timing using 4-point sinc-interpolation [39] corrected for head movement using MCFLIRT [40]. To reduce noise from spike artifacts, the data were winsorized prior to normalization [41] by exploring time courses for each voxel and finding values that were 3 standard deviations (SDs) away from the mean of that voxel's time course. Spikes that were above 3 SDs from the mean were made equal to the mean +3 SDs and spikes that were 3 SDs below the mean were made equal to the mean −3 SDs. After normalization the functional images were spatially smoothed with a Gaussian kernel of 8 mm.

Nuisance covariates were then regressed out of the data. These included the principal component of the estimated motion parameters (Berman et al., 2013), and the average global signal time course within brain voxels. Data were then low-pass filtered (cutoff of 0.08 Hz), in order to remove high-frequency noise and retain only the BOLD frequency band of interest. Finally, average ROI time courses were extracted from the data using the AAL template, generating 116 anatomically labeled ROIs of interest. These time courses were then used for cross-correlation analysis.

Task Parameters. Participants were instructed to attend to a centrally located fixation cross while in the fMRI scanner and instructed not to think about any particular memory or thought (i.e., they could think about whatever they wanted to).

Learning Dataset Details

Participants. Sixteen healthy, right-handed, native English-speaking individuals were enrolled in the study. Participants were screened for neurological, psychiatric and relevant medical conditions by a study-Medical Doctor and were also assessed by the MINI-Plus [44].

All participants provided written informed consent in accordance with the Research Ethics Boards of Baycrest Hospital, the Centre for Addiction and Mental Health and the University of Toronto, which approved this study.

The final sample was comprised of data from twelve participants (5 females, mean age: 30.8±8.2). Data from four participants were excluded due to improper task performance, technical/equipment issues and/or excessive movement artifact during fMRI scanning.

fMRI Acquisition. MRI images were acquired on a Siemens Trio 3T magnet. A T1-weighted anatomical scan was obtained using SPGR (TE = 2.6 ms, TR = 2000 ms, FOV = 256 mm, slice thickness = 1 mm). The SPGR was co-registered with the functional images and was also used to rule out any gross brain anomalies. T2* functional images (TE = 30 ms, TR = 2000 ms, flip angle = 70°, FOV = 200 mm) were obtained using an echo-planar image (EPI) acquisition sequence leading to a blood oxygenation level-dependent (BOLD) contrast. Each functional sequence consisted of twenty-eight 5-mm-thick slices in the axial-oblique plane positioned to image the entire brain.

Participants' responses were made with their right hands using the Fibre-Optic Response Pad (FORP) system, which has two four-button response pads and is designed for MR compatibility. Visual stimuli were presented on a rear projection screen placed at the foot of the MR scanner using an LCD projector. The participants viewed the stimuli using a mirror mounted on the head coil. Auditory stimuli were presented using the Silent Scan auditory presentation system (AVOTEC), which uses air conduction to transmit tones and headphones to attenuate the gradient noise. E-Prime Stimulus Presentation Software (http://www.pstnet.com) was used to control stimulus presentation, collect behavioral responses and to log the precise timing of the stimulus events.

fMRI Preprocessing Parameters. Functional images were slice-timed corrected with AFNI (http://afni.nimh.nih.gov/afni). Motion correction was completed using AIR (http://bishopw.loni.ucla.edu/AIR5/) by registering functional volumes to the 100th volume within each run. All functional volumes within each motion-corrected run were averaged to create mean functional volumes for each run. Using a rigid body transformation model, this mean functional volume was then registered with each participant's structural volume. The structural data were spatially normalized to the Common Anatomical Template previously described by [45]. Thus, the end result was a direct nonlinear transform from each initial fMRI volume into the Common Template space.

Data were smoothed using a 7 mm Gaussian kernel. The voxel time series were further adjusted by regressing out motion correction parameters, white matter (WM) time series and CSF time series. As [46], the time series of the unsmoothed data from small regions-of-interest in the corpus callosum (WM) and ventricles (CSF) of the Common Template were used as the white matter and CSF regressors respectively. This last step minimizes contamination of WM and CSF time series that can occur when signals from neighboring gray matter voxels are mixed in due to spatial smoothing or registration errors. Furthermore, we performed high-pass temporal filtering using FSL (Gaussian-weighted least-squares straight line fitting, with sigma = 75 s).

We combined four published probabilistic atlases to create a gray matter atlas with 152 Regions of Interest (ROIs). Three of these atlases are part of the FSL distribution: Harvard Oxford-Cortical, Harvard Oxford-Subcortical and Oxford Thalamic Connectivity atlases. The fourth atlas was the SUIT Cerebellar atlas (www.icn.ucl.ac.uk/motorcontrol/imaging/suit.htm). Each of the four atlases provides a thresholded maximum probability ROI mask with a threshold of 25%. This means that each voxel within the 3D image space was assigned to exactly one ROI, namely the one with the highest probability according to the sample of manually delineated single participant ROIs. If this maximum probability was below 25%, then the voxel was not assigned to any ROI. In this way each atlas provided a discrete segmentation image where voxel intensity signifies the voxel's most probable ROI membership.

All ROIs from four atlases were used, with the exception of global regions from the subcortical atlas, namely, Cerebral White Matter, Lateral Ventricles and Cerebral Cortex. To obtain consistent parcellation of thalamus we intersected a single thalamic ROI from the subcortical atlas with all thalamic subregions from the Thalamic Connectivity atlas. For a small number of voxels, there was a conflict in terms of ROI membership, such that a voxel could be a part of one ROI according to one atlas and also a part of another ROI according to another atlas (e.g. along cerebrum/cerebellum border). We resolved such conflicts by setting the following atlas precedence order from highest to lowest: Cortical, Subcortical, Thalamic, Cerebellar.

In order to create consistent left and right hemispheric subdivisions we combined ROIs from four atlases, some of which were lateralized and others which were not. For example, none of the regions within Cortical, Subcortical and Thalamic atlases are lateralized. On the other hand, the Cerebellum atlas has both lateralized and medial (non-lateralized) regions. To create a lateralization within the Cerebellum and brain stem, we used the midsaggital plane of the MNI152 template brain (x = 0 in world coordinates) and divided regions into left and right depending on the position with respect to the plane. We made an exception for medial cerebellar regions, which were left as such. The final combined gray matter ROI atlas consists of 152 regions: 48+48 cortical lateralized regions, 7+7 lateralized thalamic regions, 6+6 additional lateralized subcortical regions (pallidum, putamen, caudate, hippocampus, amygdala and accumbens), 10+10 lateralized cerebellar regions, 8 medial cerebellar regions and 1+1 lateralized brain stem regions.

For each of the 152 ROIs we extracted the time series as a weighted sum over the voxels within the region. The weighting was provided by the distance transform from the region's border, so that voxels at the core of the region would be weighted more than the voxels near region's border. The weight of each voxel was calculated as a squared distance from the region's border, normalized by the sum of all squared distances. This weighting scheme was designed to reduce artificially high correlations between small neighboring regions where signal can be smeared due to coarse resolution, and preprocessing and registration errors. This was performed separately for each condition.

Task Parameters. The overarching goal for the experiment was for participants to learn a new lexicon comprised of 30 pseudowords in an associative learning task spanning two fMRI scanning sessions. The study occurred over a three-day period. On the first day participants were trained in a MRI simulator using a parallel set of stimuli to ensure full understanding of the task to be completed during fMRI scanning. FMRI scanning then occurred on two days over the course of a one-week period.

The learning task used was developed by [47], but modified for English speakers. Participants heard a spoken pseudoword in their headphones and then briefly saw a picture of an everyday object followed by a fixation cross. Sometimes the pairings were 'correct' and sometimes 'incorrect'. Participants indicated whether or not they thought the pairings were correct by pushing one of two buttons on a response pad. The underlying learning principle was a higher co-occurrence of 'correct' pairings with a 20:1 (correct:incorrect) by the end of both scanning sessions. The learning runs across both days were additive in that the vocabulary to be learned for each participant was comprised of the same 30 words-object pairings on each of the days.

Participants also completed a reaction-time task, which was identical in structure, but used another parallel set of stimuli and lacked an underlying learning principle. In this task, participants heard a pseudoword, and were then presented with an object-picture. They were asked to simply push the first button as quickly as possible when the picture appeared on the screen.

The two scanning sessions were identically structured. The functional runs began with the reaction-time task (120 trials), followed by five learning runs (900 trials in total) and then another reaction-time run (120 trials). Each run lasted approximately 6.5 minutes. Data used in this analysis are from the second scanning day and include the first reaction-time task and the subsequent five learning runs.

Crossmodal Dataset Details

The same methods appear in [17].

Participants. Twenty-four (12 female) healthy, right-handed individuals between the ages of 19 and 35 (mean age: 23.08±3.87 years) with normal to corrected-vision were recruited for participation. All participants were screened and cleared for any neurological, psychiatric, substance abuse-related problems. All participants provided written informed consent in accordance with a joint Baycrest-University of Toronto Research Ethics Board Committee, which approved this study.

fMRI acquisition and analysis parameters. Participants were scanned in a Siemens Magnetrom TIM Trio Whole Body 3T MR scanner with a matrix 12-channel head coil. A structural MRI was obtained for each participant at the beginning of each scanning session, consisting of a 3D T1-weighted pulse sequence [echo time (TE), 2.6; 256×256 acquisition matrix, voxel size, 1.0×1.0×1.0 mm]. For functional scans, 28 oblique axial slices with full brain coverage were obtained [TR, 2 s; 64×64 acquisition matrix; voxel size, 3.125 mm×3.125 mm×5.0 mm] using T2*-weighted echo-planar image (EPI) sequence. Oblique axial slices were acquired to minimize sinus-related artifacts that occur in EPI sequences. These oblique axial slices were restored to the normal axial plane during reconstruction procedures.

Preprocessing of images was completed in Statistical Parametric Mapping (SPM5; available at http://www.fil.ion.ucl.ac.uk/spm/software/spm5/) and MELODIC [48] software packages. The images were corrected for slice timing differences in the EPI interleave acquisition, co-registered to the first EPI image in each run, corrected for gradient and residual head-motion artifacts using independent components analysis with MELODIC, spatially normalized to a standard MNI template with an affine transformation and 4d-spline interpolated and smoothed with an 8-mm Gaussian kernel. Functional data were parceled into 229 different ROIs based on sampling every 100th voxel using the AAL template as a gray matter mask.

Task Parameters. The experiment contained two types of auditory stimuli that were matched in amplitude but differed in frequency (250 Hz and 4000 Hz). The visual stimuli used in the experiment were a black and white checkerboard pattern (square) and the same checkerboard rotated 45 degrees (diamond). All stimulus presentations were controlled by Presentation software (version 10.2, Neurobehavioural Systems Inc.).

A trial was composed of a first stimulus (S1), delay, second stimulus (S2), response window and a variable inter-trial interval of 3, 5, 7, or 9 seconds. Two main task types were designed by manipulating the content of S1 and S2. For Cue 1st (C1) tasks, S1 was a cue that signaled a response compatibility rule to a subsequent lateralized target (S2). In Target 1st (C2) tasks, S1 was the lateralized target followed by the cue stimulus (S2). In a compatible trial, a cue instructed participants to press a button on the same side (left or right) as the lateralized target. In an incompatible trial, participant's pressed the button on the opposite side of the lateralized target.

Auditory and visual stimuli were presented in Cue 1st and Target 1st tasks. In auditory cue/visual target sub-tasks, the pitch of a binaural tone specified the response rule to a lateralized visual target, a square checkerboard. Low (250 Hz) and high (4000 Hz) pitch tones signaled compatible and incompatible responses, respectively. In the visual cue/auditory target sub-tasks, the shape of a visual stimulus indicated the response rule to a lateralized, monaural tone of 250 Hz. Square and diamond checkerboards corresponded to compatible and incompatible responses. In summary, modality and stimulus presentation order manipulations resulted in four tasks: auditory cue followed by visual target (C1A), visual cue followed by auditory target (C1V), visual target followed by auditory cue (C2A) and auditory target followed by visual cue (C2V).

We used a mixed event-related experimental design for collecting fMRI data. Each of the four tasks were repeated three times for a total of twelve runs (9 mins, 28 seconds in duration) with 40 trials (20 compatible, 20 incompatible) randomly presented within each run. We collected data on two scanning days (6 runs per day) and counterbalanced across task types.

MEG Dataset Details

The same methods appear in [18].

Participants. Fourteen healthy, right-handed (8 female) participants between the ages of 19 and 30 (mean age: 22±2 years) with normal or corrected-vision, were recruited for the study. All participants were screened and cleared for any neurological, psychiatric, substance abuse-related problems. All participants provided written informed consent in accordance with a joint Baycrest-University of Toronto Research Ethics Board Committee, which approved this study.

MEG acquisition and analysis parameters. MEG recordings were performed at the Rotman Research Institute at Baycrest Centre, in a dimly-lit, magnetically shielded room using a 151-channel whole-head axial gradiometer system (VSM-Med Tech Inc., Coquitlam, BC, Canada) with receiver coils uniformly spaced approximately 3 cm apart on a helmet-shaped array. Two separate blocks of MEG recordings took place, each approximately 18 minutes in length at a sampling rate of 625 Hz. The position of the participant's head in the MEG was recorded at the beginning and the end of each data session using indicator coils placed on the nasion and bilateral preauricular points. Motion tolerance was set to 0.5 cm and all participants were within this limit. MEG data was acquired with participants lying in a supine position to minimize head movements while viewing a screen above the MEG system adjusted to participants' eye level.

Independent components analysis [ICA; [49]] was used to correct for ocular and cardiac artifacts (http://sccn.ucsd.edu/eeglab/). MEG data were parsed into 150 trials per task over the range −2.0 to 1.24 s relative to scene onset, band-passed between 0.5 and 55 Hz using a bidirectional filter, and time series were down-sampled by a factor of four from the original digitization interval. The baseline interval chosen for correction was −0.5 to −1.0 s. The data were analyzed in a third-order gradient configuration for external noise correction. In addition to MEG recordings, a structural magnetic resonance image (MRI) was also acquired for each participant for co-registration with the MEG functional data. The structural image was a 3D MPRAGE T_1-weighted pulse sequence (echo time, 2.6 ms; repetition time, 2 s; 256×256 acquisition matrix; voxel size, 1.0×1.0×1.0 mm) acquired on a 3 Tesla magnet (Siemens Magnetrom TIM Trio Whole Body scanner) located at Baycrest Centre.

A data-driven approach, previously applied to electroencephalographic data [50] was employed to derive brain sources/networks that gave rise to MEG signals recorded on the scalp. Preprocessed data were concatenated into a single matrix with MEG sensors (150) on the x-axis and participants (14), conditions (2), trials (150), and time samples (407) on the y-axis. The grand data matrix was evaluated with Bayesian Information Criterion [BIC; [51]] to determine the optimal subspace that fairly expressed the complexity of the data. The complete theoretical range of models (1–150) based on the rank of the smallest dimension of the data matrix were assessed. The probability of each model was estimated by leveraging goodness of fit and model complexity. The peak probability of the distribution for all models occurred at 34. Next, Principal Component Analysis (PCA) was performed on the original data matrix with the number of principal components (PCs) restricted to 34. Subsequently, ICA replaced the orthogonal PCs with independent components (ICs) that were not necessarily uncorrelated but maximally independent in the temporal domain. 2 out of the 34 components were dropped because they contained residual artifacts. The remaining 32 group ICs were projected onto participant data by multiplying the original time series for each trial/condition with the weighting (mixing) matrix. In this way, participant-specific ICs, representing sources/networks, were calculated with weights from group analysis.

The resulting spatial maps were translated into brain locations using an event-related vector beamformer [52,53]. All 32 components showed dipolar patterns and were successfully mapped to mainly singular sources in MEG data.

For each individual, the functional maps obtained from source reconstruction were warped into a common space - the Montreal Neurological Institute (MNI) standard brain, using SPM software's (http://www.fil.ion.ucl.ac.uk/spm/software/) spatial normalization engine. To infer group-level source distributions, normalized functional images were averaged for all participants. A peak coordinate from within an activated cluster was identified from group-averaged data. Using this procedure, a spatial location was assigned to each of the 32 ICs. Functional connectivity was estimated by correlating the beamformer-reconstructed activity for all pairs of sources.

Task Parameters. Visual stimuli were eight scenes (4 indoor, 4 outdoor) taken from a repository of images used in [54]. The experiment contained two tasks: active learning and choice reaction time with no learning component, with 150 trials per task. For learning, participants linked 2 scene pairs with 2 color pairs (4 associations) through trial-and-error. The general structure of a trial consisted of scene presentation (500 ms), a delay interval (750 ms) and a color pair, after which the participants had up to 1.2 sec to record their responses. Participants received on-screen, written feedback (correct/wrong) about their response choice. After responses were made, a jittered, random, inter-trial interval between 4.5 to 6 sec ensued. In the control task, participants were instructed in advance about which colors were correct and scenes preceding these colors were shown randomly. All stimuli were unique for both tasks and were randomized for individuals. The order in which the tasks were administered was counterbalanced across participants.

PET Dataset Details

Information about the PET data set was compiled from a previously-published study by Cabeza, McIntosh, Tulving, Nyberg and Grady (1997). In that study, the authors constructed a structural equation model (SEM, also known as path analysis) to investigate how the patterns of interregional influence changed during memory encoding and memory recall, and whether these memory-related effects were modulated by aging. Specifically, data were taken from Tables 1 and 2, which show the coordinates of the nodes and the SEM-estimated beta coefficients (described in more detail below), allowing us to fully reconstruct the network for both the Encoding and Recall conditions.

The original PET data, which measured regional cerebral blood flow (rCBF), was processed in a manner analogous to "standard" BOLD signal processing, including motion correction, spatial normalization and spatial smoothing. The regional nodes of the network (n = 13) were selected from an initial exploratory analysis of the mean signal, i.e. all nodes showed a statistically significant main effect of memory task.

The data from Cabeza et al. (1997) study are unique in the sense that they represent a measure of effective connectivity, rather than functional connectivity. Thus, the connections express the direct effect one brain region has on another, above and beyond any effects of indirect connections. The values for the individual connections are the standardized path coefficients from the SEM analysis, which are analogous to regression ("beta") coefficients and represent partial correlations (McIntosh & Gonzalez-Lima, 1994).

Specifically, the path coefficients were estimated as follows. An empirical matrix of regional covariances was calculated and an initial structural network was constructed using prior empirical knowledge about the anatomical connectivity among the 13 nodes of the network. The weight of each connection or path was assigned an initial value. Through an iterative data fitting procedure, the weights were modified to find an optimal solution, which best reproduced the empirically-observed pattern of regional covariances.

Details regarding the participants, task, acquisition parameters and preprocessing parameters can be found in [31]. When analyzing data from this published report, we examined differences in effective connectivity for older adults compared to younger adults in the recall condition. Euclidean distances between brain areas was calculated using the coordinates listed in Table 1 of that publication, while the path coefficients were compiled from Table 2 of that publication.

Supporting Information

File S1 Fisher-transformed correlation matrices. Each of the Studies is represented as a MATLAB (The Mathworks, Natick, MA) cell array. Each cell represents an experimental group, and each array is organized in the following way: Conditions × Participants × Regions × Regions.

Author Contributions

Conceived and designed the experiments: BM MGB SS JJ ARM. Performed the experiments: BM MGB. Analyzed the data: BM MGB. Contributed reagents/materials/analysis tools: ZF MKA MB NC BC PJD SJ MJ MK KMKB SP PAR JJ EK. Contributed to the writing of the manuscript: BM MGB JJ ARM.

References

1. Fox MD, Snyder AZ, Vincent JL, Corbetta M, Van Essen DC, et al. (2005) The human brain is intrinsically organized into dynamic, anticorrelated functional networks. Proceedings of the National Academy of Sciences of the United States of America 102: 9673.
2. Honey CJ, Sporns O, Cammoun L, Gigandet X, Thiran JP, et al. (2009) Predicting human resting-state functional connectivity from structural connectivity. Proceedings of the National Academy of Sciences of the United States of America 106: 2035–2040.
3. Allen EA, Damaraju E, Plis SM, Erhardt EB, Eichele T, et al. (2012) Tracking whole-brain connectivity dynamics in the resting state. Cerebral Cortex.
4. Stephan KE, Marshall JC, Friston KJ, Rowe JB, Ritzl A, et al. (2003) Lateralized cognitive processes and lateralized task control in the human brain. Science 301: 384–386.
5. McIntosh AR, Rajah MN, Lobaugh NJ (1999) Interactions of prefrontal cortex in relation to awareness in sensory learning. Science 284: 1531–1533.
6. Kitzbichler MG, Henson RNA, Smith ML, Nathan PJ, Bullmore ET (2011) Cognitive Effort Drives Workspace Configuration of Human Brain Functional Networks. Journal of Neuroscience 31: 8259–8270.
7. Bassett DS, Wymbs NF, Porter MA, Mucha PJ, Carlson JM, et al. (2011) Dynamic reconfiguration of human brain networks during learning. Proceedings of the National Academy of Sciences of the United States of America 108: 7641–7646.
8. Greicius MD, Srivastava G, Reiss AL, Menon V (2004) Default-mode network activity distinguishes Alzheimer's disease from healthy aging: Evidence from functional MRI. Proceedings of the National Academy of Sciences of the United States of America 101: 4637–4642.
9. Achard S, Bullmore E (2007) Efficiency and cost of economical brain functional networks. Plos Computational Biology 3: 174–183.
10. Berman MG, Peltier S, Nee DE, Kross E, Deldin PJ, et al. (2011) Depression, rumination and the default network. Social Cognitive and Affective Neuroscience 6: 548–555.
11. Mountcastle VB (1997) The columnar organization of the neocortex. Brain 120: 701–722.
12. Tononi G, Sporns O, Edelman GM (1994) A measure for brain complexity: relating functional segregation and integration in the nervous system. Proceedings of the National Academy of Sciences 91: 5033–5037.
13. Sporns O, Tononi G, Edelman GM (2000) Theoretical neuroanatomy: Relating anatomical and functional connectivity in graphs and cortical connection matrices. Cerebral Cortex 10: 127–141.
14. Sporns O, Tononi G, Edelman GM (2000) Connectivity and complexity: the relationship between neuroanatomy and brain dynamics. Neural Networks 13: 909–922.
15. Salvador R, Suckling J, Coleman MR, Pickard JD, Menon D, et al. (2005) Neurophysiological architecture of functional magnetic resonance images of human brain. Cereb Cortex 15: 1332–1342.
16. Berman MG, Misic B, Buschkuehl M, Kross E, Deldin PJ, et al. (2014) Does resting-state connectivity reflect depressive rumination? A tale of two analyses. Neuroimage.
17. Fatima Z, McIntosh AR (2011) The interplay of cue modality and response latency in brain areas supporting crossmodal motor preparation: an event-related fMRI study. Experimental Brain Research 214: 9–17.
18. Fatima Z, Quraan MA, Kovacevic N, McIntosh AR (2013) ICA-based artifact correction improves spatial localization of adaptive spatial filters in MEG. Neuroimage 78: 284–294.
19. Toro R, Fox PT, Paus T (2008) Functional Coactivation Map of the Human Brain. Cerebral Cortex 18: 2553–2559.
20. Long XY, Zuo XN, Kiviniemi V, Yang Y, Zou QH, et al. (2008) Default mode network as revealed with multiple methods for resting-state functional MRI analysis. Journal of Neuroscience Methods 171: 349–355.
21. Zang YF, Jiang TZ, Lu YL, He Y, Tian LX (2004) Regional homogeneity approach to fMRI data analysis. Neuroimage 22: 394–400.
22. Kiebel SJ, Poline JB, Friston KJ, Holmes AP, Worsley KJ (1999) Robust smoothness estimation in statistical parametric maps using standardized residuals from the general linear model. Neuroimage 10: 756–766.
23. Krishnan A, Williams LJ, McIntosh AR, Abdi H (2011) Partial Least Squares (PLS) methods for neuroimaging: A tutorial and review. Neuroimage 56: 455–475.
24. McIntosh AR, Lobaugh NJ (2004) Partial least squares analysis of neuroimaging data: applications and advances. Neuroimage 23: S250–S263.
25. McIntosh AR, Misic B (2013) Multivariate Statistical Analyses for Neuroimaging Data. In: Fiske ST, editor. Annual Review of Psychology, Vol 64. 499-+.
26. Berman MG, Askren MK, Sook Jung M, Therrien B, Peltier S, et al. (2013) Pretreatment Worry and Neurocognitive Responses in Women With Breast Cancer. Health Psychol.
27. Askren MK, Jung MS, Berman MG, Therrien B, Peltier S, et al. (2014) Neuromarkers of Fatigue and Cognitive Complaints Following Chemotherapy for Breast Cancer: A Prospective fMRI Investigation. Breast Cancer Research and Treatment.
28. Chen KW, Reiman EM, Alexander GE, Bandy D, Renaut R, et al. (2004) An automated algorithm for the computation of brain volume change from sequential MRIs using an iterative principal component analysis and its evaluation for the assessment of whole-brain atrophy rates in patients with probable Alzheimer's disease. Neuroimage 22: 134–143.
29. Blondel VD, Guillaume J-L, Lambiotte R, Lefebvre E (2008) Fast unfolding of communities in large networks. Journal of Statistical Mechanics: Theory and Experiment 2008: P10008.
30. Rubinov M, Sporns O (2011) Weight-conserving characterization of complex functional brain networks. Neuroimage 56: 2068–2079.
31. Cabeza R, McIntosh AR, Tulving E, Nyberg L, Grady CL (1997) Age-related differences in effective neural connectivity during encoding and recall. Neuroreport 8: 3479–3483.
32. McIntosh AR, Grady CL, Ungerleider LG, Haxby JV, Rapoport SI, et al. (1994) Network Analysis of Cortical Visual Pathways Mapped with Pet. Journal of Neuroscience 14: 655.
33. Stark DE, Margulies DS, Shehzad ZE, Reiss P, Kelly AMC, et al. (2008) Regional Variation in Interhemispheric Coordination of Intrinsic Hemodynamic Fluctuations. Journal of Neuroscience 28: 13754–13764.
34. Zuo XN, Kelly C, Di Martino A, Mennes M, Margulies DS, et al. (2010) Growing Together and Growing Apart: Regional and Sex Differences in the Lifespan Developmental Trajectories of Functional Homotopy. Journal of Neuroscience 30: 15034–15043.
35. Bullmore E, Sporns O (2012) The economy of brain network organization. Nat Rev Neurosci 13: 336–349.
36. Tzourio-Mazoyer N, Landeau B, Papathanassiou D, Crivello F, Etard O, et al. (2002) Automated anatomical labeling of activations in SPM using a macroscopic anatomical parcellation of the MNI MRI single-subject brain. Neuroimage 15: 273–289.
37. Williams JB, Gibbon M, First MB, Spitzer RL (1992) The Structured Clinical Interview for DSM-III–R (SCID): II. Multisite testetest reliability. Archives of General Psychiatry 49: 630–636.
38. Smith SM, Jenkinson M, Woolrich MW, Beckmann CF, Behrens TEJ, et al. (2004) Advances in functional and structural MR image analysis and implementation as FSL. NeuroImage 23: S208.
39. Oppenheim AV, Schafer RW, Buck JR (1999) Discrete-time signal processing. Upper Saddle River, NJ: Prentice Hall.
40. Jenkinson M, Bannister P, Brady M, Smith S (2002) Improved optimization for the robust and accurate linear registration and motion correction of brain images. NeuroImage 17: 825.
41. Lazar NA, Eddy WF, Genovese CR, Welling J (2001) Statistical issues in fMRI for brain imaging. International Statistical Review 69: 105.
42. Churchill NW, Yourganov G, Spring R, Rasmussen PM, Lee W, et al. (2012) PHYCAA: Data-driven measurement and removal of physiological noise in BOLD fMRI. Neuroimage 59: 1299–1314.
43. Lund TE, Norgaard MD, Rostrup E, Rowe JB, Paulson OB (2005) Motion or activity: Their role in intra- and inter-subject variation in fMRI. NeuroImage 26: 960.
44. Sheehan DV, Lecrubier Y, Sheehan KH, Amorim P, Janavs J, et al. (1998) The Mini-International Neuropsychiatric Interview (MINI): The development and validation of a structured diagnostic psychiatric interview for DSM-IV and ICD-10. Journal of Clinical Psychiatry 59: 22–33.
45. Grady CL, Protzner AB, Kovacevic N, Strother SC, Afshin-Pour B, et al. (2010) A Multivariate Analysis of Age-Related Differences in Default Mode and Task-Positive Networks across Multiple Cognitive Domains. Cerebral Cortex 20: 1432–1447.
46. Garrett DD, Kovacevic N, McIntosh AR, Grady CL (2011) The Importance of Being Variable. Journal of Neuroscience 31: 4496–4503.
47. Breitenstein C, Knecht S (2002) Development and validation of a language learning model for behavioral and functional-imaging studies. Journal of Neuroscience Methods 114: 173–179.
48. Beckmann CF, Smith SA (2004) Probabilistic independent component analysis for functional magnetic resonance imaging. Ieee Transactions on Medical Imaging 23: 137–152.
49. Delorme A, Makeig S (2004) EEGLAB: an open source toolbox for analysis of single-trial EEG dynamics including independent component analysis. Journal of Neuroscience Methods 134: 9–21.
50. Kovacevic N, McIntosh AR (2007) Groupwise independent component decomposition of EEG data and partial least square analysis. Neuroimage 35: 1103–1112.
51. Larsen J, Hansen LK, Have AS, Christiansen T, Kolenda T (2002) Webmining: learning from the World Wide Web. Computational Statistics & Data Analysis 38: 517–532.

52. Sekihara K, Nagarajan SS, Poeppel D, Marantz A, Miyashita Y (2001) Reconstructing spatio-temporal activities of neural sources using an MEG vector beamformer technique. Ieee Transactions on Biomedical Engineering 48: 760–771.
53. Quraan MA, Cheyne D (2010) Reconstruction of correlated brain activity with adaptive spatial filters in MEG. Neuroimage 49: 2387–2400.
54. Riggs L, Moses SN, Bardouille T, Herdman AT, Ross B, et al. (2009) A complementary analytic approach to examining medial temporal lobe sources using magnetoencephalography. Neuroimage 45: 627–642.

8

Decreased Fronto-Temporal Interaction during Fixation after Memory Retrieval

Masaki Katsura[1☯], Satoshi Hirose[2,3☯], Hiroki Sasaki[1], Harushi Mori[1], Akira Kunimatsu[1], Kuni Ohtomo[1], Koji Jimura[2,3,4], Seiki Konishi[2,3]*

1 Department of Radiology, The University of Tokyo School of Medicine, Tokyo, Japan, **2** Department of Physiology, The University of Tokyo School of Medicine, Tokyo, Japan, **3** Department of Physiology, Juntendo University School of Medicine, Tokyo, Japan, **4** Precision and Intelligence Laboratory, Tokyo Institute of Technology, Yokohama, Japan

Abstract

Previous studies have revealed top-down control during memory retrieval from the prefrontal cortex to the temporal cortex. In the present functional MRI study, we investigated whether the fronto-temporal functional interaction occurs even during fixation periods after memory retrieval trials. During recency judgments, subjects judged the temporal order of two items in a study list. The task used in the present study consisted of memory trials of recency judgments and non-memory trials of counting dots, and post-trial fixation periods. By comparing the brain activity during the fixation periods after the memory trials with that during the fixation periods after the non-memory trials, we detected heightened brain activity in the lateral prefrontal cortex, the lateral temporal cortex and the hippocampus. Functional interactions during the fixation periods after the memory vs. non-memory trials as examined using a psychophysiological interaction revealed a decreased interaction from the lateral prefrontal cortex to the lateral temporal cortex, but not to the hippocampus. The functional interaction between the same frontal and temporal regions was also present during the memory trials. A trial-based functional connectivity analysis further revealed that the fronto-temporal interaction was positive and decreased during the fixation periods after the memory trials, relative to the fixation periods after the non-memory trials. These results suggest that the fronto-temporal interaction existed during the post-trial fixation periods, which had been present during the memory trials and temporally extended into the fixation periods.

Editor: Michal Zochowski, University of Michigan, United States of America

Funding: Funding was provided by the Uehara Memorial Foundation and a Grant-in-Aid for Scientific Research B (22300134). The funders had no role in study design, data collection and analysis, decision to publish, or preparation of the manuscript.

Competing Interests: The authors have declared that no competing interests exist.

* Email: skonishi@juntendo.ac.jp

☯ These authors contributed equally to this work.

Introduction

The lateral prefrontal cortex has been implicated in various types of cognitive control that guides our behavior, including memory control. The contribution of the lateral prefrontal cortex to control of memory retrieval has widely been acknowledged, such as selection or suppression of memory [1–17]. Previous studies also revealed that the memory representations in the temporal cortex were activated at the same time with the prefrontal cortex during memory retrieval [18–19], and that fiber density between prefrontal and temporal cortex predicted episodic memory performance [20], suggesting a top-down interaction from the prefrontal cortex to the temporal cortex.

Memory retrieval tasks are often designed as the alternation of memory trials and inter-trial intervals of post-trial fixation periods used as a control for memory retrieval. It is possible that memory retrieval processes and fronto-temporal interaction continue even after memory retrieval trials are completed, which may raise the possibility that the post-trial fixation periods may not be regarded as an ideal low-level control. In the present functional MRI study, we investigated whether functional interaction between the lateral prefrontal cortex and the temporal cortex exists even after memory retrieval trials. A recency judgment task was employed where two studied items were judged as to which was presented more recently [21–44]. The task consisted of recency judgment trials, non-memory trials of counting dots, and post-trial fixation periods of the same durations (3 sec each). The recency judgment task can be expected to require retrieval of greater amount of episodes for judgment of temporal order of studied items, which might resulted in greater degree of recruitment of processing related to memory retrieval even after the memory trials are completed. By comparing the brain activity during the post-trial fixation periods that followed the recency judgment trials with that during the post-trial fixation periods that followed the non-memory trials, we detected heightened brain activity. Further, a functional interaction among the brain activations identified in the

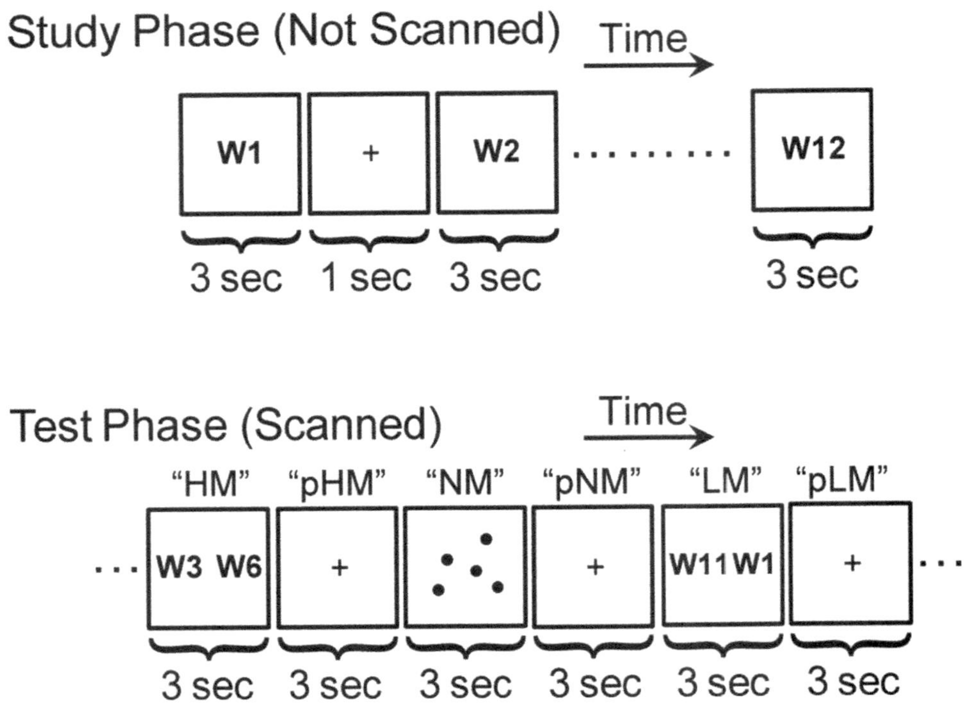

Figure 1. The memory paradigm of the present study. The task in the test phase contained memory trials of recency judgments with high and low retrieval loads (HM and LM), non-memory trials of counting dots (NM), and post-trial fixation periods (pHM, pLM and pNM) that lasted 3 sec each. W: word.

prefrontal and temporal cortex was examined using a psychophysiological interaction (PPI) [45–46] analysis. We also used resting-state data to contrast with the post-trial fixation periods where control processing was enhanced.

Materials and Methods

Subjects

Written informed consent was obtained from 31 healthy right-handed subjects (18 males; 13 females, age: 20–29 years). Three experiments were performed in a 2-hour session (Exp. 1: recency judgments; Exp. 2: dot counting and control fixation, Exp. 3: resting state). In the third experiment, 5 subjects did not complete the experiment due to the limitation of scanner time, and data from the 26 subjects were analyzed. They were scanned using experimental procedures approved by the institutional review board of the University of Tokyo School of Medicine.

MRI procedures

The experiments were conducted using a 3T fMRI system. Scout images were first collected to align the field of view centered on the subject's brain. T1-weighted images were obtained for anatomical reference (76 slices×2 mm slices; in-plane resolution = 1×1 mm). For functional imaging, a gradient echo echo-planar sequence was used (TR = 2.0 s; TE = 35 ms; flip angle = 90 degrees; 30×4 mm slices; in-plane resolution of 4×4 mm). Each run contained 36 volume images, and the first six functional images in each run were excluded from the analysis to take into account the equilibrium of longitudinal magnetization.

Behavioral Procedures

The task in Exp. 1 consisted of two main phases, study and test (Fig. 1). During the study phase, the subjects were presented with a sequence of words (list size: 12 words). Each word was presented for 3 sec, with an inter-stimulus interval (presentation of a white fixation cross) of 1 sec. Subjects were instructed to relationally encode them for later recency judgments [33,47–48]. More specifically, subjects were instructed to make up their own story from the list words, and this instruction is supposed to encourage the subjects to relate sequentially presented words that had otherwise no contexts among them. The words were concrete nouns taken from an object stimulus set [49], and were presented in strings of Japanese characters. To prevent the subjects from rehearsing the words between the study and test phases, the subjects performed a modified Wisconsin card sorting task for approximately 30 s as a distracter task [28,33,41,50].

The test phase was administered while functional images were acquired. In each of twelve runs administered to the subjects, the test phase contained four recency judgment trials with high or low mnemonic load (two "HM" and two "LM" trials) and four non-mnemonic odd/even judgment trials ("NM"), presented in a pseudorandom order. Therefore, the total numbers of HM, LM and NM trials were 24, 24 and 48, respectively. Each trial lasted for 3 sec, followed by a 3-sec fixation period, which consisted of three types of post-trial fixation periods ("pHM", "pLM" and "pNM"). During the recency judgment trials (HM and LM), two words in the studied list were simultaneously presented, one to the right and the other to the left. The subjects were instructed to choose which word had been studied more recently. The right or left word was chosen by pressing a right or left button, respectively, using the same right thumb. The word pair to be judged for LM trials included one or two end words in the study list, and the temporal distance between the paired words was greater, whereas the word pair for HM trials did not include any end words, and the temporal distance between the paired words was smaller. By contrast, during the odd/even judgment trials (NM), subjects were

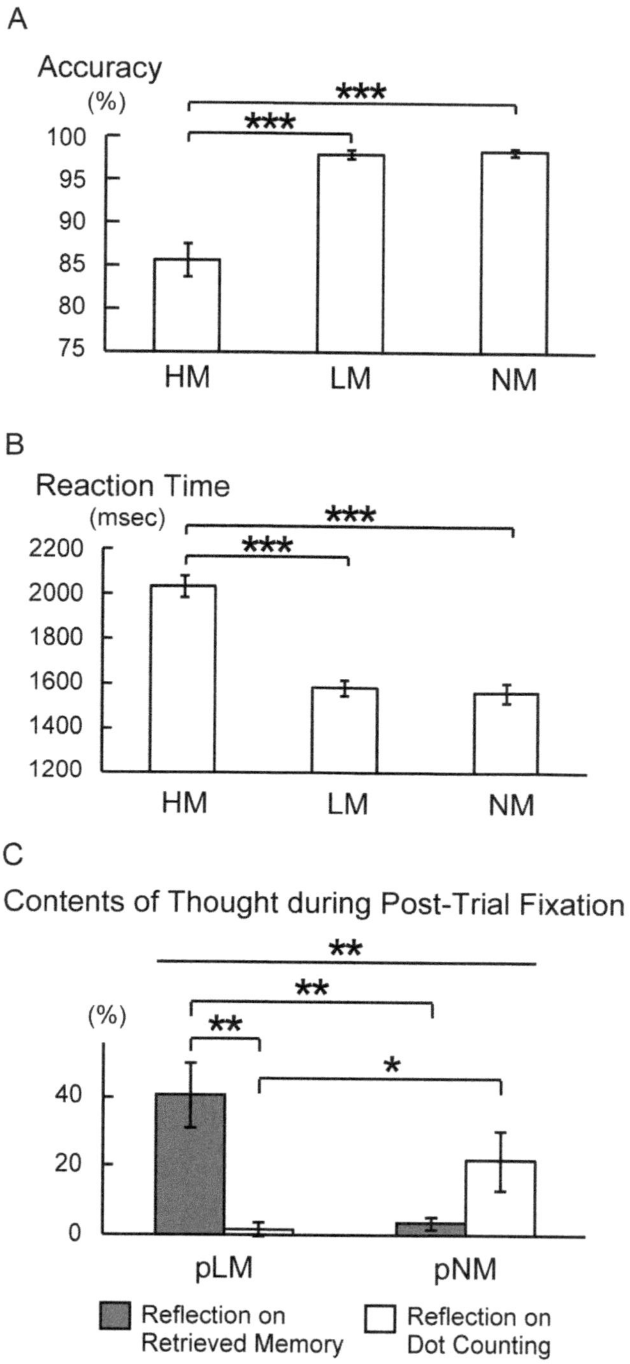

Figure 2. Behavioral data. A) Accuracy in the three types of trials, HM, LM and NM. B) Reaction time in correct trials in HM, LM and NM. C) Contents of thought during fixation periods after correct LM and NM trials. *: $p<.05$, **: $p<.01$, ***: $p<.001$.

instructed to count 3 to 8 white dots presented in the screen and to judge whether the number of the dots was even or odd. The even or odd number was chosen by pressing a right or left button, respectively, using the same right thumb. Therefore, HM and LM trials required memory retrieval processes to a greater degree than NM trials. During the post-trial fixation period, on the other hand, subjects were instructed to fixate on a cross presented at the center of the screen, but were not encouraged or discouraged to think about a particular thing. In order to avoid unwanted confound related to the difference in task performance prior to the fixation periods, the accuracy and reaction time in LM and NM trials were matched by modulating the number of dots in NM trials. Therefore, the contrast of pLM vs. pNM of central interest in the present study is expected to reveal the brain activity associated with memory-related processes after the memory trials. In other words, we focused on the pLM vs. pNM effect because, unlike the high memory conditions, this comparison was not confounded by reaction time or difficulty difference.

It is possible that a relatively weaker level of memory-related processes was recruited during the pNM presented in the runs that included recency judgment trials (HM and LM). In order to control for the possible confound, two runs of a control task were administered where five NM trials were presented in a block for 16 sec, followed by a fixation period for 16 sec, and the cycles were repeated five times for each run (Exp. 2). In addition, in order to examine the resting-state functional connectivity between the frontal and temporal regions of interest (ROIs), four runs were administered where subjects fixated on a cross hair throughout the run, approximately for 5 min (Exp. 3). The resting-state runs were not completed in 5 of the 31 subjects due to limitation in scanner time, and data from the 26 subjects were analyzed for the resting-state functional connectivity.

Data analysis

Data were analyzed using SPM8 software (http://www.fil.ion.ucl.ac.uk/spm/). Functional images were realigned, slice timing corrected, normalized to the Montreal Neurological Institute template with interpolation to a $2\times2\times2$ mm space, and spatially smoothed (full width half maximum = 8 mm). Then event timing was coded into a general linear model (GLM) [51]. The eight types of events, correct trials (HM, LM and NM), error trials, and subsequent fixation periods (pHM, pLM, pNM and post-error periods), together with run-specific regressors as effects of no interest, were coded using the canonical hemodynamic response function in SPM8, time-locked to the onset of these events. The brain activation associated with memory-related processes during the post-trial fixation periods was calculated based on the contrast of pLM vs. pNM. Group analyses were conducted using a random effects model. Significant activations were detected using a combined threshold of (1) $p<0.05$ corrected by the false discovery rate (FDR) [52,53] and (2) $p<0.001$ (uncorrected).

A psychophysiological interaction (PPI) [45,46] analysis was conducted to investigate functional interaction among brain regions during post-trial fixation periods. Based on the spherical ROIs (radius = 8 mm) determined by the post-trial contrast of pLM vs. pNM, PPIs from each of the ROIs in the left lateral prefrontal cortex to one ROI in the left temporal cortex and one ROI in the left hippocampus were calculated between two psychological conditions, pLM and pNM, in a single-subject level. A significant PPI means the regression of temporal responses depending on prefrontal top-down control processing in the low versus no-memory conditions. This regression is a simple linear form of effective connectivity and is interpreted as prefrontal influence on temporal processing. Group analyses were then conducted using a random effects model. In order to test the across-data reproducibility of the functional interaction during post-trial fixation periods, PPIs were also calculated between pHM and pNM based on the ROIs determined by the contrast of pLM vs. pNM, where PPIs had already been calculated between pLM and pNM.

Another type of a functional connectivity analysis was also performed on a trial by trial basis [54]. Briefly, each of the trials (HM/LM/NM) and post fixation periods (pHM/pLM/pNM) was

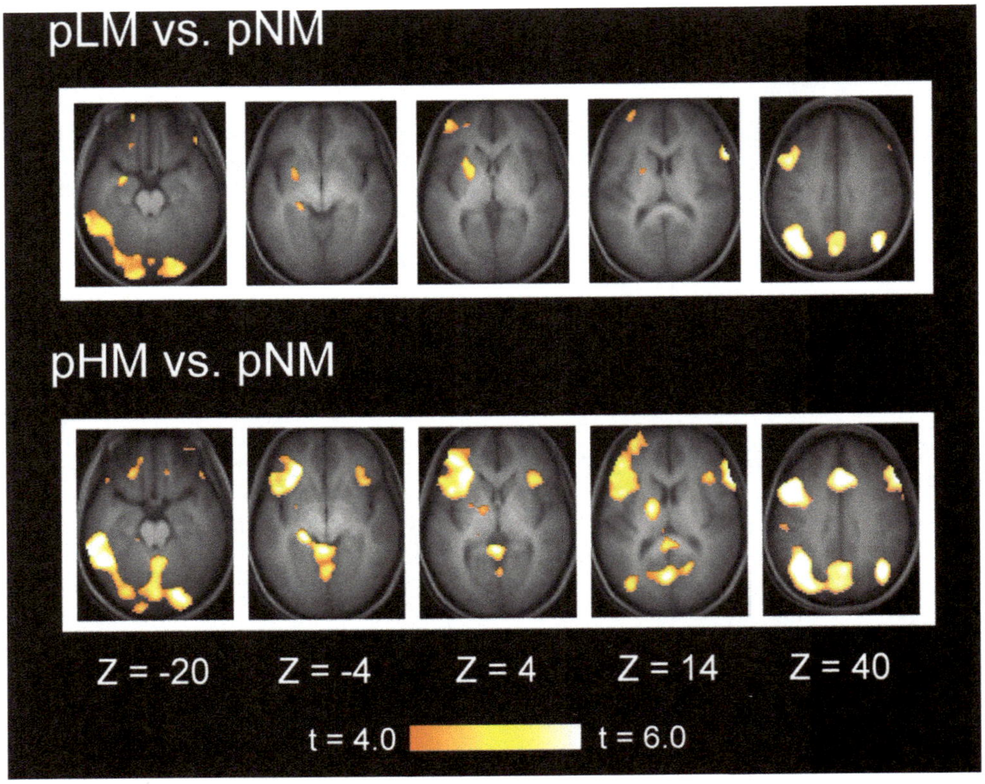

Figure 3. Statistical activation maps for signal increase in the contrast of pLM vs. pNM and pHM vs. pNM. Activation maps are displayed as transverse sections and are overlaid on top of the anatomic image averaged across subjects. Statistical significance is indicated using the color scale, and the transverse section level is indicated by the Z coordinates of Talairach space.

coded into GLM, and the parameter estimate (beta value) for each trial in these six conditions was extracted. The beta values in one condition were plotted against two ROIs, and the correlation coefficient (r) across trials was calculated. The beta values in the two ROI were averaged across all the voxels in the sphere that were selected from the frontal and temporal regions activated during pLM minus pNM. The correlation coefficient (r) was converted to Fisher's z values and then to z-score in a Gaussian distribution, and the z-score was subject to a t-test in a group analysis, to estimate a functional interaction between two ROIs in one condition.

The data analysis procedures for resting-state functional connectivity were essentially the same as those used in previous literatures [55–57]. Briefly, the acquired images were realigned, slice-timing corrected, and normalized to the standard template image. The images were subject to further preprocessing including temporal band-pass filter (0.009 Hz, f, 0.08 Hz), spatially smoothed, regression of six parameters obtained by head motion correction, whole brain signal averaged over the whole brain, ventricular signal averaged from ventricular ROI, and white matter signal averaged from white matter ROI. Functional connectivity analyses were performed on the resultant time series data, on a timepoint by timepoint basis, between a seed ROI and a

Table 1. Brain regions in the left lateral prefrontal cortex and left temporal cortex showing signal increase in the contrasts pLM vs. pNM.

	X	y	z	t	Label
Left lateral prefrontal cortex	−50	10	40	5.8	Frontal1
	−42	22	44	5.1	Frontal2
	−46	50	4	4.7	Frontal3
	−34	58	14	4.5	Frontal4
	−28	50	4	4.2	Frontal5
	−46	46	18	4.2	Frontal6
Left temporal cortex	−66	−44	−20	5.0	Lat Temporal
	−22	−32	−4	4.7	Hippocampus

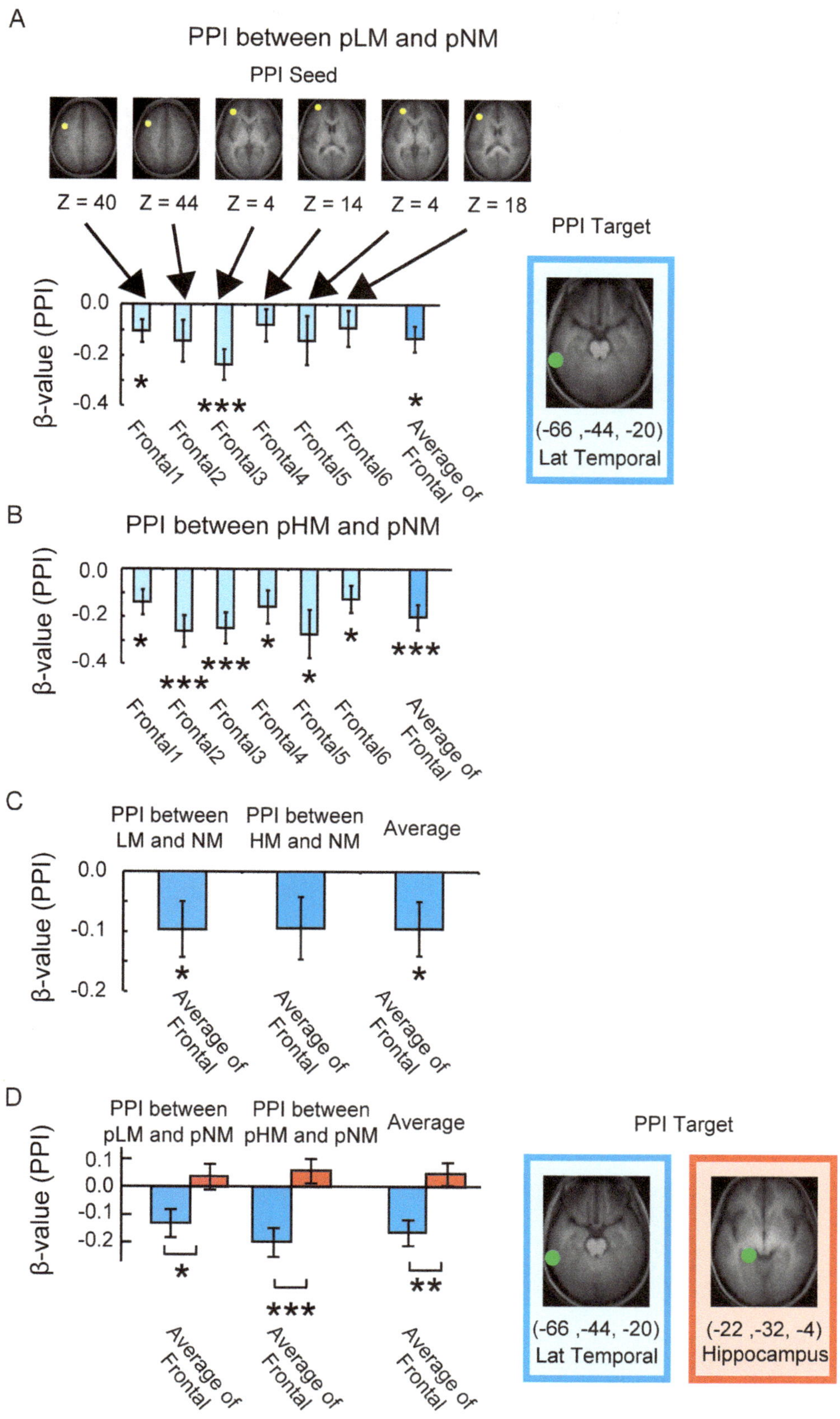

Figure 4. Inhibitory fronto-temporal interaction revealed by a PPI analysis. A) PPIs between pLM and pNM from the lateral prefrontal to the lateral temporal regions. B) PPIs between pHM and pNM from the same lateral prefrontal to the same lateral temporal regions. C) PPIs between LM/HM and NM from the same lateral prefrontal to the same lateral temporal regions. D) PPIs between pLM/pHM and pNM from the same lateral prefrontal to the lateral temporal/hippocampal regions. *: p<.05, **: p<.01, ***: p<.001.

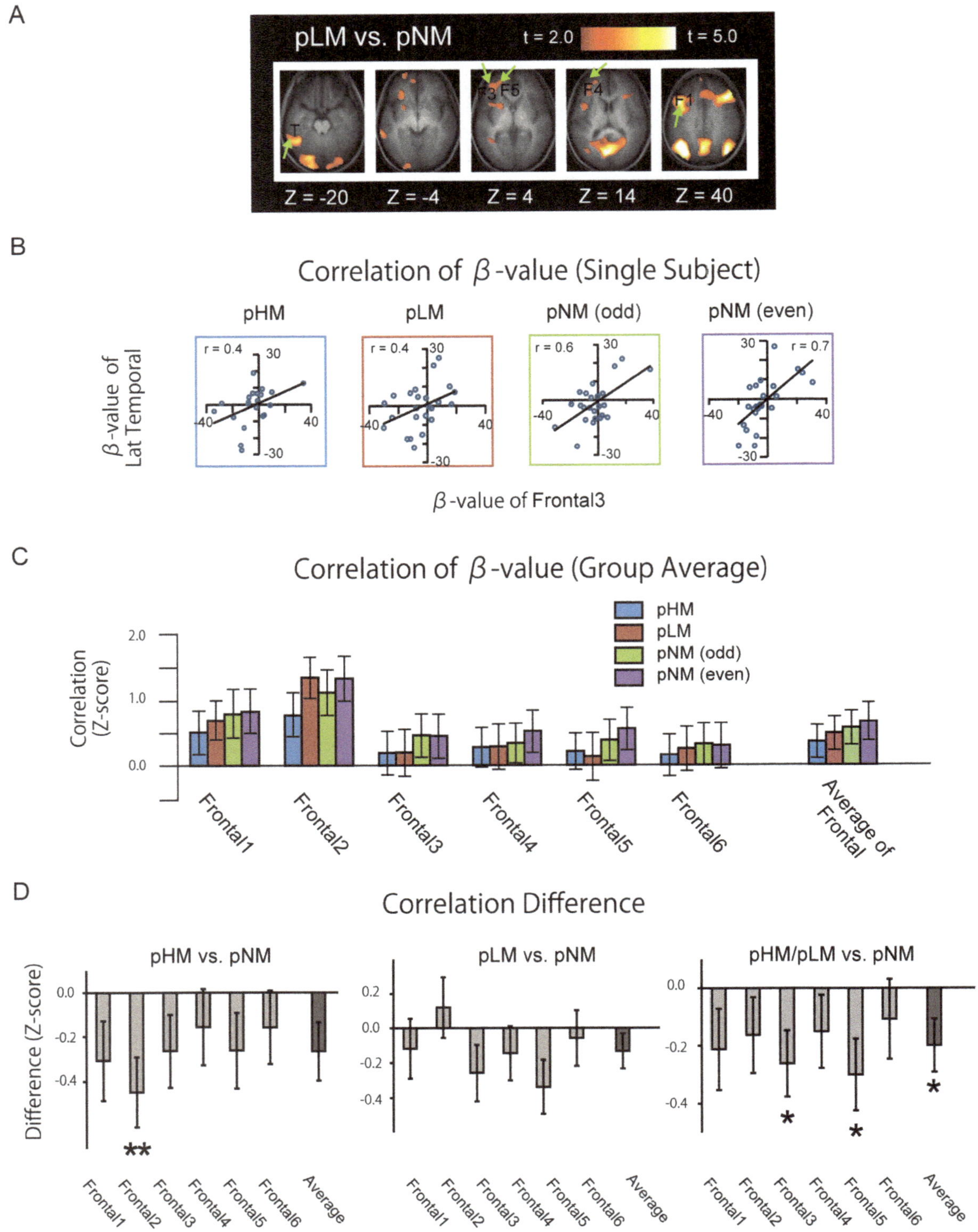

Figure 5. A functional connectivity analysis on a trial by trial basis. A) Activation maps for pLM vs. pNM generated from parameter estimates for individual events. The formats were similar to Fig. 3. B) An example of trial-based functional connectivity between frontal and temporal ROIs during pHM, pLM and pNM (odd and even) in one subject. C) Group average functional connectivity in each of the frontal and the temporal ROIs. D) The connectivity difference between pHM and pNM (left) and between pLM and pNM (middle) and between pHM/pLM and pNM (right). The formats were similar to Fig. 4. *: $p<.05$, **: $p<.01$.

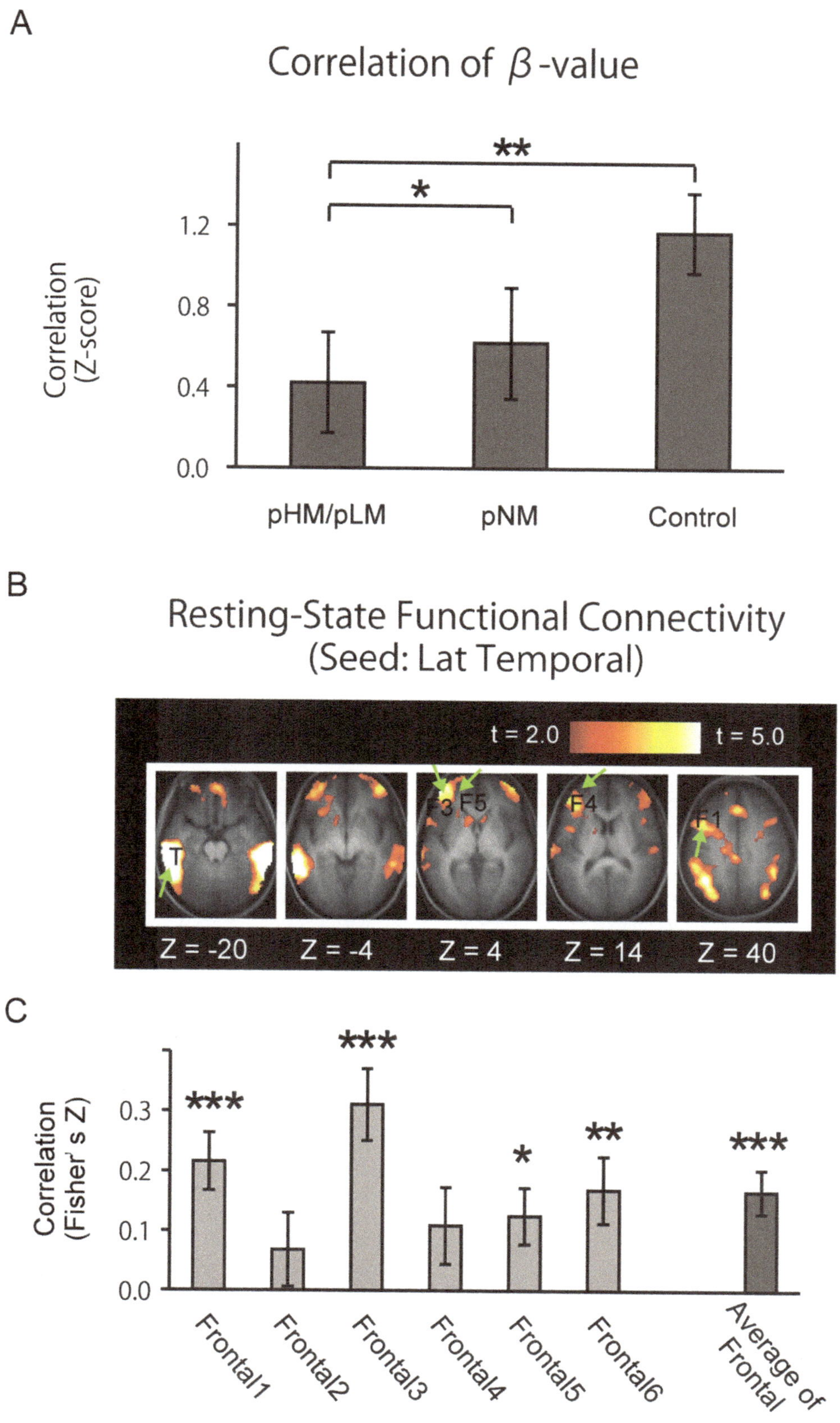

Figure 6. A) A trial-based functional connectivity during pHM/pLM, pNM and control fixation periods. B) A map of resting-state functional connectivity, with the seed placed in the lateral temporal region. The formats were similar to Fig. 3. C) The magnitude of the resting-state functional connectivity between each frontal and temporal ROIs. The formats were similar to Fig. 4. *: $p<.05$, **: $p<.01$, ***: $p<.001$.

target ROI or between a seed ROI and all the voxels in the whole brain. To estimate the statistical significance of the functional connectivity, the Fischer z transformation was applied to the correlation coefficients.

Interview on the contents of thought during post-trial fixation period

In order to ensure that memory-related processes were recruited during the post-trial fixation periods, questionnaire about the content of thought during the fixation period was administered to a different set of 11 subjects (6 males, 5 females, age: 20–29 years). The subjects performed 5 runs of 2 LM and 2 NM trials (not scanned). After the task, the subjects were asked to report the contents of thought during fixation periods that followed LM or NM trials. The task was basically the same except that the task contained only LM and NM trials. HM trials were not included in this task because subjects cannot completely discriminate HM from LM at the time of questionnaire. More specifically, in the surprise report, they were asked to classify the contents of thought into four categories: (1) reflection on previous memory trials, (2) reflection on previous counting trials, (3) others and (4) no thinking activity. The scores were provided for pLM and pNM separately. The score ranged from 0 to 10 based on the time spent in that thought, and the sum of the four scores had to be ten.

Results

Behavioral results

The correct performance was 85.6±10.9 (mean ± SD), 98.0±2.8 and 98.3±2.4% in HM, LM and NM trials, respectively (Fig. 2A). The difference was significant between HM and LM trials [t (30) = 6.4, $\underline{P}$<.001] and between HM and NM trials [t (30) = 6.4, $\underline{P}$<.001]. The reaction time was 2034±265 (mean ± SD), 1582±198 and 1563±247 ms, in HM, LM and NM trials, respectively (Fig. 2B). The difference was significant between HM and LM trials [t (30) = 14.2, $\underline{P}$<.001] and between HM and NM trials [t (30) = 10.6, $\underline{P}$<.001]. However, no significant difference in the behavioral performance was found between LM and NM. Therefore, the behavioral scores were successfully matched between LM and NM.

Post-task questionnaire administered on a different set of subjects revealed that memory-related processes were recruited more during pLM than during pNM. Subjects reflected on previous memory trials during pLM for 41%, and reflected on previous counting trials during pNM for 22% (Fig. 2C). A repeated measures two-way ANOVA revealed significant interaction between trial-type and thought-content [F (1, 10) = 14.1, $\underline{P}$< .005]. These results confirm that memory-related processes during memory trials were prolonged and were recruited during pLM.

Neuroimaging results

The brain activation associated with memory-related processes during the post-trial fixation periods was calculated based on the contrast of pLM/pHM vs. pNM. As shown in Fig. 3, significant signal increase was observed in several regions, including the regions in the left lateral prefrontal cortex, the left lateral temporal cortex and the left hippocampus. Table 1 lists the peak coordinates of the significant activations during pLM vs. pNM in the lateral prefrontal cortex and the temporal lobe that were used as regions of interest in later analyses.

To investigate functional interaction among brain regions during the post-trial fixation periods, we next conducted a psychophysiological interaction (PPI) [45,46] analysis. Six PPIs were calculated between two psychological conditions, pLM and pNM, from each of the six ROIs in the left lateral prefrontal cortex to the one ROI in the left lateral temporal cortex determined by the contrast of pLM vs. pNM (Fig. 4A). As shown in Fig. 4A, overall tendency of negative PPIs from the lateral frontal regions to the lateral temporal region was observed, suggesting decreased fronto-temporal interaction during the post-fixation periods after the memory trials. To summarize the six frontal ROIs, a PPI from the averaged frontal regions to the temporal region was significantly negative [t (30) = −2.6, $\underline{P}$<.05]. In order to test the reproducibility of the negative PPIs, PPIs were also calculated between pHM and pNM in the same ROIs based on the contrast of pLM vs. pNM (Fig. 4B). We found consistent tendency of negative PPIs, and the PPI from the averaged frontal regions to the temporal region was significantly negative [t (30) = −3.8, P<.001]. The PPI from the averaged frontal regions to the temporal region was also significantly negative when pLM and pHM were averaged [t (30) = −3.5, $\underline{P}$<.005]. Further, to test whether the functional interaction after the memory trials was also present during the memory trials, the PPIs were calculated between LM/HM and NM in the same ROIs based on the contrast of pLM vs. pNM. The negative PPI from the averaged frontal regions to the temporal region was significant between LM and NM [t (30) = −2.1, P<.05], close to significance between HM and NM [t (30) = −1.8, P = .08], and significant when HM and LM were averaged [t (30) = −2.1, P<.05].

As a reference, we also examined functional interaction between the left lateral prefrontal cortex and the left hippocampus (Fig. 4D). A PPI was calculated between pLM and pNM, from the average of the six ROIs in the lateral prefrontal cortex to the one ROI in the hippocampus determined by the contrast of pLM vs. pNM. The PPI was close to 0. When compared with the PPI to the lateral temporal cortex, the difference was significant [t (30) = 2.1, $\underline{P}$<.05]. In order to test the across-data reproducibility, PPIs were also calculated between pHM and pNM based on the same ROIs of the contrasts of pLM vs. pNM. The difference between the two PPIs was also significant [t (30) = 4.2, $\underline{P}$<.001]. When pLM and pHM are averaged, the PPI difference was also significant [t (30) = −3.3, P<.005]. These results suggest that the lateral prefrontal cortex interacted specifically with the lateral temporal cortex during post-trial fixation periods.

The fronto-temporal interaction during post-trial fixation periods was analyzed further using functional connectivity on a trial-by-trial basis [54]. To confirm that the parameter estimates for individual single events were properly calculated, the activation map was re-generated by averaging the parameter estimates for individual trials. Figure 5A demonstrates that, although the overall activation pattern appears relatively weaker, the frontal and temporal activations during pLM vs. pNM that were originally detected by the standard analysis presented in Figure 3 were successfully reproduced using the parameter estimates for individual single events. Next, the parameter estimates for individual single events were plotted against the frontal and temporal ROIs in one particular period. One example is shown in Fig. 5B, where the parameter estimates during pHM/pLM/pNM were plotted against the frontal (Frontal 3, see Table 1) and the lateral temporal ROIs in one subject. To match the number of plots in each period, pNM was divided into two halves (odd and even). The fronto-temporal interaction was investigated thoroughly, calculating the group average for every combination of the six frontal ROIs and the lateral temporal ROI during pHM, pLM and pNM (odd and even) (Fig. 5C). The difference in functional connectivity was calculated between pHM/pLM and pNM (averaged for odd and even) (Fig. 5D), to compare the results with those by the PPI analysis presented in Fig. 4. The difference between pHM/pLM and pNM when six frontal ROIs were averaged was significantly negative [t (30) = 2.2, P<.05]. Importantly, although the difference in functional connectivity was negative, the functional connectivity during each period was positive. That is, the positive fronto-temporal functional connectivity during pNM decreased during pHM/pLM.

Although the memory-related processes during pNM are expected to be minimal (Fig. 2C), we further examined control periods in two runs without any recency judgment trials, where blocks of odd/even judgment trials (NM) and fixation blocks were alternated (see Materials and Methods). Twenty-four events were individually coded in the fixation control periods, and parameter estimates were calculated using similar procedures. Figure 6A demonstrates that the fronto-temporal functional connectivity during the control period was positive, and the difference was significantly negative between pHM/pLM and pNM [t (30) = 2.2, P<.05] and between pHM/pLM and control periods [t (30) = 2.8, P<.01]. To investigate the positive functional connectivity during the control fixation periods, a resting-state functional connectivity was calculated further, using four runs where subjects fixated on a hair cross (see Materials and Methods). As shown in Figs. 6B and 6C, the resting-state functional connectivity between the frontal and temporal ROIs was significantly positive [t (25) = 4.5, P< .001].

Discussion

In the present fMRI study, we tested whether the fronto-temporal interaction that is known to occur during memory retrieval occurred even during the fixation periods where the memory trials were completed. The contrast of the post-trial fixation periods (pLM vs. pNM) in our modified recency judgment task revealed the heightened brain activity in several regions including the lateral prefrontal cortex, the lateral temporal cortex and the hippocampus. A PPI analysis revealed significant negative functional interaction from the lateral prefrontal to the lateral temporal cortex, but not to the hippocampus. The PPI was also significant during the memory retrieval trials. A trial-based functional connectivity analysis revealed positive fronto-temporal interaction that decreased during pLM relative to pNM. Moreover, a resting-state functional connectivity analysis revealed a positive fronto-temporal functional connectivity during the resting state. These results suggest that at least one part of the top-down prefrontal processing that occurred during memory retrieval was extended into the subsequent fixation periods, and raise the possibility that the post-task fixation periods may not be regarded as an ideal low-level control.

The present study revealed that the fronto-temporal functional connectivity was positive during control fixation periods, and the functional connectivity decreased during post-retrieval fixation periods. The decrease of the positive functional connectivity implies two straightforward interpretations: One is that the prefrontal control over the temporal cortex yields positive functional connectivity, and the prefrontal control is weakened during post-retrieval fixation periods, relative to the control fixation periods. The other is that the positive functional connectivity during the control fixation periods simply reflects spontaneous between-regional correlation that is irrelevant of prefrontal functioning, and the decrease of the functional connectivity reflects enhanced inhibitory prefrontal control over the temporal cortex. The present results from the resting-state functional connectivity, which is known to reflect primarily the anatomical connections [58–59], support the latter possibility. One important feature of the present observation is that the brain activity in the lateral temporal region was enhanced during pLM, but the lateral temporal activity was suppressed at the same time through enhanced inhibitory prefrontal control over the temporal cortex during pLM. One straightforward explanation for this counterintuitive pattern of brain activity and PPI would be that memory representation in the lateral temporal cortex was activated by memory retrieval processes within the non-frontal brain regions, and the brain activity surpassed the prefrontal inhibitory interaction.

The posterior lateral temporal cortex has been implicated in specific semantic knowledge [60–71]. The post-task questionnaire in the present study revealed that the subjects thought about previous memory trials during fixation after recency judgments, i.e., the stories made from the words in the study list. The stories were made of specific semantic relations between the study words, but semantic relations in the stories had to be selected from other irrelevant semantic relations. It has been proposed that the lateral prefrontal cortex is engaged during post-retrieval processing of semantic information through monitoring and decision making processes [72–75]. It has also been proposed that the lateral prefrontal cortex, especially the inferior prefrontal cortex, subserves selection of semantic information among competing alternatives [1,2,8]. Thus, the decrease of functional connectivity from the lateral prefrontal cortex to the lateral temporal cortex can be interpreted as post-retrieval processing of selecting relevant semantic representations by inhibiting irrelevant representations through monitoring and decision making processes.

Mental activity during fixation is most often associated with default mode network [76–78]. The hippocampus and the lateral temporal cortex reported in the present study appear to belong to the default mode network, and the lateral prefrontal cortex also appears to belong to the fronto-parietal control network [79,80]. The decrease of fronto-temporal functional connectivity during post-retrieval processing revealed in the present study is consistent with decreased coupling between the fronto-parietal control network and the default mode network during control processing in the pLM [81,82]. Moreover, the connectivity decrease was greater in the pHM when the control demand was heightened relative to pLM. Although full understanding of cognitive processes recruited during fixation periods needs further research, the present study suggests the fronto-temporal interaction that was extended temporally into the subsequent fixation periods.

Author Contributions

Conceived and designed the experiments: MK SK. Performed the experiments: MK HS HM AK KO KJ SK. Analyzed the data: MK SH SK. Contributed to the writing of the manuscript: MK SH SK.

References

1. Thompson-Schill SL, Swick D, Farah MJ, D'Esposito M, Kan IP, et al. (1998) Verb generation in patients with focal frontal lesions: a neuropsychological test of neuroimaging findings. Proc Natl Acad Sci USA 95: 15855–15860.
2. Thompson-Schill SL, D'Esposito M, Kan IP (1999) Effects of repetition and competition on activity in left prefrontal cortex during word generation. Neuron 23: 513–522.
3. Fletcher PC, Henson RN (2001) Frontal lobes and human memory: insights from functional neuroimaging. Brain 124: 849–881.
4. Badre D, Wagner AD (2002) Semantic retrieval, mnemonic control, and prefrontal cortex. Behav Cogn Neurosci Rev 1: 206–218.
5. Buckner RL (2003) Functional-anatomic correlates of control processes in memory. J Neurosci 23: 3999–4004.

6. Anderson MC, Ochsner KN, Kuhl B, Cooper J, Robertson E, et al. (2004) Neural Systems Underlying the Suppression of Unwanted Memories. Science 303: 232–235.
7. Aron AR, Robbins TW, Poldrack RA (2004) Inhibition and the right inferior frontal cortex. Trends Cogn Sci 8: 170–177.
8. Kan IP, Thompson-Schill SL (2004) Selection from perceptual and conceptual representations. Cogn Affect Behav Neurosci 4: 466–482.
9. Badre D, Poldrack RA, Paré-Blagoev EJ, Insler RZ, Wagner AD (2005) Dissociable controlled retrieval and generalized selection mechanisms in ventrolateral prefrontal cortex. Neuron 47: 907–918.
10. Duarte A, Ranganath C, Knight RT (2005) Effects of unilateral prefrontal lesions on familiarity, recollection, and source memory. J Neurosci 25: 8333–8337.
11. Werkle-Bergner M, Mecklinger A, Kray J, Meyer P, Düzel E (2005) The control of memory retrieval: insights from event-related potentials. Brain Res Cogn Brain Res 24: 599–614.
12. Badre D, Wagner AD (2007) Left ventrolateral prefrontal cortex and the cognitive control of memory. Neuropsychologia 45: 2883–2901.
13. Depue BE, Curran T, Banich MT (2007) Prefrontal regions orchestrate suppression of emotional memories via a two-phase process. Science 317: 215–219.
14. Davachi L, Dobbins IG (2008) Declarative Memory. Curr Dir Psychol Sci 17: 112–118.
15. Levy BJ, Anderson MC (2008) Individual differences in the suppression of unwanted memories: the executive deficit hypothesis. Acta Psychol (Amst) 127: 623–635.
16. Benoit RG, Anderson MC (2012) Opposing mechanisms support the voluntary forgetting of unwanted memories. Neuron 76: 450–460.
17. Gagnepain P, Henson RN, Anderson MC (2014) Suppressing unwanted memories reduces their unconscious influence via targeted cortical inhibition. Proc Natl Acad Sci USA 111, E1310–1319.
18. Düzel E, Cabeza R, Picton TW, Yonelinas AP, Scheich H, et al. (1999) Task-related and item-related brain processes of memory retrieval. Proc Natl Acad Sci USA 96: 1794–1799.
19. Ranganath C, Heller AS, Wilding EL (2007) Dissociable correlates of two classes of retrieval processing in prefrontal cortex. Neuroimage 35: 1663–1673.
20. Schott BH, Niklas C, Kaufmann J, Bodammer NC, Machts J, et al. (2011) Fiber density between rhinal cortex and activated ventrolateral prefrontal regions predicts episodic memory performance in humans. Proc Natl Acad Sci USA 108: 5408–5413.
21. Milner B (1971) Interhemispheric differences in the localization of psychological processes in man. Br Med Bull 27: 272–277.
22. Petrides M (1991) Functional specialization within the dorsolateral frontal cortex for serial order memory. Proc Biol Sci. 246: 299–306.
23. Zorrilla LT, Aguirre GK, Zarahn E, Cannon TD, D'Esposito M (1996) Activation of the prefrontal cortex during judgments of recency: a functional MRI study. Neuroreport. 7: 2803–2806.
24. Cabeza R, Mangels J, Nyberg L, Habib R, Houle S, et al. (1997) Brain regions differentially involved in remembering what and when: a PET study. Neuron 19: 863–870.
25. Cabeza R, Anderson ND, Houle S, Mangels JA, Nyberg L (2000) Age-related differences in neural activity during item and temporal-order memory retrieval: a positron emission tomography study. J Cogn Neurosci 12: 197–206.
26. Hintzman DL (2001) Judgments of frequency and recency: how they relate to reports of subjective awareness. J Exp Psychol Learn Mem Cogn 27: 1347–1358.
27. Dobbins IG, Foley H, Schacter DL, Wagner AD (2002) Executive control during episodic retrieval: multiple prefrontal processes subserve source memory. Neuron 35: 989–996.
28. Konishi S, Uchida I, Okuaki T, Machida T, Shirouzu I, et al. (2002) Neural correlates of recency judgment. J Neurosci 22: 9549–9555.
29. Suzuki M, Fujii T, Tsukiura T, Okuda J, Umetsu A, et al. (2002) Neural basis of temporal context memory: a functional MRI study. Neuroimage 17: 1790–1796.
30. Dobbins IG, Rice HJ, Wagner AD, Schacter DL (2003) Memory orientation and success: separable neurocognitive components underlying episodic recognition. Neuropsychologia 41: 318–333.
31. Hintzman DL (2003) Judgments of recency and their relation to recognition memory. Mem Cognit 31: 26–34.
32. Fujii T, Suzuki M, Okuda J, Ohtake H, Tanji K, et al. (2004) Neural correlates of context memory with real-world events. Neuroimage 21: 1596–1603.
33. Konishi S, Asari T, Jimura K, Chikazoe J, Miyashita Y (2006) Activation shift from medial to lateral temporal cortex associated with recency judgments following impoverished encoding. Cereb Cortex 16: 469–474.
34. Rajah MN, McIntosh AR (2006) Dissociating prefrontal contributions during a recency memory task. Neuropsychologia 44: 350–364.
35. Dudukovic NM, Wagner AD (2007) Goal-dependent modulation of declarative memory: neural correlates of temporal recency decisions and novelty detection. Neuropsychologia 45: 2608–2620.
36. Rajah MN, McIntosh AR (2008) Age-related differences in brain activity during verbal recency memory. Brain Res 1199: 111–125.
37. St Jacques P, Rubin DC, LaBar KS, Cabeza R (2008) The short and long of it: neural correlates of temporal-order memory for autobiographical events. J Cogn Neurosci 20: 1327–1341.
38. Grove KL, Wilding EL (2009) Retrieval processes supporting judgments of recency. J Cogn Neurosci 21: 461–473.
39. Lehn H, Steffenach HA, van Strien NM, Veltman DJ, Witter MP, et al. (2009) A specific role of the human hippocampus in recall of temporal sequences. J Neurosci 29: 3475–3484.
40. Greve A, Doidge AN, Evans CJ, Wilding EL (2010) Functional neuroanatomy supporting judgments of when events occurred. J Neurosci 30: 7099–7104.
41. Kimura HM, Hirose S, Kunimatsu A, Chikazoe J, Jimura K, et al. (2010) Differential temporo-parietal cortical networks that support relational and item-based recency judgments. Neuroimage 49: 3474–3480.
42. Rajah MN, Crane D, Maillet D, Floden D, Valiquette L (2011) Similarities in the patterns of prefrontal cortex activity during spatial and temporal context memory retrieval after equating for task structure and performance. Neuroimage 54: 1549–1564.
43. Rajah MN, Languay R, Grady CL (2011) Age-related changes in right middle frontal gyrus volume correlate with altered episodic retrieval activity. J Neurosci 31: 17941–1754.
44. Hirose S, Kimura HM, Jimura K, Kunimatsu A, Abe O, et al. (2013) Dissociable Temporo-Parietal Memory Networks Revealed by Functional Connectivity during Episodic Retrieval. PLoS One 8: e71210.
45. Friston KJ, Buechel C, Fink GR, Morris J, Rolls E, et al. (1997) Psychophysiological and modulatory interactions in neuroimaging. Neuroimage 6: 218–229.
46. Gitelman DR, Penny WD, Ashburner J, Friston KJ (2003) Modeling regional and psychophysiologic interactions in fMRI: the importance of hemodynamic deconvolution. Neuroimage 19: 200–207.
47. Davachi L, Wagner AD (2002) Hippocampal contributions to episodic encoding: Insights from relational and item-based learning. J Neurophysiol 88: 982–990.
48. Tubridy S, Davachi L (2011) Medial temporal lobe contributions to episodic sequence encoding. Cereb Cortex 21: 272–280.
49. Snodgrass JS, Vanderwart M (1980) A standardized set of 260 pictures: norms for name agreement, image agreement, familiarity, and visual complexity. J Exp Psychol Hum Learn 9: 164–215.
50. Jimura K, Yamashita K, Chikazoe J, Hirose S, Miyashita Y, et al. (2009) A critical component that activates the left inferior prefrontal cortex during inference resolution. Eur J Neurosci 29: 1915–1920.
51. Worsley KJ, Friston KJ (1995) Analysis of fMRI time-series revisited–again. Neuroimage 2: 173–181.
52. Genovese C, Lazar NA, Nichols T (2002) Thresholding of statistical maps in functional neuroimaging using the false discovery rate. Neuroimage 15: 870–878.
53. Chumbley JR, Friston KJ (2009) False discovery rate revisited: FDR and topological inference using Gaussian random fields. Neuroimage 44: 62–70.
54. Rissman J, Gazzaley A, D'Esposito M (2004) Measuring functional connectivity during distinct stages of a cognitive task. Neuroimage 23: 752–763.
55. Fox MD, Snyder AZ, Vincent JL, Corbetta M, Van Essen DC, et al. (2005) The human brain is intrinsically organized into dynamic, anticorrelated functional networks. Proc Natl Acad Sci USA 102: 9673–9678.
56. Fair DA, Schlaggar BL, Cohen AL, Miezin FM, Dosenbach NU, et al. (2007) A method for using blocked and event-related fMRI data to study "resting state" functional connectivity. Neuroimage 35: 396–405.
57. Hirose S, Watanabe T, Wada H, Imai Y, Machida T, et al. (2013) Functional relevance of micromodules in the human association cortex delineated with high-resolution FMRI. Cereb Cortex 23: 2863–2871.
58. Buckner RL, Andrews-Hanna JR, Schacter DL (2008) The brain's default network: anatomy, function, and relevance to disease. Ann N Y Acad Sci 1124: 1–38.
59. Honey CJ, Thivierge JP, Sporns O (2010) Can structure predict function in the human brain? Neuroimage 52: 766–776.
60. Sakai K, Miyashita Y (1991) Neural organization for the long-term memory of paired associates. Nature 354: 152–155.
61. Damasio H, Grabowski TJ, Tranel D, Hichwa RD, Damasio AR (1996) A neural basis for lexical retrieval. Nature 380: 499–505.
62. Higuchi S, Miyashita Y (1996) Formation of mnemonic neuronal responses to visual paired associates in inferotemporal cortex is impaired by perirhinal and entorhinal lesions. Proc Natl Acad Sci USA 93: 739–743.
63. Martin A, Wiggs CL, Ungerleider LG, Haxby JV (1996) Neural correlates of category-specific knowledge. Nature 379: 649–652.
64. Chao LL, Haxby JV, Martin A (1999) Attribute-based neural substrates in temporal cortex for perceiving and knowing about objects. Nature Neurosci 2: 913–919.
65. Messinger A, Squire LR, Zola SM, Albright TD (2001) Neuronal representations of stimulus associations develop in the temporal lobe during learning. Proc Natl Acad Sci USA 98: 12239–12244.
66. Tsukiura T, Fujii T, Fukatsu R, Otsuki T, Okuda J, et al. (2002) Neural basis of the retrieval of people's manes: evidence from brain-damaged patients and fMRI. J Cogn Neurosci 14: 922–937.
67. Naya Y, Yoshida M, Miyashita Y (2003) Forward processing of long-term associative memory in monkey inferotemporal cortex. J Neurosci 23: 2861–2871.
68. Takashima A, Petersson KM, Rutters F, Tendolkar I, Jensen O, et al. (2006) Declarative memory consolidation in humans: a prospective functional magnetic resonance imaging study. Proc Natl Acad Sci USA 103: 756–761.

69. Tsukiura T, Mochizuki-Kawai H, Fujii T (2006) Dissociable roles of the bilateral anterior temporal lobe in face-name associations: an event-related fMRI study. Neuroimage 30: 617–626.
70. Yamashita K, Hirose S, Kunimatsu A, Aoki S, Chikazoe J, et al. (2009) Formation of longterm memory representation in human temporal cortex related to pictorial paired associates. J Neurosci 29: 10335–10340.
71. Watanabe T, Kimura HM, Hirose S, Wada H, Imai Y, et al. (2012) Functional Dissociation between Anterior and Posterior Temporal Cortical Regions during Retrieval of Remote Memory. J Neurosci 32: 9659–9670.
72. Rugg MD, Henson RN, Robb WG (2003) Neural correlates of retrieval processing in the prefrontal cortex during recognition and exclusion tasks. Neuropsychologia 41: 40–52.
73. Hayama HR, Johnson JD, Rugg MD (2008) The relationship between the right frontal old/new ERP effect and post-retrieval monitoring: specific or non-specific? Neuropsychologia 46: 1211–1223.
74. Hayama H (2009) Functional Significance of the Neural Correlates of Post-retrieval Processing. Irvine: University of California. 254 p.
75. Hayama HR, Rugg MD (2009) Right dorsolateral prefrontal cortex is engaged during postretrieval processing of both episodic and semantic information. Neuropsychologia 47: 2409–2416.
76. Greicius MD, Krasnow B, Reiss AL, Menon V (2003) Functional connectivity in the resting brain: a network analysis of the default mode hypothesis. Proc Natl Acad Sci USA 100: 253–258.
77. Fox MD, Raichle ME (2007) Spontaneous fluctuations in brain activity observed with functional magnetic resonance imaging. Nat Rev Neurosci 8: 700–711.
78. Buckner RL, Krienen FM, Yeo BT (2013) Opportunities and limitations of intrinsic functional connectivity MRI. Nat Neurosci 16: 832–837.
79. Andrews-Hanna JR, Reidler JS, Sepulcre J, Poulin R, Buckner RL (2010) Functional-anatomic fractionation of the brain's default network. Neuron 65: 550–562.
80. Spreng RN, Sepulcre J, Turner GR, Stevens WD, Schacter DL (2013) Intrinsic Architecture Underlying the Relations among the Default, Dorsal Attention, and Fronto-parietal Control Networks of the Human Brain. J Cogn Neurosci 25: 74–86.
81. Spreng RN, Stevens WD, Chamberlain JP, Gilmore AW, Schacter DL (2010) Default network activity, coupled with the frontopari control network, supports goal-directed cognition. Neuroimage 53: 303–317.
82. Spreng RN, Schacter DL (2012) Default Network Modulation and Large-Scale Network Interactivity in Healthy Young and Old Adults. Cereb Cortex 22: 2610–2621.

9

Episodic Future Thinking in Semantic Dementia: A Cognitive and fMRI Study

Armelle Viard[1,2,3,4]*, Pascale Piolino[5,6], Serge Belliard[1,2,3,4,7], Vincent de La Sayette[1,2,3,4], Béatrice Desgranges[1,2,3,4], Francis Eustache[1,2,3,4]

1 Inserm, U1077, Caen, France, **2** Université de Caen Basse-Normandie, UMR-S1077, Caen, France, **3** Ecole Pratique des Hautes Etudes, UMR-S1077, Caen, France, **4** Centre Hospitalier Universitaire, U1077, Caen, France, **5** Université Paris Descartes, Institut de Psychologie, Memory and Cognition Lab, Paris, France, **6** Inserm UMR S894, Centre de Psychiatrie et Neurosciences, Paris, France, **7** CHU Pontchaillou, Rennes, France

Abstract

Semantic dementia (SD) is characterized by gradual loss of semantic memory. While episodic autobiographical memory seems relatively preserved, behavioral studies suggest that episodic future thinking is impaired. We used fMRI to measure brain activity in four SD patients (JPL, EP, LL, EG) while they envisioned future events and remembered personal past events. Twelve healthy elders served as controls. Episodic quality, emotion, mental imagery and level of consciousness (via remember/know judgements) were checked at debriefing. We analyzed the future compared to the past for each patient. All patients presented lateral temporal atrophy, but varied in terms of frontal and anterior hippocampal atrophy. Patient JPL presented atrophy in bilateral superior medial frontal gyri and left anterior hippocampus and was unable to engage in episodic future thinking, despite hyperactivations in frontal and occipital regions. Patient EP presented no atrophy in the anterior hippocampus, but atrophy in bilateral superior medial frontal gyrus and had difficulties to engage in episodic future thinking. Patient LL presented atrophy in left anterior hippocampus, but hyperactivated its right counterpart for future compared to past thinking, permitting her to project efficiently in the future in an episodic way. Patient EG presented no atrophy in the superior medial frontal gyri or anterior hippocampi and was able to engage in episodic future thinking. Altogether, patients' future projections differed depending on the severity and localization of their atrophy. The functional integrity of bilateral superior medial frontal gyri and anterior hippocampus appear crucial for episodic future thinking: atrophy of both structures strongly impairs future projection, while integrity of these structures or hyperactivation of residual tissue normalizes episodic future projection.

Editor: Jean-Claude Baron, INSERM U894, Centre de Psychiatrie et Neurosciences, Hopital Sainte-Anne and Université Paris 5, France

Funding: This work was supported by the University Hospital Center of Caen, Ecole Pratique de Hautes Etudes (EPHE), Fondation pour la Recherche sur le Cerveau (FRC), Inserm, UCBN (research unit U1077). The funders had no role in study design, data collection and analysis, decision to publish, or preparation of the manuscript.

Competing Interests: The authors have declared that no competing interests exist.

* Email: viard@cyceron.fr

Introduction

Semantic dementia (SD) is a variant of fronto-temporal dementia characterized by a gradual loss of semantic memory [1], with progressive anomia and deterioration of vocabulary [2]). An asymmetrical atrophy of the lateral temporal lobe is generally observed [3] with an antero-posterior gradient, the highest changes located in its anterior portion [4]. A relative preservation of episodic memory is observed [5,6], with intact recent and day-to-day memory. Episodic memory is characterized by a particular self-reflective mental state, termed autonoetic consciousness, which implies that a person recollects his/her personal events with a sense of re-experiencing, by mentally "travelling in time" in the past [7,8]. Converging lines of evidence from different fields of research indicate that remembering the past or envisioning the future share common cognitive [9,10,11] and neural underpinnings [12,13,14,15]. Indeed, past and future thinking build on similar information stored in episodic memory and rely on similar cognitive processes (i.e., self-referential processing, imagery and flexible recombination of stored details). Yet, in semantic dementia, behavioral studies have consistently shown that future thinking is impaired [16,17,18].

Duval et al. [18] examined self-representations and states of consciousness (measured via remember/know judgements) in SD patients for past, present and future periods. The future period elicited poorer performances than the past and present periods in terms of episodic self-representations and autonoetic consciousness. SD patients had difficulties in projecting themselves into the future and had an impaired level of consciousness associated to the future. These findings suggest that personal semantic memory is necessary to imagine one's future self, as confirmed by Irish et al. [16]. Indeed, Irish et al. [16] also indicated that SD patients had difficulties in episodic future simulation, despite a relative preservation of past episodic retrieval. They showed that SD patients' future thinking deficit was driven by their difficulty in providing episodic (specific) details, contrasting with elevated semantic (factual) details. SD patients' phenomenological past experiencing however (measured by subjective ratings of vividness, valence, emotional intensity, personal significance) did not differ from controls. This reveals a disconnect between objective task performances and subjective phenomenological pre-experiencing when generating future events in this population. Irish et al. [17] showed relatively intact episodic retrieval but significant impairments for episodic future thinking in their group of SD patients. Atrophy in areas of the lateral temporal cortex (left inferior temporal gyrus and bilateral temporal pole) was found to correlate with deficits in episodic future thinking. This region is known for its role in semantic processing and thus confirms previous findings that semantic knowledge is critical for the construction of novel future events [19].

Atrophy in the lateral temporal cortex is characteristic of semantic dementia and as indicated above may play a role in SD's episodic future thinking deficit, although other regions are also important (e.g., hippocampus, medial prefrontal cortex). Evidence of hippocampal atrophy is now well documented in SD, even in the early stages of the disease [20,21,22,23,24,25,26,4,27,28,29,6], although some patients were reported to have no hippocampal atrophy [30,6]. The hippocampus supports relational processing [31,32,33], including flexible recombination of details for past and future event construction [34]. Addis and Schacter [35] showed that future-associated activity in the anterior hippocampus was associated with higher demands on recombination of details. Hence, atrophy in this region may strongly affect episodic future thinking. In joint collaboration with the hippocampus, the medial prefrontal cortex is also critical in episodic future thinking. Its anterior part seems more involved in information integration and self-referential thinking, while its dorsal part has a role in generative construction [36].

Studies on future thinking in SD are scarce and no fMRI study is yet available. Neuroimaging studies on future thinking in healthy adults have shown a neural network which has striking similarities with the one recruited during episodic past remembering, including prefrontal and medial temporal cortices, medial parietal (posterior cingulate and retrosplenial cortices), posterior parietal (precuneus and temporo-parietal junction), occipital regions and the cerebellum [12,13,14,15,37,38]. We previously showed that a common network of brain regions was activated for past and future thinking in healthy older adults, reflecting the use of similar cognitive processes [19]. Our results also showed that the episodic nature of future events depended on the inferior frontal and lateral temporal gyri, involved in semantic memory retrieval.

Here, we examined episodic future thinking in four SD patients using fMRI and compared it to past remembering. A group of 12 healthy elders served as a comparison group. In the scanner, upon presentation of a cue-phrase prompting a specific past or future event (obtained by questioning a close family member), patients were asked to mentally recall specific events from the past 12 months and specific plans they intended to pursue in the next 12 months. We also collected several behavioral data to assess the degree of phenomenological (re/pre)experiencing, through ratings of episodic quality, emotional intensity, valence, mental visual imagery, level of consciousness and repetition. Beyond lateral temporal atrophy which was present in all patients and may impact episodic future thinking, each had atrophy in different regions of the episodic future thinking network. We predicted that anterior hippocampal and/or medial prefrontal atrophy would strongly impair episodic future thinking given the crucial role these regions play. We expected that, in the presence of atrophied regions within this network, different processes might arise: either activation in residual tissue, up-regulation of areas within the network or recruitment of additional brain areas.

Materials and Methods

Participants

Patient details. We studied four patients suffering from SD selected according to a codified procedure in French qualified centres by senior neurologists (VDLS & SB) whose major activity is dedicated to the diagnosis and follow-up of patients suffering from neurodegenerative disorders including semantic dementia, in addition to a neuropsychologist and a speech therapist. The four patients all presented the two core features of SD (i.e., impaired picture naming and single-word comprehension) and the three following additional criteria, as specified by Gorno-Tempini et al. [39]: impaired object knowledge, spared repetition, spared speech production (i.e., fluent) and/or surface dyslexia and severe anterior temporal atrophy (see VBM analyses). The clinical and neuropsychological follow-up of our patients, who have been re-examined between 5 to 8 years after their first consultation, has confirmed the initial diagnosis (i.e., predominant semantic memory deficits, and preserved spatial orientation and autonomy). Table 1 summarizes patients' main neuropsychological scores and z-scores. Of note, all participants were scanned within the same week as neuropsychological testing.

JPL, a 62-year-old right-handed male retired cutter with 10 years of formal education, was seen at the University Hospital Center of Caen in November 2006. JPL reported progressive memory loss, particularly involving remembering peoples' names or familiar places, difficulty in word-finding and impaired object knowledge (e.g., he would eat an orange without pealing it). His wife reported a tendency to irritability, lack of initiative and poor conversational interactions, but his day-to-day memory and spatial orientation were preserved. As a leisure activity, he played sudoku. On formal neuropsychological testing, JPL showed relatively well preserved episodic memory (good free recall, but impaired immediate recall) as measured by a procedure derived from the Grober and Buschke test [40] (see Table S9 in File S1 for brief explanation of this test and what it measures). Visuospatial abilities were good as measured by copying and delayed recall of the Rey complex figure [41]. He scored poorly on semantic memory tests, as measured by category (names of animals) and letter (words beginning by letter p) fluency tasks [42] (see Table S9 in File S1 for brief explanation of this test and what it measures). On the Semantic Knowledge Task [43] (see Table S9 in File S1 for brief explanation of this test and what it measures), he was impaired for picture naming and object knowledge, as shown by his difficulty in providing specific attributes of words. He was impaired at recognizing famous faces on the French Celebrities Questionnaire [44] (see Table S9 in File S1 for brief explanation of this test and what it measures). He performed poorly on the Mill Hill test [45], a multiple-choice synonym vocabulary questionnaire which assesses verbal knowledge. His language abilities were tested with the LEXIS battery [46] (see Table S9 in File S1 for brief explanation of this test and what it measures). He produced semantic paraphasias and presented difficulties in picture naming, word-finding, word definitions (e.g., watermelon, deer, hammock, city hall...) and single-word comprehension (e.g., when asked "what is the capital of France?", he would answer: "what does capital mean?" or when asked "in which country is Venice?", he would answer, "what is Venice?"). His speech production was fluent. Repetition, reading of a text and its restitution were spared. He presented no deficit on the Trail Making Test [47].

EP, a 77-year-old right-handed female retired general practitioner with 20 years of formal education, was seen at the University Hospital Center of Caen in April 2008. EP reported difficulties in word-finding and word comprehension, especially

Table 1. Scores on neuropsychological tests for patients JPL, EP, LL, and EG.

Neuropsychological tests	HE (mean ± s.d.)	JPL	z-score	EP	z-score	LL	z-score	EG	z-score
Episodic memory									
Grober and Buschke									
Immediate recall (/16)	15.42±0.99	**12**	**−3.455**	16	0.586	16	0.586	16	0.586
Free recall (/48)	31.75±5.36	24	−1.446	31	−0.140	29	−0.513	30	−0.326
Total recall (/48)	46.67±1.92	**38**	**−4.516**	47	0.172	48	0.693	47	0.172
Delayed recall (/16)	11±2.22	9	−0.901	14	1.351	**6**	**−2.252**	8	−1.351
Rey complex figure									
Copy (sec)	33.90±2.44	36	0.875	36	0.875	36	0.875	33	−0.375
Recall (sec)	16.93±7.33	25	1.101	18	0.146	10.5	−0.877	20	0.419
Semantic memory									
Fluency tasks									
Category fluency (/2 min)	32.64+/−7.9	**17**	**−1.980**	**9**	**−2.992**	**16**	**−2.106**	**9**	**−2.992**
Letter fluency (/2 min)	23.78+/−8.35	**7**	**−2.010**	26	0.266	**8**	**−1.890**	**5**	**−2.249**
Semantic Knowledge Task									
Picture naming (/36)	36+/−0.0	**30**	**pathological**	**32**	**pathological**	**35**	**pathological**	NA	-
Superordinate category (/54)	54+/−0.0	54	OK	54	OK	54	OK	NA	-
Specific attributes (/54)	54+/−0.0	**49**	**pathological**	**50**	**pathological**	**50**	**pathological**	NA	-
BECS-GRECO Semantic Battery									
Words/40)	39.4+/−0.9	NA	-	NA	-	NA	-	**22**	**−19.33**
Pictures (/40)	39.2+/−0.9	NA	-	NA	-	NA	-	**37**	**−2.44**
French celebrities questionnaire (%)	100+/−3.0	**39.1**	**−19.96**		NA	**34.8**	**−21.4**	**2.5**	**−31.17**
Mill Hill (/33)	25.64±5.84	**16**	**−1.651**	29	OK	20	OK	29	OK
Language									
Speech production	NA	Fluent		Fluent		Fluent		Fluent	
Repetition	NA	OK		OK		OK		OK	
Reading	NA	OK		OK		OK		OK	
LEXIS battery									
Picture naming (/80)	72.8±3.28	**55**	**−5.427**	**60**	**−3.902**	NA	-	**47**	**−7.866**
Picture naming (/64)	58.5±3.21	NA	-	NA	-	**47**	**−3.583**	NA	-
Executive functions									
TMT B-A (sec)	76±64	30	−0.719	35	−0.641	63	−0.203	66	−0.156
Other									
MMSE (/30)	28.42±1.38	27	−1.029	29	0.420	**25**	**−2.478**	28	−0.304

Table 1. Cont.

Neuropsychological tests	HE (mean ± s.d.)	JPL	z-score	EP	z-score	LL	z-score	EG	z-score
GDS (/30)	4.83±3.04	7	0.714	5	0.056	9	1.372	7	0.714
Mattis (/144)	142.17±1.34	**132**	**−7.590**	144	1.366	141	−0.873	**120**	**−16.545**

Tests: BECS GRECO Semantic Battery: Merck et al. (2011); French celebrities questionnaire: Belliard et al. (2001); GDS: Yesavage et al. (1983); Grober and Buschke (1987); Mill Hill test: Deltour (1993); Mattis: dementia rating scale (Mattis, 1976); MMSE: Mini-Mental Status Exam (Folstein et al., 1975); Rey complex figure: Rey (1970); Semantic Knowledge Task: Desgranges et al. (1996); Picture naming: LEXIS (de Partz, 2001); TMT: Trail Making Test (Reitan, 1958).
Note: The Semantic Knowledge Task was proposed to patients from Caen (JPL, EP, LL); the BECS GRECO Semantic Battery was proposed to the patient from Rennes (EG). On the Semantic Knowledge Task, performances had to be maximum to be considered unimpaired (i.e., standard deviation in control group equals zero). Hence, if patients did not obtain the maximum score, their performance was impaired (noted "pathological" in the Table). The French celebrities questionnaire was not proposed to EP at the time she participated in this fMRI study.
Results were considered as significant when $z > \pm 1.96$, $p < 0.05$. Pathological scores appear in bold and when no standard deviation was available, pathological performances were noted "pathological" in bold. HE = healthy elders; OK = performance not significantly different from healthy elders; NA = not available.

animal names and geographic locations which she once knew well. She had impaired object knowledge (e.g., for EP, zebras live in French prairies; salads and carrots grow in forests). She continued to have stimulating intellectual activities by reading and attending university senior courses, although she complained not being able to learn efficiently. She was autonomous in daily life and her day-to-day memory was preserved. On formal neuropsychological testing, EP showed relatively well preserved episodic memory on the Grober and Buschke test. Visuospatial abilities were good as measured by copying and delayed recall of the Rey complex figure. Given her high level of education, she scored poorly on semantic memory, as measured by category fluency tasks (names of animals). She produced errors on picture naming and on object knowledge, as shown by her difficulty in providing specific attributes of words on the Semantic Knowledge Task. She performed well on the Mill Hill vocabulary test. Her language abilities, tested with the LEXIS battery, confirmed her difficulties in picture naming. She produced paraphasias (semantic, visual, visuo-semantic), had difficulties on single-word comprehension and in providing word definitions (zebra, hippopotamus, elephant, kiwi…), with many specific attributes being lost. Her speech production was fluent. Repetition and reading were spared. She presented no deficit on the TMT.

LL, a 73-year-old right-handed female retired secretary with 9 years of formal education, was seen at the University Hospital Center of Caen in September 2007. LL reported difficulties in word-finding, object knowledge (e.g., she will cook cucumber and radish; she will put sugar on avocados) and recognizing people. She was fond of logical games (e.g., sudoku). She was autonomous in daily life and her day-to-day memory was preserved. On formal neuropsychological testing, LL had preserved episodic memory (on immediate and free recalls) on the Grober and Buschke test. Visuospatial abilities were good as measured by copying and delayed recall of the Rey complex figure. She scored poorly on semantic memory tests, both on category (names of animals) and letter (words beginning by letter p) fluency tasks. She produced errors on picture naming and on object knowledge (difficulty in providing specific attributes of words) on the Semantic Knowledge Task. She was impaired at recognizing famous faces on the French Celebrities Questionnaire. She performed well on the Mill Hill vocabulary test. Her language abilities, tested with the LEXIS battery confirmed her difficulties in picture naming. She also showed difficulties on single-word comprehension and made errors on word definitions (e.g., bull, kangourou, harp, volcano…). Her speech production was fluent. Repetition, reading of a text and its restitution were spared. She presented no deficit on the TMT.

EG, a 62-year-old right-handed female retired secretary with 9 years of formal education, was seen at the University Hospital Center of Rennes in October 2008. EG reported difficulties in word-finding, names of places and recognizing people. She also showed oral and written comprehension difficulties. Her spatial orientation was good and she mentioned that she frequently consulted atlases to resituate her trip itineraries. She was autonomous in daily life and her day-to-day memory was preserved. Her leisure activities consisted in playing with logical games (e.g., sudoku, video games). On formal neuropsychological testing, EG showed preserved episodic memory (on immediate, free and delayed recalls) on the Grober and Buschke test. Visuospatial abilities were good as measured by copying and delayed recall of the Rey complex figure. She scored poorly on semantic memory tests, both on category (names of animals) and letter (words beginning by letter p) fluency tasks. Being a patient from Rennes (not Caen, like the three other patients), clinicians there proposed the BECS GRECO Semantic Battery [48] to EG, instead of the Semantic Knowledge Task. On the BECS GRECO Semantic Battery, she was impaired on single-word comprehension (difficulty on semantic matching of words) and on object knowledge (difficulty on semantic matching of pictures). She was extremely impaired at recognizing famous faces on the French Celebrities Questionnaire. She presented surface dyslexia (e.g., baptism; note that in French, the [p] is not pronounced). She performed well on the Mill Hill vocabulary test. Her language abilities, tested with the LEXIS battery), confirmed her difficulties in picture naming. Her speech production was fluent. Repetition and reading were spared. She presented no deficit on the TMT.

For all patients, an indicator of disease severity was obtained with the Mini-Mental Status Exam [49] (MMSE; total score/30) which assesses both comprehension and expression abilities through eight different questions. The MMSE has already been used as an indicator of disease severity. Matuszewski et al. [50] subdivided their two groups of SD patients into a mild group (mean score on the MMSE of 26±1.91) and a moderate group (mean score of 21.29±1.07). Based on the MMSE (see Table 1), the four patients (JPL = 27; EP = 29; LL = 25; EG = 28) show high scores, indicative of an early stage of dementia (i.e., mild stage). Note that all patients were autonomous in daily life. Global cognitive functioning was assessed via the Mattis dementia rating scale [51] (total score/144; see Table S9 in File S1 for brief explanation of this test and what it measures). Signs of depression were estimated with the Geriatric Depression Scale [52] (GDS; total score/30). Table 1 summarizes patients' neuropsychological scores and z-scores according to normative data provided for each test.

Healthy elders. Twelve right-handed healthy elders (females, mean age ± s.d. = 67.2±5.2 years; ranging from 60 to 75 years old), mean years of education (11.42±2.81), with no history of psychiatric or neurological disorder were recruited through a senior university, a retirement association or a newspaper advertisement. Participants had no abnormality on their T_1-weighted high-resolution magnetic resonance imaging (MRI). They underwent a battery of neuropsychological tests to assess their cognitive abilities and all performed in the normal range (see Viard et al. [53] for a full description). Each participant resided at home and all were active in cultural pursuits, continuing education or with responsibilities in diverse associations.

The study was approved by the Regional Ethics Committee of Lower Normandy and written informed consent was obtained from all participants prior to their participation in the study. Patients understood the experiment and had full capacity to consent (i.e., no surrogate consent procedure was needed). Data on healthy elders were obtained as part of a broader experiment exploring five past periods previously published [53,54] and a future period [19]. These healthy subjects were scanned with the intention to be compared with the patients. Results of two SD patients (JPL and EP) on a task exploring episodic autobiographical memory retrieval over five past periods have been published previously [6]. Here, we present new results concerning four SD patients on the episodic future thinking task and compare them to the group of healthy elders. Of note, given the rarity of patients with semantic dementia, we were not able to perfectly match each patient to the control group. This group of healthy elders can nonetheless serve as a comparison group to our patients, given that disparities have been controlled for by adding covariates (age and years of education) in statistical analyses (see below).

Task and experimental design

Autobiographical memories from the last 12 months and future plans scheduled in the next 12 months were obtained through an interview with a close family member a week before the scanning session. The family member, in most cases the spouse, was close enough to provide specific personal past memories of the participant and actual future plans that the participant intended to pursue (i.e., events were not made up by family members, but corresponded to actual past or future events in the participant's life). Among events provided by the family member, only those which corresponded to specific (i.e., episodic) events, unique in time and space, were selected. Before scanning, participants were familiarized with the task in a training phase outside of the scanner, using different events than in the experimental task. Special care was taken to explain to the patients the tasks they had to perform. The instructions given to participants for the past period were as follows: "You will see on the screen short sentences which refer to specific past events which happened to you in the last 12 months, followed by a black screen. Press on the button as soon as you can access a specific personal past event, which lasted less than 24 hours, related to the cue and think about all the details that come to mind, until the cross appears. Try to remember the event as if you were reliving it." The instructions given to participants for the future period were as follows: "You will see on the screen short sentences which refer to future plans which you intend to pursue in the next 12 months, followed by a black screen. Press on the button as soon as you can access a specific personal future event, which will last less than 24 hours, related to the cue and think about all the details that come to mind, until the cross appears. Try to envision the event as if you were living it in advance." In the scanner, personal sentence-cues were presented visually in white on a black background, using Superlab software (3.0 version, Cedrus). During the whole experiment, participants were asked to keep their eyes open to be able to read the sentence cues. Upon presentation of the visual cue, participants were instructed to recall or envision a specific detailed event, unique in time and space, that had either occurred in the past 12 months (past period) or was scheduled in the next 12 months (future period). For both past and future events, they were asked to experience the event with as much details as possible. Past and future events were sufficiently different to refrain participants from simply recalling a similar past event when instructed to envision a future event. Two functional runs, one per period, each lasting 5 minutes, were composed of 5 experimental (i.e., 5 events) and 5 control blocks, randomly intermixed across subjects. In the experimental condition, one block consisted of a sentence-cue (5 s) followed by a blank screen (19 s) during which participants had to mentally experience the corresponding specific personal event (e.g., past: "my grandson's last birthday party"; future: "my fifty-third wedding anniversary"). In total, they had to recall five episodic past events and envision five episodic future events. They were asked to press on a button as soon as they gained access to the prompted event. In the control condition, participants were asked to detect the presence of two consecutive letters ("mb") in pseudo-words of six letters (for example, "speugr" or "mbieha") and were instructed to press on a button when "mb" was present in the pseudo-word. Five pseudowords were presented in each control block, each lasting 24 seconds (1 second for cue presentation, followed by 3.8 seconds for the response). All participants were scanned on the same scanner (1.5 tesla) at the University Hospital Center of Caen.

Following the scanning session, the debriefing took place (mean duration = 2,5 hours) in order to verify participants' engagement in the tasks and to identify the nature of the evocations experienced during scanning. Participants were asked to retrieve the five past and five future events again, using the same sentence-cues as in the scanner, but this time aloud in order to check that the events corresponded to the expected cued events and to assess their episodic nature (i.e., specificity and detail). Their episodic nature (or "episodicity") was estimated 1) with "objective" measures, using a 5-point scale (generating overall autobiographical and strictly episodic scores; see below) and 2) with "subjective" measures, by collecting participants' ratings on several behavioral scales (evaluating emotion, mental imagery, level of consciousness and effect of repetition; see below).

First, the specificity of each evocation was measured by the investigators (objective measurement of episodicity) using a fine-grained 5-point scale (0-1-2-3-4) similar to previous episodic scales used with healthy subjects and patients with cerebral diseases [55,56,57,58,59,50,53,19,6]. This scale takes into account the specificity of the content (single or repeated event), the spatiotemporal situation and the presence of details (perceptions, thoughts, feelings). A specific event, situated in time and space, with sensory details is given a score of 4. A specific event with few details, but situated in time and space, scores 3. A generic event (repeated or prolonged over time, situated in time and space) scores 2. A vague event (repeated or prolonged over time, not situated in time and space) scores 1. Absence of memory, or general information about a theme, scores 0 (see Table S10 in File S1). Two different total scores are obtained per period. First, the overall autobiographical score (AS: maximum score per period $4\times5=20$) includes all the events (specific and generic) and corresponds to the classic episodic memory score used in the well-known Autobiographical Memory Interview [56] (AMI). The AS score is expressed in terms of ratio (i.e., scores obtained for each of the five events per period were summed and divided by the maximum score per period which is 20). Second, the strictly episodic score (ES: maximum score per period $4\times5=20$) includes only the number of specific and detailed events scoring 4, using a more stringent criterion. ES is expressed in terms of ratio of strictly episodic events per period (i.e., number of strictly episodic events divided by the number of retrieved events). Two independent experts rated each event recalled at debriefing and any difference of opinion between them was discussed until a consensus was reached. A final score was calculated based on the number of episodic (past or future) events experienced by participants in the scanner (e.g., since EP experienced one episodic future event, her score was of one for the future; see Table 2).

Second, subjective measures of episodicity were used to specify the different aspects of the recollective experience. Participants rated their own evocations on several behavioral scales (10-cm lines; self-ratings) known to be crucial to control the degree of episodic (re/pre)experiencing. Emotion is an important phenomenological characteristic of vivid and persistent personal events [60]. Thus, participants were asked to rate their evocations on scales measuring emotional intensity (0 = no emotion to 10 = very strong emotion) and valence (0 = very negative to 10 = very positive). Visual mental imagery is known to increase the recall of specific details [61,62,63]. Several scales were used to measure mental visual imagery: mental strategy used (0 = verbal to 10 = visual), number of images (0 = no images to 10 = over 10 images), image quality (0 = very blurry to 10 = very clear) and perspective of mental images [64] ("field" or "observer" perspectives). Regarding perspective, three choices were proposed: observer (0), field and observer (1) or field (2). The autonoetic and noetic levels of consciousness, which characterize episodic and semantic memory respectively, can be distinguished by the remember or know (R/K) paradigm. Participants were asked to rate their evocations on a scale measuring the level of consciousness between the autonoetic and noetic states (scale range from 0 = knowing to 10 = remembering). Unlike the "knowing" state, the "remembering" state is characterized by phenomenal elements associated with (re/pre)experiencing of specific events (visual images, sensations, feelings). For the future, a "Remember" response indicates that the participant was able to pre-experience future events in advance. Recent reactivation (i.e., was an event evoked recently or not) was evaluated using two scales: (1) the frequency of rehearsal scale (0 = never to 10 = very frequent), to determine how frequently an event was rehearsed, prior to scanning and (2) the last recall scale (0 = today to 10 = over 10 years ago), to determine when each event was last recalled. Unfortunately, for JPL, subjective rating scales for the future are not available due to lost material. However, the subjective rating scales for the past and objective measures for both periods are available.

MRI data acquisition

A blocked functional MRI design was used. Lying in the scanner, participants viewed the display via a mirror to an active matrix video projector. Stimulus onset was synchronized with the acquisition of the first slice. Anatomical and functional MRIs were acquired on a General Electrics Signa 1.5 tesla MRI scanner (GE, BUC, France). First, a high-resolution T1-weighted MRI scan (T1-MRI) was acquired with a three-dimensional inversion recovery spoiled gradient echo sequence (matrix size = $256\times256\times128$; slice thickness = 1.5 mm). Second, a proton density/T2-weighted MRI scan (PD-MRI, T2-MRI) was acquired with 32 axial slices covering the entire brain and the superior part of the cerebellum (slice thickness = 3.8 mm). Finally, functional images were acquired with echo planar imaging blood oxygen level dependent (BOLD) sequence (repetition time = 6 s, echo time = 60 ms, flip angle = 90°, matrix size = $64\times64\times32$, 50 volumes, 3.8-mm-thick slices) covering the same field of view as the T2-MRI acquisition.

Construction of an old-adult template

Using voxel-based morphometry [65] (VBM5), each individual T1-MRIs of healthy elders were segmented according to the unified segmentation procedure [66] with spatial normalization included. Mean templates were calculated based on the individual segmented and normalized T1-MRIs, creating three separate old-adult templates according to tissue type (e.g. grey and white matters, cerebro-spinal fluid) which were then spatially smoothed using an 8-mm^3 full width at half maximum (FWHM) Gaussian kernel.

Functional image pre-processing

Functional images were processed and analyzed using the Statistical Parametric Mapping software (SPM5; Wellcome Trust Centre for Neuroimaging, London, United Kingdom; http://www.fil.ion.ucl.ac.uk/spml). The first six volumes of the functional acquisition were discarded, allowing for signal stabilization, and differences in slice acquisition timing were corrected. Images were realigned to correct for interscan movement with the creation of resliced mean functional volumes (mean-fMRI). For inter-modalities registration, rigid registration matrices (mean-fMRI onto T2-MRI, PD-MRI onto T1-MRI, T1-MRI onto the old-adult template) were computed, combined and then applied to fMRI volumes. Individual T1-MRIs were then segmented using the old-adult templates as priors (obtained previously, one for each tissue type; see above) and normalized. In order to set the fMRI volumes into our old-adult space, functional MRI images were resampled using the normalization parameters obtained in the segmentation step. Finally, data were spatially smoothed with an 8-mm^3 FWHM Gaussian kernel.

Table 2. Behavioral ratings for patients JPL, EP, LL, EG and healthy elders (HE) and t values comparing each patient to the control group for each period.

	HE		JPL		EP		LL		EG	
	Past	**Future**	**Past**	**Future**	**Past**	**Future**	**Past**	**Future**	**Past**	**Future**
Episodic scores										
AS score										
Mean ± sd	3.73 (±0.41)	3.17 (±0.57)	3.00	1.20	3.60	2.40	3.80	3.60	3.40	2.60
T			−1.71	**−3.32**	−0.31	−1.29	0.16	0.73	−0.77	−0.96
ES score										
Mean ± sd	3.20 (±1.08)	1.73 (±1.31)	0.80	0.00	2.40	0.80	3.20	2.40	2.40	0.00
T			−2.14	−1.27	−0.71	−0.68	0.00	0.49	−0.71	−1.27
Nb episodic events										
Mean ± sd	4.75 (±0.45)	4.00 (±1.16)	4.00	1.00	5.00	1.00	5.00	4.00	4.00	3.00
t			−1.59	−2.48	0.53	−2.48	0.53	0.00	−1.59	−0.83
Emotion										
Intensity										
Mean ± sd	5.10 (±1.59)	4.80 (±1.72)	8.73	NA	9.50	9.50	2.72	2.66	5.65	2.15
T			2.20	-	**2.66**	**2.63**	−1.44	−1.20	0.33	−1.48
Valence										
Mean ± sd	6.57 (±1.26)	6.75 (±1.05)	8.88	NA	7.80	9.00	6.32	5.70	7.90	4.20
t			1.76	-	0.94	2.06	−0.19	−0.96	1.02	−2.34
Imagery										
Mental strategy										
Mean ± sd	8.65 (±1.83)	8.86 (±1.69)	8.14	NA	10.00	10.00	9.26	5.54	9.30	6.93
t			−0.27	-	0.71	0.65	0.32	−1.89	0.34	−1.10
Image number										
Mean ± sd	5.06 (±2.12)	3.72 (±1.49)	0.80	NA	10.00	10.00	4.40	2.40	1.75	1.50
T			−1.93	-	2.24	**4.06**	−0.30	−0.85	−1.50	−1.43
Image quality										
Mean ± sd	9.13 (±1.25)	8.57 (±1.69)	9.10	NA	9.50	5.00	9.28	6.14	8.25	6.95
T			−0.02	-	0.28	−2.03	0.12	−1.38	−0.68	−0.92
Perspective										
Mean ± sd	1.40 (±0.59)	1.22 (±0.74)	0.42	NA	1.00	1.00	1.00	1.20	2.00	0.00
t			−1.60	-	−0.65	−0.29	−0.65	−0.03	0.98	−1.59
Consciousness										
R/K										
Mean ± sd	9.38 (±0.61)	6.28 (±3.47)	9.56	NA	9.90	5.00	9.24	3.22	9.23	4.15
t			0.28	-	0.82	−0.35	−0.22	−0.85	−0.24	−0.59

Table 2. Cont.

	HE		JPL		EP		LL		EG	
	Past	Future	Past	Future	Past	Future	Past	Future	Past	Future
Repetition										
Rehearsal frequency										
Mean ± sd	5.51 (±1.99)	4.39 (±2.02)	5.82	NA	0.00	9.50	6.32	4.38	3.10	3.90
t			0.15	-	**−2.66**	2.43	0.39	0.00	−1.17	−0.23
Last recall										
Mean ± sd	1.61 (±0.89)	1.46 (±1.49)	0.48	NA	0.50	1.00	2.82	1.82	3.93	4.18
t			−1.22	-	−1.20	−0.30	1.31	0.23	2.50	1.75

Note: Behavioral scales range from 0 to 10 for emotional intensity (0 = no emotion to 10 = very strong emotion), emotional valence (0 = very negative to 10 = very positive), mental strategy used (0 = verbal to 10 = visual), number of mental visual images (0 = no images to 10 = over 10 images), mental visual image quality (0 = very blurry to 10 = very clear, state of consciousness (0 = knowing to 10 = remembering), rehearsal frequency (0 = never to 10 = very frequent), last recall (0 = today to 10 = over 10 years ago). For the perspective, the maximum score is 2 (0 = observer; 1 = field and observer; 2 = field). Results were considered as significant (in bold) when t> ±2.576, p<0.01. AS = autobiographical score; ES = strictly episodic autobiographical score; NA = not available; Nb = number; sd = standard deviation; t = t statistic.

Data analyses

Behavioral data analysis. An adjusted t-test intended for single case analyses [67] was used for comparisons between each patient and healthy elders (for autobiographical scores and behavioral scales). Within-subject differences across past and future conditions were conducted using the modified t test [68] which assesses whether the difference between past and future periods in each patient differs significantly from the control group pattern. Results were considered significant at a conservative threshold of $t > \pm 2.576$, $p < 0.01$ to guard against Type 1 errors for multiple comparisons.

VBM analyses. In order to formally assess the extent of atrophy in each SD patient across the whole brain, we compared their structural MRI scans with those of the group of 12 healthy elders using voxel-based morphometry [66] (VBM5). Structural MRI images were analyzed using the optimised VBM procedure implemented in SPM5. Briefly, this involves a number of fully automated preprocessing steps including extraction of brain, spatial normalization into stereotactic (MNI) space, segmentation into grey and white matters and CSF compartments, correction for volume changes induced by spatial normalization (modulation), and smoothing with a 8-mm^3 FWHM isotropic Gaussian kernel. The preprocessing procedures used in SPM5 have been shown to produce good results when matching brains with lesions to standardised templates [69]. We used the optional "modulation of non-linear effects only" which takes into account intracranial volume, hence controlling for differences in brain sizes. Analyses focussed on grey matter. Each patient's structural scan was compared to healthy elders' scans using a two sample t-test to investigate differences in grey matter volume. The significance level was set at $p < 0.05$ FWE corrected for multiple comparisons, $k > 50$ voxels (see Tables S2 to S5 in File S1).

fMRI data analyses. fMRI time series were modelled by a general linear model (GLM) including separate regressors for each of the experimental (past and future periods) and control conditions using SPM5. All regressors were convolved with the canonical hemodynamic response function (HRF). Data were high-pass filtered (cut-off period = 96 s). Coefficients for each regressor were estimated for each participant using maximum likelihood estimates to account for serial correlations in the data. At the first level, linear contrasts of the parameter estimates for each experimental regressor of interest were calculated for each participant, subtracting the corresponding control regressor (resulting in "period minus control task" contrasts). To examine the future thinking network in each patient at the individual level, t-statistic maps were generated for the following contrasts of interest: future minus control task and future minus past period (subtracting for each period the corresponding control regressor) for each participant. The second level random effects analysis was conducted over contrast images obtained at the first level. Each patient was compared to the group of healthy elders (i.e., patients were not grouped together) using the two sample t-test model of SPM5, as recommended by Henson's guidelines (2006; http://www.mrc-cbu.cam.ac.uk//personal/rik.henson/personal/Henson_Singlecase_06.pdf) and previously used to report single case fMRI data, notably in semantic dementia [70,6]. Inter-group subtraction analyses were computed to determine which regions were differentially activated by each patient and healthy elders when comparing past and future periods. The significance level was set at $p < 0.05$ FWE corrected for multiple comparisons, $k > 10$ voxels. Coordinates of brain regions are reported in the MNI space. To control for the age difference between patients and healthy elders, age was included as covariate. EP's duration of education was higher compared to healthy elders. Since education and general intelligence are generally closely inter-related [71], variations due to differences in general intelligence between EP and healthy elders were controlled for by adding years of education as covariate for analyses comparing EP to healthy elders. Finally, to reveal pathophysiological properties of the future thinking brain network in each patient using a different method, plots of activation magnitude were obtained for each patient and average of healthy elders in several regions of interest (ROIs) of the conventional future thinking network (medial frontal gyrus, hippocampus, precuneus). For each participant, mean activation values corresponding to the difference in BOLD activation between the experimental (future period) and control tasks (for Figure S1: control task; for Figure S2: past period; see File S1), were extracted within each ROI using the "anatomical VOI analysis" of the fMRIroi SPM toolbox [54].

Results

Behavioral results

All patients were able to perform the tasks, both recalling past memories and envisioning future events, differences lay in the episodic nature of the events experienced. On the objective measures of episodicity, JPL and EP were able to pre-experience only one episodic future event (rated 3 or 4 on the episodic scale) and four semantic future events (rated 1 or 2). On the contrary, LL was able to pre-experience four episodic future events and one semantic future event. EG was able to pre-experience three episodic future events and two semantic future events. Of note, despite using verbal cues, all patients were all able to read and understand the cues.

Comparisons between each patient and healthy elders showed, on the objective measures of episodicity, significantly lower overall autobiographical score (AS) for the future and a trend for the strictly episodic score (ES) for the past for JPL (see Table 2). Based on the number of episodic events experienced, a trend showed that JPL and EP produced less episodic future events compared to healthy elders. On the subjective rating scales, main results indicated that emotional intensity was greater for the past and the future for EP compared to healthy elders. Concerning mental imagery, EP evoked a greater number of mental images for the future compared to healthy elders, although a trend showed that image quality of future mental images was less clear for EP compared to healthy elders. Within-subject comparisons, using the modified t test procedure [68], did not reveal statistical differences between past and future conditions for each patient (data not shown). Note that adding education as covariate in behavioral analyses for EP, following Crawford et al.'s [72] guidelines, did not change results (see Table S1 in File S1).

VBM results

Results depicted on Figure 1 and Tables S2 to S5 in File S1 reveal areas of grey matter volume loss in JPL, EP, LL and EG compared to healthy elders. All patients present lateral temporal atrophy, predominantly in its anterior portion (see Tables S2 to S5 in File S1). Of the four patients, three have predominant left-lateralized temporal atrophy (JPL, LL, EG) and EP has predominant right-lateralized temporal atrophy. JPL also presented atrophy in the left anterior hippocampus, left amygdala and frontal regions, in particular bilateral superior medial gyri.

Apart from predominantly right-lateralized temporal atrophy, EP also presented atrophy in frontal, in particular bilateral superior medial gyri and parietal regions (bilateral supramarginal, left inferior gyri) (see Table S3). EP showed preservation of anterior hippocampi.

Apart from predominantly left-lateralized temporal atrophy, LL also presented atrophy in left anterior hippocampus, left amygdala and bilateral inferior frontal gyri (see Table S4).

Apart from predominantly left-lateralized temporal atrophy, EG also presented atrophy in frontal regions (bilateral superior, left medial, bilateral inferior gyri) (see Table S5).

Strikingly, VBM analyses reveal that the two patients (JPL and EP) who have difficulties in envisioning the future in an episodic way present atrophy in bilateral superior medial frontal gyri which appears preserved in patients (LL and EG) who can project in the future in an episodic manner. Furthermore, the (left) anterior hippocampus, which is atrophied in JPL (and LL) may additionally explain his difficulties in episodic future projection (LL appears to compensate for this atrophy by hyperactivating the right anterior hippocampus, see below).

fMRI results

Patient JPL. At the individual level, results for the contrast future minus control task for JPL showed an essentially left-lateralized network of regions comprising the left (inferior, middle, superior) frontal gyri, middle temporal gyrus, precuneus, occipital areas and cerebellum (see Table S6). Results for the contrast future minus past period for JPL did not reveal any activation at the given threshold (see Table S7).

At the group level, the past period showed greater activations for JPL than healthy elders mainly in the left middle and inferior frontal gyri, bilateral cuneus and left insula compared to the control task (see Table 3). The future period showed greater activations for JPL than healthy elders mainly in the left calcarine sulcus, inferior and medial frontal gyri compared to the control task (see Table 4, Figure 2). Plots of activation magnitude confirm this medial frontal hyperactivation in JPL compared to healthy elders (see Figure S1). The past period showed greater activations for JPL, compared to healthy elders, in the right middle temporal gyrus compared to the future period (see Table 5). The future period showed no significant activations compared to the past period. No regions were less active in JPL compared to healthy elders.

Patient EP. At the individual level, results for the contrast future minus control task for EP showed activation in the right precuneus (see Table S6). No activation was detected for the contrast future minus past period (see Table S7).

At the group level, the past period showed greater activations for EP than healthy elders in the left middle occipital and precentral gyri compared to the control task (see Table 3). No regions were less active in EP compared to healthy elders for this contrast.

The future period showed greater activations for EP than healthy elders in the right middle temporal gyrus compared to the control task (see Table 4, Figure 2). EP showed less activation than healthy elders in the left superior occipital gyrus and right insula for the future period compared to the control task (see Table 4, Figure 2).

The past period revealed greater activations for EP than healthy elders in left middle frontal gyrus compared to the future period (see Table 5). No regions were less active in EP compared to healthy elders for this contrast.

Conversely, the future period showed greater activations in EP than healthy elders in the left parietal gyrus compared to the past period (see Table 6, Figure 3). No regions were less active in EP compared to healthy elders for this contrast.

Patient LL. At the individual level, results for the contrast future minus control task for LL showed activation in the left supplementary motor area (see Table S6). Compared to the past

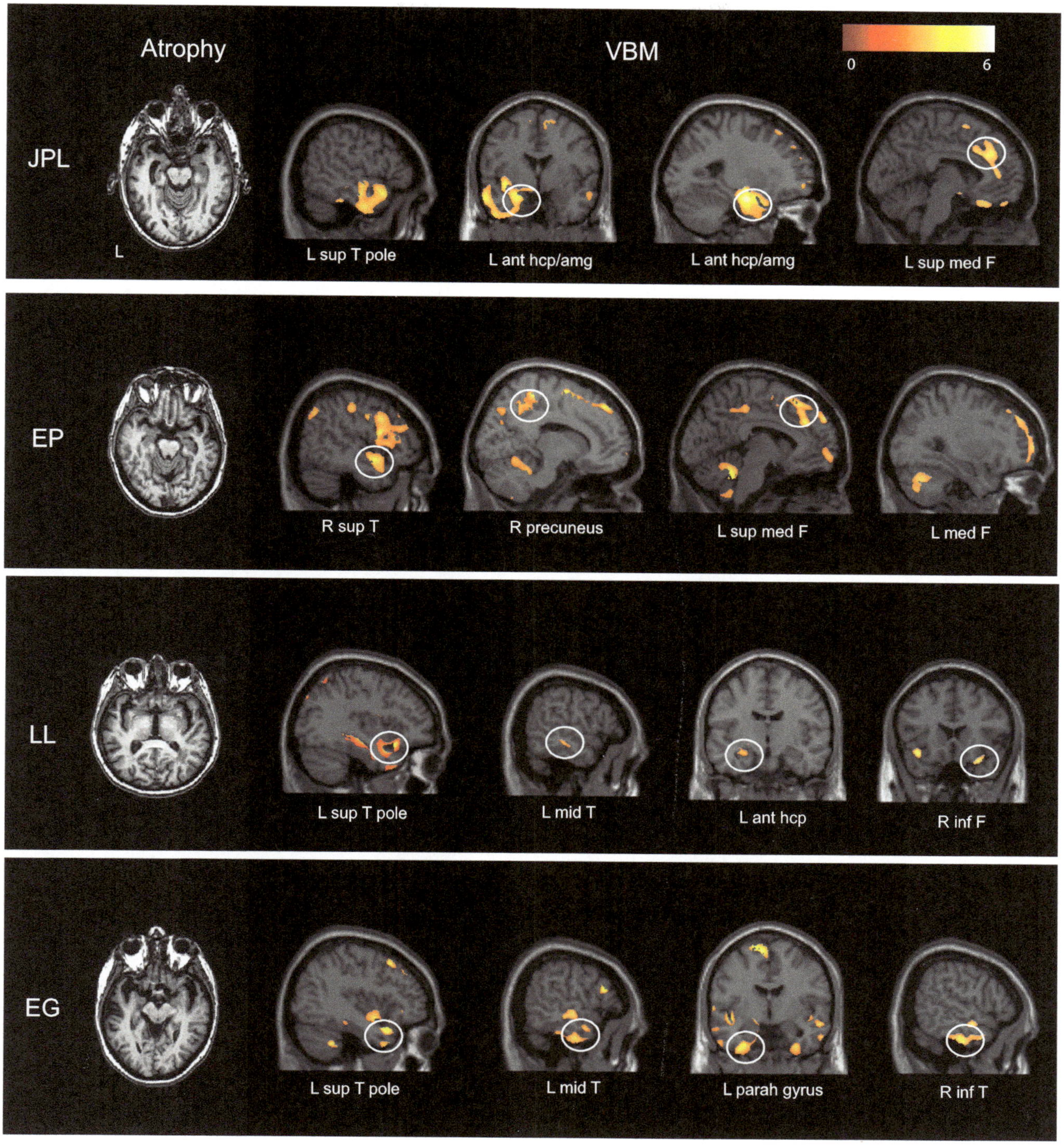

Figure 1. Structural brain scans of the four SD patients. Left panels show coronal sections through the brains of JPL, EP, LL and EG. Right panels show results of the VBM analysis superimposed on MRI scans for each patient at a corrected FWE threshold of $p<0.05$. The pronounced atrophy in superior medial frontal regions is apparent for JPL and EP and atrophy in left anterior hippocampus apparent for JPL and LL. Color scale shows voxel z-scores. See Tables S2 to S5 in File S1 for detailed VBM results. Abbreviations: amg = amygdala; ant = anterior; F = frontal; hcp = hippocampus; inf = inferior; L = left; med = medial; mid = middle; parah = parahippocampal; R = right; sup = superior; T = temporal.

period, the future period showed hyperactivation in the right middle occipital and supramarginal gyri (see Table S7).

At the group level, the past period showed greater activations for LL than healthy elders mainly in the bilateral middle temporal gyri, left middle and inferior frontal gyri, right cuneus and left caudate compared to the control task (see Table 3). LL showed less activation than healthy elders in essentially the right anterior hippocampus, left parahippocampal gyrus, lateral temporal and occipital gyri for the past period compared to the control task (see Table 3).

The future period revealed greater activations for LL than healthy elders mainly in the right supramarginal and left superior

Table 3. Results for the comparisons past>control task for JPL, EP, LL, EG compared to healthy elders (HE) with age and years of education (for EP) as covariates at a corrected FWE statistical threshold of $p<0.05$, $k>10$.

Regions	z-score	k	x	y	z
JPL>HE					
L inferior frontal gyrus	5.83	17	−34	16	28
L middle frontal gyrus	5.48	15	−44	16	40
R cuneus	5.78	21	14	−76	18
L cuneus	5.71	42	−10	−84	12
	5.40	16	−10	−72	22
L insula	5.66	24	−42	−4	−2
HE>JPL					
-	-	-	-	-	-
EP>HE					
L middle occipital gyrus	6.19	32	−46	−80	8
L precentral gyrus	5.59	47	−36	−14	46
HE>EP					
-	-	-	-	-	-
LL>HE					
R middle temporal gyrus	5.94	186	44	−58	8
L middle temporal gyrus	5.42	102	−40	−54	14
	5.13	102	−52	−58	18
L inferior frontal gyrus	5.86	67	−36	14	20
L middle frontal gyrus	5.40	67	−30	16	34
R cuneus	5.46	27	10	−86	28
L caudate	5.90	74	−16	26	2
HE>LL					
R anterior hippocampus	6.87	142	32	−4	−20
L parahippocampal gyrus	5.64	73	−30	−10	−24
R middle temporal gyrus	5.51	142	46	4	−20
R superior temporal pole	5.28	142	38	8	−20
L superior occipital gyrus	6.44	170	−20	−84	36
R superior occipital gyrus	5.66	20	26	−82	26
L middle occipital gyrus	5.37	170	−28	−76	28
	5.09	61	−24	−90	14
	5.41	19	−14	−88	−6
L cuneus	5.29	61	−10	−84	12
R inferior frontal gyrus	5.98	27	26	22	−18
R superior parietal gyrus	5.48	24	48	−38	58
R supramarginal gyrus	5.43	23	50	−34	38
	5.25	11	58	−36	30
R thalamus	5.98	81	16	−14	−2
L thalamus	5.19	64	−12	−14	−2
EG>HE					
L inferior frontal gyrus	6.66	52	−38	8	20
R middle cingulate gyrus	6.26	42	18	8	34
	5.76	29	16	−12	42
L anterior hippocampus	5.35	34	−30	−10	−22
R superior temporal pole	5.44	19	44	8	−22
HE>EG					
-	-	-	-	-	-

L: left, R: right.

Table 4. Results for the comparisons future>control task for JPL, EP, LL, EG compared to healthy elders (HE) with age and years of education (for EP) as covariates at a corrected FWE statistical threshold of $p<0.05$, $k>10$.

Regions	z-score	k	x	y	z
JPL>HE					
L calcarine sulcus	5.56	51	−10	−80	10
L inferior frontal gyrus	5.50	53	−48	20	8
L medial frontal gyrus	5.35	28	−4	10	62
HE>JPL					
-	-	-	-	-	-
EP>HE					
R middle temporal gyrus	5.35	10	52	−70	16
HE>EP					
L superior occipital gyrus	5.82	34	−20	−80	28
	5.39	34	−16	−76	36
R insula	5.36	29	36	−4	4
LL>HE					
R supramarginal gyrus	6.57	126	52	−36	38
	5.84	126	60	−36	28
	5.73	18	54	−24	32
L superior parietal gyrus	5.59	19	−26	−54	62
R medial frontal gyrus	5.66	15	10	4	56
	5.66	29	6	−14	66
	5.55	29	12	−10	70
L middle frontal gyrus	5.45	20	−34	6	54
R thalamus	5.78	13	8	−8	−8
HE>LL					
R superior frontal gyrus	5.81	233	26	4	60
L superior frontal gyrus	5.35	19	−20	4	62
	5.11	10	−16	10	58
R middle frontal gyrus	6.40	115	34	40	18
	5.64	115	26	42	22
	5.60	37	32	30	40
L middle frontal gyrus	5.77	25	−32	44	12
	5.41	54	−24	14	42
	5.33	54	−34	18	34
	5.15	54	−36	10	34
R inferior frontal gyrus	5.21	29	34	18	32
R supplementary motor area	5.31	50	8	−22	56
	5.71	31	4	−10	60
	5.28	16	14	18	58
L inferior parietal gyrus	5.79	55	−50	−24	38
R superior parietal gyrus	5.30	16	30	−66	50
L middle cingulate gyrus	5.77	50	0	−30	50
R fusiform gyrus	5.66	18	36	−42	−24
R inferior temporal gyrus	5.65	12	62	−40	−12
R superior temporal gyrus	5.55	22	56	−36	10
L posterior hippocampus	5.49	23	−30	−44	0
L posterior hippocampus	5.20	10	−24	−36	4
R precuneus	5.34	14	12	−54	66
L cuneus	5.82	36	−8	−76	18
R lingual gyrus	5.76	93	30	−48	−6
L middle occipital gyrus	5.15	10	−30	−72	20

Table 4. Cont.

Regions	z-score	k	x	y	z
R middle occipital gyrus	5.11	10	34	−76	26
R insula	5.97	54	34	−18	18
L caudate	6.04	102	−10	12	−8
	5.73	102	−4	6	−8
R caudate	5.17	102	8	10	−10
	5.91	58	14	22	10
R thalamus	5.55	19	2	−14	4
	5.45	27	12	−34	4
R vermis	5.64	36	6	−58	−16
EG>HE					
L superior temporal gyrus	5.64	45	−58	−10	0
	5.60	45	−56	−18	0
L superior parietal gyrus	5.48	16	−30	−66	52
HE>EG					
L superior occipital gyrus	6.96	118	−18	−82	54

L: left, R: right.

parietal gyri, right medial and left middle frontal gyri and right thalamus compared to the control task (see Table 4, Figure 2). LL showed less activation than healthy elders in essentially the left posterior hippocampus, frontal (bilateral superior, middle and right inferior) gyri, right precuneus, lateral parietal gyrus, right lateral temporal and occipital regions for the future period compared to the control task (see Table 4, Figure 2). Plots of activation magnitude confirm the significant lower activation in the left posterior hippocampus and right precuneus in LL compared to healthy elders (see Figure S1).

The past period showed greater activations for LL than healthy elders in the left posterior hippocampus, frontal (bilateral superior medial, middle, left superior and inferior frontal gyri), temporal (right middle, superior and left inferior temporal gyri), occipital (bilateral cuneus, middle and inferior occipital gyri) and parietal regions (angular, inferior parietal and supramarginal gyri, bilateral precuneus) compared to the future period (see Table 5). No regions were less active in LL compared to healthy elders for this contrast.

Conversely, the future period showed greater activations for LL than healthy elders in right anterior hippocampus, bilateral middle occipital gyri, right middle temporal pole and parietal regions (supramarginal and superior parietal gyri) compared to the past period (see Table 6, Figure 3). Plots of activation magnitude confirm this right anterior hippocampal hyperactivation in LL compared to healthy elders (see Figure S2). No regions were less active in LL compared to healthy elders for this contrast.

Patient EG. At the individual level, results for the contrast future minus control task for EG showed an essentially left-lateralized network of regions comprising the left middle frontal and temporal gyri (see Table S6). No activation was detected for the contrast future minus past period (see Table S7).

At the group level, the past period showed greater activations for EG than healthy elders in the left anterior hippocampus, left inferior frontal gyrus, right middle cingulate cortex and superior temporal pole compared to the control task (see Table 3). No regions were less active in EG compared to healthy elders for this contrast.

The future period showed greater activations for EG than healthy elders in the left superior temporal and superior parietal gyri compared to the control task (see Table 4, Figure 2). EG showed less activation than healthy elders in the left superior occipital gyrus for the future period compared to the control task (see Table 4, Figure 2).

The past period showed greater activations for EG than healthy elders in the left superior occipital gyrus compared to the future period (see Table 5). No regions were less active in EG compared to healthy elders for this contrast.

Conversely, the future period showed greater activations for EG than healthy elders in the right middle temporal gyrus and left calcarine sulcus compared to the past period (see Table 6, Figure 3). No regions were less active in EG compared to healthy elders for this contrast.

For sake of clarity, we also added results of the contrast future minus control task in healthy elders (see Table S8 in File S1). Results for the contrast future minus past period in healthy elders have been published previously [19].

Discussion

This work is, to our knowledge, the first fMRI study examining future projection in semantic dementia. While the sparse behavioral studies found that future projection was consistently impaired in SD [18,16,17], here we show that the capability of patients to project into their future largely depends on the structural integrity of certain brain regions, in particular the superior medial frontal cortex and anterior hippocampus. JPL presented atrophy in bilateral superior medial frontal gyri and left anterior hippocampus and had difficulties in experiencing episodic future events and to a certain extent past episodic events. Hyperactivations of neocortical (frontal and occipital) regions appeared inefficient in compensating for his deficit. EP presented atrophy in bilateral superior medial frontal gyri and, like JPL, could pre-experience only one episodic future event, but past episodic remembering was spared. However, behavioral ratings for the future were higher than those of healthy elders (in terms of

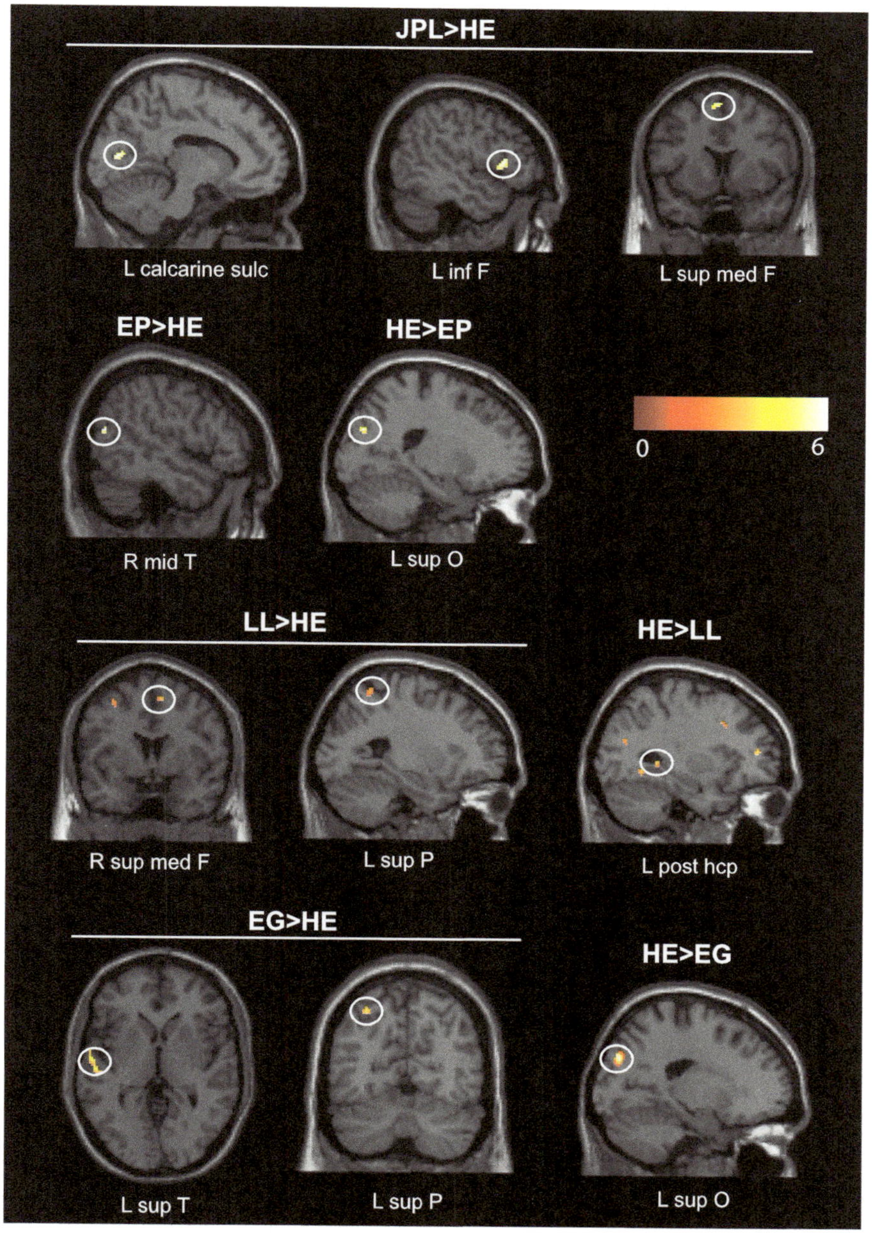

Figure 2. Results of the comparisons between the future period and the control task for EP, LL and EG depicting hyperactivations (Patient>HE) and lower activations (HE>Patient) compared to healthy elders (HE) at a corrected FWE threshold of p<0.05, k>10 voxels. Color scale shows voxel z-scores. See Table 4 for full details. Abbreviations: F = frontal; hcp = hippocampus; sup = superior; inf = inferior; L = left; med = medial; mid = middle; O = occipital; P = parietal; post = posterior; R = right; sulc = sulcus; T = temporal.

emotion and mental imagery), suggesting that EP may have overestimated her capacities to project into the future. On the contrary, LL was able to pre-experience episodic future events. Although she had left anterior hippocampal atrophy, hyperactivation of its right counterpart during future compared to past thinking compensated efficiently for this atrophy. Finally, EG who presented integrity of superior medial frontal gyri and anterior hippocampi was also able to pre-experience episodic future events. Figure 4 depicts summary representations of patients' ability to engage in episodic future thinking (disturbed or spared) depicting sites of atrophy with associated hypothesized function and brain activations for each patient compared to healthy elders. Overall, VBM analyses showed that patients who had difficulties in envisioning the future in an episodic way (JPL and EP) presented specific atrophy in superior medial prefrontal cortex, while this region was relatively preserved in LL and EG who could engage in episodic future projection. Furthermore, JPL and LL presented atrophy in (left) anterior hippocampus, a region known to be crucial for episodic past and future thinking, but LL was able to compensate efficiently by hyperactivation of its right counterpart, while JPL could not. We will mainly focus on these two key regions in the following discussion, distinguishing patients who cannot (JPL and EP) or can (LL and EG) engage in episodic future thinking.

Patients impaired in episodic future projection

JPL presented atrophy mainly in left anterior hippocampus, lateral (middle and inferior) temporal and frontal cortices, including in the bilateral superior medial frontal gyri. Behavioral ratings showed that he was impaired at episodic future projection

Table 5. Results for contrast past>future for JPL, EP, LL, EG compared to healthy elders (HE) with age and years of education (for EP) as covariates at a corrected FWE statistical threshold of $p<0.05$, $k>10$.

Regions	z-score	k	x	y	z
JPL>HE					
R middle temporal gyrus	5.62	14	44	−70	14
EP>HE					
L middle frontal gyrus	5.83	52	−34	−6	44
LL>HE					
R superior medial frontal gyrus	6.30	65	10	62	26
	5.46	83	4	66	4
L superior medial frontal gyrus	5.53	142	−4	64	28
	5.15	142	−6	62	20
	5.43	83	−8	62	0
L superior frontal gyrus	5.73	151	−16	58	16
	5.27	151	−20	60	24
	5.48	12	−18	36	52
	5.04	39	−20	48	16
L medial frontal gyrus	5.16	33	−12	50	−6
R medial frontal gyrus	5.41	12	2	−20	56
L middle frontal gyrus	6.19	161	−30	16	36
	6.11	151	−36	58	14
	6.08	52	−30	44	10
	5.45	29	−46	30	30
	5.40	39	−20	48	26
R middle frontal gyrus	6.00	34	32	16	54
	5.99	162	42	14	42
	5.69	34	32	10	48
L inferior frontal gyrus	5.15	17	−56	18	30
	5.26	12	−46	28	16
L posterior hippocampus	6.07	108	−26	−40	−2
	5.83	108	−24	−38	6
R parahippocampal gyrus	5.82	308	36	−38	−12
R middle temporal gyrus	5.66	51	54	−54	8
	5.23	51	44	−56	10
	5.39	42	18	−74	58
R superior temporal gyrus	5.56	40	58	−34	10
L inferior temporal gyrus	5.35	21	46	−68	8
	5.29	12	−46	−60	−12
R fusiform gyrus	5.34	35	26	−78	−6
R cuneus	6.08	59	12	−88	30
L cuneus	5.72	21	−10	−78	20
L middle occipital gyrus	5.98	48	−36	−74	24
	5.35	55	−24	−58	32
	5.14	80	−38	−78	36
R inferior occipital gyrus	5.43	35	34	−86	−4
	5.15	12	38	−76	−4
R angular gyrus	6.55	180	40	−62	40
	6.01	180	46	−72	36
L angular gyrus	5.57	55	−34	−54	36
L inferior parietal gyrus	5.67	60	−52	−24	38
	5.51	80	−32	−78	42
R inferior parietal gyrus	5.39	39	56	−52	46

Table 5. Cont.

Regions	z-score	k	x	y	z
	5.19	39	56	−44	44
R supramarginal gyrus	5.55	19	52	−22	22
R precuneus	5.74	35	12	−50	44
	5.48	13	8	−56	56
L precuneus	5.62	66	−12	−56	40
L anterior cingulate gyrus	5.43	20	−6	44	6
L middle cingulate gyrus	5.76	58	−4	−42	46
R thalamus	5.64	29	12	−32	4
	5.44	20	18	−20	14
R cerebellum	6.44	205	12	−62	−16
	5.75	205	18	−64	−22
	5.53	13	34	−42	−26
EG>HE					
L superior occipital gyrus	6.29	28	−16	−84	34

No regions were less active by patients compared to healthy elders for this contrast. L: left, R: right.

and past remembering. The overall autobiographical score (AS) for the future and a trend for the strictly episodic autobiographical score (ES) for the past were significantly lower compared to healthy elders, indicating that JPL had difficulties in providing episodic details for future and past periods. A trend also showed that he produced less episodic future events compared to healthy elders. Irish et al. [16] showed that the future thinking deficit in SD was driven by a difficulty to provide "internal" details (i.e., episodic details, central to the event), while "external" details (i.e., semantic facts) were more numerous. With JPL, we confirm behavioral studies showing that SD patients are impaired at projecting into the future in an episodic way [18,16,17] and provide the neural correlates of these cognitive findings. JPL presented atrophy in bilateral superior medial frontal gyri (approximately corresponding to Brodmann areas 8 and 9). This area has been previously reported in episodic prospection studies [73,74,75,36] and has a role in processing coherent contexts [36] (BA9), manipulating processes in working memory [76] (BA8),

Table 6. Results for contrast future>past for JPL, EP, LL, EG compared to healthy elders (HE) with age and years of education (for EP) as covariates at a corrected FWE statistical threshold of $p<0.05$, $k>10$.

Regions	z-score	k	x	y	z
JPL>HE					
-	-	-	-	-	-
EP>HE					
L inferior parietal cortex	6.90	91	−52	−34	46
	6.54	91	−44	−42	52
LL>HE					
L middle occipital gyrus	6.77	130	−22	−82	36
R middle occipital gyrus	5.72	12	26	−92	6
R supramarginal gyrus	6.68	262	52	−36	38
	6.28	262	60	−36	30
	6.11	262	54	−22	32
L superior parietal gyrus	5.44	15	−24	−54	60
R posterior hippocampus	5.80	23	24	−44	4
R anterior hippocampus	5.42	21	30	−4	−20
R middle temporal pole	5.28	15	46	4	−18
EG>HE					
R middle temporal gyrus	5.52	21	60	−52	8
L calcarine sulcus	5.35	14	−6	−90	−6

No regions were less active by patients compared to healthy elders for this contrast. L: left, R: right.

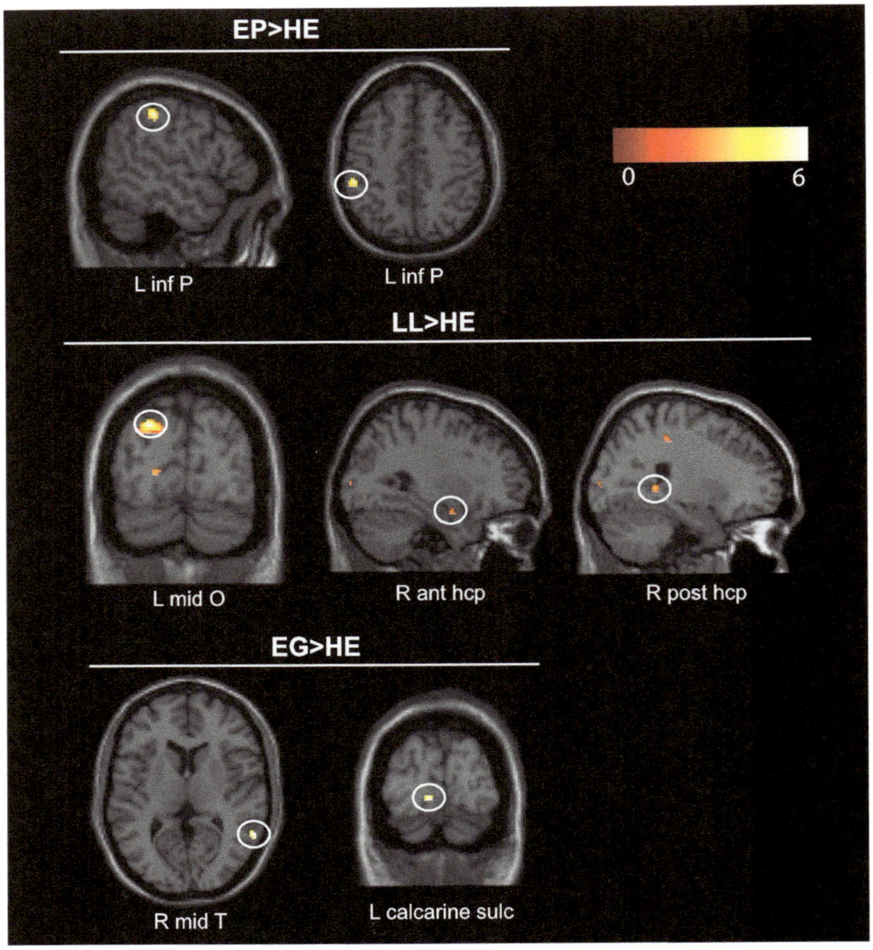

Figure 3. Results of the comparisons between the future and past periods for JPL, EP, LL and EG compared to healthy elders (HE) at a corrected FWE threshold of $p<0.05$, $k>10$ voxels. See Table 6 for full details. Abbreviations: ant = anterior; hcp = hippocampus; inf = inferior; L = left; mid = middle; O = occipital; P = parietal; post = posterior; R = right; sulc = sulcus; T = temporal.

creative story generation [77] (BA8) and autonoetic consciousness [8,37], essential to pre-experience episodic future events. Bilateral atrophy in this region may also have been responsible for JPL's inability to project into the future. JPL also presents atrophy in the left anterior hippocampus. We previously showed that anterior hippocampal integrity in SD is crucial for episodic past remembering [6,70]. Here, we expand these findings to episodic future thinking which also requires anterior hippocampal integrity. The anterior hippocampus supports relational processing [31,32,33], including flexible recombination of details for past and future event construction [34]. Addis and Schacter [35] showed that future-associated activity in the anterior hippocampus was associated with higher demands on recombination of details. Left atrophy in this region may be in part responsible for JPL's inability to project into the future in an episodic way. Thus, we confirm that atrophy in crucial regions of the future thinking network (e.g., superior medial frontal gyrus and anterior hippocampus), overlapping with the autobiographical memory network, impairs episodic future projection. Examination of activation patterns at the individual level indicated that JPL failed to activate the core episodic future thinking network observed in healthy elders (reported in Table S8 and Viard et al. [19]), although several regions may show similar activation patterns across patient and healthy elders (e.g., precuneus, middle cingulate gyrus). Compared to healthy elders, JPL hyperactivated left (medial and inferior) frontal and occipital regions during future thinking compared to the control task. Plots of activation magnitude confirmed hyperactivation in the medial frontal gyrus in JPL compared to healthy elders. Yet, these hyperactivations did not efficiently compensate for atrophied regions, since he was unable to pre-experience episodic future events, as shown by behavioral results.

EP also presented atrophy in frontal cortices, including bilateral superior medial frontal gyri, and lateral (middle and superior) temporal cortices, but sparing of anterior hippocampi. EP was able to pre-experience only one episodic future event, most being semantic. Indeed, like JPL, a trend showed that EP produced less episodic future events compared to healthy elders. She was however not impaired at episodic past remembering. It appears that integrity of anterior hippocampi may have permitted EP to remember episodic past memories, but atrophy of bilateral superior medial frontal gyri may have been in part responsible for EP's deficit in episodic future thinking. Examination of activation patterns at the individual level indicated that, except for the right precuneus, EP failed to activate the core future thinking network observed in healthy elders (Table S8; [19]). Direct comparisons with healthy elders showed that EP hyperactived the inferior parietal and middle temporal cortices for the

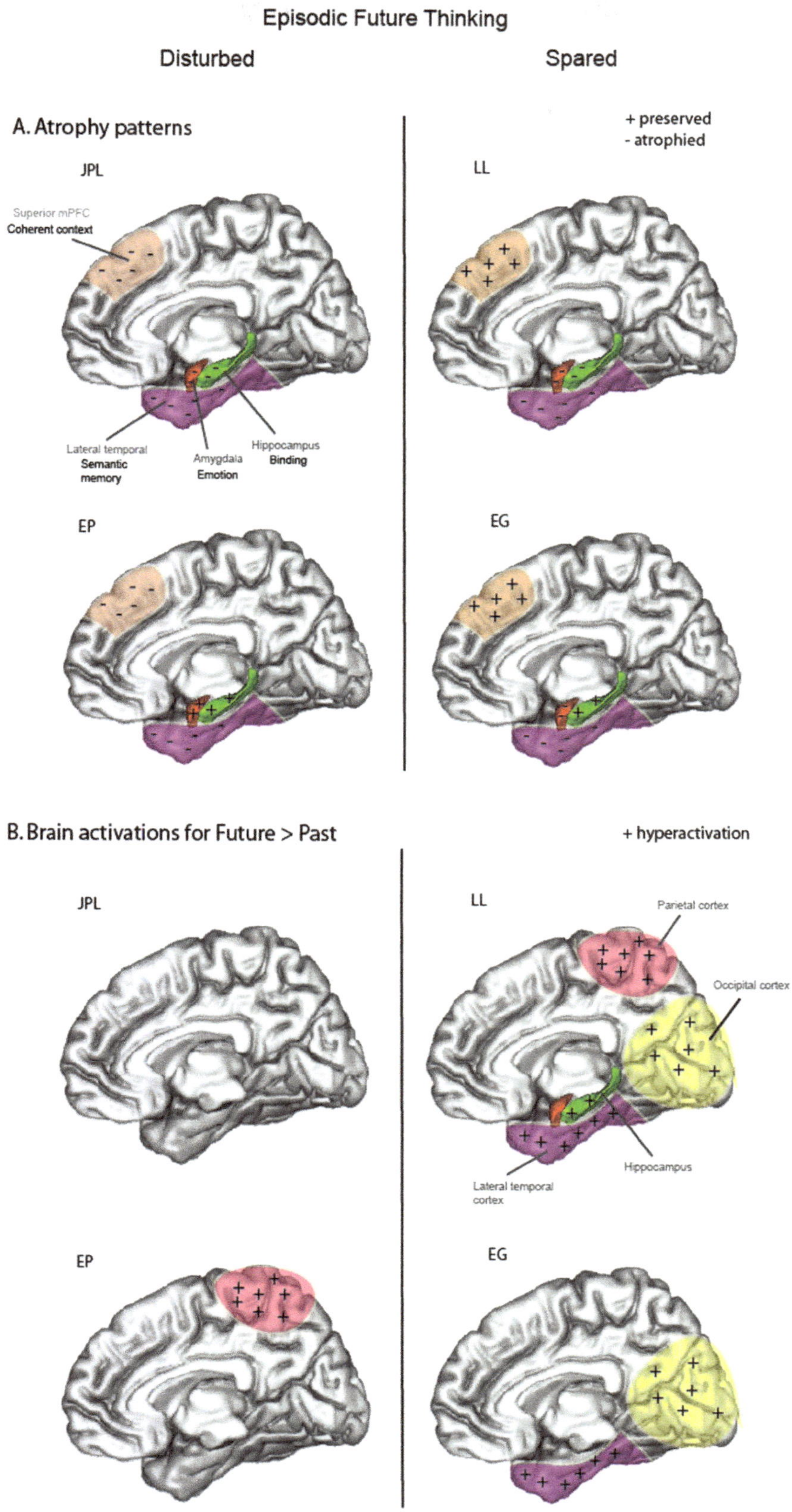

Figure 4. Summary representations of patients' ability to engage in episodic future thinking (left: disturbed; right: spared) depicting (A) localization of preserved (+) or atrophied (−) brain regions and associated hypothesized function (superior medial prefrontal cortex (mPFC): coherent context processing; hippocampus: binding; amygdala: emotional processing; lateral temporal cortex: semantic processing) and (B) brain activations for each patient compared to healthy elders for the contrast Future>Past thinking (see results on Table 6).

future compared to the past period, or to the control task, which appeared inefficient in compensating for her deficit, since she could pre-experience only one episodic future event.

EP had higher ratings on the scale of emotional intensity compared to healthy elders for the past and the future. Conversely, Irish et al. [78] found impaired emotion processing in a group of SD patients during past remembering and suspected that atrophy in the amygdala, generally reported in such patients, might explain their emotional processing deficit. Here, EP's bilateral amygdala were not atrophied compared to healthy elders, but she showed less activation than healthy elders in the right insula for the future compared to the control task, a region known to be implicated in emotional processing [79,80,81]. Hence, EP seems to evaluate the phenomenological nature of her mental evocations inadequately and may tend to exaggerate or overestimate her emotions on behavioral self-ratings. This may be paralleled with Irish et al.'s [16] findings of a disconnect between "objective" task performances (as shown here by scores on the episodic scale) and "subjective" phenomenological pre-experiencing (as shown here by self-ratings) when generating future events in SD. An early report by Snowden et al. [82] had already indicated that SD patients showed "exaggerated reactions to sensory stimuli" which fits with the present results.

Decreased activity in the occipital cortex for the future period compared to the control task was observed for EP compared to healthy elders. This decreased activity in a visuospatial area for the future contradicts EP's behavioral self-ratings on visual imagery which indicate a greater number of mental images for the future for EP compared to healthy elders. Yet, a trend showed that EP's image quality of future events was less clear compared to healthy elders. Overall, as for ratings of emotional intensity, EP may have overestimated the number of images she visualized.

Overall, JPL and EP both presented atrophy in bilateral superior medial prefrontal cortices, in addition to their lateral temporal atrophy, and were impaired at projecting into the future in an episodic way. JPL, unlike EP, was also impaired at remembering the past and presented atrophy in left anterior hippocampus. Thus, joint atrophy in bilateral superior medial prefrontal cortices and anterior hippocampi may have prevented episodic thinking in the past and the future (as observed in JPL). Atrophy in bilateral superior medial prefrontal cortices, but preservation of anterior hippocampal structures, appear to preserve past episodic recollection, at least to a certain extent, but impairs episodic future thinking (as observed in EP).

Patients capable to engage in episodic future thinking

LL presented atrophy mainly in left anterior hippocampus, frontal (superior, inferior) and lateral (middle and superior) temporal cortices. LL was able to pre-experience episodic future events. Examination of activation patterns at the individual level showed that LL failed to activate the core future thinking network observed in healthy elders (Table S8; [19]), although several regions (e.g., occipital and parietal cortices) showed similar activation patterns across her and healthy elders. Nevertheless, she was able to engage in episodic future thinking and pre-experience future plans. Thus, at the neural level, she was able to develop different strategies from those of healthy elders which proved successful at the behavioral level since she was able to perform the future thinking task by envisionning several episodic future events. Indeed, hyperactivation in the right anterior hippocampus was detected for future compared to past thinking, confirmed by plots of activation magnitude. This right anterior hippocampal activation probably compensated for atrophy in its left counterpart. Addis et al. [74] showed that future event construction uniquely engaged the right hippocampus, possibly as a response to the novelty of these events. Beyond its role in relational processing in memory [83], this structure also has the capacity to bind disparate event details for novel future scenarios. Of note, out of the four patients, LL was the one who showed the most reductions in the pattern of neural activity compared to healthy adults, essentially in occipital regions for the past and occipital and frontal regions for the future. These reductions, however, appeared to be sufficiently compensated by hyperactivations in LL (in occipital cortex for the past and frontal cortex for the future) compared to healthy adults, since she was able to efficiently engage in episodic past and future thinking.

EG was able to engage in episodic past and future thinking in spite of atrophy in lateral temporal areas (superior, middle, inferior) gyri and poles and frontal (superior, middle) regions. Irish et al. [17] showed that atrophy in lateral temporal (inferior temporal cortex and temporal pole) correlated with deficits in episodic future thinking in their group of SD patients. Here, although correlations were not possible since we report single cases, we show that EG and LL, who were both able to engage in episodic future thinking, hyperactivated remnant tissue in lateral temporal lobes for the future compared to the past. Hence, our results corroborate Irish et al.'s [17] findings which suggest that lateral temporal cortex, strongly implicated in semantic memory, is critical for the construction of novel future events. Altogether, we extend Irish et al.'s [17] findings by showing that lateral temporal hyperactivation in addition to the integrity of superior medial frontal cortex and anterior hippocampus promote episodic future thinking in SD patients.

Overall, two patients out of four (LL and EG) were able to engage in episodic future thinking, unlike what has been reported in the behavioral literature [16,17,18]. Methodological differences may explain these discrepancies. Here, we used highly personalized cues derived from an interview with the spouse. These personally-relevant stimuli directly point to a specific event. Previous studies, instead, used single words which the patient should use to imagine a plausible future event. These stimuli may not immediately direct to a unique personally-relevant event which has already been planned by the participant. Hence, constructing personally-relevant sentences may be more helpful to trigger episodic future thinking in patients with semantic dementia who present integrity of superior medial prefrontal cortices and anterior hippocampus. Moreover, the group analysis approach used in previous studies may have obscured preservation of function that might have been evident in some (but not all) patients, which we highlighted here by using a case study approach.

Limits

Albeit the clinical and theoretical relevance of the present findings, some potential limits should be mentioned. Given the rarity of patients with semantic dementia, we were not able to perfectly match each patient to the control group. Thus, results may have been influenced by differences in age and years of education (only EP) between each patient and the group of healthy elders. Yet, these variables were added as covariates in the analyses to attenuate any confound between patients and healthy elders. Adding a second covariate to control for differences in education between EP and healthy elders may have underestimated brain activations in EP. Yet, even with a higher education level compared to healthy elders, EP had difficulties in episodic future thinking. Hence, brain activations which may have been underestimated in the analyses (due to the addition of covariates) could not have been sufficient anyway to compensate for EP's deficit in episodic future thinking, since she was able to pre-experience only one episodic future event.

Another potential bias is that a male (JPL) was compared to a group of healthy females. Semantic dementia affects similarly males and females [84,85] and no studies have shown a gender effect in this pathology. However, some studies have observed gender differences favouring women on episodic-memory tasks requiring verbal processing, but favouring men when requiring visuospatial processing [86,87,88]. Yet, the gender difference between JPL and the group of healthy elders may have played only a marginal role in the present results as mental retrieval of past memories and future projection involve both verbal and visuo-spatial processing.

Finally, unlike some studies in the future thinking field that use the cue-word technique with generic stimuli [16,17,74], the task used here was not to simulate or imagine a plausible fictitious future event, but to pre-experience an actual future event that was really supposed to happen in the next twelve months, prompted from a personally-relevant cue. In other words, future events had not happened yet, but were going to happen. Hence, since future events were actual projects that participants really intended to pursue in the future, these were planned in the past. Of note, in everyday life, this kind of future thinking is very frequent, probably the most frequent concerning the recent future. Thus, retrieval processes may have happened in the future thinking condition. Results from behavioral scales evaluating recent reactivation can indicate if each event was evoked recently or not. On the frequency of rehearsal scale, LL and EG obtained scores below 4.5 indicating that they did not frequently rehearse their future plans in the past. EP obtained a score of 9.5, suggesting that she frequently rehearsed her future plans. Yet, EP envisioned only one episodic future event (the four other events being semantic). Thus, she was probably able to envision this unique future plan in an episodic way because she had frequently rehearsed it. On the last recall scale, EP, LL and EG obtained scores indicating that, on average, they last recalled their future plans a sufficiently long time ago, minimizing a possible retrieval effect. It is nevertheless possible that by presenting cues referring to actual future plans, a retrospective thinking effect may have happened. However, unlike some future thinking studies in which participants are asked to imagine plausible future events (which are not necessarily going to happen) using generic cues, here we chose to study the self-projecting aspect of future thinking in which future actions are planned beforehand [12]. It would be interesting to study the purely imaginative aspect, as some studies have already explored [89].

Conclusion

Altogether, this study aimed at examining the neural correlates of future projection in SD compared to past remembering. Main results indicated that episodic future projection in patients with lateral temporal atrophy largely depends on the integrity of superior medial prefrontal cortices and anterior hippocampi. With atrophy in the bilateral superior medial frontal gyri and left anterior hippocampus, JPL was unable to engage into past or future episodic thinking, in spite of neocortical hyperactivity which appeared inefficient in compensating for atrophy within these key regions. EP presented atrophy in bilateral superior medial frontal gyri and was, like JPL, able to pre-experience only one episodic future event, but past remembering appeared relatively preserved. On the contrary, LL despite atrophy in the left anterior hippocampus, was able to efficiently compensate for the deficit by hyperactivating its right counterpart during episodic future thinking. EG, who did not show atrophy in the superior medial frontal gyrus nor anterior hippocampus, was able to envision episodic future events. Altogether, these findings suggest that patients' ability to envision the future in an episodic way largely depends on the severity and localization of their atrophy, in addition to their lateral temporal atrophy. Our results indicate that the integrity of the superior medial frontal gyri and anterior hippocampi, in addition to the use of personally-relevant cues, are essential to trigger episodic future thinking.

Supporting Information

File S1 Contains the following files: **Table S1**: Behavioral ratings comparing EP and healthy elders (HE) for past and future periods with years of education added as covariate. Significant results appear in bold ($p<0.05$). AS = autobiographical score; ES = strictly episodic autobiographical score; Nb = number; p = probability; sd = standard deviation. **Table S2**: Areas of grey matter volume loss in JPL vs. 12 healthy elders at a corrected FWE statistical threshold of $p<0.05$. L: left, R: right. **Table S3**: Areas of grey matter volume loss in EP vs. 12 healthy control participants at a corrected FWE statistical threshold of $p<0.05$. L: left, R: right. **Table S4**: Areas of grey matter volume loss in LL vs. 12 healthy elders at a corrected FWE statistical threshold of $p<0.05$. L: left, R: right. **Table S5**: Areas of grey matter volume loss in EG vs. 12 healthy control participants at a corrected FWE statistical threshold of $p<0.05$. L: left, R: right. **Table S6**: Results for the contrast future>control task for JPL, EP, LL and EG at a corrected FWE statistical threshold of $p<0.05$, $k>10$. **Table S7**: Results for the contrast future>past period for JPL, EP, LL and EG at a corrected FWE statistical threshold of $p<0.05$, $k>10$. L: left, R: right. **Table S8**: Results for the contrast future>control task for healthy elders at a corrected FWE statistical threshold of $p<0.05$, $k>10$. L: left, R: right. SMA = supplemental motor area. **Figure S1**: plots of activation magnitude for each patient (JPL, EP, LL and EG) and average of healthy elders (Ctl) in the bilateral medial frontal gyri, hippocampi and precuneus for the contrast future>control task. **Table S9**: Brief explanation of the neuropsychological tests used to test participants and what they measure. **Table S10**: Specificity scoring chart of past and future episodic tasks, performed at debriefing.

Acknowledgments

Thanks to Brigitte Landeau, Karine Lebreton, Vanessa Matuszewski, Alice Pélerin and Alan Young for their help in this study.

Author Contributions

Conceived and designed the experiments: AV PP BD FE. Performed the experiments: AV PP VdLS. Analyzed the data: AV. Contributed reagents/materials/analysis tools: AV. Wrote the paper: AV. Patient recruitment: VdLS SB.

References

1. Snowden JS, Goulding PJ, Neary D (1989) Semantic dementia: A form of circumscribed cerebral atrophy. Behav Neurol 2: 167–182.
2. Neary D, Snowden JS, Gustafson L, Passant U, Stuss D, et al. (1998) Frontotemporal lobar degeneration: a consensus on clinical diagnostic criteria. Neurology 51: 1546–1554.

3. Hodges JR, Patterson K (2007) Semantic dementia: a unique clinicopathological syndrome. Lancet Neurol 6: 1004–1014.
4. Desgranges B, Matuszewski V, Piolino P, Chételat G, Mézenge F, et al. (2007) Anatomical and functional alterations in semantic dementia: a voxel-based MRI and PET study. Neurobiol of Aging 28: 1904–1913.
5. Hodges JR, Graham KS (2001) Episodic memory: insights from semantic dementia. Philos Trans R Soc Lond B Biol Sci 356: 1423–1434.
6. Viard A, Desgranges B, Matuszewski V, Lebreton K, Belliard S, et al. (2013) Autobiographical memory in semantic dementia: New insights from two patients using fMRI. Neuropsychologia 51: 2620–2632.
7. Tulving E (2001) Episodic memory and common sense: how far apart? Philos Trans R Soc Lond B Biol Sci 356: 1505–1515.
8. Wheeler MA, Stuss DT, Tulving E (1997) Toward a theory of episodic memory: the frontal lobes and autonoetic consciousness. Psychol Bull 121: 331–354.
9. D'Argembeau A, Van der Linden M (2004) Phenomenal characteristics associated with projecting oneself back into the past and forward into the future: influence of valence and temporal distance. Conscious Cogn 13: 844–858.
10. D'Argembeau A, Van der Linden M (2006) Individual differences in the phenomenology of mental time travel: The effect of vivid visual imagery and emotion regulation strategies. Conscious Cogn 15: 342–350.
11. Gamboz N, Brandimonte MA, De Vito S (2010) The role of past in the simulation of autobiographical future episodes. Exp Psychol 57: 419–428.
12. Buckner RL, Carroll DC (2007) Self-projection and the brain. Trends Cogn Sci 11: 49–57.
13. Hassabis D, Maguire EA (2007) Deconstructing episodic memory with construction. Trends Cogn Sci 11: 299–306.
14. Hassabis D, Maguire EA (2009) The construction system of the brain. Philos Trans R Soc Lond B Biol Sci 364: 1263–1271.
15. Schacter DL, Addis DR (2007) The cognitive neuroscience of constructive memory: remembering the past and imagining the future. Philos Trans R Soc Lond B Biol Sci 362: 773–786.
16. Irish M, Addis DR, Hodges JR, Piguet O (2012a) Exploring the content and quality of episodic future simulations in semantic dementia. Neuropsychologia 50: 3488
17. Irish M, Addis DR, Hodges JR, Piguet O (2012b) Considering the role of semantic memory in episodic future thinking: evidence from semantic dementia. Brain 135: 2178
18. Duval C, Desgranges B, de La Sayette V, Belliard S, Eustache F, et al. (2012) What happens to personal identity when semantic knowledge degrades? A study of the self and autobiographical memory in semantic dementia. Neuropsychologia 50: 254–265.
19. Viard A, Chételat G, Lebreton K, Desgranges B, Landeau B, et al. (2011) Mental time travel into the past and the future in healthy aged adults: an fMRI study. Brain Cogn 75: 1–9.
20. Chan D, Fox NC, Scahill RI, Crum WR, Whitwell JL, et al. (2001) Patterns of temporal lobe atrophy in semantic dementia and Alzheimer's disease. Ann Neurol 49: 433–442.
21. Good CD, Scahill RI, Fox NC, Ashburner J, Friston KJ, et al. (2002) Automatic differentiation of anatomical patterns in the human brain: validation with studies of degenerative dementias. NeuroImage 17: 29–46.
22. Rosen HJ, Gorno-Tempini ML, Goldman WP, Perry RJ, Schuff N, et al. (2002) Patterns of brain atrophy in frontotemporal dementia and semantic dementia. Neurology 58: 198–208.
23. Boxer AL, Rankin KP, Miller BL, Schuff N, Weiner M, et al. (2003) Cinguloparietal atrophy distinguishes Alzheimer disease from semantic dementia. Arch Neurol 60: 949–956.
24. Davies RR, Graham KS, Xuereb JH, Williams GB, Hodges JR (2004) The human perirhinal cortex and semantic memory. Eur J Neurosci 20: 2441–2446.
25. van de Pol LA, Hensel A, van der Flier WM, Visser PJ, Pijnenburg YA, et al. (2006) Hippocampal atrophy on MRI in frontotemporal lobar degeneration and Alzheimer's disease. J Neurol Neurosurg Psychiatry 77: 439–442.
26. Nestor PJ, Fryer TD, Hodges JR (2006) Declarative memory impairments in Alzheimer's disease and semantic dementia. NeuroImage 30: 1010–1020.
27. Lehmann M, Douiri A, Kim LG, Modat M, Chan D, et al. (2010) Atrophy patterns in Alzheimer's disease and semantic dementia: a comparison of FreeSurfer and manual volumetric measurements. NeuroImage 49: 2264–2274.
28. Acosta-Cabronero J, Patterson K, Fryer TD, Hodges JR, Pengas G, et al. (2011). Atrophy, hypometabolism and white matter abnormalities in semantic dementia tell a coherent story. Brain 134: 2025–2035.
29. La Joie R, Perrotin A, de La Sayette V, Egret S, Doeuvre L, et al. (2013) Hippocampal subfield volumetry in mild cognitive impairment, Alzheimer's disease and semantic dementia. NeuroImage Clin 3:155–162.
30. Mummery CJ, Patterson K, Price CJ, Ashburner J, Frackowiak RS, et al. (2000) A voxel-based morphometry study of semantic dementia: relationship between temporal lobe atrophy and semantic memory. Ann Neurol 47: 36–45.
31. Chua EF, Schacter DL, Rand-Giovannetti E, Sperling RA (2007) Evidence for a specific role of the anterior hippocampal region in successful associative encoding. Hippocampus 17: 1071–1080.
32. Davachi L, Mitchell JP, Wagner AD (2003) Multiple routes to memory: distinct medial temporal lobe processes build item and source memories. Proc Natl Acad Sci U S A 100: 2157–2162.
33. Jackson O 3rd, Schacter DL (2004) Encoding activity in anterior medial temporal lobe supports subsequent associative recognition. NeuroImage 21: 456–462.
34. Preston AR, Shrager Y, Dudukovic NM, Gabrieli JD (2004) Hippocampal contribution to the novel use of relational information in declarative memory. Hippocampus 14: 148–152.
35. Addis DR, Schacter DL (2008) Constructive episodic simulation: temporal distance and detail of past and future events modulate hippocampal engagement. Hippocampus 18: 227–237.
36. Abraham A, Schubotz RI, von Cramon DY (2008) Thinking about the future versus the past in personal and non-personal contexts. Brain Res 1233: 106–119.
37. Nyberg L, Kim AS, Habib R, Levine B, Tulving E (2010) Consciousness of subjective time in the brain. Proc Natl Acad Sci U S A 107: 22356–22359.
38. Viard A, Desgranges B, Eustache F, Piolino P (2012) Factors affecting medial temporal lobe engagement for past and future episodic events: an ALE meta-analysis of neuroimaging studies. Brain Cogn 80: 111–125.
39. Gorno-Tempini ML, Hillis AE, Weintraub S, Kertesz A, Mendez M, et al. (2011) Classification of primary progressive aphasia and its variants. Neurology 76:1006–1014.
40. Grober E, Buschke H (1987) Genuine memory deficits in dementia. Dev Neuropsychol 3: 13–36.
41. Rey A (1970) Test de mémorisation d'une série de 15 mots. In: Rey A, editor. L'examen clinique en psychologie. Paris: PUF.
42. Cardebat D, Doyon B, Puel M, Goulet P, Joanette Y (1990) [Formal and semantic lexical evocation in normal subjects. Performance and dynamics of production as a function of sex, age and educational level]. Acta Neurol Belg 90: 207–217.
43. Desgranges B, Eustache F, Rioux P, de La Sayette V, Lechevalier B (1996) Memory disorders in Alzheimer's disease and the organization of human memory. Cortex 32: 387–412.
44. Belliard S, Perron M, Rouyer F, Golfier V, Sartori E, et al. (2001) [Présentation d'une batterie franç aise de personnes célèbres. Résultats auprès de patients atteints de démence sémantique]. Revue Neurologique 157:10–14.
45. Deltour JJ (1993) Echelle de vocabulaire de Mill Hill de JC Raven. Adaptation française et normes européennes du Mill Hill et du Standard Progressive Matrices de Raven. Braine-le-Chateau: Editions l'application des techniques modernes.
46. de Partz MP, Bilocq V, De Wilde V, Seron X, Pillon A (2001) LEXIS: Tests pour l'évaluation des troubles lexicaux chez la personne aphasique. Marseille: Solal.
47. Reitan R (1958) Validity of the Trail Making Test as an indicator of organic brain damage. Percept Mot Skills 8: 271–276.
48. Merck C, Charnallet A, Auriacombe A, Belliard S, Hahn-Barma V, et al. (2011) The GRECO neuropsychological semantic battery (BECS GRECO): Validation and normative data. Rev Neuropsychol 3: 235–255.
49. Folstein MF, Folstein SE, McHugh PR (1975) Mini -mental state. A practical method for grading the cognitive state of patients for the clinician. J Psychiatr Res 12: 189–198.
50. Matuszewski V, Piolino P, Belliard S, de la Sayette V, Laisney M, et al. (2009) Patterns of autobiographical memory impairment according to disease severity in semantic dementia. Cortex 45: 456–472.
51. Mattis S (1976) Mental status examination for organic mental symptoms in elderly patients. In: Bellak L, Karatsu TB, editors. Geriatric psychiatry: a handbook for psychiatrists and primary care physicians. New York: Grune et Stratton. pp. 77–121.
52. Yesavage JA, Brink TL, Rose TL, Lum O, Huang V, et al. (1983) Development and validation of a geriatric depression screening scale: a preliminary report. J Psychiatr Res 17: 37–49.
53. Viard A, Piolino P, Desgranges B, Chételat G, Lebreton K, et al. (2007) Hippocampal activation for autobiographical memories over the entire lifetime in healthy aged subjects: An fMRI study. Cereb Cortex 17: 2453–2467.
54. Viard A, Lebreton K, Chételat G, Desgranges B, Landeau B, et al. (2010) Patterns of hippocampal-neocortical interactions in the retrieval of episodic autobiographical memories across the entire life-span of aged adults. Hippocampus 20: 153–165.
55. Graham KS, Hodges JR (1997) Differentiating the roles of the hippocampal complex and the neocortex in long-term memory storage: evidence from the study of semantic dementia and Alzheimer's disease. Neuropsychology 11: 77–89.
56. Kopelman MD, Wilson BA, Baddeley AD (1989) The autobiographical memory interview: a new assessment of autobiographical and personal semantic memory in amnesic patients. J Clin Exp Neuropsychol 11:724–744.
57. Piolino P, Desgranges B, Belliard S, Matuszewski V, Lalevée C, et al. (2003a) Autobiographical memory and autonoetic consciousness: triple dissociation in neurodegenerative diseases. Brain 126: 2203–2219.
58. Piolino P, Belliard S, Desgranges B, Perron M, Eustache F (2003b) Autobiographical memory and autonoetic consciousness in a case of semantic dementia. Cogn Neuropsychol 20: 619–639.
59. Piolino P, Giffard-Quillon G, Desgranges B, Chételat G, Baron JC, et al. (2004) Re-experiencing old memories via hippocampus: a PET study of autobiographical memory. NeuroImage 22: 1371–1383.
60. Brewer W (1988) Memory for randomly sampled autobiographical events. In: Neisser U, Winograd E, editors. Remembering reconsidered: ecological and

traditional approaches to the study of memory. Cambridge: Cambridge University Press. pp. 21–90.
61. Dewhurst SA, Conway MA (1994) Pictures, images, and recollective experience. J Exp Psychol Learn Mem Cogn 20: 1088–1098.
62. Brewer W (1996) What is recollective memory? In: Rubin DC, editor. Remembering our past: studies in autobiographical memory. Cambridge: Cambridge University Press. pp. 19–66.
63. Rubin DC, Schrauf RW, Greenberg DL (2003) Belief and recollection of autobiographical memories. Mem Cognit 31: 887–901.
64. Nigro G, Neisser U (1983) Point of view in personal memories. Cogn Psychol 15: 467–482.
65. Good CD, Johnsrude IS, Ashburner J, Henson RN, Friston KJ, et al. (2001) A voxel-based morphometric study of ageing in 465 normal adult human brains. NeuroImage 14: 21–36.
66. Ashburner J, Friston KJ (2005) Unified segmentation. NeuroImage 26: 839–851.
67. Crawford JR, Garthwaite PH, Azzalini A, Howell DC, Laws KR (2006) Testing for a deficit in single-case studies: effects of departures from normality. Neuropsychologia 44: 666–677.
68. Crawford JR, Garthwaite PH (2002) Investigation of the single case in neuropsychology: confidence limits on the abnormality of test scores and test score differences. Neuropsychologia 40:1196–1208.
69. Crinion J, Ashburner J, Leff A, Brett M, Price C, et al. (2007) Spatial normalization of lesioned brains: performance evaluation and impact on fMRI analyses. Neuroimage 37:866–875.
70. Maguire EA, Kumaran D, Hassabis D, Kopelman MD (2010) Autobiographical memory in semantic dementia: a longitudinal fMRI study. Neuropsychologia 48: 123–136.
71. Deary IJ, Johnson W (2010) Intelligence and education: causal perceptions drive analytic processes and therefore conclusions. The International Journal of Epidemiology 39:1362–9.
72. Crawford JR, Garthwaite PH, Ryan K (2011) Comparing a single case to a control sample: testing for neuropsychological deficits and dissociations in the presence of covariates. Cortex 47: 1166–1178.
73. Okuda J, Fujii T, Ohtake H, Tsukiura T, Tanji K, et al. (2003) Thinking of the future and past: the roles of the frontal pole and the medial temporal lobes. NeuroImage 19: 1369–1380.
74. Addis DR, Wong AT, Schacter DL (2007) Remembering the past and imagining the future: common and distinct neural substrates during event construction and elaboration. Neuropsychologia 45: 1363–1377.
75. Szpunar KK, Watson JM, McDermott KB (2007) Neural substrates of envisioning the future. Proc Natl Acad Sci U S A 104: 642–647.
76. Cabeza R, St Jacques P (2007) Functional neuroimaging of autobiographical memory. Trends Cogn Sci 11: 219–227.
77. Howard-Jones PA, Blakemore SJ, Samuel EA, Summers IR, Claxton G (2005) Semantic divergence and creative story generation: an fMRI investigation. Brain Res Cogn Brain Res 25: 240–250.
78. Irish M, Hornberger M, Lah S, Miller L, Pengas G, et al. (2001) Profiles of recent autobiographical memory retrieval in semantic dementia, behavioural-variant frontotemporal dementia, and Alzheimer's disease. Neuropsychologia 49: 2694–26702.
79. Ochsner KN, Gross JJ (2005) The cognitive control of emotion. Trends Cogn Sci 9: 242–249.
80. Holland AC, Kensinger EA (2010) Emotion and autobiographical memory. Phys Life Rev 7: 88–131.
81. Craig AD (2009) How do you feel now? The anterior insula and human awareness. Nat Rev Neurosci 10: 59–70.
82. Snowden JS, Bathgate D, Varma A, Blackshaw A, Gibbons ZC, et al. (2001) Distinct behavioural profiles in fronto temporal dementia and semantic dementia. J Neurol Neurosurg Psychiatry 70:323–332.
83. Eichenbaum H (2001) The hippocampus and declarative memory: cognitive mechanisms and neural codes. Behav Brain Res 127:199–207.
84. Belliard S, Bon L, LeMoal S, Jonin PY, Vercelletto M, et al. (2007) [Démence sémantique]. Psychol Neuropsychiatr Vieil 5:127–138.
85. Thompson SA, Patterson K, Hodges JR (2003) Left/right asymmetry of atrophy in semantic dementia: behavioral-cognitive implications. Neurology 61: 1196–1203.
86. Herlitz A, Nilsson LG, Bäckman L (1997) Gender differences in episodic memory. Mem Cognit 25: 801–811.
87. St Jacques PL, Conway MA, Cabeza R (2011) Gender differences in autobiographical memory for everyday events: retrieval elicited by SenseCam images versus verbal cues. Memory 19: 723–732.
88. Andreano JM, Cahill L (2009) Sex influences on the neurobiology of learning and memory. Learn Mem 16: 248–266.
89. Summerfield JJ, Hassabis D, Maguire EA (2009) Cortical midline involvement in autobiographical memory. Neuroimage 44:1188–1200.

10

Comparison of Total Variation with a Motion Estimation Based Compressed Sensing Approach for Self-Gated Cardiac Cine MRI in Small Animal Studies

Juan F. P. J. Abascal[1,2*¶], **Paula Montesinos**[1,2¶], **Eugenio Marinetto**[1,2], **Javier Pascau**[1,2], **Manuel Desco**[1,2,3]

1 Departamento de Bioingeniería e Ingeniería Aeroespacial, Universidad Carlos III de Madrid, Madrid, Spain, **2** Instituto de Investigación Sanitaria Gregorio Marañón (IiSGM), Madrid, Spain, **3** Centro de Investigación en Red de Salud Mental (CIBERSAM), Madrid, Spain

Abstract

Purpose: Compressed sensing (CS) has been widely applied to prospective cardiac cine MRI. The aim of this work is to study the benefits obtained by including motion estimation in the CS framework for small-animal retrospective cardiac cine.

Methods: We propose a novel B-spline-based compressed sensing method (SPLICS) that includes motion estimation and generalizes previous spatiotemporal total variation (ST-TV) methods by taking into account motion between frames. In addition, we assess the effect of an optimum weighting between spatial and temporal sparsity to further improve results. Both methods were implemented using the efficient Split Bregman methodology and were evaluated on rat data comparing animals with myocardial infarction with controls for several acceleration factors.

Results: ST-TV with optimum selection of the weighting sparsity parameter led to results similar to those of SPLICS; ST-TV with large relative temporal sparsity led to temporal blurring effects. However, SPLICS always properly corrected temporal blurring, independently of the weighting parameter. At acceleration factors of 15, SPLICS did not distort temporal intensity information but led to some artefacts and slight over-smoothing. At an acceleration factor of 7, images were reconstructed without significant loss of quality.

Conclusion: We have validated SPLICS for retrospective cardiac cine in small animal, achieving high acceleration factors. In addition, we have shown that motion modelling may not be essential for retrospective cine and that similar results can be obtained by using ST-TV provided that an optimum selection of the spatiotemporal sparsity weighting parameter is performed.

Editor: Wang Zhan, University of Maryland, College Park, United States of America

Funding: JFPJ Abascal and P Montesinos were funded by the Cardiovascular Research Network (RIC, RD12/0042/0057) from the Ministerio de Economía y Competitividad (www.mineco.gob.es/). The funder had no role in study design, data collection and analysis, decision to publish, or preparation of the manuscript.

Competing Interests: The authors have declared that no competing interests exist.

* Email: jabascal@hggm.es

¶ These authors contributed equally to this work.

Introduction

Cardiac cine magnetic resonance imaging (MRI) has proved very useful for assessing heart motility and cardiac function. Cine imaging involves an intrinsic tradeoff between the acquisition time, spatiotemporal resolution, and signal-to-noise ratio (SNR) of the reconstructed images. Therefore, this application greatly benefits from acceleration techniques that reduce acquisition time. Traditional acceleration techniques were based on parallel imaging [1,2]. The next generation of accelerating techniques—UNFOLD [3], k-t BLAST, and k-t SENSE [4]—exploited temporal redundancy. In the last few years, compressed sensing has achieved even higher acceleration factors [5–11].

Compressed sensing generates accurate image reconstructions from highly undersampled data obtained using randomized sampling and a nonlinear reconstruction algorithm that forces the image to be sparse in a transformed domain. Among the possible transform domains, one of the most widely used is the image gradient domain that leads to the minimization of the so-called total variation (TV). Reconstruction involves the solution of a convex constrained optimization problem, which can be accurately solved with classic optimization methods [12]. However, these are generally computationally expensive, and a common strategy is to approximate the problem by adopting an equivalent unconstrained optimization formulation. A new approach based on the Split Bregman method can accurately and efficiently resolve constrained optimization problems including L1-norm and TV penalty functions [13–15]. Split Bregman has been validated with static MRI [14] and cardiac cine data, in which the spatiotemporal TV (ST-TV) method is applied [16].

Motion-based reconstruction methods have been proposed as a generalization of temporal TV methods [17–19]. While temporal TV imposes sparsity by ensuring that few pixels change over time, a sparser transform can be achieved by incorporating knowledge of the motion across frames into the reconstruction algorithm. The above mentioned studies [17,18,19] focused on prospective cardiac cine and proved to be superior to previously used methods, such as kt-FOCUSS for human data [17] and to ST-TV for small-animal data [19].

Prospective cardiac cine requires the use of ECG recording and detection of R waves, which may be challenging in small animals at high field strengths, especially in the presence of pathologies such as myocardium infarction. This can be overcome by using retrospective cine, which relies on navigators to classify the data into different time frames [16,20].

Substantial differences might be found in the behaviour of motion-based CS algorithms between its use in prospective human data and retrospective data applied to small animal. As opposite to humans, in the case of small animal, a higher heartbeat rate, lower SNR, different number of frames, and higher presence of artefacts motivate the repetition and averaging of several experiments. The repetition and averaging of data can be used to increase the acceleration achievable with CS, as the potential of CS depends on the level of randomization of the undersampling, which can be increased with randomization across repetitions in addition to the more usual encoding direction and temporal dimension [16].

All the aforementioned differences between prospective human data and retrospective animal data may influence the performance of CS methodologies. The aim of this work is to study the benefit of incorporating motion estimation within the compressed sensing framework into retrospective cardiac cine MRI for small-animal studies. To this purpose, we propose a novel B-spline-based compressed sensing method (SPLICS) based on motion estimation, which is evaluated by comparing with ST-TV using retrospective cardiac cine data from both healthy and infarcted rats. In addition, we assess the effect of an optimum weighting between spatial and temporal sparsity to further improve results with both SPLICS and ST-TV.

Methods

Compressed sensing

Compressed sensing enables accurate image reconstructions from randomly undersampled data [21,22] by using convex optimization and imposing sparsity of the image in a transform domain, subject to a data fidelity constraint. Sparsity can be enforced by minimizing the L1-norm of the solution in the transform domain. With f as the measured k-space, F the undersampled Fourier operator, and u the image assumed to be sparse under the transform Ψ, compressed sensing formulates the following constrained optimization problem

$$\min_u \|\Psi u\|_1 \text{ such that } \|Fu-f\|_2^2 \leq \rho \quad (1)$$

where ρ depends on the variance in signal noise as $\rho = N\sigma^2$, being N is the number of data points, for independent and identically distributed noise.

For static image reconstruction, the transformed domain chosen is usually the spatial gradient, $\Psi = \nabla_{x,y}$, such that $\|\Psi u\|_1 = \|\nabla_{x,y} u\|_1$ is the spatial TV.

Compressed sensing for cardiac cine MRI

Dynamic cardiac applications are generally sparser in the temporal domain than in the spatial domain. In this work, we examine the effect of a spatiotemporal weighting parameter, α, that allows us to control the amount of sparsity enforced in one domain with respect to the other ($0 \leq \alpha \leq 1$). With this approach, a general compressed sensing reconstruction method that combines spatial and temporal sparsity can be written as

$$\min_u (1-\alpha)\|\nabla_{x,y} u\|_1 + \alpha\|Tu\|_1 \text{ such that } \|Fu-f\|_2^2 \leq \rho \quad (2)$$

where both the image and raw data are represented by column vectors that comprise all frames, such that $u = [u_1^T, \ldots, u_I^T]^T$, $f = [f_1^T, \ldots, f_I^T]^T$, I is the number of cardiac phases, F and $\nabla_{x,y}$ are operators that act frame by frame, and T is a sparsifying operator along the temporal dimension. Hereafter, we use isotropic spatial TV for the spatial sparsity transform $\|\nabla_{x,y} u\|_1 = \sqrt{(\nabla_x u)^2 + (\nabla_y u)^2}$.

ST-TV reconstruction. Spatiotemporal-total variation imposes sparsity on both spatial and temporal gradient domains [16]. As temporal gradient ensures that few pixels change over time, it is suitable for dynamic processes in which the background is static. By letting $T = \nabla_t$ in equation (2), ST-TV becomes

$$\min_u (1-\alpha)\|\nabla_{x,y} u\|_1 + \alpha\|\nabla_t u\|_1 \text{ such that } \|Fu-f\|_2^2 \leq \rho \quad (3)$$

where the temporal gradient ∇_t relates a pixel in a frame to the same pixel in the next frame, assuming a cyclic condition.

A compressed sensing approach using B-spline motion estimation (SPLICS). Motion-based reconstruction methods are based on simultaneous or alternating reconstruction of both motion and images from the data. If T in equation (2) represents an operator that encodes the motion between frames, thus relating pixels across frames, the compressed sensing problem for joint estimation of motion and images can be written as

$$\min_{u,T} (1-\alpha)\|\nabla_{x,y} u\|_1 + \alpha\|Tu\|_1 \text{ such that } \|Fu-f\|_2^2 \leq \rho \quad (4)$$

where both images u and the encoded motion T between frames are unknown. Modelling the motion across frames can be considered an extension of ST-TV that leads to a much sparser representation in the temporal domain. This is shown in figure 1 where full data reconstruction is represented on spatial gradient domain, $|\nabla_{x,y} u_1|$, temporal-gradient domain, $|\nabla_t u_1|$, and motion-corrected domain, $|Tu_1|$. Thus, in the case of a sparser temporal representation, one could increase the weight α enforcing temporal sparsity over spatial sparsity.

In our case, motion was estimated using a free-form deformation (FFD) model, which represents the motion in terms of cubic B-spline bases in order to preserve smoothness [23,24]. B-splines have interesting properties such as positivity, symmetry, compact support and maximal order of approximation [25–27]. These properties make B-splines to be computationally efficient during interpolation and differentiation. FFD uses a sparse mesh of control points to model motion, which is interpolated using spline functions. A hierarchical approach enables the mesh of control points to be increased using multiresolution.

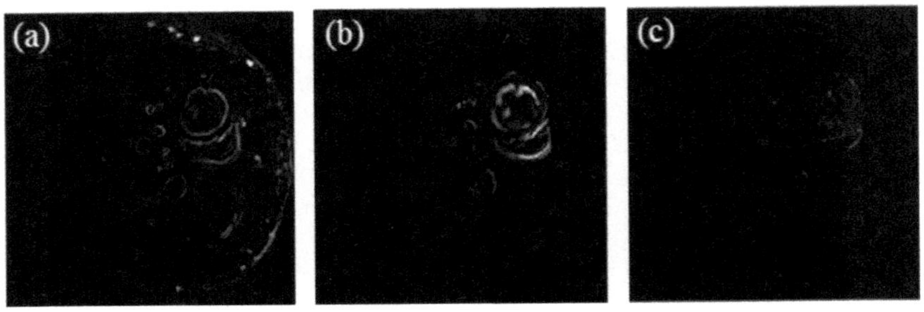

Figure 1. Full data reconstruction for end-diastole represented on the different transform domains. Sparsity of full data reconstruction on (a) spatial-gradient domain, $|\nabla_{xy}u_1|$, (b) temporal-gradient domain, $|\nabla_t u_1|$, and (c) motion-corrected domain, $|Tu_1|$. Images are shown with the same window/level.

FFD has been widely used in medical image-registration to model deformation. The nonrigid registration problem searches for the spatial transformation R_i:(x,y,z)→(x',y',z'), which maps any point from the image u_i at the ith-frame to a point on the image at the following frame u_{i+1}. Interpolation is then applied to relate pixel intensity between frames, with the result that $R_i(u_i)$ comprises both registration and interpolation. The registration problem can be written as

$$\min_{R_i} \| R_i(u_i) - u_{i+1} \|_2^2 + \lambda C_{\text{smooth}}(R_i) \quad (5)$$

where C_{smooth} is a smoothness penalty function, generally in the form of a thin plate of metal bending energy [24]. For the implementation of the FFD-based registration method, we used the software available in MATLAB Central (Dirk-Jan Kroon; B-spline grid, image and point based registration; 2012, retrieved from <http://www.mathworks.com/matlabcentral/fileexchange/20057-b-spline-grid-image-and-point-based-registration>), which is based on the Quasi Newton L-BFGS optimization method. This approach requires selection of a threshold for the stopping criterion, the number of grid points, and the number of refinement grids within the hierarchical approach.

Given the registered images, the temporal sparsity transformation is obtained as

$$Tu = \begin{bmatrix} R_1 u_1 - u_2 \\ R_2 u_2 - u_3 \\ \cdots \\ R_I u_I - u_1 \end{bmatrix} \quad (6)$$

With regard to implementation of the SPLICS method, instead of solving equation (4), we propose an alternating two-step approach that estimates the motion in a first step and reconstructs the images using the estimated motion in a second step (pseudo-code is shown in Table 1). For the first estimate, u_{estimate}, we used the solution given by ST-TV, which is only used to estimate the motion. It is important to remember that both registration and reconstruction steps are iterative processes. For the registration step, we used the nonrigid registration method from equation (5); for the reconstruction step, we used the Split Bregman method, as shown in the next section.

Implementation of ST-TV and SPLICS based on the Split Bregman formulation. We implemented ST-TV (equation (3)) and SPLICS (Table 1) using the Split Bregman method, which is computationally efficient for solving constrained optimization problems with L1-norm functionals [14]. The Split Bregman formulation separates L2- and L1-norm functionals in such a way that they can be solved analytically in two alternating steps. Constraints are imposed using the Bregman iteration as explained below. As motion-based reconstruction can be written as a generalization of the ST-TV, we develop the formulation for the general case and then provide details for an efficient computation in both ST-TV and SPLICS.

For solving equation (2) for a general operator T we generalize the Split Bregman formulation presented in [14,16]. To allow for splitting, we include new variables, d_x, d_y, and w, and formulate a new problem equivalent to equation (2), as follows:

$$\min_{u,d_x,d_y,w} (1-\alpha)\|(d_x,d_y)\|_1 + \alpha\|w\|_1 \text{ such that } \|Fu - f\|_2^2 \le \rho, \\ d_x = \nabla_x u, d_y = \nabla_y u, w = Tu \quad (7)$$

Using the Bregman iteration, this problem can now be easily handled by applying the equivalent unconstrained optimization problem and imposing constraints by adding a Bregman iteration b_i for each constraint. Thus,

$$\min_{u,d_x,d_y,w} (1-\alpha)\|(d_x,d_y)\|_1 + \alpha\|w\|_1 + \frac{\mu}{2}\|Fu - f^k\|_2^2 \\ + \frac{\lambda}{2}\|d_x - \nabla_x u - b_x^k\|_2^2 + \frac{\lambda}{2}\|d_y - \nabla_y u - b_y^k\|_2^2 + \frac{\lambda}{2}\|w - Tu - b_w^k\|_2^2 \quad (8)$$

where k is the iteration number and the Bregman iterations are given by

$$\begin{aligned} b_x^{k+1} &= b_x^k + \nabla_x u^{k+1} - d_x^{k+1} \\ b_y^{k+1} &= b_y^k + \nabla_y u^{k+1} - d_y^{k+1} \\ b_w^{k+1} &= b_w^k + Tu^{k+1} - w^{k+1} \\ f^{k+1} &= f^k + f - Fu^{k+1} \end{aligned} \quad (9)$$

The Bregman iterations impose the constraints iteratively by adding the error back into the unconstrained formulation given in equation (8), thus making its solution converge to the solution of the constrained problem in equation (2). The last line in equation (9) enforces the data constraint, producing a sequence of solutions such that the solution error norm and the data fidelity term

Table 1. Pseudo-code for the SPLICS method.

$n=0, \hat{u}^0 = u_{\text{estimate}}$
while $\|u^n - u^{n-1}\|_2 / \|u^{n-1}\|_2 < \varepsilon$
$u^n = \hat{u}^n$
Registration step : $R_i^n = \min_{R_i} \|R_i(u_i^n) - u_{i+1}^n\|_2^2 + \lambda C_{\text{smooth}}(R_i), i = 1, \ldots, I$
Reconstruction step : $\hat{u}^n = \min_u (1-\alpha)\|\nabla_{x,y} u\|_1 + \alpha \|T^n u\|_1$ such that $\|Fu - f\|_2^2 \le \rho$
$n \to n+1$
end

decrease monotonically. This framework is more robust than equivalent approximated unconstrained problems or continuation methods that impose constraints iteratively by slowly increasing the regularization parameters (for more details see [14]).

Note that u and the auxiliary variables are independent of each other; therefore, (8) can be split into several equations, one for each variable, and solved sequentially

$$\begin{aligned} u^{k+1} &= \min_u \frac{\mu}{2}\|Fu - f^k\|_2^2 + \frac{\lambda}{2}\|d_x^k - \nabla_x u - b_x^k\|_2^2 \\ &\quad + \frac{\lambda}{2}\left\|d_y^k - \nabla_y u - b_y^k\right\|_2^2 + \frac{\lambda}{2}\|w^k - Tu - b_w^k\|_2^2 \\ d_x^{k+1}, d_y^{k+1} &= \min_{d_x, d_y} (1-\alpha)\|(d_x, d_y)\|_1 + \frac{\lambda}{2}\|d_x - \nabla_x u^{k+1} - b_x^k\|_2^2 \\ &\quad + \frac{\lambda}{2}\left\|d_y - \nabla_y u^{k+1} - b_y^k\right\|_2^2 \\ w^{k+1} &= \min_w \alpha\|w\|_1 + \frac{\lambda}{2}\|w - Tu^{k+1} - b_w^k\|_2^2 \end{aligned} \quad (10)$$

Since the solution of u only involves L2-norm functionals, it can be found exactly by differentiating the cost function and equating it to zero. The resulting linear system, which corresponds to a Gauss-Newton step, is given by

$$\begin{aligned} &Ku^{k+1} = r \\ &K = \mu F^T F + \lambda \nabla_x{}^T \nabla_x + \lambda \nabla_y{}^T \nabla_y + \lambda T^T T \\ &r = \mu F^T f^k + \lambda \nabla_x{}^T (d_x - b_x^k) + \lambda \nabla_y{}^T \left(d_y - b_y^k\right) + \lambda T^T (w - b_w^k) \end{aligned} \quad (11)$$

Note that the solution u is obtained analytically from a quadratic penalty function; therefore, an estimation of the step-size is not required. The linear system constitutes a very large scale problem, where $K = N^2 \times N^2$ ($N = 192$), yet it can be efficiently solved using a Krylov solver, which involves only matrix-vector multiplications, as follows:

$$\mu F^T(Fu) + \lambda \nabla_x{}^T(\nabla_x u) + \lambda \nabla_y{}^T(\nabla_y u) + \lambda T^T(Tu) = r \quad (12)$$

Here, we used the biconjugate gradient stabilized as the Krylov solver. This methodology has been applied in SPLICS, where F, ∇_i, and T can be treated as general operators.

For ST-TV, all operators, $T = \nabla_t$, F, ∇_x, ∇_y, and ∇_t, and the variables, u, d, and w, can be expressed in the Fourier domain, with dimension N×N. In this case, solving equation (12) in the Fourier domain is much faster than the equivalent Krylov solver in the image domain. In the case of SPLICS T cannot be represented in the Fourier domain and thus the problem has to be solved in the image domain [14,16].

For both ST-TV and SPLICS, d_x, d_y, and w are solved analytically using shrinkage formulas, which are thresholding operations [14,28]

$$\begin{aligned} d_j^{k+1} &= \max\left(s^k - (1-\alpha)/\lambda, 0\right) \frac{\left|\nabla_j u^{k+1} + b_j^k\right|}{s^k}, \\ s^k &= \sqrt{\left|\nabla_x u^{k+1} + b_x^k\right|^2 + \left|\nabla_y u^{k+1} + b_y^k\right|^2} \\ w^{k+1} &= \text{shrink}(Tu^{k+1} + b_w^k, \alpha/\lambda) \\ &= \max\left(\left|Tu^{k+1} + b_w^k\right| - \alpha/\lambda, 0\right) \text{sign}\left(Tu^{k+1} + b_w^k\right), j = x, y. \end{aligned} \quad (13)$$

Test data set and undersampling

Test data set. Self-gated rat cardiac cine sequences, IntraGateFLASH, were acquired with a 7T Bruker Biospec 70/20 scanner using a linear coil resonator for transmission and a dedicated four-element cardiac phased array coil for reception. Acquisition parameters were: TE = 2.43 ms, TR = 8 ms, number of total repetitions = 200, number of frames = 8, matrix size = 192×192, FOV = 5×5 cm, slice thickness = 1.2 mm, and acquisition time = 5 min 7 s. Four Wistar male rats (weight 300 g to 350 g) were used in this study divided in healthy animals (wild type) and infarct animals (figure 2). Two out of four animals were induced with isoflurane (4%), intubated and place on isoflurane (2%) anaesthesia with mechanical ventilation for the duration of the surgical procedure. We induced a myocardial infarction by permanent left anterior descending artery occlusion as described previously [29]. The animals were exposed to 12/12 light/dark circle and allowed access to food and water ad libitum. Animals were handled according to the European Communities Council Directive (2010/63/UE) and national regulations (RD 53/2013) and under the approval of the Animal Experimentation Ethics Committee of Hospital General Universitario Gregorio Marañón.

Undersampling pattern. In order to reduce acquisition time, it is necessary to skip phase encoding lines in the acquisition scheme. One of the requirements of the compressed sensing

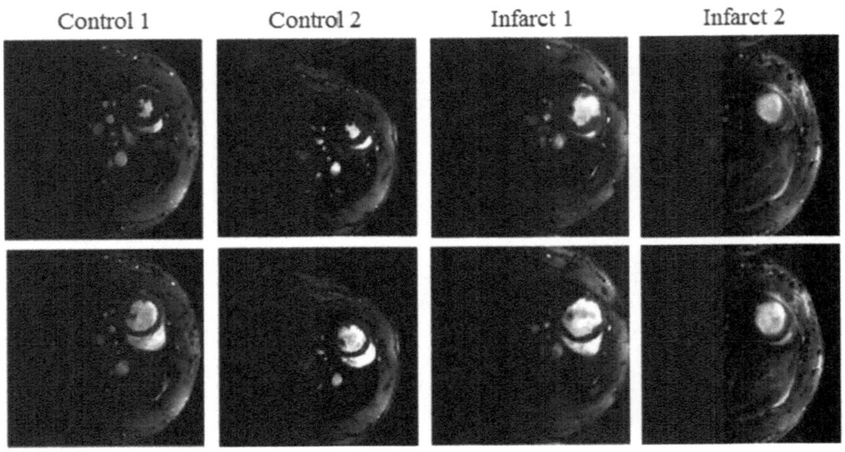

Figure 2. End-systole (first row) and end-diastole (second row) from fully-sampled data reconstruction.

technique is that the undersampling pattern should be random in order to produce incoherent artifacts [22]. By adapting the methodology proposed by Lustig *et al.* [22], in our work, we create quasi-random undersampling patterns in which randomization is performed in the phase encoding direction and through the temporal dimension.

A polynomial probability density function (figure 3(a)) that assigns sampling probabilities to different regions of k-space was used to generate undersampling patterns that are random in the phase encoding direction (figure 3(b)). Then, changing the undersampling pattern for each time point leads to an undersampling acquisition scheme that is random in both phase encoding and temporal directions (figure 3(c)).

Undersampling patterns were simulated using the fully sampled dataset. After the undersampling process, each of the remaining phase encoding lines is binned into a specific cardiac frame (8 final frames), where coincident phase encoding lines are averaged. This averaging step, in combination with randomization over time, results in that the percentage of non-zero data in the final k-spaces is higher than the percentage of data actually acquired [15]. To avoid confusion, two different terms are defined: 'acceleration factor' (indicated with an x), which represents the speed up rate with respect to the fully sampled data, and 'percentage of filled k-space' (FS), which corresponds to the percentage of nonzero lines after the averaging step. For example, a given undersampling pattern can preserve only 7% of the acquired data, providing an acceleration factor of ×15; however, after the classification and averaging step, FS = 26%.

The reconstruction process was performed separately for each element of the phased array antenna and combined with a sum of squares operation.

Evaluation

For an acceleration factor ×7 (FS = 60%) from the complete data (percentage of filled k-space shown within parenthesis), the effect of the spatiotemporal weighting parameter α was analyzed in the range 0.99 to 0.01 (α = 0.99, 0.9, 0.7, 0.5, 0.3, 0.1, 0.01), for the data set 1. SPLICS and ST-TV results were compared to better understand the benefit of including motion estimation. The number of iterations (k in equation (10)) had to be selected for both ST-TV and SPLICS. To ensure the best result for each method, we chose the iteration numbers that provided minimum solution error, adopting the full data reconstruction (figure 2) as the gold standard.

We analyzed the results obtained by both methods for acceleration factors ×7 (FS = 60%), ×10 (FS = 40%), ×15 (FS = 26%), ×20 (FS = 22%) for all data sets.

Reconstructed images were evaluated in terms of the relative solution error norm within a region-of-interest (ROI) that comprised the whole heart. The presence of artifacts in reconstructed images was analyzed by visual inspection, and temporal blurring was evaluated by measuring temporal intensity changes on a circular ROI located in the inner part of the myocardium (diameter = 6 pixels).

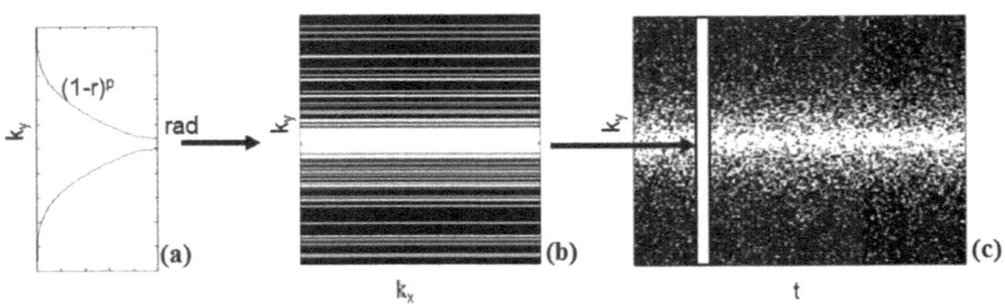

Figure 3. Undersampling pattern strategy used in this study in which randomization is performed along both phase encoding and temporal directions. Probability density function in (a) is used to generate undersampling patterns that are random in the phase encoding direction (b). Time randomization is achieved by changing the undersampling pattern for each temporal instant (c).

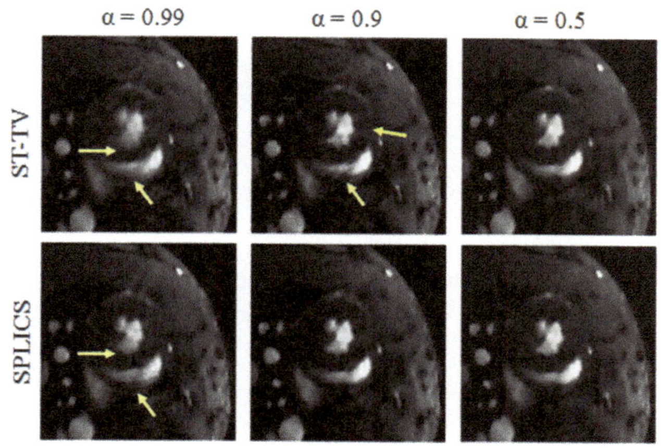

Figure 4. Image zoom corresponding to an acceleration factor ×7 (FS = 60%) reconstructed with ST-TV and SPLICS for three different values of the spatiotemporal weighting parameter α (0.99, 0.9, 0.5). The arrows indicate locations where temporal blurring and artifacts are more noticeable. All images have the same window/level.

Results

Effect of the spatiotemporal weighting parameter

We show reconstructed images for 3 different values of the spatiotemporal weighting parameter α ($\alpha = 0.99$, 0.9, and 0.5) for ST-TV and SPLICS. The outcome of ST-TV proved to be similar to that of SPLICS for a wide range of the weighting parameter ($\alpha \leq 0.5$) (figure 4). From $\alpha = 0.99$ to $\alpha = 0.9$ (large temporal weight), ST-TV led to significant temporal blurring effects and motion artifacts. SPLICS was more robust against the selection of α. SPLICS corrected for temporal blurring effects and motion artifacts for $\alpha = 0.9$ and $\alpha = 0.5$ and reduced them for $\alpha = 0.99$. The best results were obtained with ST-TV for $\alpha = 0.5$ and with SPLICS for $\alpha = 0.9$ and $\alpha = 0.5$, with no noticeable differences between these results. For values of α lower than 0.5, images remain similar to those obtained with $\alpha = 0.5$ (images not shown).

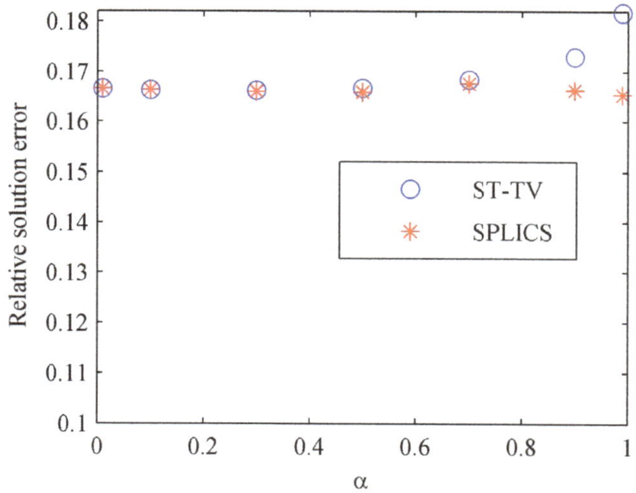

Figure 5. Relative solution error norm corresponding to an acceleration factor ×7 (FS = 60%) reconstructed with ST-TV and SPLICS (images in figure 4) for different values of the spatiotemporal weighting parameter α.

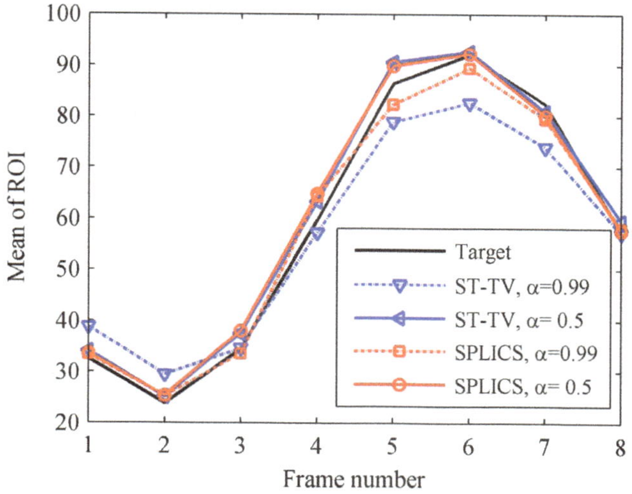

Figure 6. Temporal intensity changes, corresponding to a circular ROI located within the myocardium, for the images reconstructed with ST-TV and SPLICS (see also figure 4).

Visual findings are in agreement with the normalized solution error norm shown in figure 5. For ST-TV, $\alpha \leq 0.5$ yielded the lowest solution error, and increasing α from 0.7 to 0.99 increased the solution error. On the other hand, SPLICS maintained low solution error for all values of α.

Figure 6 shows temporal intensity changes for ST-TV and SPLICS. For $\alpha = 0.5$ both methods recovered the temporal data; for $\alpha = 0.99$, ST-TV presented higher temporal blurring than SPLICS.

As for the reconstruction parameters, the initial image was estimated using ST-TV with parameters $\lambda = 1$ and $\mu = 2$. For the registration step, we used three meshes of control points and a

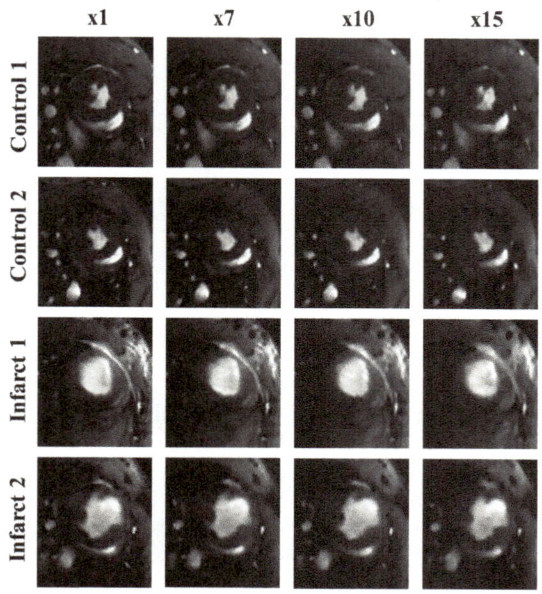

Figure 7. Image zoom of the end-systole corresponding to acceleration factors ×7 (FS = 60%), ×10 (FS = 40%) and ×15 (FS = 26%) reconstructed with SPLICS for a spatiotemporal weighting parameter α = 0.5. Images show different window/level for each subject, in order to make them look similar.

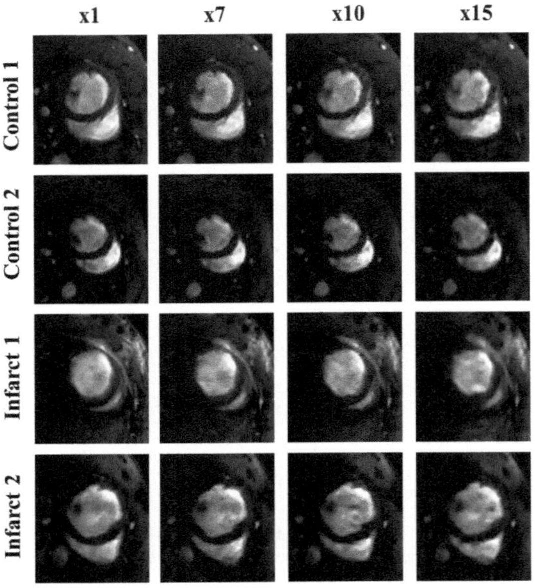

Figure 8. Image zoom of end-diastole corresponding to acceleration factors ×7 (FS = 60%), ×10 (FS = 40%) and ×15 (FS = 26%) reconstructed with SPLICS for a spatiotemporal weighting parameter $\alpha = 0.5$. Images show different window/level for each subject, in order to make them look similar.

hierarchical approach (8×8, 12×12, and 20×20), with a convergence tolerance of 10^{-4}. For the reconstruction step, we empirically chose $\lambda = 1$ and $\mu = 2$. We applied only one iteration of the alternating method ($n = 1$ in Table 1), as further iterations did not significantly improve these data.

Analysis of acceleration factor achieved

Figure 7 shows the end-systole reconstructed with SPLICS for acceleration factors ×7 (FS = 60%), ×10 (FS = 40%) and ×15 (FS = 26%), for $\alpha = 0.5$ (due to the similarities between SPLICS and ST-TV, we only show results given by SPLICS). For acceleration factors up to ×7, image quality is close to that of the fully-sampled data. Decreasing the percentage of data acquired resulted in a slight increase in artefacts and in the smoothing effect from ×10 (FS = 40%) to ×15 (FS = 26%). For ×20 (FS = 22%), reconstructed images were strongly over-smoothed (results not shown).

Figure 8 shows the end-diastole (equivalent to figure 7) reconstructed with SPLICS for acceleration factors ×7 (FS = 60%), ×10 (FS = 40%) and ×15 (FS = 26%). Like in systole, decreasing the percentage of acquired data results in an increase in artefacts together with some smoothing effect. However, the diastole is more prone to motion and flow artefacts than the systole. This effect is more clear in control subjects.

Temporal intensity changes are shown in figure 9. For acceleration factors ×10 (FS = 40%) and ×15 (FS = 26%), temporal intensity changes are similar to those in the fully sampled data; for ×20 (FS = 22%), temporal smoothing becomes more significant.

Regarding convergence, the iteration number that provided best results varied in the range from 105 to 380 iterations for the different subjects and undersampling factors, with larger variation across subjects than across undersampling factors. As in a real compressed sensing acquisition the target image is not available, we tested the effect of reconstructing all data sets with a fixed number of iterations, comparing results given by 100, 200 and 300 iterations, and found images to be similar (data not shown).

Computation time for ST-TV was 0.12 s per iteration (Intel Core i7-3770 CPU 3.40 GHz, 8 GB RAM, 64-bit operating system), and it took 1.5 minutes to reconstruct all the images with 200 iterations (eight frames, four array elements). In each iteration, the heavier part of the computation was two 3D FFT and two 2D FFT image frame-by-image frame, which were required for inversion of the linear system in the Fourier domain. In the case of SPLICS, the registration step took 1.5 minutes and the computation time for the reconstruction step depended on the tolerance of the Krylov solver used for the inversion of the linear system in the image domain: 2.4 s per iteration for a tolerance of 10^{-4} and 1.2 s per iteration for a tolerance of 10^{-2}. As the linear system does not need to be solved with high precision, a tolerance of 10^{-2} was sufficient and gave the same solution as 10^{-4}. In this case, SPLICS took 15.5 minutes to reconstruct all the images with 200 iterations. A straightforward parallelization over the four phase arrays reduced computation times to 55.5 s for ST-TV and 6.6 minutes for SPLICS (35 seconds for the registration step and 6 minutes for the reconstruction step).

Discussion

We studied the influence of incorporating motion estimation in the compressed sensing framework for retrospective cardiac MRI in small animal. To this end, we proposed a new motion-based reconstruction method (SPLICS) and compared it with ST-TV, as SPLICS can be considered as a generalization of ST-TV that also models motion. In addition, we investigated the effect of the spatiotemporal weighting parameter intended to control the relative degree of spatial and temporal sparsity.

Previous works have combined spatial and temporal sparsifying operators [16,19,30]. In our work we compared the effect of the spatiotemporal weighting parameter on both ST-TV and motion-based reconstruction. We found that ST-TV with low relative temporal weighting ($\alpha \leq 0.5$) led to similar results than SPLICS. When temporal weighting was increased ($\alpha > 0.5$) ST-TV led to images with temporal blurring effects and motion artifacts on the moving parts of the image. On the other hand, SPLICS appeared more robust for all α values, as it also takes into account the motion information of the moving parts of the images. Hence, from our results it seems that for retrospective cardiac cine in small animal ST-TV with an optimum weighting parameter provides good results and does not require motion modelling.

A motion-based reconstruction method has been shown to improve k-t FOCUSS for prospective human cine [17] and ST-TV for prospective small-animal cine [19]. In [19] it was found that ST-TV led to temporal blurring while motion-based reconstruction corrected these effects. In contrast, for retrospective data we obtained that ST-TV with optimum selection of the spatiotemporal weighting parameter did not lead to temporal blurring artifacts, providing a solution similar to that of SPLICS. Thus, motion-based reconstruction would provide an improvement only in those cases where other methods lead to temporal blurring effects.

While motion-based reconstruction has led to better results than k-t FOCUSS and ST-TV for prospective data, we found similar results between SPLICS and ST-TV for retrospective data. These discrepancies between our results and previous ones may be due to differences in the acquisition process and in the way the undersampling process was applied. In our case, for retrospective small-animal cine, we have taken advantage of the repetition and averaging step by also randomizing the undersampling pattern

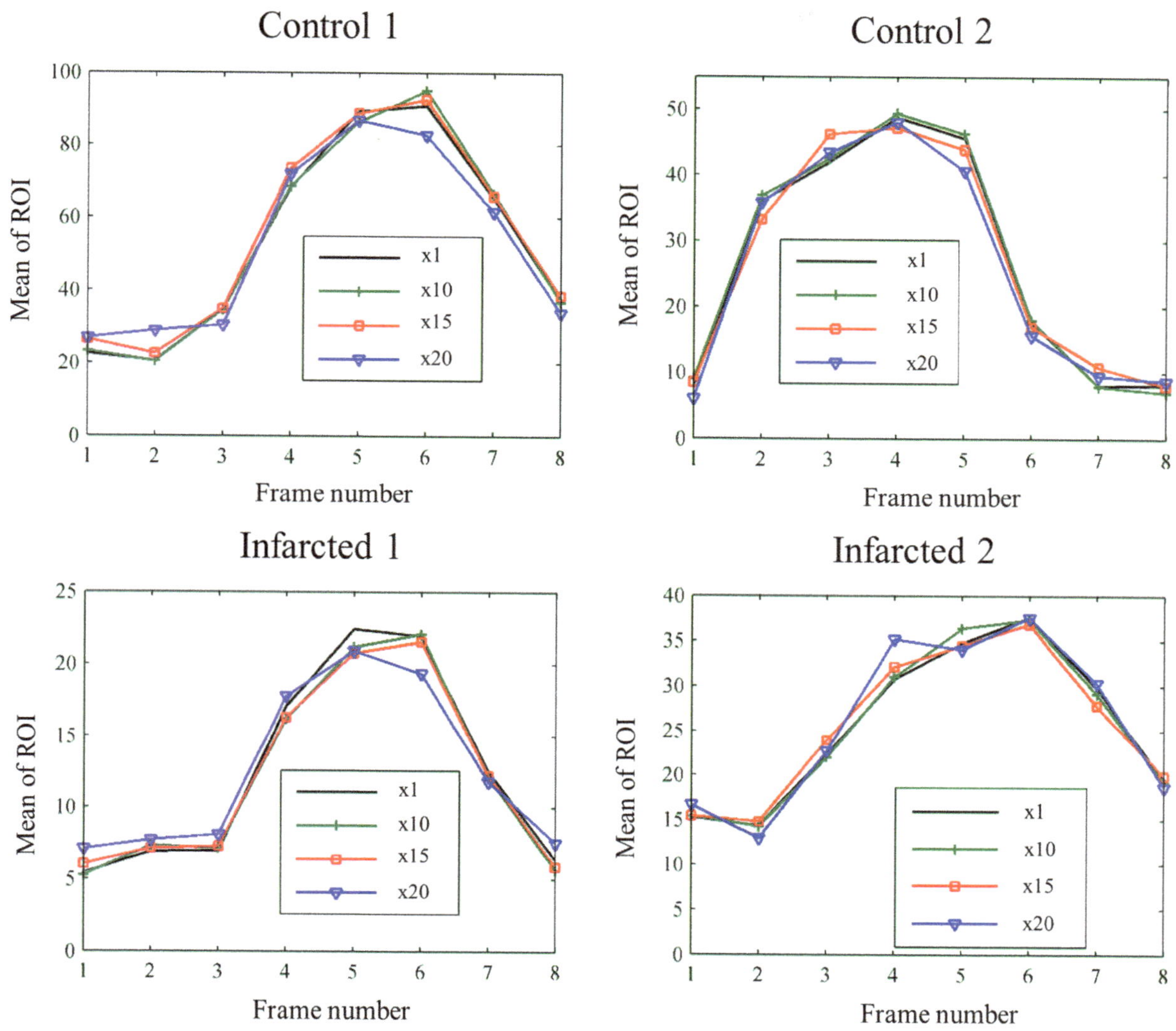

Figure 9. Temporal intensity changes for the images shown in figure 8 for all data sets, measured on a circular ROI (diameter = 6 pixels) located at the inner part of the myocardium.

across repetitions. With the prospective cine dataset the undersampling scheme led to a number of different undersampling patterns (figure 3(b)) equal to the number of frames. However, with the retrospective case the undersampling scheme used produced a number of different undersampling patterns equal to the number of repetitions (figure 3(c)), which is 17 times higher than the number of frames. In this way, the retrospective acquisition benefits from higher randomization. The same strategy could be also applied to prospective sequences by changing the undersampling pattern across different averages during the acquisition, but, to the best of our knowledge, no previous works have addressed this strategy for motion-based reconstruction. However, although randomization across repetitions can be applied to the prospective sequence, some differences still remain between prospective and retrospective undersampling processes. While the prospective acquisition scheme allows us to decide in advance which undersampling pattern will be applied to each frame, this is not possible for retrospective cine. In the retrospective case once the acquisition has finished, acquired phase-encoding lines are binned into cardiac frames based on the recorded navigator data, making it impossible to determine in advance the undersampling pattern on each frame [16].

The claimed acceleration factor depends on the quality criterion and the tolerance to artefacts. Adopting the criterion of preservation of image quality, for acceleration factors up to ×7 (FS = 60%), image quality is close to that of the fully-sampled data. Higher accelerations resulted in an increase of the smoothing artifact. However, adopting the criterion of temporal intensity changes in an ROI in the myocardium and the presence of artefacts at end-systole/diastole, which are the frames used to extract functional measurements such as ejection fraction and left-ventricle mass [31], results showed that accelerations up to ×10 (FS = 40%) – ×15 (FS = 26%) are feasible. For an acceleration factor ×10 the important features in the image were preserved and images presented high resolution. An acceleration factor ×15 led to a slight increase in artefacts and over-smoothing effect, without distorting temporal intensity information. Higher accelerations led to over-smoothed images that affected both resolution and temporal intensity changes. However, we remark that image quality in both the fully sampled and undersampled data sets is variable across frames. End of systole and end of diastole showed good quality in all cases but some intermediate frames presented some motion artefacts that became more conspicuous as the acceleration increased. Comparing to previous works, a wide range of acceleration factors can be found in the literature. However, most works focused on prospective clinical applications and only two included retrospective reconstruction [6,32]. Of the few studies addressing preclinical small-animal applications [16,33–36], only two used retrospective self-gated cine sequences, obtaining acceleration factors of 3 [36] and 15 [16] with a ST-TV method similar to the one used in this paper.

To our knowledge, our work is the first one that studies motion estimation not only in normal cases [19] [17] but also in rats with myocardial infarction. We found small differences between infarcted and healthy animals. Temporal intensity changes were slightly better recovered in infarcted animals because the myocardium motion is compromised in this case. Motion artefacts were more apparent for healthy animals.

Previous work that proposed motion-based reconstruction methods modeled motion using optical flow methods [18], block-matching algorithms and phase-based motion estimation [37]. The latter was found to be more robust than block-matching algorithms and optical flow methods [17]. Our motion estimation step consisted of free-form deformation, which is a widely used nonrigid registration method in medical imaging, based on hierarchical B-splines [23,38]. However, further work would be required to better understand the differences among motion estimation methods for cardiac cine compressed sensing MRI.

Our study is subject to a series of limitations. Our conclusions were drawn from an undersampled dataset made from fully sampled data instead of being directly acquired. Further work will focus on validation with real-time undersampled data and analysis of the effect of randomization across repetitions for prospective cine, which may further increase the potential of CS. In this work we focused on the comparison between SPLICS and ST-TV, assessing the quality of the reconstruction based on local image quality criteria. To determine acceleration factors achievable in real scenarios, a much larger dataset including both patients and control datasets and the evaluation of global metrics, such as ejection fraction, will be required. It is possible that a given method, even being better in technical terms, does not increase clinical usefulness, but this issue is out of the scope of our work.

Conclusion

We studied the benefit of motion-based reconstruction for retrospective cardiac cine in small-animal studies, using SPLICS, a new motion-based reconstruction method. We also compared SPLICS to ST-TV and analyzed the effect of the spatiotemporal sparsity parameter. We found that ST-TV with optimum α leads to results similar to those of SPLICS. On the other hand, SPLICS is more robust for the selection of the weighting parameter and provided similar or superior results in all our cases. Hence, we have validated SPLICS and found that for retrospective cardiac cine ST-TV with optimum spatiotemporal weighting parameter is a good methodology for accelerating retrospective cardiac cine MRI in small animals.

Author Contributions

Conceived and designed the experiments: JA PM. Performed the experiments: PM. Analyzed the data: JA PM. Contributed reagents/materials/analysis tools: JA PM EM JP MD. Wrote the paper: JA PM EM JP MD.

References

1. Griswold MA, Jakob PM, Heidemann RM, Nittka M, Jellus V, et al. (2002) Generalized autocalibrating partially parallel acquisitions (GRAPPA). Magn Reson Med 47: 1202–1210.
2. Pruessmann KP, Weiger M, Scheidegger MB and Boesiger P (1999) SENSE: sensitivity encoding for fast MRI. Magn Reson Med 42: 952–962.
3. Madore B, Glover GH and Pelc NJ (1999) Unaliasing by fourier-encoding the overlaps using the temporal dimension (UNFOLD), applied to cardiac imaging and fMRI. Magn Reson Med 42: 813–828.
4. Tsao J, Boesiger P and Pruessmann KP (2003) k-t BLAST and k-t SENSE: dynamic MRI with high frame rate exploiting spatiotemporal correlations. Magn Reson Med 50: 1031–1042.
5. Lustig M, Santos JM, Donoho D and Pauly JM (2006) k-t SPARSE: High frame rate dynamic MRI exploiting spatio-temporal sparsity. Proceedings of the 14th Annual Meeting of ISMRM, Seattle, Washington, USA: 2420.
6. Jung H, Sung K, Nayak KS, Kim EY and Ye JC (2009) k-t FOCUSS: a general compressed sensing framework for high resolution dynamic MRI. Magn Reson Med 61: 103–116.
7. Usman M, Prieto C, Schaeffter T and Batchelor PG (2011) k-t Group sparse: a method for accelerating dynamic MRI. Magn Reson Med 66: 1163–1176.
8. Montefusco LB, Lazzaro D, Papi S and Guerrini C (2011) A fast compressed sensing approach to 3D MR image reconstruction. IEEE transactions on medical imaging 30: 1064–1075.
9. Goud S, Yue H and Jacob M (2010) Real-time cardiac MRI using low-rank and sparsity penalties. Biomedical Imaging: From Nano to Macro, 2010 IEEE International Symposium on: 988–991.
10. Zhao B, Haldar JP and Liang ZP (2010) PSF Model-Based Reconstruction with Sparsity Constraint: Algorithm and Application to Real-Time Cardiac MRI. Annual International Conference of the IEEE Engineering in Medicine and Biology Society: 3390–3393.
11. Brinegar C, Haosen Z, Wu YJL, Foley LM, Hitchens TK, et al. (2009) Real-time cardiac MRI using prior spatial-spectral information. Engineering in Medicine and Biology Society, 2009 EMBC 2009 Annual International Conference of the IEEE: 4383–4386.
12. Nocedal J and Wright SJ (2006) Numerical Optimization. Springer Series in Operations Research and Financial Engineering. 664 p.
13. Osher S, Burger M, Goldfarb D, Xu JJ and Yin WT (2005) An iterative regularization method for total variation-based image restoration. Multiscale Model Simul 4: 460–489.
14. Goldstein T and Osher S (2009) The Split Bregman Method for L1-Regularized Problems. SIAM J Imaging Sci 2: 323–343.
15. Abascal J, Chamorro-Servent J, Aguirre J, Arridge S, Correia T, et al. (2011) Fluorescence diffuse optical tomography using the split Bregman method. Med Phys 38: 6275–6284.
16. Montesinos P, Abascal JFPJ, Cussó L, Vaquero JJ and Desco M (2014) Application of the compressed sensing technique to self-gated cardiac cine sequences in small animals. Magn Reson Med 72: 369–380.
17. Asif MS, Hamilton L, Brummer M and Romberg J (2013) Motion-adaptive spatio-temporal regularization for accelerated dynamic MRI. Magn Reson Med 70: 800–812.
18. Bilen C, Selesnick I, Yao W, Otazo R and Sodickson DK (2011) A motion compensating prior for dynamic MRI reconstruction using combination of compressed sensing and parallel imaging. Signal Processing in Medicine and Biology Symposium (SPMB), 2011 IEEE: 1–6.
19. Abascal JFPJ, Montesinos P, Marinetto E, Pascau J, Vaquero JJ, et al. (2013) A Prior-Based Image Variation (PRIVA) Approach Applied to Motion-Based Compressed Sensing Cardiac Cine MRI. XIII Mediterranean Conference on Medical and Biological Engineering and Computing 2013. Springer International Publishing. pp. 233–236.
20. Bovens SM, Boekhorst B, den Ouden K, van de Kolk KWA, Nauerth A, et al. (2011) Evaluation of infarcted murine heart function: comparison of prospectively triggered with self-gated MRI. NMR Biomed 24: 307–315.
21. Candes EJ, Romberg J and Tao T (2006) Robust uncertainty principles: Exact signal reconstruction from highly incomplete frequency information. IEEE Trans Inf Theory 52: 489–509.
22. Lustig M, Donoho D and Pauly JM (2007) Sparse MRI: The application of compressed sensing for rapid MR imaging. Magn Reson Med 58: 1182–1195.
23. Hill DL, Batchelor PG, Holden M and Hawkes DJ (2001) Medical image registration. Phys Med Biol 46: R1–45.
24. Rueckert D, Sonoda LI, Hayes C, Hill DLG, Leach MO, et al. (1999) Nonrigid registration using free-form deformations: application to breast MR images. Medical Imaging, IEEE Transactions on 18: 712–721.
25. Blu T, Thevenaz P and Unser M (2003) Complete parameterization of piecewise-polynomial interpolation kernels. IEEE Trans Image Process 12: 1297–1309.
26. Blu T, Thevenaz P and Unser M (2001) MOMS: maximal-order interpolation of minimal support. IEEE Trans Image Process 10: 1069–1080.
27. De Boor C (1972) On calculating with B-splines. Journal of Approximation Theory 6: 50–62.
28. Wang YL, Yang JF, Yin WT and Zhang Y (2008) A New Alternating Minimization Algorithm for Total Variation Image Reconstruction. SIAM J Imaging Sci 1: 248–272.

29. Tarnavski O, McMullen JR, Schinke M, Nie Q, Kong S, et al. (2004) Mouse cardiac surgery: comprehensive techniques for the generation of mouse models of human diseases and their application for genomic studies. Physiol Genomics 16: 349–360.
30. Lingala SG, Hu Y, DiBella E and Jacob M (2011) Accelerated dynamic MRI exploiting sparsity and low-rank structure: k-t SLR. IEEE transactions on medical imaging 30: 1042–1054.
31. Yang Z, Berr SS, Gilson WD, Toufektsian M-C and French BA (2004) Simultaneous Evaluation of Infarct Size and Cardiac Function in Intact Mice by Contrast-Enhanced Cardiac Magnetic Resonance Imaging Reveals Contractile Dysfunction in Noninfarcted Regions Early After Myocardial Infarction. Circulation 109: 1161–1167.
32. Moghari MH, Akcakaya M, O'Connor A, Basha TA, Casanova M, et al. (2011) Compressed-Sensing Motion Compensation (CosMo): A Joint Prospective-Retrospective Respiratory Navigator for Coronary MRI. Magn Reson Med 66: 1674–1681.
33. Wech T, Lemke A, Medway D, Stork LA, Lygate CA, et al. (2011) Accelerating Cine-MR Imaging in Mouse Hearts Using Compressed Sensing. J Magn Reson Imaging 34: 1072–1079.
34. Wech T, Lygate C, Neubauer S, Kostler H and Schneider J (2012) Highly accelerated cardiac functional MRI in rodent hearts using compressed sensing and parallel imaging at 9.4T. Journal of Cardiovascular Magnetic Resonance 14: P65.
35. Christodoulou AG, Bo Z and Zhi-Pei L (2011) Regularized image reconstruction for PS model-based cardiovascular MRI. Biomedical Imaging: From Nano to Macro, 2011 IEEE International Symposium on: 57–60.
36. Motaal AG, Coolen BF, Abdurrachim D, Castro RM, Prompers JJ, et al. (2013) Accelerated high-frame-rate mouse heart cine-MRI using compressed sensing reconstruction. NMR Biomed 26: 451–457.
37. Asif MS, Hamilton L, Brummer M and Romberg J (2013) Motion-adaptive spatio-temporal regularization for accelerated dynamic MRI. Magn Reson Med 70: 800–812.
38. Xie Z and Farin GE (2004) Image registration using hierarchical B-splines. Visualization and Computer Graphics, IEEE Transactions on 10: 85–94.

11

Deep White Matter in Huntington's Disease

Owen Phillips[1], Ferdinando Squitieri[2]*, Cristina Sanchez-Castaneda[3], Francesca Elifani[2], Carlo Caltagirone[1,4], Umberto Sabatini[3], Margherita Di Paola[1]*

1 Clinical and Behavioural Neurology Dept, IRCCS Santa Lucia Foundation, Rome, Italy, **2** IRCSS Neuromed, Pozzilli, Italy, **3** Radiology Dept, IRCCS Santa Lucia Foundation, Rome, Italy, **4** Neuroscience Dept, University of Rome "Tor Vergata", Rome, Italy

Abstract

White matter (WM) abnormalities have already been shown in presymptomatic (Pre-HD) and symptomatic HD subjects using Magnetic Resonance Imaging (MRI). In the present study, we examined the microstructure of the long-range large deep WM tracts by applying two different MRI approaches: Diffusion Tensor Imaging (DTI) -based tractography, and T2*weighted (iron sensitive) imaging. We collected Pre-HD subjects (n = 25), HD patients (n = 25) and healthy control subjects (n = 50). Results revealed increased axial (AD) and radial diffusivity (RD) and iron levels in Pre-HD subjects compared to controls. Fractional anisotropy decreased between the Pre-HD and HD phase and AD/RD increased and although impairment was pervasive in HD, degeneration occurred in a pattern in Pre-HD. Furthermore, iron levels dropped for HD patients. As increased iron levels are associated with remyelination, the data suggests that Pre-HD subjects attempt to repair damaged deep WM years before symptoms occur but this process fails with disease progression.

Editor: David Blum, Inserm U837, France

Funding: This work was supported by the Italian Ministry of Health grant 204/GR-2009-1606835. Also, support was provided by the European Commission: Marie Curie Fellowship for career development to CS (FP7-PEOPLE-2011-IEF). The authors are grateful for the support they received from the Italian Ministry of Health (Ricerca Corrente), European Huntington's Disease Network for the Registry Study, by the "Italian League for Huntington and related diseases onlus (www.lirh.it)" to FS. The funders had no role in study design, data collection and analysis, decision to publish, or preparation of the manuscript. The authors are grateful to all patients for contributing to the work.

Competing Interests: The authors have declared that no competing interests exist.

* Email: m.dipaola@hsantalucia.it (MDP); ferdinando.squitieri@lirh.it (FS)

Introduction

Huntington's disease (HD) is a neurodegenerative autosomal dominate disorder caused by increased CAG repeats, this leads to increased accumulation of mutant huntingtin, and formation of intranuclear inclusions and eventually to brain damage. Damage has long been thought to start in the striatum (for review see: [1]), however, most areas of the brain show abnormalities. Of the abnormalities found in the HD brain, the changes to white matter in particular have been become a major focus of research.

A model for the white matter changes in HD has been formulated [2], which suggests that the pathogenesis of HD begins with a deleterious effect of the mutant huntingtin on myelin. Indeed mutant huntingtin is not found in higher levels in the neurons that degenerate first, rather the mutated protein is expressed throughout the nervous system and periphery [3]. This implies that its primary impact may not be on neurons. The myelin breakdown is, in turn, associated with increased density of oligodendrocytes in the brain, which are involved in repairing myelin damage. As the oligodendrocytes have the highest iron content, when they increase in number, iron content increases [2].

Abnormalities in white matter cause downstream effects through a complex physiological process that is still being uncovered (see [4] for a summary). In short, oligodendrocytes and myelin abnormalities can slow or stop fast axon transport, which can result in synaptic loss and eventually axonal degeneration in a retrograde, ("Dying back") fashion [5].

In the last decades in-vivo Magnetic Resonance Imaging (MRI) investigations have revealed the extent of changes to white matter in HD. MRI research has reported extensive white matter volume loss in the whole brain [6], in the frontal lobe [7] and across the total cerebrum [8], as well as changes to white matter microstructure; the motor cortico-striatal circuit [9–12], sensorimotor cortex, [10], corpus callosum [11,13], and across extensive distributed white matter fibers (corpus callosum, superior and inferior longitudinal fasciculi and external capsule) [12]) years before symptoms occur.

The increasing evidence that white matter is negatively impacted in HD even before disease onset (Pre-HD) has led us to investigate the changes in the large white matter tracts in Pre-HD and HD and how these changes were related to the iron content. We first investigated the corpus callosum and found that early callosal white matter demyelination damage characterizes HD in the pre-symptomatic stage [11]. At that clinical stage, the myelin breakdown starts at the level of the early and heavily myelinated callosal fibres [14]. Changes in iron content (reduction) manifest in the early stages of HD, likely indicating a failure of the remyelination processes at that time. Then we focused on the cortical spinal tract, which is the brain's main motor fiber [15]. We found that a likely active repair mechanism (as indicated by increased iron) helps keep the cortical spinal tract at a normal functional level in the presymptomatic stage. However, this repair seems to fail with disease progression and cortical spinal white matter tract damage becomes extensive in HD patients. The damage to the cortical spinal white matter tract appears to occur in a retrograde ("Dying back") fashion, similar to what happens in striatal and cortical projection neurons [5,16].

In the present study we were interested in making a step forward, by investigating the whole deep white matter in HD, definable as the large easily identifiable association white matter tracts, i.e. the arcuate fasciculus (AF), the superior longitudinal fasciculus (SLF), the cingulate (Cing), the inferior longitidinal fasciculus (ILF), the inferior occipital fasciculus (IFO), the anterior thalamic radiation (ATR) and the uncinate fasciculus (UF). We studied the deep white matter tracts both as a combined whole (called from now on "total deep white matter") in order to investigate the disease effect on deep white matter in general and as single tracts (AF, SLF, Cing, ILF, IFO, ATR, and UF; we will refer to them as "individual deep white matte tracts") in order to identify possible regional variations in the disease process.

With the white matter model in mind, we adopted two different MRI approaches to investigate the deep white matter in HD: Diffusion Tensor Imaging (DTI)-based tractography and T2*weighted imaging.

DTI is the MRI technique most frequently used to study white matter fiber changes. It is a non-invasive technique that uses local water diffusion in the brain tissue. Although the biological determinants of diffusion parameters (fractional anisotropy-FA, axial diffusivity-AD and radial diffusivity-RD) are not yet fully understood (for a discussion on diffusion imaging see [17], it is agreed that this approach is sensitive to microstructural tissue properties. Indeed, it has been used in numerous studies to investigate everything from the effects of age on white matter in healthy subjects [18] to disease effects in Alzheimer's disease [19] and schizophrenia [20].

T2* weighted volumes, which are sensitive to iron/ferritin [21,22] are useful to investigate the iron content that is associated with the remyelination process [2]. The few studies present in literature show a non-univocal picture of the regional white matter iron content changes in HD, with no iron level differences in the callosal splenium, but decreased iron levels in the frontal lobe white matter [2], the callosal isthmus [14] and the cortical spinal white matter tract [15]. However, no studies to date in HD have combined the sensitivity of DTI tractography to identify the deep white matter in-vivo with T2* weighted volume images. By combining these imaging methods in a large cohort of subjects (25 HD patients, 25 Pre-HD and 50 healthy subjects), we can assess the effect HD has on the deep white matter tissue microstructure (total and individual tracts).

The main aims of our study were the following: 1) to examine total deep white matter microstructure in Pre-HD subjects and HD patients; 2) to investigate whether variations in connectivity parameters (FA, AD, RD) and in iron level within the deep white matter provide evidence for the white matter demyelination and remyelination model in HD; 3) to explore whether white matter microstructural properties vary by individual deep white matter tract in a particular manner.

Methods

Subjects

Subject demographics and clinical assessments are outlined in Table 1. HD patients (n = 25) and Pre-HD subjects (n = 25), underwent a genetic test (abnormal CAG repeats ≥36) and were examined clinically by the same neurologist (FS) with expertise in HD. All individuals were assessed using the Unified Huntington's Disease Rating Scale (UHDRS), which includes motor, cognitive, behavioral, and functional subscales [23]. Each section consists of a multistep subscale. The motor section measures eye movements, limb coordination, tongue impersistence and movement disorders (such as rigidity, bradykinesia, dystonia, chorea, and gait disturbances). A higher score means more motor impairment. The cognitive scale mainly evaluates executive function. A higher score means better cognitive performance. The behavioral section investigates the presence of depression, aggressiveness, obsessions/compulsions, delusions/hallucinations and apathy. A higher score means more impairment. The functional assessments include the HD functional capacity scale (HDFCS), the independence scale and a checklist of common daily tasks. All three scales mainly investigate independence in daily life activities. The HDFCS is reported as the total functional capacity (TFC) score (range 0–13) and is the only functional subscale with established psychometric properties (including inter-rater reliability and validity), which are based on radiographic measures of disease progression. Thus, the TFC score is used worldwide to determine patients' HD stage. On the independence scale, the investigator indicates whether the patient can perform the task that evaluates independence level (range 10–100). The checklist (functional assessment) is summed by giving a score of 1 to all "yes" answers (range 0–25). Pre-HD are defined as those subjects whom the suspected clinical diagnosis is confirmed by DNA analysis, which revealed (CAG)(n) expansion into the range characteristic of Huntington disease (>36 or repeats), but who do not have manifested Huntington's disease symptoms yet defined by a total motor score of <5 in the UHDRS and cognitive and behavioral assessment within the normality. The Disease Burden index, a measure of disease severity, was used according to the already described formula (age × [CAG-35.5]), where CAG is the number of CAG repeats [24]. A higher score reflects increased disease severity. The Mini Mental State Examination (MMSE) [25], which measures global cognitive functioning, was administered to Pre-HD subjects and HD patients. A lower score reflects greater impairment.

Fifty individually healthy subjects were recruited from the community. Patients in the advanced stages of disease (Stages III and IV) and/or with traumatic brain injury or focal lesions were excluded.

Ethics Statement

Presymptomatic test, genetic diagnosis and clinical exams were performed at Neurological Research Institute IRCCS Neuromed. All participants had the cognitive capacity to understand the research protocol and gave their oral and written consent. Cognitive capacity to consent was determined the MMSE. No subjects had cognitive impairment (see score on Table 1). In no case was there a surrogate consent procedure consented on the behalf of participants. Consent was obtained according to the Declaration of Helsinki and the Santa Lucia Foundation Research Ethics Committee approved the study.

MRI Data Acquisition

All MRI data was acquired on a 3T Allegra MRI system (Siemens, Germany) using a birdcage head coil. Scans were collected in a single session, with the following pulse sequences: 1) proton density and T2-weighted double turbo spin echo (SE) acquired in transverse planes (time repetition [TR]: 4500 ms, time echo [TE]: 12 ms, time to inversion [TI]: 112 ms, field of view [FOV]: 230×172 mm, matrix: 320×240, slice thickness: 5 mm, number of slices: 24); 2) fluid-attenuated inversion recovery in the same planes as the SE sequence (TR/TE/TI: 8500/109/

Table 1. Sociodemographic and clinical characteristics of patients and control subjects.

	Pre-HD (n = 25)	HD (n = 25)	Controls (n = 25)	Fisher's Exact Test; F or T Test	df	p
Characteristics						
Gender male/female	16/9	14/11	30/20	0.367	2	0.833
Age (years ± SD)	37.44±7.01	47.40±14.53	42.88±12.48	4.349	2	0.012[a††]
CAG repetition length	43.28±2.17	46.68±6.80	NA	−2.380	48	0.021[a††]
MMSE	27.82±1.24	24.97±3.23	NA	3.682	38	0.001[b††]
UHDRS Motor	8.00±9.28	37.22±13.18	NA	−8.695	44	0.001[a††]
UHDRS Cognitive	257.80±42.34	142.65±50.35	NA	8.046	41	0.001[b††]
UHDRS Behavioural	7.67±7.84	18.39±9.13	NA	−4.160	42	0.001[a††]
UHDRS Functional	25±0	17.91±5.68	NA	5.984	44	0.001[b††]
TFC	13±0	8.39±2.37	NA	9.329	44	0.001[b††]
Independence scale	99.8±1.04	78.04±12.49	NA	8.312	44	0.001[b††]
Disease burden	292.3±87.52	458.6±104.75	NA	−6.091	48	0.001[a††]

Legend. HD = Huntington's disease; Pre-HD = gene-positive, without motor symptoms; SD = standard deviation; df = degrees of freedom; CAG, trinucleotide repeat number; MMSE = Mini Mental State Examination; UHDRS = Unified Huntington's Disease Rating Scale; TFC = Total Functional Capacity; NA = Not Available;
[††]T-student, Bonferroni correction.
[a]Pre-HD<HD (when referred to a cognitive scale comparison or CAG repetition, higher punctuations mean greater impairment).
[b]Pre-HD>HD (when referred to a cognitive scale comparison, higher punctuations mean lesser impairment).
*MMSE: Missing data for 5 Pre-HD & 5 HD subjects.
*UHDRS Motor: Missing data for 2 Pre-HD & 2 HD subjects.
*UHDRS Cognitive: Missing data for 5 Pre-HD & 2 HD subjects.
*UHDRS Behavioral: Missing data for 4 Pre-HD & 2 HD subjects.
*UHDRS Functional: Missing data for 2 Pre-HD & 2 HD subjects.
*TFC: Missing data for 2 Pre-HD & 2 HD subjects.

2000 ms; FOV: 230×168 mm, matrix: 256×256, slice thickness: 5 mm, number of slices: 24); 3) T1-weighted 3D images, with partitions acquired in the sagittal plane, using a modified driven equilibrium Fourier transform [26] sequence (TE/TR/TI: 2.4/7.92/910 ms, flip angle: 15°, 1 mm3 isotropic voxels); and 4) diffusion-weighted volumes were also acquired using SE echo-planar imaging (TE/TR: 89/8500 ms, bandwidth: 2126 Hz/voxel, matrix: 128×128, 80 axial slices, voxel size: 1.8×1.8×1.8 mm) with 30 isotropically distributed orientations for the diffusion sensitizing gradients at a b value of 1000 s/mm2 and 6 b = 0 images. Scanning was repeated 3 times to increase the signal-to-noise ratio.

Six consecutive T2*-weighted gradient echo-planar whole-brain volumes were acquired at different time of echo (TE) (TEs: 6, 12, 20, 30, 45 and 60 ms; TR = 5000; bandwidth = 1116 Hz/vx; matrix size 128×128×80; flip angle 90°; voxel size of 1.5×1.5×2 mm3).

Images were visually inspected for gross anatomical abnormalities by 2 experienced observers (a neuropsychologist expert in neuroimaging and a neuroradiologist) blind to participant identities.

Images were also visually inspected for movement artifacts, which are a common source of concern while studying HD. Since movement can compromise tracking, we excluded subjects who had excessive movement in their scans.

DTI Processing

Diffusion-weighted images were processed with FMRIB's Software Library (FSL 4.1 www.fmrib.ox.ac.uk/fsl/). Images were corrected for eddy current distortion. The non-diffusion-weighted images were skull stripped using FSL's Brain Extraction Tool (BET) (http://www.fmrib.ox.ac.uk/fsl/bet2/index.html), and used to mask all diffusion-weighted images. A diffusion tensor model was fitted at each voxel using Diffusion Toolkit, generating FA, AD, and RD maps. RD was defined as the average of the second and third eigenvalues of the diffusion tensor, while AD corresponded to the first eigenvalue.

T2*weighted images processing

T2*weighted volumes were post processed accordingly to previously published methods [21,27]. Briefly the six T2*weighted volumes were averaged in order to generate a mean T2*-weighted volume. A full affine 3D alignment was calculated between each of the six T2*-weighted volumes and the mean T2*-weighted volume. For each subject we performed a voxel-by-voxel nonlinear least-squares fitting of the data acquired at the six TEs to obtain a mono-exponential signal decay curve. In order to facilitate analysis of relaxation results, we considered the inverse of relaxation times, i.e. relaxation rates R2* = 1/T2*×1000.

Iron images (R2*) were registered into subject DTI space using FSL Flirt 12 degree of freedom transformation with the DTI B0 image used as the reference image. Registrations were visually inspected for accuracy.

Tractography

Tractography methods are outlined in more detail in [28], however, the tractography and ROI drawing was modified to use TrackVis, an interactive environment for fiber tracking reconstruction, display and analysis developed at the Harvard Medical School Martinos Center for Biomedical Imaging at Massachusetts General Hospital (www.trackvis.org). The FACT approach was used to reconstruct fiber paths. A track angle threshold of 35° was used as well as an image mask based on the B0 image to restrict tracking to biologically plausible results.

Tractography of the total deep white matter was performed by manually drawing regions of interest on each individuals FA color map by a single expert (O.P.) who was blinded to subject age, gender, and diagnosis. To determine intra-rater reliability, fiber tracts were identified in 10 randomly chosen brain volumes. Reliability was assessed using the intraclass correlation coefficient (2-way mixed for intra-rater). The advantage of DTI-based tractography is that the tracts can be precisely mapped within subjects without the reliance on registration prodedures to align imaging data across subjects [28].

Region of interest placement for the AF, SLF, Cing, ILF, IFO, ATR, and UF was based on Wakana, et al [28]. The total deep white matter was for the present study considered to be the combined white matter of the individual tracts (AF, SLF, Cing, ILF, IFO, ATR, and UF). FA, AD, RD, and iron were calculated for each subject by averaging all voxels over the total deep white matter and separately for each individual tract, counting each voxel only once. Excellent intra-reliability was achieved for ROI placement, as determined by computing the intra-class correlation coefficients for tract volume and mean FA, AD, RD and Iron (Table S1). It is important to note, that the specific anatomical delineations for the deep white matter tracts are still emerging. For example, the ILF in [28], may include the middle longitudinal fasciculus (see [29] and the specific delineations of the SLF and AF (temporal component of the SLF) has been a source on contention, [30].

Statistical Analysis

Demographic differences were assessed using chi-square, independent sample t-tests or Anova as appropriate. All statistical analyses were performed using SPSS 14.0.

To test for total deep white matter differences among groups, a Multivariate Analysis of Variance (Manova) was applied to all three groups (healthy controls, HD patients and Pre-HD subjects). Sex and age were included as covariates in the model. After that, contrasts were run to individuate the significant difference between groups.

In order to localize differences in individual deep white matter tracts between groups, a Multivariate Analysis of Variance (Manova) was applied to all three groups (healthy controls, HD patients and Pre-HD subjects). Sex and age were included as covariates in the model. After that, contrasts were run to individuate the significant difference between groups.

All results were corrected using a False Discovery Rate (FDR) correction, where order ranked p-values less than the resulting q-value were considered significant. Practically, results with a p-value less than 0.03 were considered significant.

Results

Subject demographics are reported in Table 1. Pre-HD subjects and HD patients differed in age and CAG repetition length, but not in gender. Additionally, as expected, HD patients had significantly poorer performances with respect to all measures assessed by the UHDRS, and also a significantly higher score of Disease Burden.

Total Deep White Matter Findings

Results are shown in Figure 1.

Statistical details are outlined in Table 2.

FA: Pre-HD subjects did not have significantly reduced FA. HD patients had reduced FA compared to Pre-HD subjects and controls.

AD: Pre-HD subjects had increased AD compared to controls. HD patients had increased AD compared to Pre-HD and control subjects.

RD: Pre-HD subjects showed increased RD compared to controls. HD patients also had increased RD compared to Pre-HD subjects and controls.

R2*: R2* values were elevated in Pre-HD subjects both compared to controls and HD patients. HD patients did not have different values of R2* compared to controls.

We explored the individual covariates' effect on white matter parameters, we found that age has an impact on diffusivity differences (AD and RD) between Controls and Pre-HD subjects, that results in the loss of statistical significance. All other results remain significant in the same direction. We did not find any effect of gender on the white matter parameters.

Hemisphere Deep White Matter

Results are shown in Figure 2.

Hemisphere deep white matter is the combined total of the deep white matter tracts for the left and, separately, for the right hemisphere. Statistical details are outlined in Table 2.

FA: Pre-HD subjects had reduced FA in the right hemisphere deep white matter and HD patients had reduced FA in both the left and right hemisphere deep white matter compared to both Pre-HD and control subjects.

AD: Pre-HD subjects had increased right hemisphere AD compared to controls. HD patients had increased AD compared to Pre-HD and control subjects in both hemispheres.

RD: Pre-HD subjects showed bilateral increases in RD compared to controls and HD patients had elevated bilateral RD compared to Pre-HD subjects and controls.

R2*: R2* values were elevated in both hemispheres within Pre-HD subjects compared to both controls and HD patients. HD patients did not have different values of R2* compared to controls.

Individual Deep White Matter tract Findings

Results are shown in Figure 2 and Figure 3.

Statistical details of tractography analysis of the individual deep white matter tracts are in Table 3 and Table S2.

FA: Pre-HD subjects revealed, compared to controls, lower FA in the right SLF, IFO and UF for Pre-HD subjects. In comparisons to controls, HD patients had lower FA bilaterally in the AF, SLF, Cing, IFO, ILF, and UF. Finally, FA analyses between Pre-HD subjects and HD patients revealed reductions in HD patients bilaterally in the AF, SLF, Cing, IFO as well as the right ILF.

AD: Pre-HD subjects exhibited, compared to controls, increased AD bilaterally in the SLF and ATR. AD analysis between HD patients and controls revealed increased AD bilaterally in the AF, SLF, IFO, and ATR as well as the left ILF and right UF. Furthermore, when comparing Pre-HD subjects with HD patients, HD patients had increased AD bilaterally in AF, SLF, IFO, and ATR as well as the left ILF.

RD: Pre-HD subjects, compared to healthy controls, showed significant increased RD in the SLF, and ATR bilaterally, as well as the right IFO. HD patients also showed increased RD compared to healthy controls bilaterally in the AF, SLF, Cing, ILF, IFO, ATR, and UF. Finally, Pre-HD subjects had lower RD compared to HD patients bilaterally in the AF, SLF, Cing, ILF, IFO, ATR and right UF.

R2*: The analysis between Pre-HD subjects and controls revealed increased R2* values in Pre-HD subjects in the left AF and right Cing and IFO. There were no differences in R2* values between HD patients and controls. However, when comparing

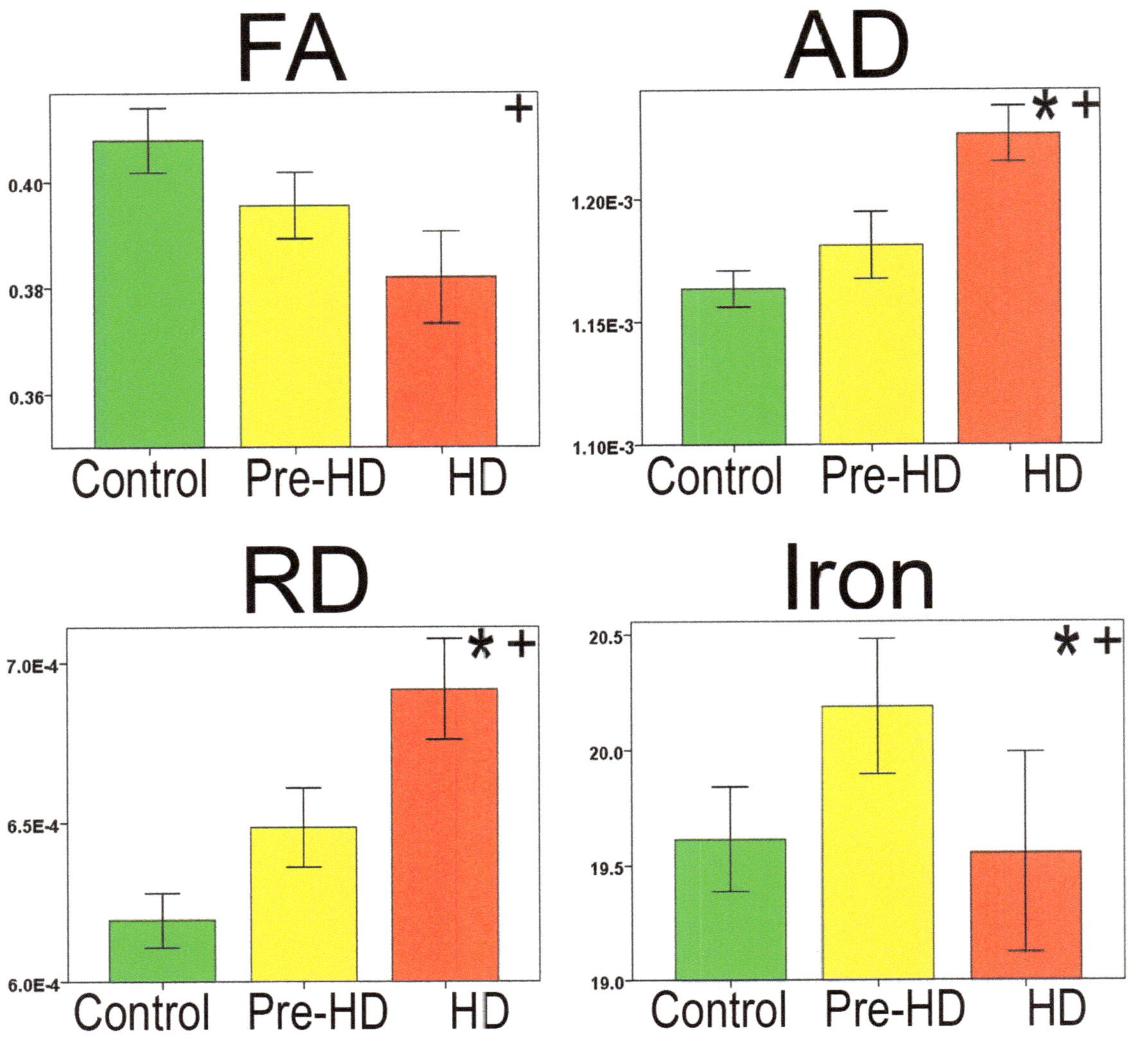

Figure 1. Total Deep White Matter Tractography and Group Comparison. Bar graphs show differences between Total Deep White Matter FA, AD, RD, and Iron. The error bars represent the Standard Error Mean (SEM). Legend. FA = Fractional Anisotropy; AD = Axial Diffusivity; RD = Radial Diffusivity. (AD/RD Mean units: 10^{-3} mm^2/s, R2* (10^{-3} mm^1/s). * Significant difference between Pre-HD and Controls+ Significant difference between Pre-HD and HD.

Pre-HD subjects and HD patients, Pre-HD subjects had increased R2* values bilaterally in the IFO as well as in the left AF, SLF and right Cing, ILF and ATR.

Discussion

This study sought to identify variations in the deep white matter (total and individual tracts) of Pre-HD subjects and HD patients compared to each other and to healthy controls. A number of major findings emerged from the results: (1) increases in AD and RD in total deep white matter are present in Pre-HD subjects before disease onset; (2) Pre-HD subjects show increased total deep white matter iron content (R2* values) compared to both controls and HD patients; (3) changes in individual white matter tracts in Pre-HD are pervasive and become worse as the disease progresses.

Postmortem studies have repeatedly demonstrated the striking myelin breakdown and white matter atrophy in HD [31]. Furthermore, a HD mouse model [32], found thinner myelin sheaths and increased myelin periodicity (that is less compacted the white matter). Also, an increasing number of white matter DTI studies on human subjects have found extensive distributed changes to white matter microstructure both in Pre-HD and HD subjects [9–13,33–36]

Our current findings on total deep white matter are in line with these previous works. We found an increase in AD and RD in Pre-HD subjects compared to healthy controls and abnormalities become significantly worse in HD. The precise biological meaning of the DTI parameters is still unclear [17] and caution should be used in interpreting the results. However, AD a measure of how fast diffusion occurs in the preferred direction, has been shown to be sensitive to the number of axons, as well as their coherence [37]. Increased AD is related to white matter axonal atrophy likely associated with Wallerian degeneration [38]. RD is a measure of how fast diffusion occurs in the perpendicular direction. Increased RD is thought to reflect reductions in myelination [39].

These white matter changes can be interpreted as a manifestation of the pathology's evolution. Indeed, our data suggests that the deep white matter incurs early axonal atrophy (increased AD) and myelin damage (increased RD) even before measurable symptoms appear (Pre-HD stage), and this insult to deep white

Table 2. Total Deep White Matter Tractography Group Comparisons.

Region		Pre-HD	HD	Control	MANOVA F	MANOVA df	MANOVA P	Control vs Pre-HD P	Control vs HD P	Pre-HD vs HD P
	FA	0.399±0.017	0.378±0.022	0.408±0.023	14.81	2,95	0.001	0.048	**0.001**	**0.005**
Total Deep White Matter	AD	1.118E-03±3.00E-05	1.234E-03±3.00E-05	1.116E-03±3.00E-05	41.52	2,95	0.001	**0.013**	**0.001**	**0.001**
(mean value ± SD)	RD	6.38E-04±4.00E-0	7.01E-04±4.00E-05	6.19E-04±3.00E-05	42.132	2,95	0.001	**0.002**	**0.001**	**0.001**
	R2*	20.19±0.75	19.54±1.08	19.62±0.71	4.383	2,85	0.011	**0.010**	0.676	**0.010**

Legend. FA = Fractional Anisotropy; AD = Axial Diffusivity; RD = Radial Diffusivity. (AD/RD Mean units: 10^{-3} mm^2/s, R2* (10^{-3} mm^1/s).
*Significant FDR corrected results are in **BOLD**.

matter increases progressively as the disease progresses (stage I and II). However, it is important to keep in mind the hypothesis that abnormal brain development may contribute to the pathogenesis of HD, as a precursor to the more global neurodegeneration process [40]. Future longitudinal studies are needed to examine if deep white matter changes are already in place in young Pre-HD subjects.

In order to explore the underlying mechanism of deep white matter abnormalities in HD, we examined the iron content. We found a significant increase in iron content within Pre-HD subjects compared to both healthy controls and HD patients. This suggests that a repair mechanism is active in Pre-HD subjects, and it may lead to an increase in oligodendrocytes before disease onset. The data is in line with previous reports on iron levels in Pre-HD subjects. In fact, extremely elevated numbers of oligodendrocytes have been reported years before symptom appearance [41–43]. The ability to repair appears to keep the brain working with minimal symptoms early in the disease and may be why white matter damage has not been identified to be a central part of HD. The repair mechanism may mask the downstream effects the damage causes.

Furthermore, because HD patients have substantially impaired total deep white matter compared to Pre-HD subjects, it may indicate that the repair process is failing. There are two likely reasons for this. One, the oligodendrocytes themselves may be abnormal and thus they do not function correctly and/or the accumulation of oligodendrocytes could be helpful at first, but may be harmful once the levels become too high by causing neuronal excitotoxicity and promoting free radical toxicity [2]. Either of these possibilities fit with the idea that the HD brain is continually trying to remyelinate in a losing attempt to compensate for the disease-related myelin loss [2]. In HD, these remyelination processes may successfully compensate during younger years, which usually correspond to the beginning of the pathology or to the years before onset (Pre-HD stage), but eventually begin failing in older years as brain myelin volume continues to grow and the maintenance of this expanding volume becomes increasingly difficult. This is similar to what happens in healthy older individuals [44] and likely explains the decrease in iron content that we found between Pre-HD and HD subjects.

Interestingly, myelin may play a role in producing adenosine triphosphate (ATP) [46], if this is the case, damage to the total deep white matter could have a substantial impact on the brain's available energy, however, future studies will be needed to verify this.

The R2* measurement has some limitations. Indeed it is sensitive to increases in tissue iron, which increases the R2* value [45] but it is not a specific measure of iron. In fact, many other tissue changes, including myelination, calcifications, blood flow, and increased tissue water, can influence the R2* measure.

Although R2* is not an exclusive measure of iron, combined with diffusivity parameters it helps us reach a conclusion regarding the data. This is because as our DTI findings in Pre-HD subjects indicate tissue damage with more water and myelin damage (see changes in diffusivity Figure 1 and 2), both factors should lower the R2* values in our data. However, we still found higher R2* values in Pre-HD group (Figure 2). This suggests that higher R2* values reflect greater iron in our Pre-HD group.

Furthermore, shimming effects were controled for using the protocol outlined in Peran et al. [27].

However, in the future, higher Tesla strengths, such as 7T or above, and phase images (more related to the iron content) or quantitative susceptibility mapping should be investigated to confirm this data.

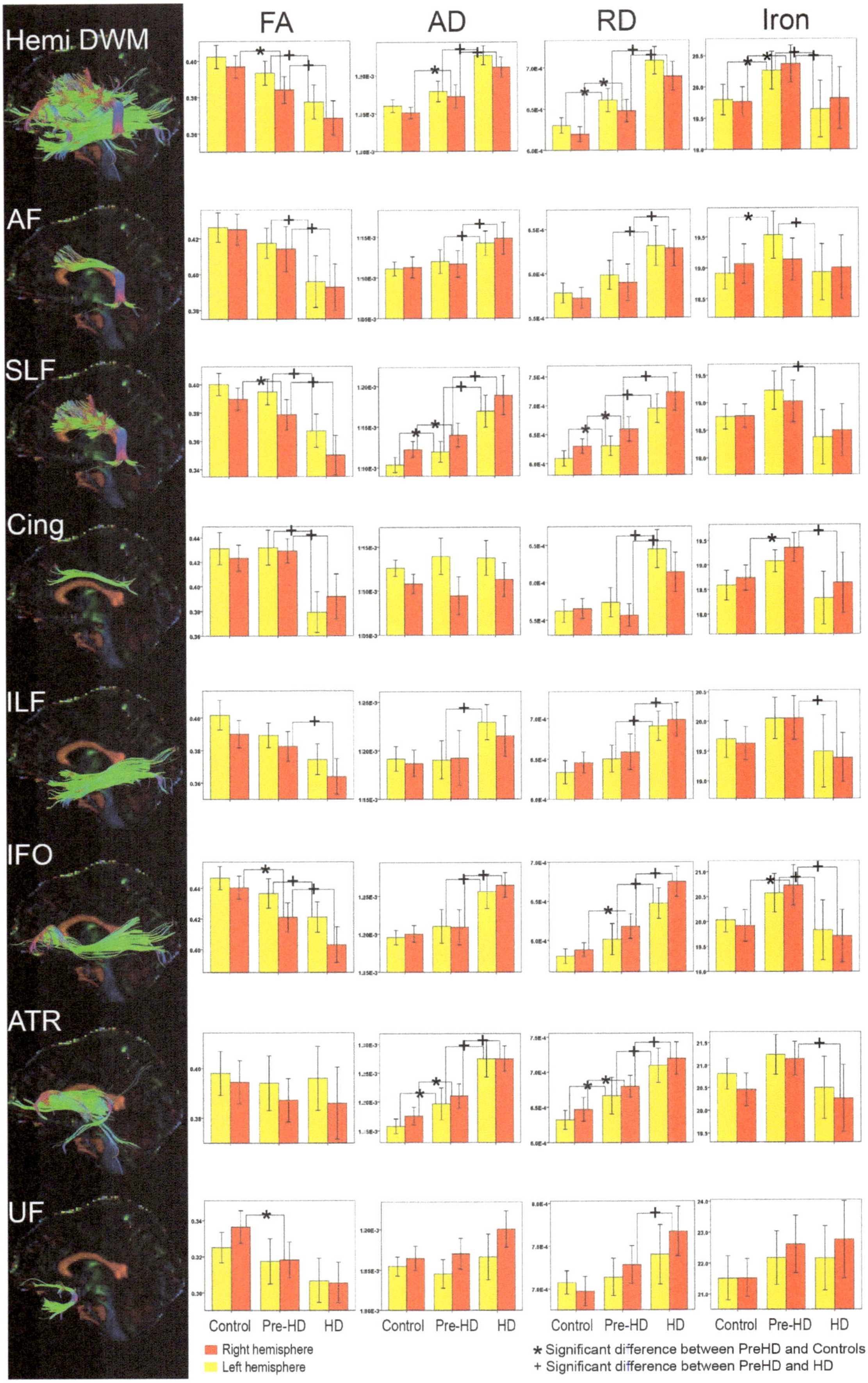

Hemi DWM
AF
SLF
Cing
ILF
IFO
ATR
UF
FA
AD
RD
Iron
Control Pre-HD HD
Right hemisphere
Left hemisphere
* Significant difference between PreHD and Controls
+ Significant difference between PreHD and HD

Figure 2. Individual Deep White Matter Tractography and Group Comparison. Bar graphs show differences between Deep White Matter Tracts FA, AD, RD, and Iron. The error bars represent the Standard Error Mean (SEM). Legend. FA = Fractional Anisotropy; AD = Axial Diffusivity; RD = Radial Diffusivity. (AD/RD Mean units: 10^{-3} mm^2/s, R2* (10^{-3} mm^1/s) Tracts are from a representative single subject. Legend. Hemi DWM = total Deep White Matter for each hemisphere, it is the result of the individual white matter tracts combined, AF = Arcuate Fasciculus, SLF = Superior Longitudinal Fasciculus, Cing = Cingulate, ILF = Inferior Longitudinal Fasciculus, IFO = Inferior Frontal Occipital fasciculus, ATR = Anterior Thalamic Radiation, UF = Uncinate Fasciculus.

In order to identify whether the changes in the deep white matter were localized to individual tracts or presented in a pattern, we examined each tract's microstructure. When comparing controls and Pre-HD subjects, we found the ILF tract was spared in Pre-HD subjects (no difference in FA, AD, RD and iron level). We also found that the AF and Cing did not show any microstructure changes (no difference in FA, AD, RD) but they present a higher level of iron unilaterally (left side for the AF, right side for the Cing) which indicates that the repair mechanism is working in these fibers, hiding the microstructural damage. We further found the IFO and UF were damaged unilaterally (decreased right FA, and increased RD for the IFO, decreased right FA for the UF) and increased iron level in the right IFO which indicates that the repair mechanism is at a breaking point, with both high level of iron and microstructural damage detectable. Finally, we found that the SLF and the ATR were the most damaged tracts at the microstructural level (increased of AD and RD bilaterally) and no difference in iron, which indicates that the repair mechanism already failed in those fibers, and the damage progressed to impair both sides of the tracts.

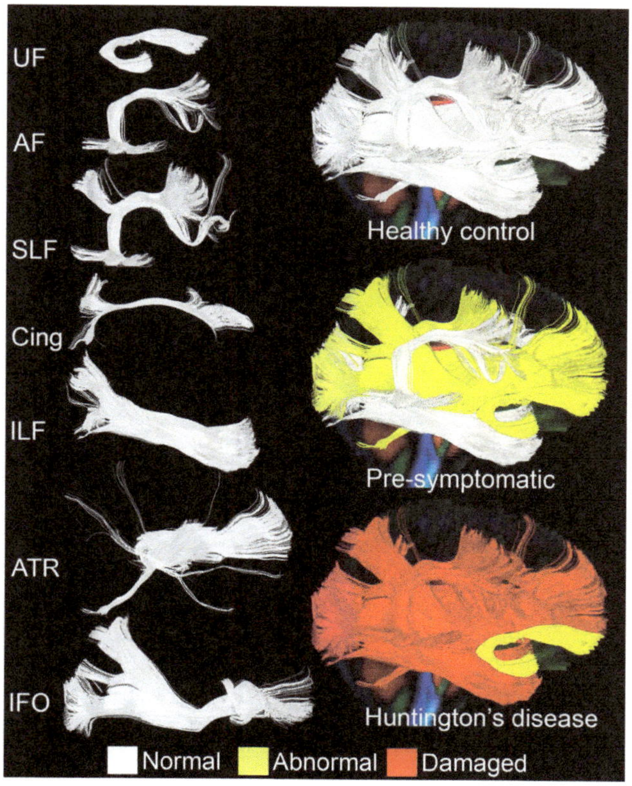

Figure 3. Deep White Matter Microstructure for Each Group. Tracts shown use colour to represent the overall microstructure for each tract within each group. White = Normal, Yellow = Abnormal, Red = - Damaged. Tracts Legend. AF = Arcuate Fasciculus, SLF = Superior Longitudinal Fasciculus, Cing = Cingulate, ILF = Inferior Longitudinal Fasciculus, IFO = Inferior Frontal Occipital fasciculus, ATR = Anterior Thalamic Radiation, UF = Uncinate Fasciculus.

Thus, it seems that individual white matter tracts are impaired in a specific manner in Pre-HD subjects, and it is possible to describe a pattern in the tract damage, going from spared (ILF), to more damaged (SLF and ATR), passing through those only partially damaged (IFO and UF) to those damaged and under repair (AF and Cing).

When we compare Pre-HD subjects with HD patients, the fibers already damaged in the Pre-HD phase, proceed in a peculiar way. The ILF, initially spared in Pre-HD, becomes impaired in HD (increased AD on the left side; increased RD bilaterally; increased iron on the right side); the AF and Cing, initially with a spared microstructure in Pre-HD, show bilateral microstructural changes in HD; the IFO, damaged unilaterally in Pre-HD, becomes impaired bilaterally in HD; the UF remains stable and relatively spared in both Pre-HD and HD; the SLF and the ATR, already damaged in the Pre-HD phase, become increasingly impaired. We found a high level of iron in Pre-HD compared to HD at the level of the SLF and the ATR, which was not present when Pre-HD subjects were compared with controls, which suggests a repair mechanism was active but is no longer working in HD patients.

Thus it seems that in our sample group: the SLF and ATR are fibers involved in the early phase of the pathology (Pre-HD) while the IFO is relatively spared early but worsens quickly unlike the UF which is more spared throughout the course of the pathology.

The difference in the individual white matter tracts damage (i.e. unilateral or bilateral involvement, early or late involvement in the course of the pathology) may be due to their different function and/or structure. As for the function, it seems there is a link between the fibers we have found damaged or spared (as the UF) and some aspects of the disease. For example, the ATR is involved in executive function and planning complex behaviours and working memory and encoding of new stimuli [47]. The SLF, with its three subcomponents SLFI SLFII and SFLII, is involved in regulation of higher aspects of motor behavior, in spatial attention and in gesture [48,49]. The IFO is involved in the awareness and use of visual information for the purpose of guiding movements and in the preparation and release of reaching-grasping arm movement [50] as well as the execution of language processing [49]. The UF, which is the spared one, is linked with the regulation of auditory stimuli and recognition memory [50] and likely plays a role in the language network [49]. However, despite our growing understanding of the deep white matter tracts, there is still much we do not yet know about their function thus, cautious consideration is warranted before drawing conclusions between the HD symptomology and specific tracts.

As for the structure, there is some evidence that HD might preferentially damage large early myelinating fibers such as those in the isthmus/splenium of the corpus callosum, which connect to the occipital lobe [13,14,33]. Large fibers can be advantageous because they encode more information but even a simple doubling in firing rate appears to more than quadruple an axon's energy use [51]. Large early myelinating high caliber fibers might thus be particularly susceptible. However, all the tracts had significantly worse microstructure as the disease progressed, with changes in

Table 3. Individual Deep White Matter Tractography Group Comparisons.

Region	Parameters		MANOVA		Control vs Pre-HD	Control vs HD	Pre-HD vs HD
		F	df	P	P	P	P
	FA	11.72	2,95	0	0.128	**0.001**	**0.007**
Hemi DWM L	AD	41.226	2,95	0	0.033	**0.001**	**0.001**
	RD	42.081	2,95	0	**0.002**	**0.001**	**0.001**
	R2*	3.956	2,85	0.023	**0.027**	0.392	**0.009**
	FA	15.459	2,95	0	**0.025**	**0.001**	**0.008**
Hemi DWM R	AD	32.857	2,95	0	**0.013**	**0.001**	**0.001**
	RD	33.854	2,95	0	**0.004**	**0.001**	**0.001**
	R2*	4.217	2,85	0.018	**0.007**	0.945	**0.023**
	FA	9.489	2,95	0.000	0.284	**0.001**	**0.008**
AF L	AD	7.662	2,95	0.001	0.358	**0.001**	**0.014**
	RD	12.412	2,95	0.001	0.097	**0.001**	**0.007**
	R2*	4.184	2,85	0.018	**0.009**	0.921	**0.018**
	FA	9.259	2,95	0.001	0.204	**0.001**	**0.013**
AF R	AD	5.869	2,95	0.004	0.832	**0.001**	**0.011**
	RD	12.739	2,95	0.001	0.183	**0.001**	**0.003**
	R2*	0.106	2,85	0.899	0.773	0.809	0.647
	FA	10.908	2,95	0	0.132	**0.001**	**0.010**
SLF L	AD	25.772	2,95	0	**0.007**	**0.001**	**0.001**
	RD	26.074	2,95	0	**0.003**	**0.001**	**0.001**
	R2*	5.118	2,85	0.008	0.035	0.133	**0.002**
	FA	14.621	2,95	0	**0.023**	**0.001**	**0.013**
SLF R	AD	18.941	2,95	0	**0.020**	**0.001**	**0.002**
	RD	22.77	2,95	0	**0.002**	**0.001**	**0.004**
	R2*	2.184	2,85	0.119	0.194	0.276	0.040
	FA	11.218	2,95	0	0.453	**0.001**	**0.001**
Cing L	AD	1.282	2,95	0.282	0.131	0.366	0.603
	RD	18.397	2,95	0	0.052	**0.001**	**0.001**
	R2*	2.331	2,85	0.103	0.092	0.499	0.042
	FA	5.607	2,95	0.005	0.852	**0.002**	**0.006**
Cing R	AD	0.573	2,95	0.566	0.343	0.850	0.339
	RD	7.015	2,95	0.001	0.904	**0.001**	**0.003**
	R2*	3.669	2,85	0.03	**0.018**	0.721	**0.019**
	FA	8.587	2,95	0	0.089	**0.001**	0.050
ILF L	AD	7.036	2,95	0.001	0.768	**0.001**	**0.002**
	RD	12.574	2,95	0	0.218	**0.001**	**0.002**
	R2*	1.804	2,85	0.171	0.193	0.395	0.064
	FA	7.896	2,95	0.001	0.337	**0.001**	**0.014**
ILF R	AD	2.333	2,95	0.102	0.764	0.035	0.129
	RD	10.176	2,95	0	0.381	**0.001**	**0.003**
	R2*	3.79	2,85	0.027	0.056	0.235	**0.008**
	FA	8.716	2,95	0	0.146	**0.001**	**0.027**
IFO L	AD	15.865	2,95	0	0.277	**0.001**	**0**
	RD	23.041	2,95	0	0.064	**0.001**	**0**
	R2*	3.781	2,85	0.027	0.050	0.262	**0.008**
	FA	17.85	2,95	0	**0.006**	**0.001**	**0.014**
IFO R	AD	19.794	2,95	0	0.595	**0.001**	**0**
	RD	47.271	2,95	0	**0.005**	**0.001**	**0**
	R2*	7.113	2,85	0.001	**0.003**	0.327	**0.001**

Table 3. Cont.

Region	Parameters	MANOVA			Control vs Pre-HD	Control vs HD	Pre-HD vs HD
		F	df	P	P	P	P
	FA	0.148	2,95	0.862	0.593	0.803	0.810
ATR L	AD	32.937	2,95	0	**0.022**	**0.001**	**0.001**
	RD	16.961	2,95	0	**0.022**	**0.001**	**0.005**
	R2*	2.368	2,85	0.100	0.160	0.283	0.033
	FA	0.848	2,95	0.431	0.344	0.263	0.887
ATR R	AD	30.096	2,95	0	**0.019**	**0.001**	**0.001**
	RD	15.608	2,95	0	**0.025**	**0.001**	**0.008**
	R2*	3.577	2,85	0.032	0.032	0.463	**0.014**
	FA	3.174	2,95	0.046	0.352	**0.014**	0.193
UF L	AD	1.214	2,95	0.302	0.413	0.306	0.124
	RD	2.577	2,95	0.081	0.757	**0.027**	0.110
	R2*	0.893	2,85	0.413	0.274	0.282	0.997
	FA	10.228	2,95	0	**0.017**	**0.001**	0.114
UF R	AD	4.421	2,95	0.015	0.753	**0.004**	0.032
	RD	10.889	2,95	0	0.064	**0.001**	**0.024**
	R2*	2.673	2,85	0.075	0.087	0.046	0.785

Legend. AF = Arcuate Fasciculus, SLF = Superior Longitudinal Fasciculus, Cing = Cingulate, ILF = Inferior Longitudinal Fasciculus, IFO = Inferior Frontal Occipital fasciculus, ATR = Anterior Thalamic Radiation, UF = Uncinate Fasciculus; Hemi DWM = total left and right Deep White Matter, it is the result of the individual white matter tracts combined for each hemisphere; FA = Fractional Anisotropy; AD = Axial Diffusivity; RD = Radial Diffusivity; R = Right; L = Left.
*Significant FDR corrected results are in **BOLD**.

FA, AD and RD involving the tracts bilaterally. In particular though, across the DTI parameters (FA, AD, RD), the parameter that was most sensitive to disease effects was RD, indeed each individual tract (AF, SLF; Cing, ILF, IFO and UF) presented an increase in RD for HD patients.

Again our data is in line with the accumulating number of DTI studies of Pre-HD and HD subjects that have looked at white matter. For example, a very recent paper showed extensive alterations to white matter in HD that effects many different anatomical regions [12] and others are rapidly uncovering similar findings [9–11]. Because these abnormalities in white matter are being reliably found despite different populations and different methodological approaches, it strongly suggests that there may be a common mechanism damaging white matter across the whole brain in HD. This is important because damage to white matter is extremely detrimental to the brain. There are extensive reasons for this and they are covered in detail by Bartzokis [16]). In short, 1) synapses depends on axonal transport for survival and this is disrupted when white matter is damaged; 2) repair is extremely energetically expensive; 3) repaired myelin is not as good (thinner sheaths, increased number of internodes) as the original undamaged one.

Conclusions

White matter is critical to the human brain's complexity [16] and we have shown that it is damaged in Pre-HD years before symptoms occur in a specific pattern. Furthermore, Pre-HD subjects attempt to repair this damage but fail as the disease progresses. Finally, the data presented supports the conclusion that changes to deep white matter are a central component of HD.

Supporting Information

Table S1 Intra-rater Reliability Coefficient.

Table S2 Tract Measures.

Author Contributions

Analyzed the data: OP. Wrote the paper: OP. Interpreted the data: OP MDP. Revised the manuscript: MDP US FS CC. Performed the experiment: CSC FE. Collected the data: CSC FE.

References

1. Esmaeilzadeh M, Ciarmiello A, Squitieri F (2011) Seeking brain biomarkers for preventive therapy in Huntington disease. CNS Neurosci Ther 17: 368–386.
2. Bartzokis G, Lu PH, Tishler TA, Fong SM, Oluwadara B, et al. (2007) Myelin breakdown and iron changes in Huntington's disease: pathogenesis and treatment implications. Neurochem Res 32: 1655–1664.
3. Ehrlich ME (2012) Huntington's disease and the striatal medium spiny neuron: cell-autonomous and non-cell-autonomous mechanisms of disease. Neurotherapeutics 9: 270–284.
4. Bartzokis G (2012) Neuroglialpharmacology: myelination as a shared mechanism of action of psychotropic treatments. Neuropharmacology 62: 2137–2153.
5. Han I, You Y, Kordower JH, Brady ST, Morfini GA (2010) Differential vulnerability of neurons in Huntington's disease: the role of cell type-specific features. J Neurochem 113: 1073–1091.
6. Squitieri F, Cannella M, Simonelli M, Sassone J, Martino T, et al. (2009) Distinct brain volume changes correlating with clinical stage, disease progression rate, mutation size, and age at onset prediction as early biomarkers of brain atrophy in Huntington's disease. CNS Neurosci Ther 15: 1–11.
7. Aylward EH, Anderson NB, Bylsma FW, Wagster MV, Barta PE, et al. (1998) Frontal lobe volume in patients with Huntington's disease. Neurology 50: 252–258.

8. Paulsen JS, Magnotta VA, Mikos AE, Paulson HL, Penziner E, et al. (2006) Brain structure in preclinical Huntington's disease. Biol Psychiatry 59: 57–63.
9. Kloppel S, Draganski B, Golding CV, Chu C, Nagy Z, et al. (2008) White matter connections reflect changes in voluntary-guided saccades in pre-symptomatic Huntington's disease. Brain 131: 196–204.
10. Dumas EM, van den Bogaard SJ, Ruber ME, Reilman RR, Stout JC, et al. (2012) Early changes in white matter pathways of the sensorimotor cortex in premanifest Huntington's disease. Hum Brain Mapp 33: 203–212.
11. Di Paola M, Luders E, Cherubini A, Sanchez-Castaneda C, Thompson PM, et al. (2012) Multimodal MRI analysis of the corpus callosum reveals white matter differences in presymptomatic and early Huntington's disease. Cereb Cortex 22: 2858–2866.
12. Novak MJ, Seunarine KK, Gibbard CR, Hobbs NZ, Scahill RI, et al. (2013) White matter integrity in premanifest and early Huntington's disease is related to caudate loss and disease progression. Cortex.
13. Phillips O, Sanchez-Castaneda C, Elifani F, Maglione V, Di Pardo A, et al. (2013) Tractography of the Corpus Callosum in Huntington's Disease. PLoS One 8: e73280.
14. Di Paola M, Phillips OR, Sanchez-Castaneda C, Di Pardo A, Maglione V, et al. (2014) MRI measures of corpus callosum iron and myelin in early Huntington's disease. Hum Brain Mapp 35: 3143–3151.
15. Phillips O, Squitieri F, Sanchez-Castaneda C, Elifani F, Griguoli A, et al. (2014) The Corticospinal Tract in Huntington's Disease. Cereb Cortex.
16. Bartzokis G (2011) Alzheimer's disease as homeostatic responses to age-related myelin breakdown. Neurobiol Aging 32: 1341–1371.
17. Jones DK, Knosche TR, Turner R (2012) White matter integrity, fiber count, and other fallacies: The do's and don'ts of diffusion MRI. Neuroimage.
18. Phillips OR, Clark KA, Luders E, Azhir R, Joshi SH, et al. (2013) Superficial white matter: effects of age, sex, and hemisphere. Brain Connect 3: 146–159.
19. Di Paola M, Luders E, Di Iulio F, Cherubini A, Passafiume D, et al. (2010) Callosal atrophy in mild cognitive impairment and Alzheimer's disease: different effects in different stages. Neuroimage 49: 141–149.
20. Phillips OR, Nuechterlein KH, Asarnow RF, Clark KA, Cabeen R, et al. (2011) Mapping corticocortical structural integrity in schizophrenia and effects of genetic liability. Biol Psychiatry 70: 680–689.
21. Cherubini A, Peran P, Caltagirone C, Sabatini U, Spalletta G (2009) Aging of subcortical nuclei: microstructural, mineralization and atrophy modifications measured in vivo using MRI. NeuroImage 48: 29–36.
22. Cherubini A, Peran P, Hagberg GE, Varsi AE, Luccichenti G, et al. (2009) Characterization of white matter fiber bundles with T2* relaxometry and diffusion tensor imaging. Magn Reson Med 61: 1066–1072.
23. Kieburtz K, Penney JB, Como P, Ranen N, Shoulson I, et al. (1996) Unified Huntington's disease rating scale: Reliability and consistency. Movement Disorders 11: 136–142.
24. Penney JB Jr, Vonsattel JP, MacDonald ME, Gusella JF, Myers RH (1997) CAG repeat number governs the development rate of pathology in Huntington's disease. Ann Neurol 41: 689–692.
25. Folstein MF, Folstein SE, McHugh PR (1975) "Mini-mental state". A practical method for grading the cognitive state of patients for the clinician. J Psychiatr Res 12: 189–198.
26. Deichmann R, Schwarzbauer C, Turner R (2004) Optimisation of the 3D MDEFT sequence for anatomical brain imaging: technical implications at 1.5 and 3 T. Neuroimage 21: 757–767.
27. Peran P, Hagberg G, Luccichenti G, Cherubini A, Brainovich V, et al. (2007) Voxel-based analysis of R2* maps in the healthy human brain. J Magn Reson Imaging 26: 1413–1420.
28. Wakana S, Caprihan A, Panzenboeck MM, Fallon JH, Perry M, et al. (2007) Reproducibility of quantitative tractography methods applied to cerebral white matter. Neuroimage 36: 630–644.
29. Makris N, Preti MG, Asami T, Pelavin P, Campbell B, et al. (2013) Human middle longitudinal fascicle: variations in patterns of anatomical connections. Brain Struct Funct 218: 951–968.
30. Dick AS, Bernal B, Tremblay P (2013) The Language Connectome: New Pathways, New Concepts. Neuroscientist.
31. de la Monte SM, Vonsattel JP, Richardson EP Jr (1988) Morphometric demonstration of atrophic changes in the cerebral cortex, white matter, and neostriatum in Huntington's disease. J Neuropathol Exp Neurol 47: 516–525.
32. Xiang Z, Valenza M, Cui L, Leoni V, Jeong HK, et al. (2011) Peroxisome-proliferator-activated receptor gamma coactivator 1 alpha contributes to dysmyelination in experimental models of Huntington's disease. J Neurosci 31: 9544–9553.
33. Rosas HD, Lee SY, Bender AC, Zaleta AK, Vangel M, et al. (2010) Altered white matter microstructure in the corpus callosum in Huntington's disease: implications for cortical "disconnection". Neuroimage 49: 2995–3004.
34. Bohanna I, Georgiou-Karistianis N, Sritharan A, Asadi H, Johnston L, et al. (2011) Diffusion tensor imaging in Huntington's disease reveals distinct patterns of white matter degeneration associated with motor and cognitive deficits. Brain Imaging Behav 5: 171–180.
35. Marrakchi-Kacem L, Delmaire C, Guevara P, Poupon F, Lecomte S, et al. (2013) Mapping cortico-striatal connectivity onto the cortical surface: a new tractography-based approach to study Huntington disease. PLoS One 8: e53135.
36. Matsui JT, Vaidya JG, Johnson HJ, Magnotta VA, Long JD, et al. (2013) Diffusion weighted imaging of prefrontal cortex in prodromal huntington's disease. Hum Brain Mapp.
37. Takahashi M, Ono J, Harada K, Maeda M, Hackney DB (2000) Diffusional anisotropy in cranial nerves with maturation: quantitative evaluation with diffusion MR imaging in rats. Radiology 216: 881–885.
38. Hasan KM, Sankar A, Halphen C, Kramer LA, Brandt ME, et al. (2007) Development and organization of the human brain tissue compartments across the lifespan using diffusion tensor imaging. Neuroreport 18: 1735–1739.
39. Schmierer K, Wheeler-Kingshott CA, Tozer DJ, Boulby PA, Parkes HG, et al. (2008) Quantitative magnetic resonance of postmortem multiple sclerosis brain before and after fixation. Magn Reson Med 59: 268–277.
40. Nopoulos PC, Aylward EH, Ross CA, Johnson HJ, Magnotta VA, et al. (2010) Cerebral cortex structure in prodromal Huntington disease. Neurobiol Dis 40: 544–554.
41. Gomez-Tortosa E, MacDonald ME, Friend JC, Taylor SA, Weiler LJ, et al. (2001) Quantitative neuropathological changes in presymptomatic Huntington's disease. Ann Neurol 49: 29–34.
42. Myers RH, Vonsattel JP, Paskevich PA, Kiely DK, Stevens TJ, et al. (1991) Decreased neuronal and increased oligodendroglial densities in Huntington's disease caudate nucleus. J Neuropathol Exp Neurol 50: 729–742.
43. Sotrel A, Paskevich PA, Kiely DK, Bird ED, Williams RS, et al. (1991) Morphometric analysis of the prefrontal cortex in Huntington's disease. Neurology 41: 1117–1123.
44. Bartzokis G, Lu PH, Heydari P, Couvrette A, Lee GJ, et al. (2012) Multimodal magnetic resonance imaging assessment of white matter aging trajectories over the lifespan of healthy individuals. Biol Psychiatry 72: 1026–1034.
45. Browne SE (2008) Mitochondria and Huntington's disease pathogenesis: insight from genetic and chemical models. Ann N Y Acad Sci 1147: 358–382.
46. Ravera S, Panfoli I, Calzia D, Aluigi MG, Bianchini P, et al. (2009) Evidence for aerobic ATP synthesis in isolated myelin vesicles. Int J Biochem Cell Biol 41: 1581–1591.
47. Zoppelt D, Koch B, Schwarz M, Daum I (2003) Involvement of the mediodorsal thalamic nucleus in mediating recollection and familiarity. Neuropsychologia 41: 1160–1170.
48. Makris N, Kennedy DN, McInerney S, Sorensen AG, Wang R, et al. (2005) Segmentation of subcomponents within the superior longitudinal fascicle in humans: a quantitative, in vivo, DT-MRI study. Cereb Cortex 15: 854–869.
49. Muthusami P, James J, Thomas B, Kapilamoorthy TR, Kesavadas C (2013) Diffusion tensor imaging and tractography of the human language pathways: Moving into the clinical realm. J Magn Reson Imaging.
50. Schmahmann JD, Pandya DN (2006) Fiber pathways of the brain. Oxford; New York: Oxford University Press. xviii, 654 p. p.
51. Perge JA, Niven JE, Mugnaini E, Balasubramanian V, Sterling P (2012) Why do axons differ in caliber? J Neurosci 32: 626–638.

12

Greater BOLD Variability in Older Compared with Younger Adults during Audiovisual Speech Perception

Sarah H. Baum[1,2]*, **Michael S. Beauchamp**[1]

1 Department of Neurobiology and Anatomy, University of Texas Medical School at Houston, Houston, Texas, United States of America, **2** Vanderbilt Brain Institute, Vanderbilt University, Nashville, Tennessee, United States of America

Abstract

Older adults exhibit decreased performance and increased trial-to-trial variability on a range of cognitive tasks, including speech perception. We used blood oxygen level dependent functional magnetic resonance imaging (BOLD fMRI) to search for neural correlates of these behavioral phenomena. We compared brain responses to simple speech stimuli (audiovisual syllables) in 24 healthy older adults (53 to 70 years old) and 14 younger adults (23 to 39 years old) using two independent analysis strategies: region-of-interest (ROI) and voxel-wise whole-brain analysis. While mean response amplitudes were moderately greater in younger adults, older adults had much greater within-subject variability. The greatly increased variability in older adults was observed for both individual voxels in the whole-brain analysis and for ROIs in the left superior temporal sulcus, the left auditory cortex, and the left visual cortex. Increased variability in older adults could not be attributed to differences in head movements between the groups. Increased neural variability may be related to the performance declines and increased behavioral variability that occur with aging.

Editor: Evan Stuart Balaban, McGill University, Canada

Funding: Funding was provided by National Institutes of Health (NIH) (http://www.nih.gov/) 1T32EB006350-04, to SHB; and NIH (http://www.nih.gov/) R01NS065395, TL1RR024147, to MSB. The funders had no role in study design, data collection and analysis, decision to publish, or preparation of the manuscript.

* Email: Sarah.H.Baum@vanderbilt.edu

Introduction

The ability of older adults to understand both auditory-only and audiovisual speech declines with age [1–4]. This decline extends to other important cognitive functions, such as memory, visuospatial abilities, and speed of information processing [5–8]. Interestingly, performance declines with age are not uniform across multiple trials of the same task. Older adults exhibit much greater variability in performance: on some trials, older adults perform as well as younger adults, but on other trials, older adults perform much worse [9–11]. This type of performance decline, referred to as increased intrasubject variability, may be a particularly sensitive measure of age-related changes [12].

We hypothesized that the increased intrasubject variability with age observed in behavioral paradigms should have a neural counterpart. For example, *in vivo* electrophysiology investigations of the visual cortex of experimental animals show increased variability and decreased stimulus specificity with age during viewing of simple visual stimuli [13–15]. Increased neural variability in the auditory brain stem response of healthy older adults has been related to deficits in speech in noise perception [16]. Variability on a cognitive motor task has been tied to individual differences in activation and functional connectivity of the dorsal pre-motor cortex [17]. Wide variability has also been observed in the network activation and functional connectivity of posterior default mode and frontal executive networks in a large cohort (1000BRAINS) of healthy older subjects, which may be related to differences in neuropsychological tests of cognitive and motor function [18]. Conversely, other investigations of variability in healthy aging have pointed to the possibility of *decreased* variability with age [19–21]. This necessitates continued research to investigate to fully understand the role of response variability in healthy aging.

We used rapid event-related blood-oxygen level dependent magnetic resonance imaging (BOLD fMRI) to measure brain responses to passively-presented audiovisual speech syllables. This allowed us to focus on perceptual processing differences between young and old rather than differences in higher cognitive function and performance. We predicted that repeated presentations of identical speech stimuli would evoke fMRI responses that were more variable in older adults than in younger adults. Neural responses to audiovisual speech were examined using two complementary methods. First, we used a region-of-interest (ROI) analysis focused on the three core areas of the multisensory speech perception network: auditory cortex, visual cortex, and the superior temporal sulcus (STS). Second, we used a voxel-wise analysis to search for differences between older and younger subjects outside of our predefined ROIs.

Materials and Methods

2.1. Ethics Statement

All subjects provided written informed consent and were compensated for their time in accordance with an experimental

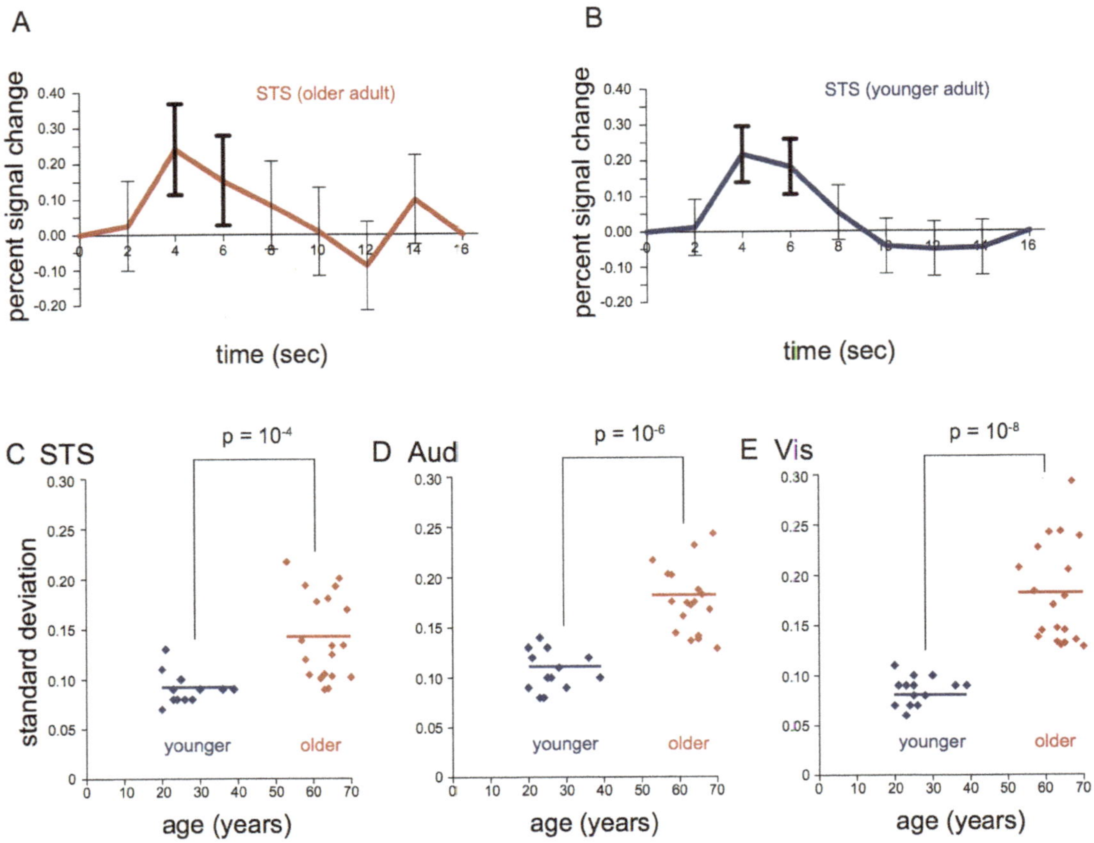

Figure 1. Mean and standard deviation of BOLD responses to audiovisual speech within subjects. A: Hemodynamic response in the left STS of a single older adult (subject JI). Error bars indicate standard deviation of the response within that subject (intrasubject variability) at each time point. The variability at the 4-second and 6-second time points (bold error bars) was used for group analysis. Representative single subject chosen as the subject whose standard deviation was closest to the mean standard deviation for all older subjects. B: Hemodynamic response in the left STS of a single younger adult (subject HU). Representative single subject chosen as the subject whose standard deviation was closest to the mean standard deviation for all younger subjects. C: Scatter plot of age vs. within-subject standard deviation of the STS response. Blue symbols represent younger adults ($n = 14$), red symbols represent older adults ($n = 19$). The lines show the mean of the within-subject standard deviation across each group. The brackets show the results of an unpaired t-test between the within-subject standard deviation in each group. D: Scatter plot of age vs. within-subject standard deviation of the left auditory cortex response. E: Scatter plot of age vs. within-subject standard deviation of the left visual cortex response.

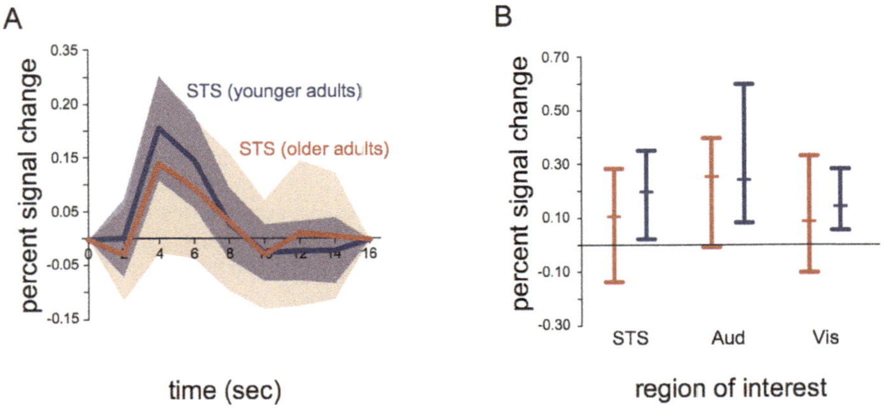

Figure 2. Mean and standard deviation of BOLD responses to audiovisual speech across subjects. A: Average hemodynamic response to audiovisual syllables in the left STS for older adults (red) and younger adults (blue). Shaded region indicates standard deviation of the group response (intersubject variability). B: Response amplitudes in the left STS (STS), left auditory cortex (Aud), and left visual cortex (Vis) across all older adults (red) and younger adults (blue). Error bars show the complete range of data (subjects with maximum and minimum response); middle bar shows median subject.

protocol approved by the Committee for the Protection of Human Subjects of the University of Texas Health Science Center at Houston.

2.2. Subjects and exclusion criteria

The young adult cohort consisted of 14 subjects (20–39 years, 6 female, mean age 26.1 years). 24 older subjects were recruited for the study. Five older adult subjects were excluded (two for poor speech identification scores, three for MRI data quality concerns, see details below), leaving 19 total subjects whose data are reported here (53–70 years, 12 female, mean age 63.0 years).

Vision in the older subjects was assessed using a Snellen eye chart. Each eye was tested separately. The range of acuities was 20/20 to 20/70. Hearing in the older subjects were evaluated using a modified Bekesy threshold test at 500 and 2000 Hz [22]. Our subjects had a range of 6.7 dB–30.9 dB for 500 Hz and 7.3–39.4 dB for 2000 Hz, within the normal range (two standard deviations from the mean) for hearing thresholds based on their age [23]. However, speech abilities decline at a different rate than pure audiometric measures later in life [24]. Therefore, we also tested identification of auditory-only and audiovisual syllables. Most subjects scored near ceiling on auditory-only syllable identification (83%–100%, average performance 93%) and audiovisual syllables. Two subjects scored poorly on auditory-only syllable identification (<70%) and were excluded from the analysis. Cognitive function was assessed using the standardized Mini Mental State Examination (MMSE) [25]. All subjects' scores indicated no decline in cognitive function (scores ranged from 26–30, mean MMSE 28.4, scores 25 out of 30 points or greater indicate normal cognitive function). Two older subjects were excluded for large head movements during fMRI data acquisition (standard deviation of motion regressor >3 mm). One older subject was excluded because an initial analysis of the fMRI data showed response amplitudes more than 3 standard deviations greater than the mean.

2.3. Overview of fMRI experiment and analysis

We used two independent methods for fMRI analysis: region-of-interest (ROI) and voxel-wise whole-brain analysis, which give complementary information about brain activity [26,27]. ROI analysis allows us to examine areas for which we have an *a priori* hypothesis and does not require that data be transformed to a brain template, thus allowing for differences in individual anatomy. Furthermore, it limits Type I errors by limiting the number of statistical tests to a handful of ROIs [28]. However, ROI analyses are blind to effects outside of the predefined ROIs and to functional specialization within ROIs. Therefore, we also performed a voxel-wise analysis to examine activity across the entire brain.

2.4. Block-design localizer

A block-design localizer was used to generate the regions-of-interest (ROIs). Each block contained 10 two-second trials, one word per trial, followed by 10 seconds of fixation baseline. Each trial contained a single word from a bank of digital video recordings of 105 single-syllable words (*e.g.* "view", "door", "make") spoken by a female native English speaker. Words were selected from the MRC Psycholinguistic Database [29]. Auditory-only words consisted of the auditory component of each video with a white visual fixation crosshairs and visual-only words consisted of only the visual component of the video recording.

In older adults, the localizer scan series contained six blocks (two auditory-only, two visual-only and two audiovisual blocks in random order). Each block contained a target trial (the word "press") of the same type (auditory-only, visual-only, or audiovisual) as the other stimuli in the block; subjects were instructed to pay attention to each stimulus and press a response button only during target trials. In younger adults, ten blocks were presented (five auditory-only and five visual-only in random order) with no target trials.

2.5. fMRI responses to audiovisual speech syllables

For the main experiment, stimuli were presented in two-second trials in a rapid event-related design. Each trial contained a single audiovisual syllable, consisting of McGurk (auditory "ba"+visual "ga", auditory "pa"+visual "ka"), non-McGurk incongruent (auditory "ga"+visual "ba", auditory "ka"+visual "pa"), congruent ("ba", "ga", "da", "pa", "ka" and "ta"), target (audiovisual "press" in older adults, audiovisual "ma" in younger subjects) and fixation trials (fixation crosshairs only). There was only a single exemplar of each audiovisual syllable, meaning that subjects were exposed to identical stimuli repeatedly. This allowed us to isolate the effects of neural variability. Subjects were instructed to respond with a button press only to target trials and to make no response to all other trials. Behavioral data in the scanner was not collected for two younger subjects. Subjects performed near ceiling on this task (18/19 older adults at 100% accuracy; 10/12 younger adults at 100% accuracy) suggesting a high degree of alertness (no significant difference between groups, $t_{29} = 0.6$, $p = 0.57$).

Table 1. Regions of activation in response to audiovisual speech in both older and younger adults.

Label	Area (mm^2)	Peak t-value
R fusiform gyrus, inferior occipital gyrus, middle occipital gyrus *(26, −71, −6)*	4593	6.2
R fusiform gyrus, inferior occipital gyrus, middle occipital gyrus *(55, −21, 2)*	3054	4.3
R superior temporal sulcus and gyrus *(55, −21, 2)*	2361	7.4
L superior temporal gyrus *(−46, −33, 16)*	2315	5.8
L middle occipital gyrus *(−23, −93, 5)*	560	4.9
R supramarginal gyrus and subcentral gyrus *(49, −6, 44)*	219	3.9
Total	13102	

Regions are ranked by area (only clusters greater than 160 mm^2 are reported) and Talairach coordinates following anatomical label in *(x, y, z)* format are the weighted center of mass of the cluster.

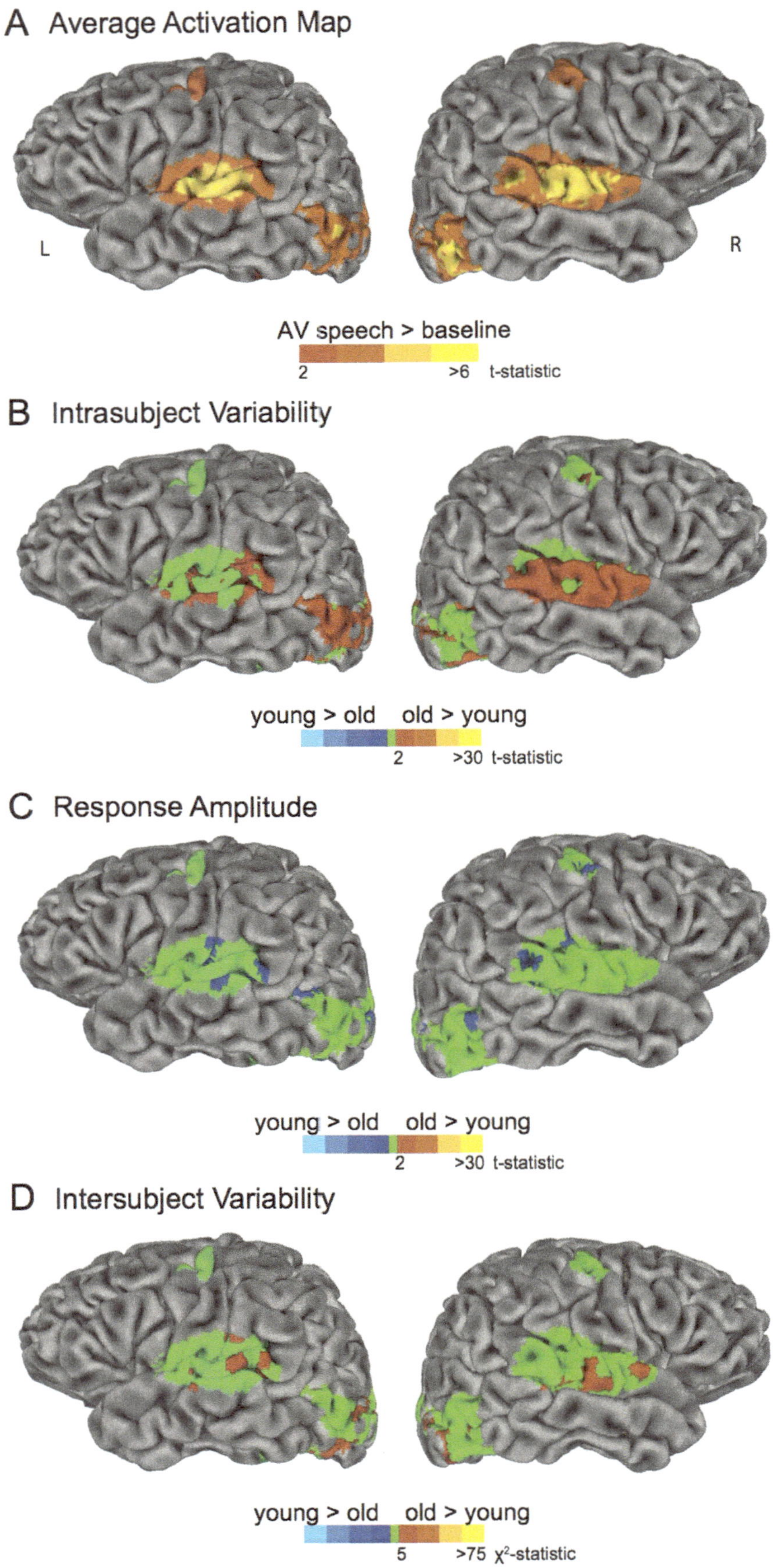
A Average Activation Map
L
R
AV speech > baseline
2
>6 t-statistic
B Intrasubject Variability
young > old old > young
2
>30 t-statistic
C Response Amplitude
young > old old > young
2
>30 t-statistic
D Intersubject Variability
young > old old > young
5
>75 χ^2-statistic

Figure 3. Whole-brain analysis of differences in intrasubject variability, response amplitude, and intersubject variability in older and younger adults. A: Regions that show a significant positive response ($t > 2$ for all audiovisual syllables *vs.* baseline) to audiovisual speech in both older and younger adults. L: left hemisphere, R: right hemisphere. B: Differences in intrasubject variability (variability of the amplitude of the BOLD response to audiovisual speech within each subject) between older and younger subjects, masked by active regions in (A). Orange regions indicate areas with greater intrasubject variability in older adults. C: Differences in response amplitude. Green regions indicate no difference in response amplitude; blue regions indicate areas of greater response amplitude in younger adults. D: Differences in intersubject variability (variability of the amplitude of the BOLD response *across* subjects). Orange regions indicate areas with greater response variability in older adults.

The total length of each video was cropped with digital video editing software (iMovie, Apple Computer) such that each clip started and ended in a neutral, mouth-closed position. Each video stimulus varied in length from 1.7 to 1.8 seconds followed by fixation crosshairs for the remainder of the trial (the crosshairs were always presented in the same screen location as the mouth of the talker visible during other trials in order to minimize eye movements). Prior to the scan, a volume check was conducted for each subject outside the scanner without the presence of scanner noise. Sample videos from the experiment were played and the volume was adjusted so that the volume was "as loud as possible without being uncomfortable or hurting in any way". After each scan series subjects were asked if they could hear the stimuli presented and if any volume adjustments were necessary.

Subjects viewed audiovisual stimuli presented in a rapid event-related design with slight variations in the number of trials, as follows: older subjects, $n = 6$:150 audiovisual syllables, 40 target trials; older subjects, $n = 13$:160 audiovisual syllables, 50 target trials; younger subjects, $n = 5$:220 audiovisual syllables, 70 target trials; younger subjects, $n = 9$:200 audiovisual syllables, 80 target trials.

2.6. MRI and fMRI analysis

Two T1-weighted MP-RAGE anatomical MRI scans were collected at the beginning of each scanning session with a 3 Tesla whole-body MR scanner (Phillips Medical Systems). The two anatomical scans were aligned to each other and averaged in order to provide maximal gray-white matter contrast. These scans were then used to create a cortical surface model using FreeSurfer [30,31] for visualization in SUMA [32]. For the fMRI scan series, T2* weighed images were collected using gradient echo-planar imaging (TR = 2000 ms, TE = 30 ms, flip angle = 90°) with in-plane resolution of 2.75×2.75 mm. Auditory stimuli were presented through MRI-compatible in-ear headphones (Sensimetrics, Malden, MA) which were covered with ear muffs to reduce the amount of noise from the scanner. Visual stimuli subtending approximately 20×30 degrees of visual angle were presented on a projection screen with an LCD projector and viewed through a mirror attached to the head coil. Responses to the target trials were collected using a fiber-optic button response pad (Current Designs, Haverford, PA). Analysis of the functional scan series was conducted using Analysis of Functional NeuroImages (AFNI) [33].

2.6.1. fMRI analysis: response amplitude and variability. In order to generate whole brain maps of the amplitude and standard deviation measures at each voxel, we carried out a voxel-wise analysis using the AFNI function *3dDeconvolve*, which uses maximum-likelihood estimation in the context of the generalized linear model (GLM). TENTzero functions were used to estimate the individual hemodynamic response function (using the option – *iresp*) and standard deviation of each response function (using the option – *sresp*) in each voxel for each stimulus type, beginning at stimulus onset and ending 16 seconds later for single syllables and 26 seconds later for blocks of words (the response was constrained to begin and end at zero amplitude). The model functions consisted of independent, piecewise linear impulse response functions (also known as stick functions) that independently estimated the amplitude of the hemodynamic response at each time point following stimulus presentation. This methodological point is important because it allowed us to estimate the amplitude and standard deviation from the actual response in each individual voxel, not from a fixed hemodynamic response function such as a gamma variate. The use of a fixed function could introduce a confound because of differences in hemodynamic response functions; for instance, if older people had slightly broader hemodynamic response functions, then their deviation from a fixed function would be greater, unrelated to trial-to-trial variability.

For single syllables, we estimated the amplitude of the response as the mean of the response at 4 seconds and 6 seconds after stimulus onset (the peak of the hemodynamic response function). To estimate BOLD variability within each subject for single syllables, the standard deviation at the 4-second and 6-second time points of each impulse response function were averaged to produce a single value per voxel. The brain response to all audiovisual syllables (both response amplitude and variability) was similar, so they were combined for further analysis and only the average across stimulus types (excluding target trials) is reported.

2.6.2. Region-of-interest selection. Data from the whole-brain voxel-wise analysis (*2.6.1*) was first grouped using regions of interest created for each subject individually in native image space. ROIs were selected to target brain areas that are reliably active during multisensory speech perception [34]. A combination of anatomical and functional criteria was used. The anatomic parcellation of the cortical surface was constructed from each individual subject's structural scans with FreeSurfer [35,36]. Functional criteria were constructed from the independent localizer runs (see section 2.4 for details), eliminating bias [37].

We considered three contrasts when constructing the three regions of interest: auditory words vs. fixation baseline, visual words vs. fixation baseline, and audiovisual words vs. fixation baseline. The STS ROI was defined by finding all voxels in the posterior half of the anatomically parcellated STS that showed a significant response ($t > 2$, $p < 0.05$) during the localizer ($t > 2$ for auditory-only word blocks *vs.* baseline and $t > 2$ for visual-only word blocks *vs.* baseline). For 5 out of 19 older adults, no voxels in the left STS met this criterion, so an alternative criterion was used ($t > 2$ for audiovisual word blocks *vs.* baseline). The auditory cortex ROI was defined by finding voxels in the anatomically parcellated transverse temporal gyrus, lateral superior temporal gyrus and planum temporale that were significantly active during the auditory-only blocks ($t > 2$ for auditory-only word blocks *vs.* baseline). The extrastriate visual cortex ROI was defined by finding voxels in the anatomically parcellated extrastriate lateral occipitotemporal cortex that were active during the visual-only blocks ($t > 2$ for visual-only word blocks *vs.* baseline).

2.6.3. Whole-brain analysis. For the whole-brain voxel-wise analysis, subjects' individual data were first aligned to the N27 atlas brain [38] using the AFNI function *auto_tlrc*. Blurring kernels of approximately 3–6 mm have been found to be the most sensitive for detecting activation clusters [39]. We chose a 3×3×3 mm FWHM Gaussian kernel to minimize blurring between adjacent ROIs.

Table 2. Regions with greater intrasubject variability in older adults compared to younger adults.

Label	Area (mm^2)	Peak t-value
R superior temporal gyrus *(54, −19, 1)*	2341	5.0
L middle and inferior occipital gyri *(−38, −69, −3)*	1943	5.8
L planum temporale *(−47, −29, 13)*	1697	4.9
R inferior occipital gyrus *(37, −61, −13)*	882	4.2
R superior temporal sulcus *(45, −56, 5)*	163	5.3
Total	7026	

Regions are ranked by area (only clusters greater than 160 mm^2 are reported) and Talairach coordinates following anatomical label in *(x, y, z)* format are the weighted center of mass of the cluster.

To conduct a voxel-wise search for any differences in response amplitude, the average response amplitude (average of the response to all non-target audiovisual speech stimuli relative to fixation baseline at the 4 and 6 second time points) was calculated in each voxel in each subject. *3dttest++* was used to perform an unpaired t-test for every voxel in standard space between the old and young adult groups. The results were mapped from the MRI volume to the cortical surface with *3dSurf2Vol* and masked with the group t-statistic ($t > 2$ for the contrast of all audiovisual syllables *vs.* baseline). After the voxel-wise t-test we preformed a clustering technique [40]. This finds only voxels that are significantly active above a particular threshold and spatially contiguous. The probability of finding two voxels above a particular threshold *and* being adjacent is much smaller than the chance of a single voxel above that threshold [41]. Using the AFNI program *slow_surf_clustsim.py*, we estimated that a cluster with a size of 160 mm^2 would have a corrected p-value of 0.045. A clusterizing filter on the surface (*SurfClust*) was applied and only regions larger than 160 mm^2 (and $t > 2$ for the contrast of all audiovisual syllables *vs.* baseline) are reported.

To conduct a voxel-wise search for differences in intersubject variability, the MATLAB function *vartestn* was used to perform a Bartlett's multiple sample test for equal variances on the response amplitudes, followed by clusterizing.

To conduct a voxel-wise search for differences in intrasubject variability, an unpaired t-test between groups was performed on the standard deviation of the response at each voxel (*3dttest++*) followed by clusterizing.

2.6.4. Motion correction. Functional data for each subject was first aligned to the averaged anatomical dataset for that subject and then motion-corrected using local Pearson correlation with the AFNI script *align_epi_anat.py* [42]. For each volume, an estimate of the amount of motion in each direction, relative to the reference, was produced. These estimates were used as regressors of no interest in the fMRI analysis. To capture a single value describing the amount of head motion in each subject, the standard deviation of each motion direction across time was averaged across motion directions.

In addition to the standard motion correction steps described above, we also performed the "motion scrubbing" procedure developed by Power and colleagues [43] to further investigate if motion was a potential confound in our main finding of increased intrasubject variability in older adults. First, motion estimates at each time point were calculated in each of the six motion directions (rotational measures: roll, pitch, yaw, and displacement measures: superior, left, and posterior directions). Rotational displacement measures were converted to millimeters using the formula $d = R*(\pi/180)*r$, where R is the rotation in degrees and r is the radius (we used $r = 50$ mm as prescribed by Power). To express the total amount of motion for each time point in a single value, the absolute value of the displacement in each direction was summed, where the total displacement at the *i*th data point was $D_i = |d_\alpha|+|d_\beta|+|d_\gamma|+|d_x|+|d_y|+|d_z|$. Then the framewise displacement for the *i*th time point was calculated as $FD_i = D_{(i-1)} - D_i$ to express instantaneous head motion. The scrubbing threshold was half of the smallest voxel dimension, as recommended by Power (EPI volumes were collected using a 2.75 mm isotropic voxel, therefore we used a threshold = 1.375 mm). The GLM analysis was then completed a second time, excluding the data points with a framewise displacement exceeding this threshold.

Results

3.1 Responses in the ROIs to audiovisual speech

Our initial analysis focused on three ROIs implicated as critical nodes in the network for multisensory speech perception: the left

Table 3. Regions with greater response amplitude in younger adults compared to older adults.

Label	Area (mm^2)	Peak t-value
R occipital pole *(13, −94, 5)*	302	3.3
R superior temporal sulcus *(47, −36, 4)*	273	3.8
L occipital pole *(−17, −93, 5)*	223	4.3
L subcentral sulcus *(−53, −21, 13)*	202	3.6
Total	1000	

Regions are ranked by area (only clusters greater than 160 mm^2 are reported) and Talairach coordinates following anatomical label in *(x, y, z)* format are the weighted center of mass of the cluster.

Table 4. Regions with greater intersubject variability in older adults compared to younger adults.

Label	Area (mm^2)	Peak χ^2
L inferior occipital gyrus *(−30, −75, −12)*	1819	29
R inferior occipital gyrus *(24, −81, −8)*	1552	27
R superior temporal gyrus *(62, −8, 2)*	438	15
R transverse temporal gyrus *(44, −24, 10)*	200	7.8
R fusiform gyrus *(34, −49, −19)*	194	9.7
L superior frontal gyrus *(−1, 0, 56)*	164	27
Total	4367	

Regions are ranked by area (only clusters greater than 160 mm^2 are reported) and Talairach coordinates following anatomical label in *(x, y, z)* format are the weighted center of mass of the cluster.

superior temporal sulcus (STS), the left auditory cortex, and the left extrastriate visual cortex.

3.1.1. Variability of the hemodynamic response in ROIs within subjects. The left STS showed a robust hemodynamic response to audiovisual syllables that was similar in amplitude in individual older and younger subjects. An important behavioral difference in many behavioral paradigms between older and younger subjects is the variability across trials *within* individual subjects (intrasubject variability). To search for a neural correlate of this phenomenon, we calculated the hemodynamic response function in each subject in every voxel and then measured the standard deviation across trials at each time point in the hemodynamic response within each subject (plotting them as error bars around the mean at each time point). As shown in Figure 1A and 1B, while the response amplitudes were similar for individual older and younger subjects, the variability at each time point of the response was much larger in the older subject.

To quantify this difference, we averaged the standard deviation from the peak of the response (4 and 6 seconds after stimulus onset) to produce a single number for intrasubject variability for each ROI for each subject (Figure 1C–E). For each ROI, there was much greater within-subject standard deviation in older subjects (STS: 0.14% in older adults *vs.* 0.09% in younger adults, $t_{31} = 4.2$, $p = 2\times10^{-4}$; auditory cortex: 0.18% *vs.* 0.11%, $t_{31} = 5.9$, $p = 10^{-6}$; visual cortex: 0.18% *vs.* 0.08%, $t_{31} = 7.0$, $p = 10^{-8}$).

3.1.2. Mean and standard deviation of the hemodynamic response in ROIs across subjects. An unpaired t-test with percent signal change in the left STS as the dependent measure revealed slightly greater amplitude of mean response in younger adults (0.19% in younger adults *vs.* 0.12% in older adults, $t_{31} = 2.1$, $p = 0.048$). There were no significant differences in auditory cortex (0.26% *vs.* 0.24%, $t_{31} = 0.5$, $p = 0.63$) or visual cortex (0.16% *vs.* 0.10%, $t_{31} = 1.5$, $p = 0.15$).

The standard deviation of the response across subjects was also similar between groups (Figure 2; left STS: SD of 0.08% for younger adults *vs.* 0.12% for older adults, Bartlett's multiple sample test for equal variances $\chi^2_1 = 2.5$, $p = 0.12$; left auditory cortex: 0.14% *vs.* 0.12%, $\chi^2_1 = 0.7$, $p = 0.41$; left visual cortex: 0.08% *vs.* 0.12%, $\chi^2_1 = 2.3$, $p = 0.13$).

3.2. Whole-brain analysis

Our first set of analyses was limited to our three *a priori* ROIs created using block-design localizers. To overcome this limitation, and to prevent any biases introduced by slight differences in the localizers between old and young subjects, our second set of analyses examined the entire brain. First, we selected all voxels that showed a significant positive response ($t > 2$ for all audiovisual syllables *vs.* baseline) to audiovisual syllables across old and young subjects (Table 1 and Figure 3A).

3.2.1. Variability of the whole-brain hemodynamic response within subjects. We calculated the variability of the response *within* each subject at each voxel, and then compared the two groups. Many brain regions showed greater intrasubject variability in older adults (Table 2 and Figure 3B), including left auditory cortex and bilateral extrastriate visual cortex (total area on the cortical surface = 7026 mm^2; peak t-statistic = 5.8, $p = 2\times10^{-6}$). There were no regions where intrasubject variability was greater in younger adults.

3.2.2. Mean and standard deviation of the whole-brain hemodynamic response across subjects. We compared the amplitude and standard deviation of the response across subjects. Younger adults had greater amplitude of response in right and left visual cortex and right superior temporal sulcus (Table 3 and Figure 3C; total area = 1000 mm^2; peak t-statistic = 4.3, $p = 2\times10^{-5}$; there were no regions where response amplitude was greater in older subjects). Older adults had greater standard deviation of response in bilateral visual cortex and right superior temporal cortex (Table 4 and Figure 3D; total area = 4367 mm^2; peak Bartlett's $\chi^2_1 = 29$, $p = 9\times10^{-8}$; no regions with greater standard deviation in younger adults).

3.3. Potential confound: differences in head movements between younger and older adults

Our initial analysis used standard techniques for estimation and correction of head motion in the functional data, and our GLM included motion estimates as regressors of no interest. Estimated head motion was small in both groups but greater in older than younger adults (0.48 mm *vs.* 0.32 mm, $p = 0.004$). The finding of increased BOLD signal variability in older adults remained unchanged after applying a "motion scrubbing" procedure [43]: STS: 0.13% *vs.* 0.09%, $t_{31} = 3.4$, $p = 0.002$; auditory cortex: 0.18% *vs.* 0.10%, $t_{31} = 5.3$, $p = 8\times10^{-6}$; visual cortex: 0.17% *vs.* 0.09%, $t_{31} = 5.5$, $p = 1.6\times10^{-5}$. There was no correlation in either group between amount of head motion and intrasubject variability (older adults: $r = 0.04$, $p = 0.88$; younger adults: $r = 0.16$, $p = 0.59$). An ANCOVA with age group as one factor, head motion as a covariate, and standard deviation of the fMRI response as the dependent variable and revealed no interaction between age group and head motion in any ROI ($p > 0.68$), and the finding of increased intrasubject variability in older adults remained significant (STS: $F_{1,29} = 13$, $p = 0.001$; auditory cortex: $F_{1,29} = 25$, $p = 3\times10^{-5}$; visual cortex: $F_{1,29} = 34$, $p = 2\times10^{-6}$). A whole-brain ANCOVA that included the amount of head motion in each subject as a covariate gave results nearly identical to the analysis without the head motion covariate. Discarding the six older adults with the greatest amount of head motion rendered group differences in head movements insignificant (0.39 mm *vs.* 0.32 mm, $p = 0.10$), but left the main finding of increased intrasubject variability intact (left STS: 0.14% *vs.* 0.09%, $t_{25} = 3.7$, $p = 0.001$; left auditory cortex: 0.18% *vs.* 0.11%, $t_{25} = 5.4$, $p = 10^{-4}$; visual cortex: 0.17% *vs.* 0.08%, $t_{25} = 6.7$, $p = 5 \times 10^{-7}$).

Discussion

We compared brain responses to repeated presentations of identical audiovisual speech in healthy older and younger adults using fMRI. The most important finding was greater intrasubject variability in the older adults: across multiple presentations of identical stimuli, older adults had greater variability in their brain responses than younger adults. This was true across all of the brain areas that responded to audiovisual speech and was confirmed with two independent types of analysis (ROI and whole-brain). We also observed two less robust effects: older adults had smaller mean response amplitudes than younger adults, and the older adult group had a greater standard deviation of the response amplitude (intersubject variability) than younger adults.

What is the relationship between variability and perception/processing?

Across a variety of behavioral tasks, older adults have worse performance and increased intrasubject variability compared with young adults [11,44–47]. Older adults with mild dementia show more intrasubject variability than healthy age-matched controls [48] and healthy older adults with more trial-to-trial variability showed greater cognitive declines over time [12].

While a link between increased neural (BOLD fMRI) variability and increased behavioral variability is sensible on its face, the precise link between the two is a matter of speculation. With increased neural variability the distribution of responses in a population of neurons to a given stimulus would become wider, which in turn would make it harder for the brain to differentiate between the possible stimuli that evoked the response [49]. Consistent with this idea, decreased stimulus specificity has been observed in single cell recordings of older cats and non-human primates [13–15]. Older adults are particularly impaired in perceiving speech if it is embedded in artificially generated noise [2,4,50,51]. The increased noise in the stimulus could exacerbate the effects of increased neural variability, which could be considered "neural noise". We did not test older subjects using noisy audiovisual speech, the type of speech on which they are most impaired. Therefore, we could not directly compare the increased neural variability we observed in older subjects with the decreased performance of recognizing speech in noise that they are known to have. Future studies using noisy stimuli would be expected to produce poorer performance and reveal differences between subjects correlated with BOLD variability.

Neural variability at early stages of cortical sensory processing might be compounded by neural variability at decision layers higher in the cortical hierarchy. Speech perception involves categorical judgments about the identity of each syllable. Neuronal variability could impair these decisions, an effect that may be even more important than added sensory noise [52]. Neuronal variability may also differentially affect the ability to make both fine and coarse discriminations. Low levels of neuronal variability favor fine discriminations performed at locations in stimulus space in which neuronal selectivity changes rapidly, while high levels of neuronal variability favor coarse discriminations performed at locations in stimulus space where neuronal responses are maximal [53]. Therefore, increased neuronal variability with aging might impair fine discrimination while leaving coarse discriminations relatively intact. Within individual trials, variability in neural responses can allow a population of neurons to encode multiple stimulus attributes. For instance, the mean of the population response may encode the stimulus estimate, while the variability of the population response encodes the uncertainty [54,55].

Previous fMRI studies showing greater inter/intrasubject variability in older adults

There have been a number of fMRI studies comparing young and older adults in other tasks, and the preponderance of these studies have reported more variability in older adults, as we observed in our dataset. D'Esposito et al. [56] measured BOLD responses in motor cortex to a bilateral button press cued by the appearance of a briefly presented white circle. Greater intrasubject variability in older adults compared to younger adults was observed; there were no differences in response amplitude and only a small increase in intersubject variability. Huettel et al. [57] measured responses in visual cortex to checkerboard stimuli with no behavioral task. Greater intrasubject and intersubject variability in older adults was observed, with no difference in amplitude of response. Samanez-Larkin et al. [58] found that healthy older adults exhibited suboptimal decision-making on a financial investment task compared to younger adults and also exhibited greater temporal variability in the nucleus accumbens. In contrast to these studies that reported more variability in older adults, Garrett et al. [21] reported *less* neural variability in older adults using a variety of complex cognitive tasks. One possible explanation for this result is that the analysis of Garrett et al. used a measure derived from multivariate voxel pattern analysis (MVPA) to measure variability across all brain voxels. MVPA analyses and traditional univariate analyses such as ours may give conflicting or even contradictory results. The explanation for these discrepancies is a matter of debate [59].

Potential Confounds

A potential confound in BOLD fMRI studies of older populations is vascular changes with age [60]. However, studies that directly measure neuronal activity also find age-related increases in variability. Anderson et al. [61] presented auditory syllables to healthy older adults and measured the auditory brain stem response, an electrophysiological measure of neuronal activity that is not influenced by the vasculature, and found greater variability in older adults. In a study of non-human primates, single neuron responses in V1 and MT of older monkeys had greater variability than in younger monkeys [62]. These findings suggest that the variability differences in our study have a neuronal component in addition to any possible vascular sources.

Intergroup differences in fMRI studies may also be driven by differences in head movements, especially in studies of resting state functional connectivity [43,63]. In a task-based study such as ours, averaging the response to multiple stimuli reduces movement effects, since head movements and stimulus presentation are independent. We used five different methods to account for differences in head motion, and found no effect on our main results. Consistent with these analyses, two previous studies (Huettel et al. [57] and D'Esposito et al. [56]) did not find a correlation between head motion and BOLD signal variability.

Conclusion

Our most robust finding was of greater intrasubject variability in older adults. This finding was true in both the ROI and whole-brain analysis. Among the physical changes to the aging brain, a decrease in myelination has been observed [64,65]. These decreases in white matter integrity could lead to increases in neuronal variability by preventing neurons from firing consistently even with the same sensory input. Better understanding the neural sources of this variability and its behavioral consequences may help in designing strategies to ameliorate declines in speech perception, one of our most important cognitive functions.

Acknowledgments

We thank Vips Patel for assistance with MR data collection.

Author Contributions

Conceived and designed the experiments: SHB MSB. Performed the experiments: SHB. Analyzed the data: SHB. Contributed reagents/materials/analysis tools: SHB MSB. Contributed to the writing of the manuscript: SHB MSB.

References

1. Sumby WH, Pollack I (1954) Visual contribution to speech intelligibility in noise. Journal of the Acoustic Society of America 26: 212–215.
2. Dubno JR, Dirks DD, Morgan DE (1984) Effects of age and mild hearing loss on speech recognition in noise. The Journal of the Acoustical Society of America 76: 87–96.
3. Grant KW, Seitz PF (2000) The use of visible speech cues for improving auditory detection of spoken sentences. Journal of the Acoustical Society of America 108: 1197–1208.
4. Gosselin PA, Gagne JP (2011) Older adults expend more listening effort than young adults recognizing audiovisual speech in noise. International journal of audiology 50: 786–792.
5. Peich MC, Husain M, Bays PM (2013) Age-related decline of precision and binding in visual working memory. Psychology and aging 28: 729–743.
6. Cerella J, Hale S (1994) The rise and fall in information-processing rates over the life span. Acta psychologica 86: 109–197.
7. Jenkins L, Myerson J, Joerding JA, Hale S (2000) Converging evidence that visuospatial cognition is more age-sensitive than verbal cognition. Psychology and aging 15: 157–175.
8. Hedden T, Gabrieli JD (2004) Insights into the ageing mind: a view from cognitive neuroscience. Nature reviews Neuroscience 5: 87–96.
9. Bielak AA, Cherbuin N, Bunce D, Anstey KJ (2013) Intraindividual Variability Is a Fundamental Phenomenon of Aging: Evidence From an 8-Year Longitudinal Study Across Young, Middle, and Older Adulthood. Developmental psychology.
10. Vandermorris S, Murphy KJ, Troyer AK (2013) Age-related elevations in intraindividual variability on associative memory tasks. Neuropsychology, development, and cognition Section B, Aging, neuropsychology and cognition.
11. Lovden M, Schmiedek F, Kennedy KM, Rodrigue KM, Lindenberger U, et al. (2013) Does variability in cognitive performance correlate with frontal brain volume? NeuroImage 64: 209–215.
12. Lovden M, Li SC, Shing YL, Lindenberger U (2007) Within-person trial-to-trial variability precedes and predicts cognitive decline in old and very old age: longitudinal data from the Berlin Aging Study. Neuropsychologia 45: 2827–2838.
13. Schmolesky MT, Wang Y, Pu M, Leventhal AG (2000) Degradation of stimulus selectivity of visual cortical cells in senescent rhesus monkeys. Nature Neuroscience 3: 384–390.
14. Hua T, Li X, He L, Zhou Y, Wang Y, et al. (2006) Functional degradation of visual cortical cells in old cats. Neurobiology of aging 27: 155–162.
15. Liang Z, Yang Y, Li G, Zhang J, Wang Y, et al. (2010) Aging affects the direction selectivity of MT cells in rhesus monkeys. Neurobiology of aging 31: 863–873.
16. Anderson S, Parbery-Clark A, Yi, Kraus N (2011) A neural basis of speech-in-noise perception in older adults. Ear and hearing 32: 750–757.
17. Stewart JC, Tran X, Cramer SC (2014) Age-related variability in performance of a motor action selection task is related to differences in brain function and structure among older adults. Neuroimage 86: 326–334.
18. Caspers S, Moebus S, Lux S, Pundt N, Schutz H, et al. (2014) Studying variability in human brain aging in a population-based German cohort-rationale and design of 1000BRAINS. Front Aging Neurosci 6: 149.
19. Grady CL, Garrett DD (2014) Understanding variability in the BOLD signal and why it matters for aging. Brain Imaging Behav 8: 274–283.
20. Garrett DD, Kovacevic N, McIntosh AR, Grady CL (2011) The importance of being variable. J Neurosci 31: 4496–4503.
21. Garrett DD, Kovacevic N, McIntosh AR, Grady CL (2012) The Modulation of BOLD Variability between Cognitive States Varies by Age and Processing Speed. Cerebral Cortex 23: 684–693.
22. Price LL (1963) Threshold testing with Bekesy audiometer. Journal of speech and hearing research 6: 64–69.
23. Brant LJ, Fozard JL (1990) Age changes in pure-tone hearing thresholds in a longitudinal study of normal human aging. The Journal of the Acoustical Society of America 88: 813–820.
24. Divenyi PL, Stark PB, Haupt KM (2005) Decline of speech understanding and auditory thresholds in the elderly. The Journal of the Acoustical Society of America 118: 1089–1100.
25. Folstein MF, Folstein SE, McHugh PR (1975)"Mini-mental state". A practical method for grading the cognitive state of patients for the clinician. Journal of psychiatric research 12: 189–198.
26. Saxe R, Brett M, Kanwisher N (2006) Divide and conquer: a defense of functional localizers. Neuroimage 30: 1088–1096; discussion 1097–1089.
27. Friston KJ, Rotshtein P, Geng JJ, Sterzer P, Henson RN (2006) A critique of functional localisers. Neuroimage 30: 1077–1087.
28. Poldrack RA (2007) Region of interest analysis for fMRI. Social cognitive and affective neuroscience 2: 67–70.
29. Wilson M (1988) MRC psycholinguistic database: Machine-usable dictionary, version 2.00. Behavioral Research Methods, Instruments, & Computers 20: 6–10.
30. Dale AM, Fischl B, Sereno MI (1999) Cortical surface-based analysis. I. Segmentation and surface reconstruction. Neuroimage 9: 179–194.
31. Fischl B, Sereno MI, Dale AM (1999) Cortical surface-based analysis. II: Inflation, flattening, and a surface-based coordinate system. Neuroimage 9: 195–207.
32. Argall BD, Saad ZS, Beauchamp MS (2006) Simplified intersubject averaging on the cortical surface using SUMA. Human Brain Mapping 27: 14–27.
33. Cox RW (1996) AFNI: Software for analysis and visualization of functional magnetic resonance neuroimages. Computers and Biomedical Research 29: 162–173.
34. Nath AR, Beauchamp MS (2011) Dynamic changes in superior temporal sulcus connectivity during perception of noisy audiovisual speech. Journal of Neuroscience 31: 1704–1714.
35. Destrieux C, Fischl B, Dale A, Halgren E (2010) Automatic parcellation of human cortical gyri and sulci using standard anatomical nomenclature. NeuroImage 53: 1–15.
36. Fischl B, van der Kouwe A, Destrieux C, Halgren E, Segonne F, et al. (2004) Automatically parcellating the human cerebral cortex. Cerebral Cortex 14: 11–22.
37. Kriegeskorte N, Simmon WK, Bellgowan PS, Baker CI (2009) Circular analysis in systems neuroscience: the dangers of double dipping. Nature Neuroscience 12: 535–540.
38. Mazziotta J, Toga A, Evans A, Fox P, Lancaster J, et al. (2001) A probabilistic atlas and reference system for the human brain: International Consortium for Brain Mapping (ICBM). Philosophical Transactions of the Royal Society B: Biological Sciences 356: 1293–1322.
39. Skudlarski P, Constable RT, Gore JC (1999) ROC analysis of statistical methods used in functional MRI: individual subjects. NeuroImage 9: 311–329.
40. Xiong J, Gao J, Lancaster J, Fox P (1995) Clustered pixels analysis for functional MRI activation studies of the human brain. Human Brain Mapping 3: 287–301.
41. Forman SD, Cohen JD, Fitzgerald M, Eddy WF, Mintun MA, et al. (1995) Improved assessment of significant activation in functional magnetic resonance imaging (fMRI): use of a cluster-size threshold. Magnetic resonance in medicine : official journal of the Society of Magnetic Resonance in Medicine/Society of Magnetic Resonance in Medicine 33: 636–647.
42. Saad ZS, Glen DR, Chen G, Beauchamp MS, Desai R, et al. (2009) A new method for improving functional-to-structural MRI alignment using local Pearson correlation. NeuroImage 44: 839–848.
43. Power JD, Barnes KA, Snyder AZ, Schlaggar BL, Petersen SE (2012) Spurious but systematic correlations in functional connectivity MRI networks arise from subject motion. NeuroImage 59: 2142–2154.
44. Murphy KJ, West R, Armilio ML, Craik FI, Stuss DT (2007) Word-list-learning performance in younger and older adults: intra-individual performance variability and false memory. Neuropsychology, development, and cognition Section B, Aging, neuropsychology and cognition 14: 70–94.
45. MacDonald SW, Karlsson S, Rieckmann A, Nyberg L, Backman L (2012) Aging-related increases in behavioral variability: relations to losses of dopamine D1 receptors. The Journal of neuroscience : the official journal of the Society for Neuroscience 32: 8186–8191.
46. Hultsch DF, MacDonald SW, Dixon RA (2002) Variability in reaction time performance of younger and older adults. The journals of gerontology Series B, Psychological sciences and social sciences 57: P101–115.

47. West R, Murphy KJ, Armilio ML, Craik FI, Stuss DT (2002) Lapses of intention and performance variability reveal age-related increases in fluctuations of executive control. Brain and cognition 49: 402–419.
48. MacDonald SW, Nyberg L, Backman L (2006) Intra-individual variability in behavior: links to brain structure, neurotransmission and neuronal activity. Trends in Neurosciences 29: 474–480.
49. Li SC, Lindenberger U, Sikstrom S (2001) Aging cognition: from neuromodulation to representation. Trends in cognitive sciences 5: 479–486.
50. Stephan KE, Marshall JC, Friston KJ, Rowe JB, Ritzl A, et al. (2003) Lateralized cognitive processes and lateralized task control in the human brain. Science 301: 384–386.
51. Jones AK, Friston K, Frackowiak RS (1992) Localization of responses to pain in human cerebral cortex. Science 255: 215–216.
52. Beck JM, Ma WJ, Pitkow X, Latham PE, Pouget A (2012) Not noisy, just wrong: the role of suboptimal inference in behavioral variability. Neuron 74: 30–39.
53. Butts DA, Goldman MS (2006) Tuning curves, neuronal variability, and sensory coding. PLoS biology 4: e92.
54. Ma WJ, Beck JM, Latham PE, Pouget A (2006) Bayesian inference with probabilistic population codes. Nature Neuroscience 9: 1432–1438.
55. Knill DC, Pouget A (2004) The Bayesian brain: the role of uncertainty in neural coding and computation. Trends in Neurosciences 27: 712–719.
56. D'Esposito M, Zarahn E, Aguirre GK, Rypma B (1999) The effect of normal aging on the coupling of neural activity to the bold hemodynamic response. NeuroImage 10: 6–14.
57. Huettel SA, Singerman JD, McCarthy G (2001) The effects of aging upon the hemodynamic response measured by functional MRI. Neuroimage 13: 161–175.
58. Samanez-Larkin GR, Kuhnen CM, Yoo DJ, Knutson B (2010) Variability in nucleus accumbens activity mediates age-related suboptimal financial risk taking. The Journal of neuroscience : the official journal of the Society for Neuroscience 30: 1426–1434.
59. Jimura K, Poldrack RA (2012) Analyses of regional-average activation and multivoxel pattern information tell complementary stories. Neuropsychologia 50: 544–552.
60. Fang HCH (1976) Observations on aging characteristics of cerebral blood vessels, macroscopic and microscopic features. In: Terry RD, Gershon S, editors. Neurobiology of aging. New York: Raven Press. 155–166.
61. Anderson S, Parbery-Clark A, White-Schwoch T, Kraus N (2012) Aging affects neural precision of speech encoding. The Journal of Neuroscience 32: 14156–14164.
62. Yang Y, Liang Z, Li G, Wang Y, Zhou Y (2009) Aging affects response variability of V1 and MT neurons in rhesus monkeys. Brain Research 1274: 21–27.
63. Van Dijk KR, Sabuncu MR, Buckner RL (2012) The influence of head motion on intrinsic functional connectivity MRI. NeuroImage 59: 431–438.
64. Lu PH, Lee GJ, Raven EP, Tingus K, Khoo T, et al. (2011) Age-related slowing in cognitive processing speed is associated with myelin integrity in a very healthy elderly sample. Journal of clinical and experimental neuropsychology 33: 1059–1068.
65. Kerchner GA, Racine CA, Hale S, Wilheim R, Laluz V, et al. (2012) Cognitive processing speed in older adults: relationship with white matter integrity. PloS one 7: e50425.

13

Distribution of Mesenchymal Stem Cells and Effects on Neuronal Survival and Axon Regeneration after Optic Nerve Crush and Cell Therapy

Louise Alessandra Mesentier-Louro[1,2], Camila Zaverucha-do-Valle[1,2], Almir Jordão da Silva-Junior[1,2], Gabriel Nascimento-dos-Santos[1,2], Fernanda Gubert[1,2], Ana Beatriz Padilha de Figueirêdo[1,2], Ana Luiza Torres[1,2], Bruno D. Paredes[1,2], Camila Teixeira[3], Fernanda Tovar-Moll[3,4,5], Rosalia Mendez-Otero[1,2], Marcelo F. Santiago[1,2]*

1 Instituto de Biofísica Carlos Chagas Filho, Universidade Federal do Rio de Janeiro, Rio de Janeiro, Brazil, **2** Instituto Nacional de Ciência e Tecnologia de Biologia Estrutural e Bioimagem, INBEB, Rio de Janeiro, Brazil, **3** National Center of Structural Biology and Bioimaging (CENABIO), Universidade Federal do Rio de Janeiro, Rio de Janeiro, Brazil, **4** D'Or Institute for Research and Education (IDOR), Rio de Janeiro, Brazil, **5** Institute of Biomedical Sciences (ICB), Universidade Federal do Rio de Janeiro, Rio de Janeiro, Brazil

Abstract

Bone marrow-derived cells have been used in different animal models of neurological diseases. We investigated the therapeutic potential of mesenchymal stem cells (MSC) injected into the vitreous body in a model of optic nerve injury. Adult (3–5 months old) Lister Hooded rats underwent unilateral optic nerve crush followed by injection of MSC or the vehicle into the vitreous body. Before they were injected, MSC were labeled with a fluorescent dye or with superparamagnetic iron oxide nanoparticles, which allowed us to track the cells *in vivo* by magnetic resonance imaging. Sixteen and 28 days after injury, the survival of retinal ganglion cells was evaluated by assessing the number of Tuj1- or Brn3a-positive cells in flat-mounted retinas, and optic nerve regeneration was investigated after anterograde labeling of the optic axons with cholera toxin B conjugated to Alexa 488. Transplanted MSC remained in the vitreous body and were found in the eye for several weeks. Cell therapy significantly increased the number of Tuj1- and Brn3a-positive cells in the retina and the number of axons distal to the crush site at 16 and 28 days after optic nerve crush, although the RGC number decreased over time. MSC therapy was associated with an increase in the FGF-2 expression in the retinal ganglion cells layer, suggesting a beneficial outcome mediated by trophic factors. Interleukin-1β expression was also increased by MSC transplantation. In summary, MSC protected RGC and stimulated axon regeneration after optic nerve crush. The long period when the transplanted cells remained in the eye may account for the effect observed. However, further studies are needed to overcome eventually undesirable consequences of MSC transplantation and to potentiate the beneficial ones in order to sustain the neuroprotective effect overtime.

Editor: Niels Olsen Saraiva Câmara, Universidade de Sao Paulo, Brazil

Funding: This study was supported by grants from the Conselho Nacional de Desenvolvimento Científico e Tecnológico (www.cnpq.br), Coordenação de Aperfeiçoamento de Pessoal de Nível Superior (www.capes.gov.br), Fundação Carlos Chagas Filho de Amparo à Pesquisa do Estado do Rio de Janeiro (www.faperj.br), and the Brazilian Ministry of Health (www.saude.gov.br). The study was supported from grants from the Instituto Nacional de Ciência e Tecnologia de Biologia Estrutural e Bioimagem, INBEB. The funders had no role in study design, data collection and analysis, decision to publish, or preparation of the manuscript.

Competing Interests: The authors have declared that no competing interests exist.

* Email: marcelo.santiago@biof.ufrj.br

Introduction

Diseases that affect the optic nerve, such as glaucoma and diabetic retinopathy, are common causes of blindness worldwide [1]. In addition, traumatic optic neuropathy leads to visual impairment and frequently to irreversible blindness [2]. Visual loss occurs because, in mammals, injury to the optic nerve, e.g., crush or transection, results in the progressive retrograde degeneration of axons and the death of retinal ganglion cells (RGC), mainly by apoptosis [3–5].

Strategies developed to enhance survival and regeneration of RGC include the inhibition of myelin-derived proteins and blockage of rho kinase [6–9], deletion of PTEN [10] and/or SOCS-3 [11,12], macrophage activation and delivery of oncomodulin [13–18], delivery and stimulation of ciliary neurotrophic factor [8,19,20], regulation of KLF family members [21], cell therapy [22–24] and a combination of multiple approaches [14,25]. Despite the remarkable progress in the understanding of the mechanisms and pathways involved in neuronal survival and regeneration, at present there are no clinically and currently applicable therapies to sustain RGC survival and/or to promote long-distance axon regeneration. Injection of trophic factors into the vitreous body prevents neuronal loss, but the effect is transitory [26], and even after peripheral-nerve grafting, which provides a permissive environment for regeneration of central neurons, RGC survival decreases overtime [27].

Cell therapy with bone marrow-derived cells is a potentially useful approach since these cells can be used as a source of trophic factors [28], have immunomodulatory properties [29], and can be transfected to enhance the production of specific factors [30]. The bone marrow is the best-characterized source of adult stem cells [31], which have been widely used in models of neurological diseases [32], such as brain ischemia [33–36], spinal cord injury [37], peripheral nerve injury [38], and in the visual system, in models of glaucoma [22] and optic nerve injury [23,24,39].

Of importance, homing of bone marrow cells after transplantation might be crucial, since they are attracted to damaged areas of the nervous system [40]. Several studies have analyzed short-term engrafting of mesenchymal stem cells (MSC) after transplantation into the eye, using *in vitro* and *ex vivo* approaches [41–44]; but, to our knowledge, there are no reports of long-term *in vivo* tracking of MSC injected into the eye after optic nerve injury.

In this study, we investigated whether MSC can protect RGC from death and increase axonal regeneration in a model of optic nerve crush. In addition, for the first time, we followed transplanted MSC labeled with superparamagnetic iron oxide nanoparticles (SPION) *in vivo* during several weeks, using magnetic resonance imaging (MRI).

Materials and Methods

Animals and ethics statement

A total of 61 adult (3-5-month-old) Lister Hooded rats were used in this study. Animals were used in accordance with the ARVO Statement for the Use of Animals in Ophthalmic and Vision Research, and the protocols were approved by the Committee for the Use of Experimental Animals of the Centro de Ciências da Saúde from the Universidade Federal do Rio de Janeiro (reference number: DAHEICB 052). Seven rats were used for extraction of bone marrow cells, and 54 for optic nerve crush. All procedures were performed under anesthesia with ketamine and xylazine or isofluorane, and every effort was made to minimize suffering.

Bone marrow extraction and cell culture

Adult Lister Hooded rats were deeply anesthetized by inhalation of isofluorane and euthanized by cervical dislocation. Bone marrow was extruded from femurs and tibias and seeded into plastic culture flasks at a density of 1×10^6 cells/cm^2 in DMEM-F12 containing 10% fetal bovine serum (FBS), penicillin (100U/mL) and streptomycin (100 μg/mL, all from Invitrogen Inc., Carlsbad, CA, USA) and kept in an incubator at 37°C and 5%/95% CO_2/air. After 48 h, non-adherent cells were removed by washing with phosphate-buffered saline (PBS) and the medium was completely changed every 2–3 days. Cells were grown until approximately 90% confluent and then passaged (0.25% trypsin 1 mM EDTA, Invitrogen Inc.) and plated at a density of 7×10^3 cells/cm^2. For cryopreservation, cells were frozen at the first or second passages in FBS with 10% dimethyl sulfoxide (DMSO; Merck KGaA, Darmstadt, Germany), using a Bio-Cool Controlled Rate Freezer (SP Scientific, Warminster, PA, USA), and then stored in liquid nitrogen. For all the experiments, thawed cells were cultured and used from the third to fifth passages.

Multipotent mesenchymal stem cell characterization

MSC identity was analyzed by the induction of adipogenesis, osteogenesis and chondrogenesis, and also by immunophenotyping.

MSC differentiation assays were performed as described previously [45]. Briefly, to evaluate the adipogenic differentiation, ~50% confluent cells were cultivated for 16 days in DMEM F-12 supplemented with 1 μM dexamethasone, 10 μg/mL insulin, 0.5 μM isobutylmethylxanthine and 200 μM indomethacin. Cells were stained with 0.2% Oil Red O for 30 min to reveal the intracellular accumulation of lipid-rich vacuoles. Osteogenic differentiation was performed with medium supplemented with 1 μM dexamethasone, 10 mM b-gly-cerolphosphate, and 0.5 μM ascorbic phosphate. Calcium deposits were revealed by 1% Alizarin Red staining for 30 min in water. All reagents used for both assays were from Sigma (Sigma-Aldrich Co., St Louis, MO, USA). To investigate the chondrogenic differentiation potential, labeled MSCs were trypsinized and resuspended in culture medium at 1.6×10^7 cells/mL. To form micromass cultures, cells were seeded in 7-μL droplets in the center of 24-well plates and cultured under high-humidity conditions. After 2 h chondrogenic medium (Invitrogen Inc.) was added to the culture plates and the cells were cultured for 2 weeks. The micromass formed was embedded in paraffin, sectioned, and the presence of proteoglycans was evaluated by staining with 1% Alcian Blue (Sigma-Aldrich Co.) in 3% acetic acid (Sigma-Aldrich Co.) solution for 30 min.

MSC immunophenotyping was determined by the presence or absence of characteristic surface markers [31,46]. For flow cytometry analysis, 5×10^6 cells were suspended in 500 μL saline and incubated with rat immunoglobulins and 5% FBS for 20 min at room temperature, to block unspecific binding. Aliquots of 1×10^6 cells were incubated for 20 min in the dark, at 4°C, with the following antibodies: anti-CD34-PE (1:100, Santa Cruz Biotechnology, Santa Cruz, CA, USA), anti-CD45-FITC, anti-CD11b-FITC (1:100, both from Invitrogen Inc.), anti-CD90-PE and anti-CD29-FITC (1:100, both from BD Biosciences, San José, CA, USA). Aliquots of 5×10^5 cells were incubated without antibodies as a control, or with propidium iodide to evaluate cell viability. Cells were washed twice in PBS and analyzed in a BD FACS Aria II flow cytometer (BD Biosciences). Acquired data were analyzed by FlowJo v.7.6.4 software (FlowJo, USA).

Preparation of MSC for transplantation

On the day of the transplantation, MSC were detached from the plates using trypsin-EDTA and centrifuged at 300×g for 5 min, with medium containing 10% FBS. Precipitated cells were suspended in PBS containing DNAse (625 ng/mL, dornase alpha-rhDNase, Pulmozyme, Roche), to avoid aggregation of DNA released by disrupted cells, and centrifuged again. Cells were counted in an Automated Cell Counter (Countess Automated Cell Counter, Invitrogen Inc.) and suspended at a concentration of 1×10^5 cells/μL in saline containing DNAse prior to administration.

MSC labeling

Cells were labeled before transplantation to allow tracking by confocal microscopy or by MRI. For the short period of evaluation of the transplant, cells were incubated in suspension with CellTrace FarRed DDAO-SE (2.5 μg/mL) for 40 min at 37°C and 5%/95% CO_2/air. CellTrace strongly binds to primary amines inside and outside the cell, according to the manufacturer. Cells were washed three times in PBS and prepared for administration as described previously. For long-term and *in vivo* tracking of the transplanted cells, they were incubated with superparamagnetic iron oxide (SPION) particles (FeraTrack Contrast Particles, Milteny Biotec, Bergisch Gladbach, Germany), as previously described [45]. Briefly, particles were prepared as described by the manufacturer and incubated with the cells in culture for 4 h, at 37°C and 5%/95% CO_2/air. The medium was removed, and the cells were washed with PBS, detached with trypsin-EDTA and prepared for administration as described above.

Incorporation of FeraTrack nanoparticles by the MSC was analyzed by immunocytochemistry to identify the dextran-coating of the particles, and/or by Prussian blue reaction to detect iron within the cells, as described previously [45]. For these analyses the labeled cells were plated on glass coverslips coated with 0.1% gelatin, rinsed in PBS and fixed in 4% paraformaldehyde.

For immunocytochemistry, coverslips were rinsed in 0.1% Triton X-100 in PBS (PBST) and incubated in 5% normal goat serum (Sigma-Aldrich Co) for 30 min at room temperature. The cells were incubated in primary antibody (anti-dextran, 1:500, StemCell Technologies, Vancouver, BC, Canada) overnight at 4°C. Cells were then washed in 0.1% PBST and incubated with the secondary antibody (Alexa Fluor 488 goat anti-mouse IgG, 1:1000, Invitrogen Inc.) and TO-PRO-3 stain to label nuclei (1:1000, Invitrogen Inc.) for 2 h at room temperature. Coverslips were rinsed in PBS and mounted with Vectashield (Vector Laboratories, Burlingame, CA). Fluorescent samples were analyzed under a confocal microscope (Zeiss LSM 510 Meta). For the Prussian blue reaction, cells were washed twice with PBS and incubated with Perls' reagent (20% potassium ferrocyanide and 20% hydrochloric acid in water) for 20 min at room temperature. Cultures were then washed once in PBS, dehydrated through a graded ethanol series and mounted with Entellan (Merck KGaA). The samples were observed by light microscopy.

Optic-nerve crush and intraocular injections

A total of 54 animals were submitted to optic nerve crush, performed as previously described [39]. Briefly, adult Lister-hooded rats were anesthetized by intraperitoneal injection of ketamine (50 mg/Kg) and xylazine (15 mg/Kg). Under a stereoscopic microscope, the left optic nerve was accessed by making an incision in the skin covering the orbital bone. The nerve was exposed and the dura mater surrounding it was cut longitudinally. Nerve crush was performed by compression with tweezers for 15 s, at 1 mm behind the eye, with care to avoid damage to the blood vessels. Immediately after the crush, a 5 µL suspension of 5×10^5 MSC or vehicle (0.9% saline with DNAse) was injected into the vitreous, in the intersection between the sclera and the cornea at the upper temporal side of the eye, with care to avoid lens injury. The same volume of vitreous was aspirated before injection of cells or vehicle, in order to avoid increasing the pressure inside the eye. Before and after the procedure, the back of the eye was observed through the operating dissecting microscope as previously described [23,39] to assess the integrity of the retinal blood flow. Animals with damage to the lens or to the retinal blood vessels were excluded from the experiment. After the procedure, the incision in the skin was sutured and topical anesthetic was applied. Animals were kept under supervision and warmed by a lamp until they recovered from the anesthesia.

In vivo magnetic resonance imaging (MRI)

Cells were tracked in vivo by MRI measurements at 2, 14 and 18 weeks after optic nerve crush and cell transplantation. MRI experiments were performed in the National Center of Structural Biology and Bioimaging (CENABIO/UFRJ). The right eye was used as a control and was injected intravitreously with the vehicle of the cells. For MRI, animals were anesthetized by intraperitoneal injection of ketamine (50 mg/Kg) and xylazine (15 mg/Kg) and positioned in the MRI coil. Images were acquired in a 7-T magnetic resonance scanner (7T/210 horizontal Varian scanner, Agilent Technologies, Palo Alto, CA, USA), using fast spin echo (FSE) proton density (PD) sequences (matrix: 192×192, slice thickness: 0.5 mm; 15 continuous slices) in the axial (TR/TE: 1500/11 ms; field of view: 30×30 cm), coronal (TR/TE: 2100/11 ms; field of view: 30×30.5 cm) and sagittal (TR/TE: 1500/11 ms; field of view: 30×30.5 cm) planes. Data were processed with the use of VnmrJ Software (Agilent Technologies).

RGC survival analysis

Animals were euthanized with an overdose of anesthetics and perfused through the heart with ice-cold saline, followed by 4% paraformaldehyde in 0.1 M phosphate buffer. Eyes were removed and retinas were dissected in PBS. Free-floating retinas were frozen in 0.5% PBST for 15 min at −80°C. Retinas were thawed and washed twice in the same solution for 10 min at room temperature. Primary antibodies anti-Brn3a produced in goat (1:250, Santa Cruz Biotechnology) and anti-Tuj1 produced in mouse (1:250, Covance, Berkeley, CA, USA) were diluted in 0.2% PBST and 5% normal donkey serum and incubated overnight at 4°C. Retinas were washed three times in PBS and incubated with the secondary antibodies Cy3 donkey anti-goat IgG (1:1000, Jackson Immunoresearch Laboratories, West Grove, PA) and Alexa Fluor 488 donkey anti-mouse IgG (1:500, Invitrogen Inc.) in the same solution of the primaries for 2 h at room temperature. Retinas were washed three times in PBS, flat-mounted, and covered with Vectashield (Vector Laboratories). All steps were performed under gentle shaking, except the freezing procedure.

Retinas were imaged under a Zeiss Axiovert 200 M microscope equipped with epi-fluorescence optics and a Zeiss MRM digital camera, at 1.0 and 3.5 mm from the optic disc, in all quadrants of the retina. For Brn3a, 5 images of 0.135 mm^2 were taken at each distance, and for Tuj1, 10 images of 0.032 mm^2 were taken at each distance. Tuj1 images were manually counted by a blinded observer. Brn3a images were automatically counted using the Analyze Particles function of Image J software (NIH); before opting for the automatic cell count, we compared manual and automatic counts and found no statistically significant difference (data not shown). The mean number of cells was divided by the area of the image to estimate the number of RGC per square millimeter of retina. The number of cells in each experimental group was normalized to the control group (contralateral eyes) and expressed as a percentage of the control. To estimate the total number of cells per retina, the mean number of cells at 1.0 and 3.5 mm from the optic disc was multiplied by the mean area of the retina. Five flat-mounted retinas with well-preserved borders were imaged under an EVOS Microscope (AMG); the area was measured using Image J software and averaged to obtain a mean value of retinal area.

RGC axon labeling and counting

Cholera Toxin B subunit conjugated to Alexa488 (CTB-488, Invitrogen Inc.) was used as an anterograde tracer of RGC axons. Briefly, 4 µl of CTB-488 (0.2% diluted in PBS with 1% DMSO) was injected into the vitreous body two days before euthanasia. Animals were euthanized and perfused as described above, and the nerve segments were dissected to the level of the optic chiasm, and transferred to increasing sucrose solutions until 30%. Tissue was embedded in optimal cutting temperature (OCT, Tissue-Tek) and sectioned longitudinally on a cryostat (Leica Microsystems, Wetzlar, Germany) at 14 µm thickness. Optic nerve sections were rinsed with PBS, nuclei were counterstained with DAPI (4′,6-diamidino-2-phenylindole, 2.7 mg/ml, Sigma) and slides were mounted with Vectashield (Vector Laboratories). Nerve sections were observed under a Zeiss Axiovert 200 M microscope, and axon growth was analyzed by counting the number of axons labeled with CTB-488 extending from 0.25 to 2.0 mm from the crush site. Values were normalized by the formula described by Leon and colleagues [15] and expressed as the total number of axons per nerve at each distance from the lesion site.

Histochemistry

Animals were perfused, and the eyes with attached nerves were dissected and transferred to sucrose solutions as in the previous item. Tissue was embedded in OCT and sectioned at 20 μm thickness. Tissue sections were rinsed with 0.1% PBST and incubated in 5% normal goat serum (Sigma-Aldrich Co) for 1 h at room temperature, followed by incubation with primary antibodies overnight at 4°C. Sections were then washed in 0.1% PBST and then incubated with secondary antibodies and TO-PRO-3 (1:1000, Invitrogen Inc.) for 2 h at room temperature. Slides were rinsed in PBS and mounted with VectaShield (Vector Laboratories). Primary antibodies used were anti-dextran (mouse, 1:500, StemCell Technologies), anti-IBA1 (rabbit, 1:400, Wako Pure Chemical Industries, Osaka, Japan), anti-IL-1β (rabbit, 1:100, Peprotech, London, UK) and anti-FGF-2 (mouse, 1:200, Millipore). Secondary antibodies used were Alexa Fluor 488 goat anti-mouse IgG and Alexa Fluor 555 goat anti-rabbit IgG. Fluorescent samples were analyzed under a confocal microscope (Zeiss LSM 510 Meta). For the Prussian blue reaction and documentation, the procedure was similar to that described for cells on coverslips.

Fluorescence intensity quantification

Fluorescence intensity quantification was performed two weeks after optic nerve crush. Briefly, retinal sections were immunostained with FGF-2 and IL-1β specific antibodies, and TO-PRO was used to stain nuclei, as described above. Three retinas from the untreated group and 3 retinas from the treated group were analyzed. For each retina, 9 Z stack images (1.3 μm thickness) from at least 3 different sections were randomly acquired with a confocal microscope (Zeiss LSM 510 Meta, ZEN 2009 software) under identical parameters for all the slides (microscope objective lens 40×1.3 NA, 16 bits images with a resolution of 512×512 pixels). Individual slices of each stack were analyzed using ZEN 2009 software. The area of the ganglion cell layer was outlined in each image, in the FGF-2 or IL-1β channel; the TO-PRO signal was used only for localization of the retinal layers. The average mean gray value per stack normalized by the vehicle injected group was used for statistical analysis.

Statistical Analysis

For RGC survival analysis, the results for the crushed groups were expressed as a percentage of the mean of contralateral eyes and compared using an unpaired t-test. For analysis of axon regeneration, the number of axons in crushed groups was compared using an unpaired t-test at each distance from the crush site analyzed. For FGF-2 and IL-1β expression, the average mean gray value was normalized by vehicle injected group and an unpaired t-test was performed to compare vehicle and MSC injected groups. Results are displayed as the mean ± SEM. GraphPad Prism software was used for all statistical analyses.

Results

Characterization and distribution of MSC

The MSC phenotype was confirmed by the analysis of its differentiation potential in adipocytes, osteocytes and chondrocytes (Figure 1), as well as by the expression of CD90 and CD29 (Figure 2B), and the lack of expression of CD45, CD11b/c and CD34 (Figure 2C-D). For distribution analysis, MSC were labeled with CellTrace (Figure 3) and transplanted intravitreously after optic nerve crush. One day after the procedure, numerous labeled cells were found mainly in the vitreous body (Figure 3), in close proximity to the retina. Because fluorescent dyes can lose intensity with time, we used an additional method to track the transplanted cells *in vivo* and *ex vivo* for extended times, which is important information before the translation to a clinical therapy.

MSC were labeled with SPION (FeraTrack), which can be visualized *in vivo* by MRI and also *ex vivo* by histochemical methods in the ocular tissues. In order to localize the MSC graft in the eye, we analyzed the presence of FeraTrack-labeled cells *ex vivo* at 2 and 18 weeks after nerve crush and cell transplantation. Figure 4A-D shows the presence of SPION in the MSC before transplantation. Since the particles are coated with dextran, it is possible to reveal them with a specific antibody (Figure 4A). In addition, the iron is easily seen as pigmented dots by transmitted light (Figure 4B) and is perfectly spatially correlated with dextran staining (Figure 4C). The iron in the SPION can also be revealed in FeraTrack-labeled MSC by the Prussian blue reaction (Figure 4D). Furthermore, we made cryostat sections of crushed nerves attached to MSC-injected eyes for dextran or Prussian blue staining. Pigmented cells positive for dextran were found in the vitreous body 2 weeks after cell transplantation (Figure 4E-G). A large amount of iron was also detected in the vitreous by the Prussian blue reaction (Figure 4H). After 18 weeks, iron-positive cells were still found in the vitreous (Figure 4I-K) and most of them were in the proximity of the optic disc, as revealed by Prussian blue staining (Figure 4L-M). To exclude the possibility of phagocytosis of iron-labeled MSC by inflammatory cells, we immunostained neighboring eye sections from the animals shown in Figure 4 with anti-IBA1 antibody, that identifies macrophages and microglia. IBA1 was expressed in the inner retinal layers, probably by resident microglia, but the vast majority of the cells

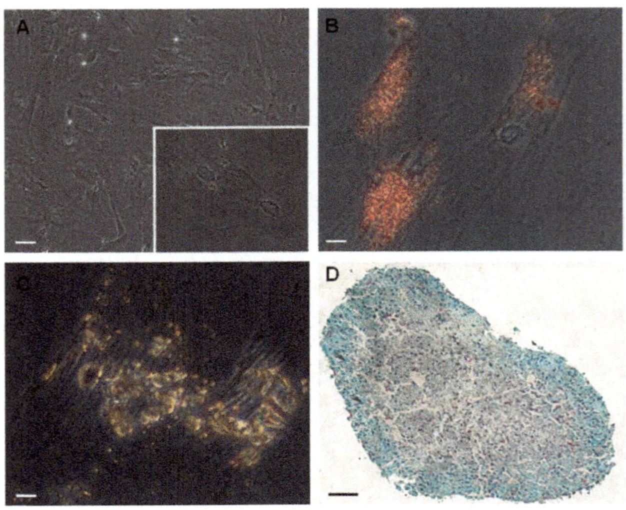

Figure 1. MSC differentiation in adipocytes, osteocytes and chondrocytes. (A) Cultured MSC have fibroblastoid morphology under phase contrast; inset shows adherent MSC in higher magnification. (B) Cells were cultivated in adipogenic medium, fixed and incubated with Oil Red O to identify lipid vacuoles (red staining). (C) Cells were cultured in osteogenic medium and calcium deposits were revealed with alizarin red (yellowish-brown staining). (D) Cells were cultivated in chondrogenic medium, forming a micromass; proteoglycans were stained with alcian blue and nuclei counterstained with Nuclear Fast Red. Scale bar: 50 μm (A), 12.5 μm (B,C), 50 μm (D).

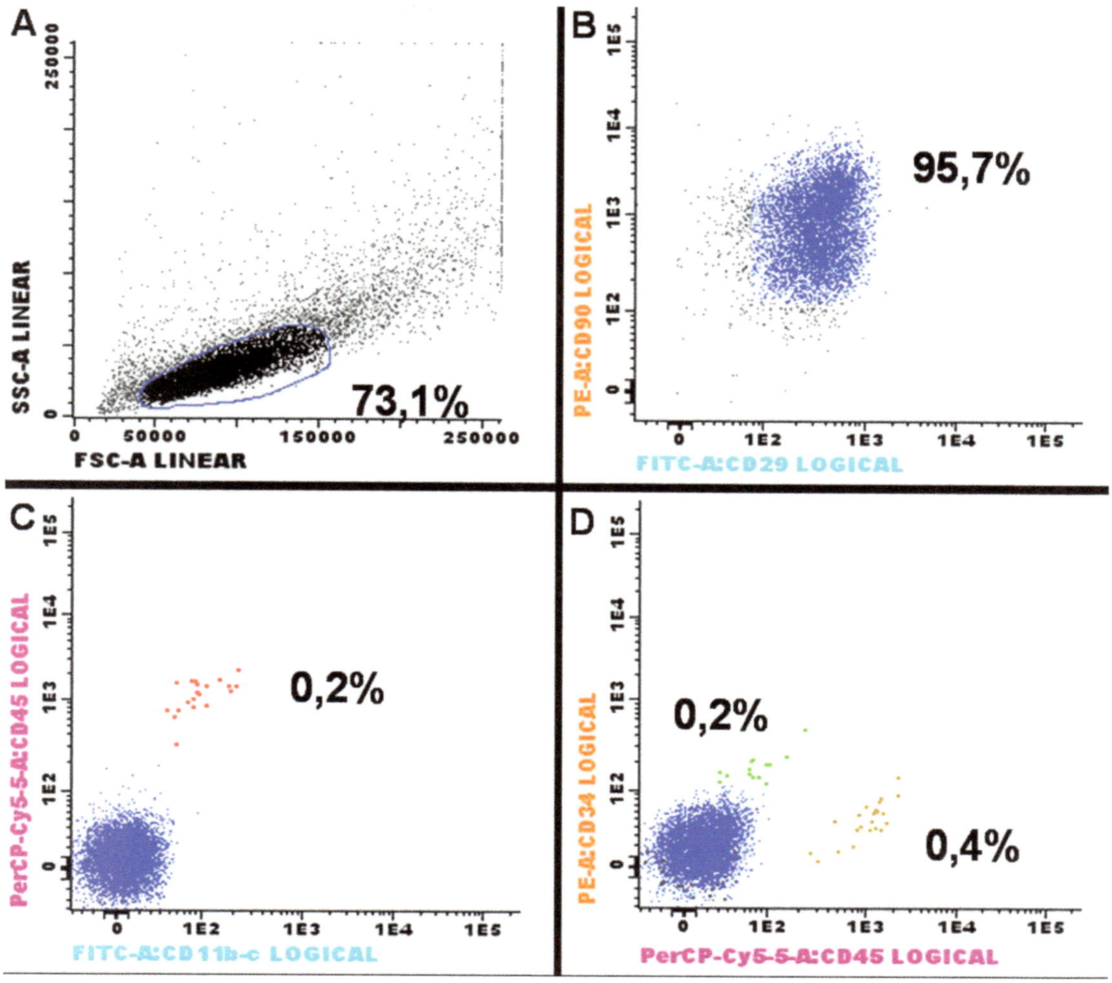

Figure 2. MSC immunophenotyping by flow cytometry. MSC were analyzed from passages 3 to 5, after being frozen and thawed. (A) Forward Scatter (FSC) and Side Scatter (SC) profiles of MSC. The gate in (A) was drawn to exclude doublets of cells. Ninety-five percent of the analyzed cells were positive for CD90 and CD29 (B), 99.8% were negative for CD45 and CD11b-c (C), 99.8% were negative for CD34, and 99.6% were negative for CD45 (D). These results are consistent with the phenotype of multipotent mesenchymal stem cells.

found in the vitreous body were negative to IBA1 (Figure S2 in File S1). A small amount of iron was also found in the optic nerve in the vicinity of the crush site (Figure 4N).

Figure 5 A-D shows MRI images two weeks after unilateral optic nerve crush (left) and injection of FeraTrack-labeled MSC. The right eye was injected with the washing solution of the last cell centrifugation/washing. No signal of the washing solution injected in the right eye was detected. In contrast, the signal of the labeled cells was visible as a dark stain next to the lens in the left eye (arrow in Figure 5A-C). Furthermore, the signal of labeled cells remained in the left eye over time, up to 18 weeks after nerve crush and cell transplantation (Figures 5E-G and 5I-K). There was no evident reduction of the signal over the weeks analyzed, suggesting that the cells remained inside the eye for at least 18 weeks (compare Figures 5C, 5G and 5K).

Taken together, these results imply a long-term permanence of the MSC graft in the eye, mainly in the vitreous body. To assess the potential therapeutic effect of the transplanted cells, we analyzed RGC survival and axonal regeneration over time.

MSC were neuroprotective after optic nerve crush

RGC survival was analyzed 16 and 28 days after optic nerve crush, quantifying the number of RGC immunostained with Tuj1 and Brn3a, at both 1.0 and 3.5 mm from the optic disc.

Tuj1 recognizes neuronal βIII tubulin (Figure 6A) and is widely used as a RGC marker [10,11,17,19,27]. Indeed, one study demonstrated a correlation higher than 95% between Tuj1-positive cells in the ganglion cell layer and RGC retrogradely labeled with Fluorogold, after different experimental procedures [47].

Sixteen days after optic nerve crush, we observed a reduction in the number of cell bodies immunostained with Tuj1 (inset in Figure 6B) and also degeneration of the nerve fibers inside the retina (arrows in Figure 6B), compared to the control retina (Figure 6A). The reduction in the number of RGC after optic nerve crush was less evident after MSC transplantation (6C). In addition, the optic fibers in the retina were more preserved (arrows in Figure 6C) and qualitatively similar to those observed in the control retinas (Fig 6A). Quantitative analyses showed that the number of Tuj1-positive cells in the vehicle-injected group was reduced to 10.34% and 16.16% of the number in the control group, at 1.0 and 3.5 mm from the optic disc, respectively.

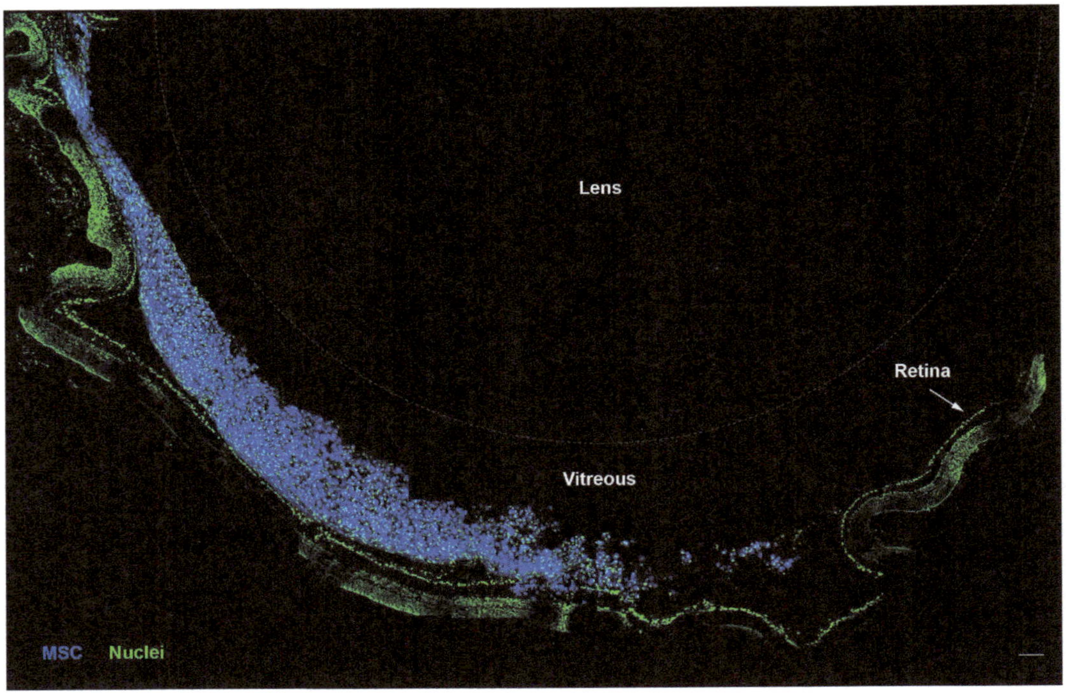

Figure 3. MSC are located in the vitreous body 1 day after optic nerve crush and cell transplantation. Photomontage of confocal images of a cryostat section through the eye. MSC (blue) were labeled with CellTrace prior to injection in the vitreous body, and were located mainly in this region 1 day after transplantation. Nuclei (green) in the retina and in the vitreous body were stained with Sytox Green. The lens is outlined with a dashed line. Scale bar: 100 μm.

Treatment with MSC increased these percentages to 23.61% (Figure 6G) and 51.09% (Figure 6H), respectively, which represent 1.3- and 2.2-fold increases of the MSC-treated group over the group treated with the vehicle alone.

We also studied the survival of RGC using immunostaining for Brn3a, a transcription factor that is a member of the class Brn3 of POU-homeodomain factors [48]. Brn3a has been reported as a reliable marker of adult rat RGC in both naïve and injured retinas [49–51]. Sixteen days after lesion, there was a very large decrease in the number of Brn3a-positive cells in the retina (Figure 6E), compared to control retinas (Figure 6D). In the MSC-treated group, the decrease in RGC number was less dramatic than in the untreated group (Figure 6F). The quantitative analyses revealed that in the vehicle-injected group, the number of Brn3a-positive cells was reduced to 5.78% and 9.31% of the control, at 1.0 and 3.5 mm from the optic disc, respectively. MSC injection increased these percentages to 26.5% (Figure 6I) and 26.4% (Figure 6J), respectively, which represents 3.5- and 1.8-fold increases of the MSC-treated group over the group treated with the vehicle alone.

Twenty-eight days after optic nerve crush, we observed a very large reduction in the number of Tuj1-positive cells and thinning of nerve fibers in the retina in the vehicle-injected group (arrows in Figure 7B), compared to the control (Figure 7A). In the MSC-injected group the number of Tuj1-positive cells (Figure 7C) was also reduced compared with the control but was larger than in the vehicle-injected group. Axon bundles are also more preserved in the MSC treated than in the vehicle injected group (arrows in Figure 7B-C). The quantitative analyses revealed that the percentage of Tuj1-positive cells in the vehicle-injected group was 6.28% and 11.0% of control, at 1.0 and 3.5 mm from the optic disc, respectively. MSC injection increased these percentages to 18.4% (Figure 7G) and 24.3% (Figure 7H), respectively, which represent 1.9- and 1.2-fold increases of the MSC-treated group over the group treated with the vehicle alone.

The number of Brn3a-positive cells was dramatically reduced 28 days after nerve crush in the vehicle-injected group (Figure 7E), compared to the control (Figure 7D). This reduction was attenuated when the animals were treated with MSC (Figure 7F). The quantitative analysis showed that the percentage of Brn3a-positive cells in the vehicle-injected group was only 2.03% and 2.73% of the number in the control, at 1.0 and 3.5 mm from the optic disc, respectively. MSC injection increased these percentages to 4.24% (Figure 7I) and 6.61% (Figure 7J), respectively, which represent 1.1- and 1.4-fold increases of the MSC-treated group over the group treated with the vehicle alone. The quantification of Tuj1- and Brn3a-positive cells and the estimated number of RGC per retina are summarized in Table S1 in File S1. These results clearly indicate that intravitreous MSC transplantation significantly promoted long-term neuroprotection of RGC after a severe optic nerve crush.

MSC promoted axonal regeneration after optic nerve crush

To assess the number of axons that are able to regenerate after the crush site, we labeled them with CTB-488 injected into the vitreous body. The toxin is anterogradely transported from the retinal ganglion cells to the superior colliculus, through undamaged nerves (Figure 8A). In the crushed nerves, we counted the positive fibers at 0.25, 0.50, 0.75, 1.00, 1.50 and 2.00 mm distal from the crush site (Figure 9). In our model, optic nerve crush damages all axons; four days after the lesion, virtually all axons had CTB-488 transport interrupted at the injury site (Figure 8B). Sixteen days after injury, a few axons were able to regenerate farther from the crush site in the vehicle-injected animals

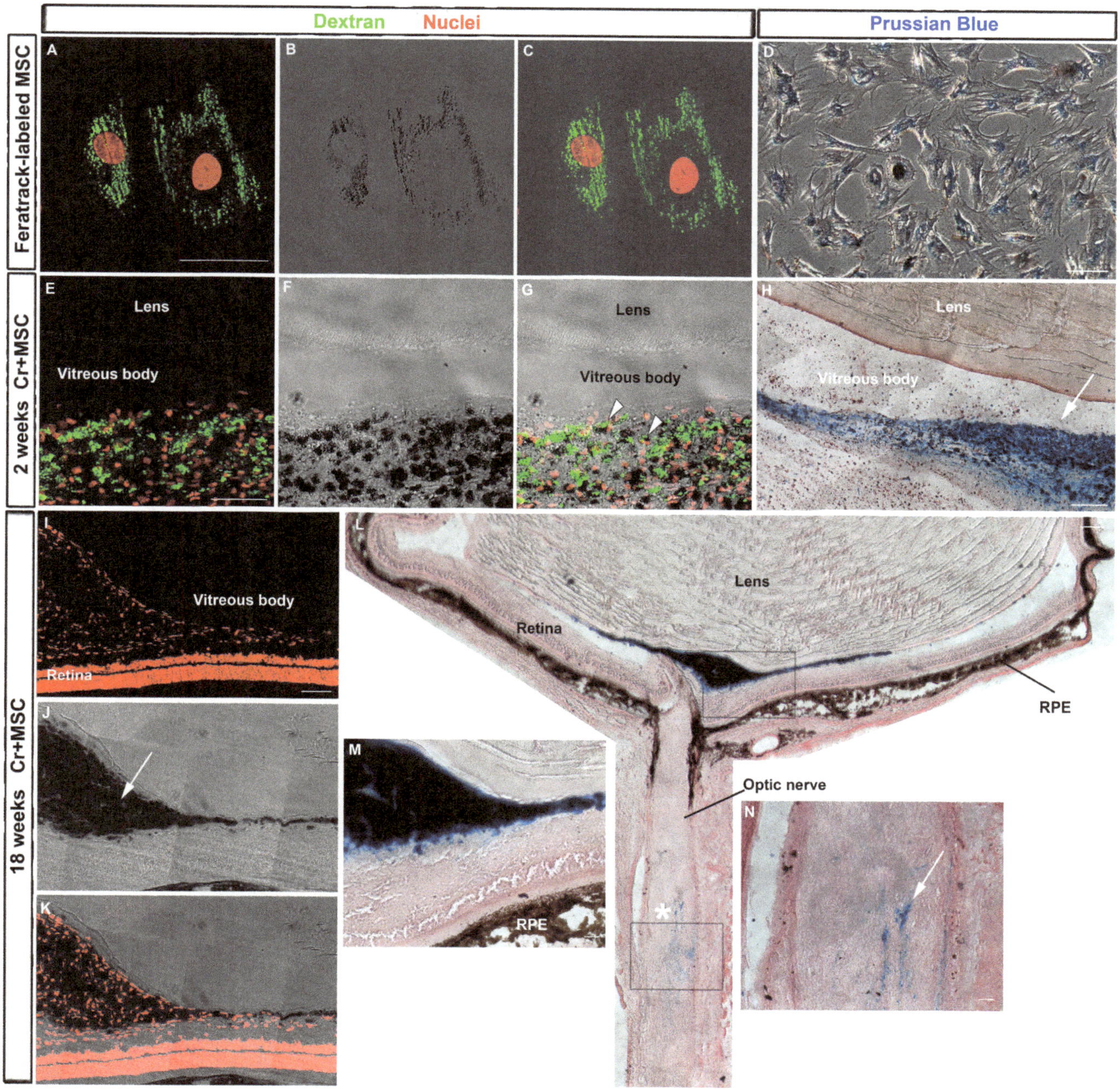

Figure 4. Detection of FeraTrack-labeled MSCs *in vitro* and after transplantation. A: Cells were labeled with FeraTrack for 4 h, fixed, and immunostained with anti-dextran antibody (green) to identify dextran-coated particles and nuclei stained with TOPRO (red) (A and C). Iron from SPION is visible as dark spots inside the cell (B-C) or after Prussian blue reaction (D). E-G: Sixteen days after nerve injury and MSC injection, these cells are found in the vitreous body as dextran-positive cells (green) with dark spots (arrowheads in G). Nuclei were stained with TOPRO (red, in E and F). H: Photomontage of transmitted light images of a cryostat section through the eye reacted with Prussian blue. Labeled cells are found mostly in the vitreous body (arrow). I-N: Eighteen weeks after nerve injury and cell transplantation, SPION are visible as dark spots by transmitted light (arrow in J) and also after Prussian blue reaction (L-N). I-K: Photomontage of confocal images from the eye; nuclei stained with TOPRO (red, in I and K). L: Photomontage of transmitted light images of the eye and proximal optic nerve after Prussian blue reaction. Iron was detected mainly in the vitreous body (blue in M), but a small amount was found also in the optic nerve (blue in N), close to the crush site (asterisk). (M,N) Higher magnification of upper (M) and lower (N) boxes in L. RPE, retinal pigmented epithelium. Scale bar: 50 μm.

(Figure 9A), and MSC treatment significantly increased (by 3.2 fold) the number of axons extending up to 0.75 mm from the injury site (Figure 9B, E; $P<0.001$; 94.82±21.54 axons/nerve in the vehicle-injected group and 401.9±109.1 axons/nerve in the MSC-injected group). After 28 days, the axons had grown further in both groups (Figure 9C-D), but the MSC-injected group showed a 2.0-fold increase in the number of axons extending up to 1.00 mm from the crush site (Figure 9F; $P<0.05$; 59.37±17.00 axons/nerve in the vehicle-injected group and 176.8±38.95 axons/nerve in the MSC-injected group). The mean of axons per nerve at each distance is given in Table S2 in File S1. These results suggest that MSC therapy increased the number of axons

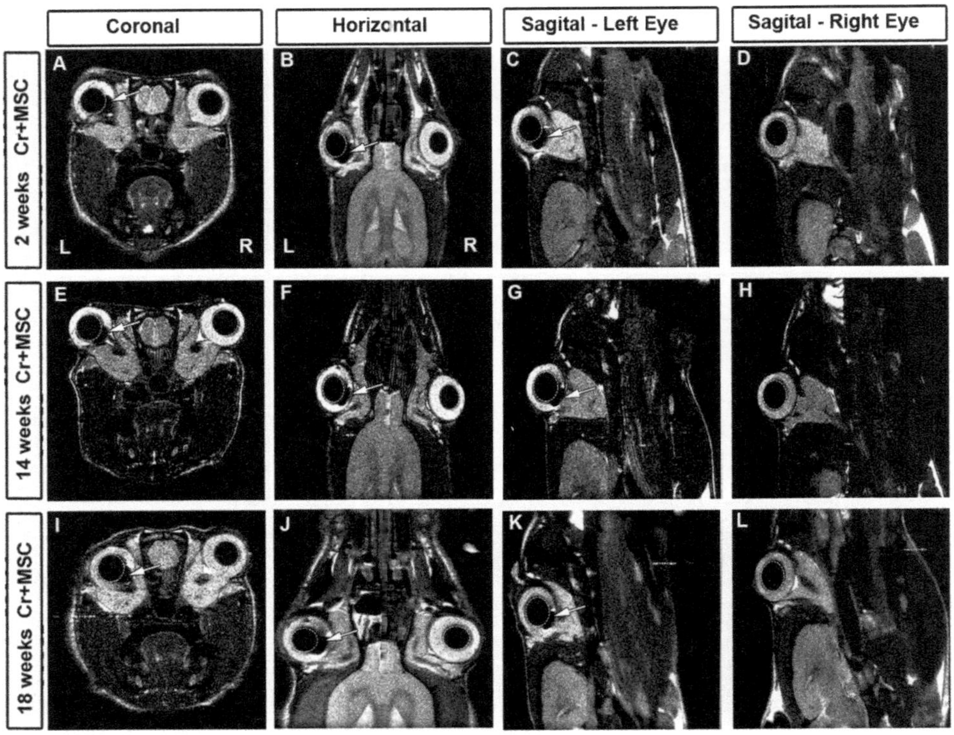

Figure 5. Detection of FeraTrack-labeled MSCs by *in vivo* MRI. MSC were labeled with Fera Track for 4 h and injected in the vitreous body of the left eye after optic nerve crush. (A-L) Representative images of *in vivo* MRI at coronal (A,E,I), horizontal (B,F,J), and sagittal planes (C,G,K; at left eye level and D,H,L; at right eye level) at different survival times. Arrows indicate hypointense (black) spots corresponding to FeraTrack-labeled cells in the vitreous body of the left eye. Labeled cells were found at 2 (A-C), 14 (E-G) and 18 weeks (I-K) after optic nerve crush and cell transplantation. The right eye was injected with the washing solution of the cells; no signal was detected (D,H,L and right hemisphere of coronal and horizontal images). The lenses are circled with dashed lines; right (R) and left (L) hemispheres.

that cross the injury site and stimulated them to regenerate over longer distances compared with vehicle-treated eyes. In addition, this regenerative effect of the cell therapy was sustained overtime, as seen at 16 and 28 days after injury.

MSC injection upregulated FGF-2 and IL-1β in the ganglion cell layer

We analyzed the expression of FGF-2 (Figure 10A-D) and IL-1β (Figure 10E-H) in the retinal ganglion cell layer of the saline injected ($n = 3$) and MSC treated ($n = 4$) groups, using specific antibodies. FGF-2 expression increased significantly ($P<0.05$, Figure 10I) in the MSC treated group (1.827 ± 0.2767, ratio to vehicle injected group). IL-1β was also significantly more expressed ($P<0.05$, Figure 10J) in the MSC treated group ($1.854 \pm 0{,}2278$, ratio to vehicle injected group).

Discussion

Optic nerve crush induced drastic RGC degeneration, which has been widely associated to programmed cell death [52,53]. Several apoptotic effectors such as caspase-3 and -9, Bax, Bcl-2 and p38 MAP kinase are modulated in the retina after optic nerve injury [54–58] and active caspase-3 is expressed by terminal transferase-mediated dUTP nick-end labelling (TUNEL)-positive rat RGC after axotomy [55]. We observed a more than 90% reduction in the number of Tuj1 and Brn3a positive cells in the retina after optic nerve crush, corroborating the results of several other studies on RGC degeneration after axonal damage [51,59,60].

In previous studies we have shown that treatment with bone marrow mononuclear cells (BMMC) reduces RGC death and increases nerve regeneration 2 weeks after optic nerve crush [23]. BMMC are a mixed population containing different types of myeloid and lymphoid cells and also stem/progenitor cells such as MSC [31,61]. One could argue that cell therapies with mixed populations of cells have the advantage of affecting several potential targets at the same time. On the other hand, identifying the possible therapeutic effects of each transplanted cell type is an intricate task. Here we investigated the long-term effects of MSC therapy, a purified population of bone marrow-derived cells, in the same model of optic nerve injury that we have studied previously. All cells used in this study were once frozen and thawed, which facilitates their translation into a putative clinical therapy. Another advantage of the MSC is that it is possible to increase their numbers in order to obtain uniform populations of well-characterized cells, and therefore, any therapy-derived effect can be narrowed to a single cell type.

Furthermore, during the last 10 years, preclinical studies have shown that MSC transplantation is a promising approach to treat several neurological diseases [62], such as amyotrophic lateral sclerosis [63,64], Alzheimer's disease [65,66], Parkinson's [67], spinal cord injury [68], stroke [69,70] and multiple sclerosis [71,72]. In experimental models of these diseases, the administration of MSC through different routes was able to increase the survival of motor neurons [73,74], reduce the accumulation of amyloid-β (Aβ) in the brain [65], reduce the loss of dopaminergic neurons [75], improve functional outcome [76,77] and reduce demyelination [78,79]. Some studies have associated the beneficial

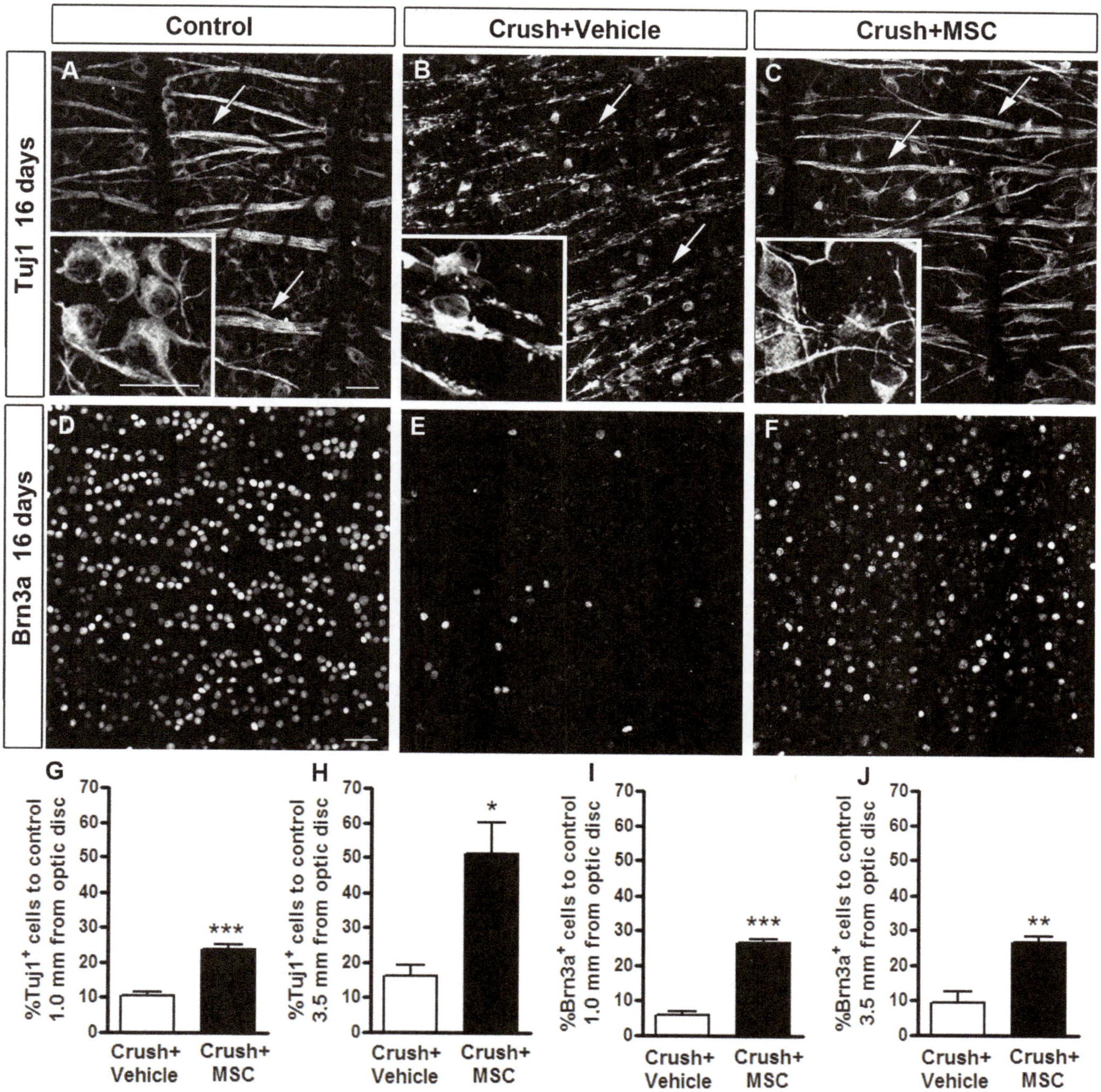

Figure 6. MSC transplantation increased RGC survival 16 days after optic nerve crush. A-F: Confocal images of flat-mounted retinas labeled with Tuj1 (A-C) or anti-Brn3a (D-F) antibodies. Insets in A-C are higher magnifications of the images to illustrate the morphology of the Tuj1-positive cells. In the control retina (contralateral eye) numerous cells are labeled with Tuj1 (A) and Brn3a (D), and axon bundles are intact (arrows in A). Sixteen days after optic nerve crush, there was a large reduction in the number of RGCs (B and E) and axon bundles were notably compromised, as revealed by Tuj1 staining (arrows in B). In the MSC-injected animals (C and F) the number of surviving RGCs was increased compared to the vehicle-injected ones, and Tuj1 staining in axon bundles was similar to the control (arrows in C). G-J: Quantification of RGC survival 16 days after nerve crush using Tuj1 (G, H) or Brn3a labeling (I, J). Results are displayed as mean ± SEM of the percentage of Tuj1+ or Brn3a+ cells relative to the control retina (contralateral eye). $^*P<0.05$; $^{**}P<0.01$; $^{***}P<0.001$. Scale bar in A-F: 50 μm.

effects with the increase of neurotrophins in the injured tissue [80,81], and, importantly, many of them have suggested that MSC can control the inflammatory activity associated with tissue degeneration [62], e.g., by promoting an alternative microglial activation [82,83] or controlling the infiltration of inflammatory cells into the central nervous system [71].

In general, intraocular transplanted cells do not migrate inside the neural retina [42–44] and we found that several weeks after Feratrack-labeled MSC transplantation, the iron from Feratrack was localized in the vitreous body, which is free of resident cells. The MRI signal intensity was not decreased overtime and several nuclei were identified in the regions with iron up to 18 weeks after crush and cell transplantation (the longest period of time that we

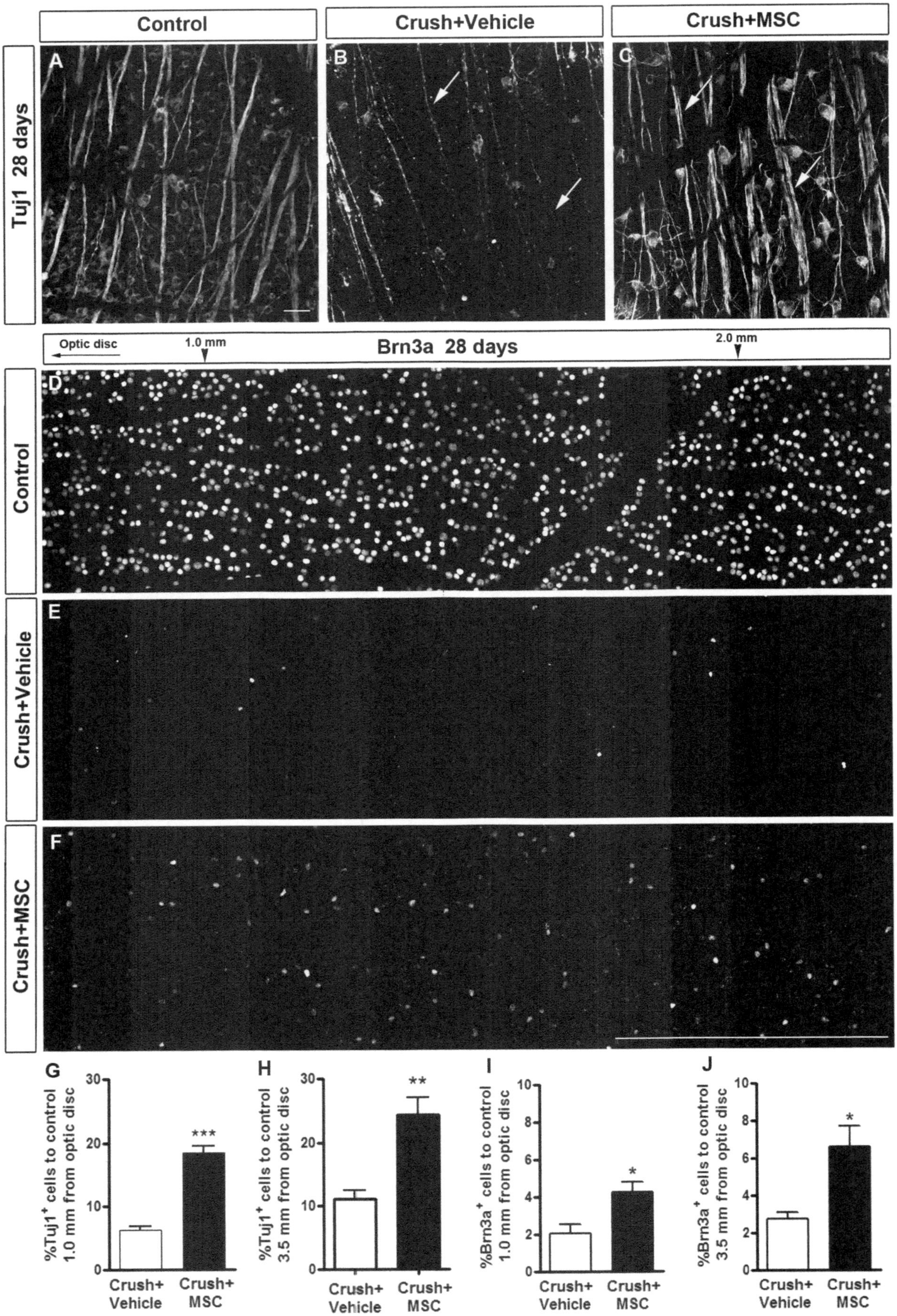
Control
Crush+Vehicle
Crush+MSC
Tuj1 28 days
A
B
C
Optic disc
1.0 mm
Brn3a 28 days
2.0 mm
D
Control
E
Crush+Vehicle
F
Crush+MSC
G
%Tuj1+ cells to control 1.0 mm from optic disc
***
Crush+ Vehicle
Crush+ MSC
H
%Tuj1+ cells to control 3.5 mm from optic disc
**
I
%Brn3a+ cells to control 1.0 mm from optic disc
*
J
%Brn3a+ cells to control 3.5 mm from optic disc
*

Figure 7. MSC transplantation increased RGC survival 28 days after optic nerve crush. A-C: Confocal images of flat-mounted retinas labeled with Tuj1 antibody (A-C). D-F: Photomontage of confocal images of flat-mounted retinas labeled with Brn3a antibody. A, D: Control retina (contralateral eye). B, E: Twenty-eight days after optic nerve injury, there was a large reduction in the number of RGCs, and axon bundles were thinner (arrows in B) in the vehicle-treated group compared to control. C, F: In MSC-injected animals, the number of surviving RGCs increased compared to vehicle-injected animals, and axon bundles were similar to control (arrows in C). G-J: Quantification of RGC survival 28 days after nerve crush at 1.0 mm or 3.5 mm from the optic disc, using Tuj1 (G, H) or Brn3a labeling (I, J). Results are displayed as mean ± SEM of the percentage of Tuj1+ or Brn3a+ cells relative to the control retina (contralateral ye). *P<0.05; **P<0.01; ***P<0.001. Scale bar: 50 μm (A-C); 500 μm (D-F).

have analyzed). Although we cannot exclude the possibility that monocytes/macrophages invade the vitreous, these cells have a very short life span and for that reason it is very unlikely that the iron signal and nuclei could be associated to inflammatory cells and not to the transplanted MSC. Indeed, the vast majority of the cells found in the vitreous did not express IBA1, supporting the permanence of the MSC graft. This suggests that MSC may exert a more continuous and long-term effect than canonical transitory approaches, e.g., a single injection of a drug or trophic factor. Furthermore, we also expected to have a sustained effect compared to BMMC transplantation, since these cells are no longer found in the eye two weeks after they were injected [39].

The presence of MSC in the eye for several days could be directly responsible for the therapeutic effect observed in our study. We have found that in the treated group, the number of RGC revealed with either Tuj1 or Brn3a was at least twice as large as in the vehicle group, at both 16 and 28 days after injury. Notably, the percentage of Brn3a-positive cells was smaller than that of Tuj1-positive cells in the crushed groups. This difference can be explained by the rapid loss of Brn3a in injured RGC [51] and the presence of displaced amacrine cells [84] labeled with Tuj1 in the ganglion cell layer. In addition, in both experimental groups there was a decrease in RGC survival from 16 to 28 days after injury (Figure S1 in File S1), which was expected, since the degeneration is progressive; but suggests that not all of the cells that were protected by cell therapy at 16 days were effectively rescued. However, both Tuj1 and Brn3a markers had significantly different percentages between the MSC- and vehicle-injected groups, indicating a higher RGC survival due to cell therapy. Together with the increase in the number of regenerating axons beyond the crush site, our data also suggests that in the MSC-treated group there is a large number of RGC and/or that the protected RGC were capable of extending longer axons than in the vehicle-injected group. A longer follow-up period after injury would reveal whether these beneficial MSC effects are sustained.

The mechanisms of action of MSC after transplantation are still elusive but it is important to consider that intravitreally delivered MSC are confined to the site of injection and their effect is rather local than systemic, which would be the case if the cells were injected intravenously. In the vitreous body, MSC are in close proximity to the damaged retina, favoring paracrine activity and the modulation of host cells. Indeed, we have seen that MSC *in vitro* express trophic factors such as fibroblast growth factor 2 (FGF-2), vascular endothelial growth factor (VEGF) and ciliary neurotrophic factor (CNTF) (data not shown), and it was shown that MSC produce VEGF, brain-derived neurotrophic factor

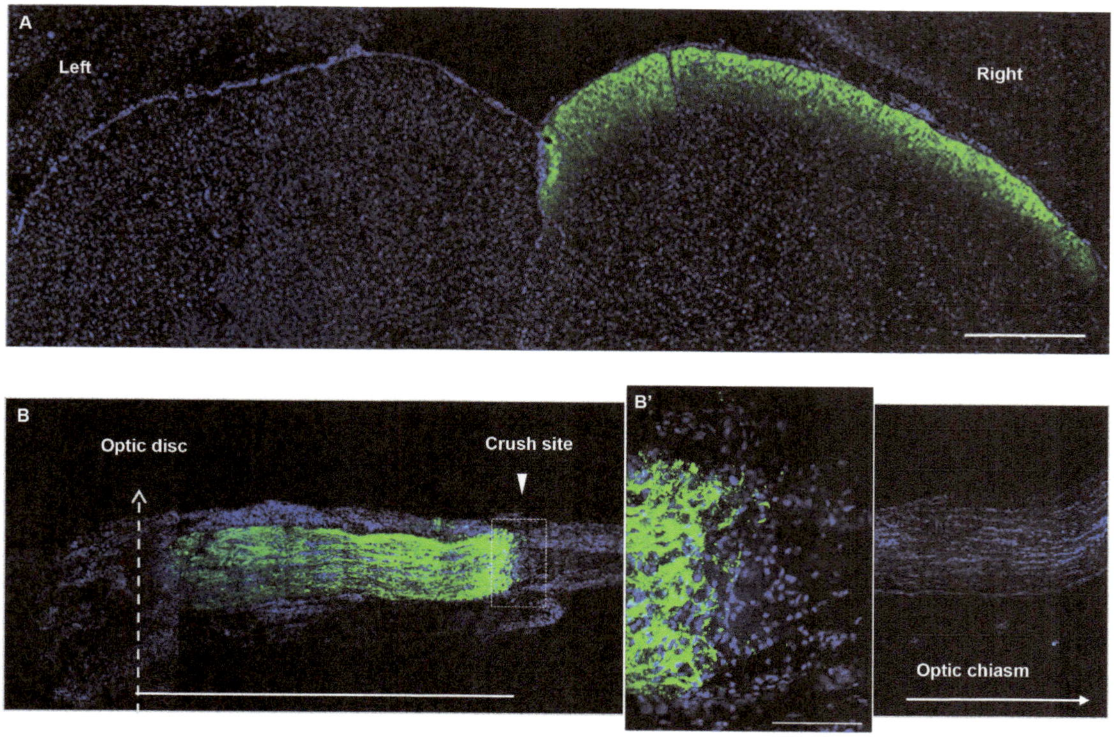

Figure 8. Anterograde labeling with CTB-488. (A) Photomontage of images of the superior colliculus of a rat 2 days after intravitreous injection of CTB-488 (green). In the absence of optic nerve injury, the tracer is transported from the left eye through the optic nerve until it reaches the right superior colliculus. (B) Photomontage of images of a nerve 4 days after injury. CTB-488 positive axons (green) do not extend farther into the crush site; B′ shows higher magnification. Nuclei (blue) were stained with DAPI. Scale bars: 250 (A), 1000 (B) and 100 (B′) μm.

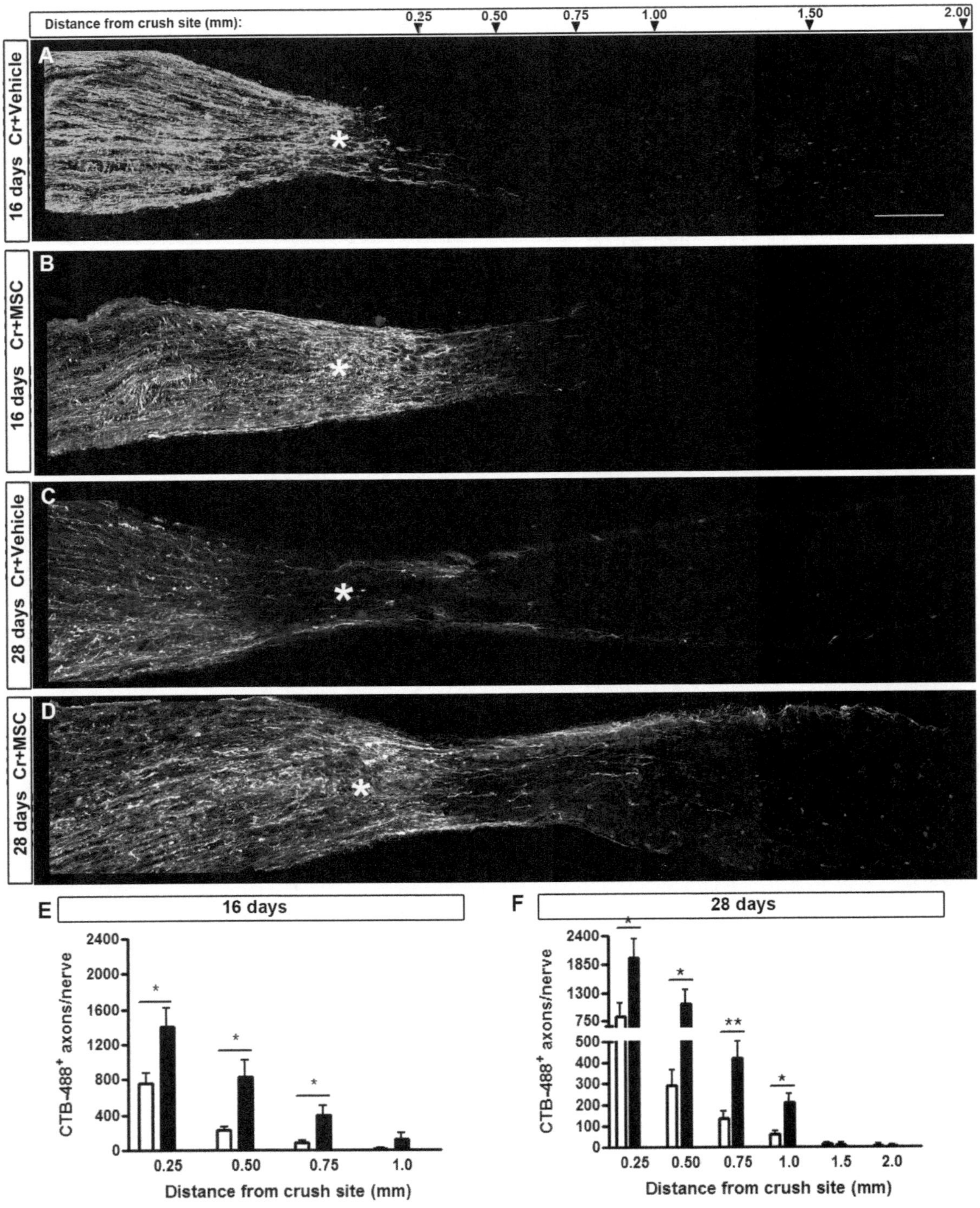

Figure 9. MSC transplantation increased RGC axon regeneration 16 and 28 days after optic nerve crush. A-D: Photomontage of confocal images of optic nerve sections to illustrate axonal outgrowth. CTB-488 was injected into the vitreous body 2 days prior to euthanasia to label the axons. Sixteen days after nerve crush (A,B,E) only a few axons had crossed the lesion site (asterisk) in the vehicle-injected animals (A) and this number was larger in the MSC-injected animals (B). Twenty-eight days after optic nerve injury (C,D,F), the MSC-injected group had an even larger number of axons regenerating beyond the crush site, compared to the vehicle-injected group. E, F: Quantification of CTB-488$^+$ axons per nerve at different distances from the crush site (from 0.25 to 2.0 mm). Results are displayed as mean ± SEM. *$P<0.05$; **$P<0.01$. Scale bar: 200 μm.

(BDNF), nerve growth factor (NGF) and hepatocyte growth factor (HGF) when cultured with injured brain extracts [85,86]. In a glaucoma model and after ischemia/reperfusion of the retina, MSC increase RGC survival and the expression of CNTF and FGF-2 in the retina [42,43]. FGF-2 is one of the most studied growth factors from the point of view of its neuroprotective effects[87] and our results showed that MSC upregulated FGF-2 in the retinal ganglion cell layer, similar to what we observed after therapy with bone marrow mononuclear cells[23].

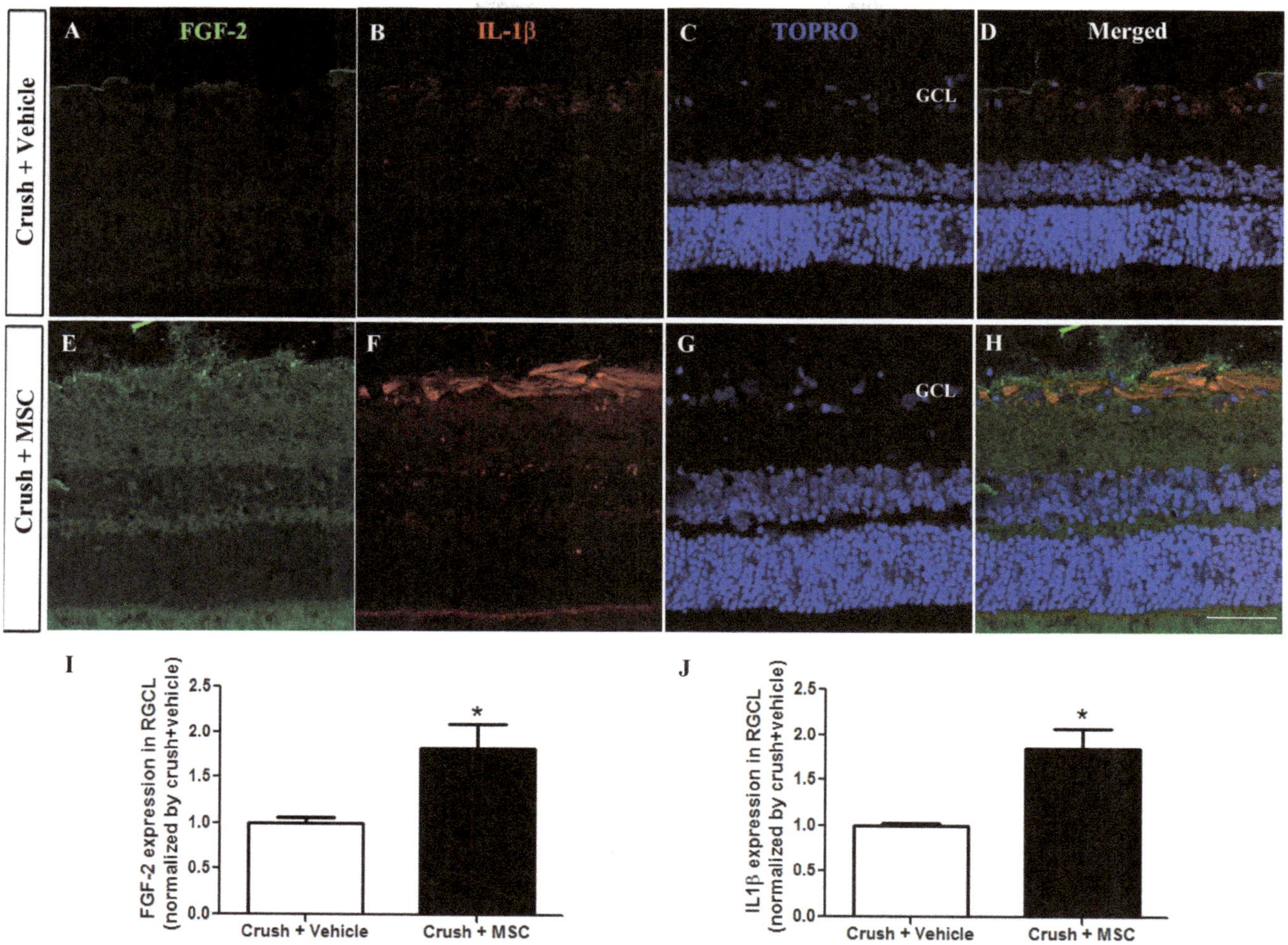

Figure 10. MSC transplantation increases FGF-2 and IL-1β expression in the retinal ganglion cell layer. (A-H) Confocal images of FGF-2 and IL-1β expression in retinas from vehicle injected (A-D) and MSC treated (E-H) groups. TOPRO (C, G) was used for nuclei staining. Images are representative of 3 animals per experimental condition. Scale Bar: 20 µm. (I, J) Graphs show the average mean gray value of Z stack images normalized by the vehicle injected group. *$p<0.05$, unpaired t-test. RGCL: retinal ganglion cell layer. Scale bar: 50 µm.

In addition to the modulation of trophic factors, MSC have immunomodulatory properties that were identified with reports that MSC could arrest T cell proliferation [88,89] and this characteristic has been increasingly explored as a potential approach to treat neuroinflammatory disorders [90]. Indeed, intravenous or intracerebral injection of MSC ameliorated the clinical course of experimental autoimmune encephalomyelitis (EAE) in mice by inducing T cell anergy and reducing lymphocytic infiltration [71,91]. MSC have been suggested to inhibit not only T lymphocytes but also other immune cells such as B cells, dendritic cells and natural killer cells [92]. There are also evidences that MSC induce an alternative activation of microglia into an anti-inflammatory phenotype, decreasing neuronal death after ischemia and favoring the clearance of Aβ in a transgenic model of Alzheimer's disease [36,66]. Importantly, when cultivated with T cell blasts or T cell hybridomas that do not produce inflammatory cytokines in the absence of antigen stimulation, MSC were not immunosuppressive [93]. Indeed, there are cumulative evidences that MSC must be activated or "licensed" by inflammatory pro-cytokines, in particular IL-1β, interferon (IFN)-γ and TNF-α, in order to exert their immunosuppressive effects [92–94]. In this study, we observed that animals treated with MSC had an increased expression of IL-1β in the retina, specifically in the RGC layer, suggesting that MSC created a pro-inflammatory environment. It is possible that phagocytosis of eventually dead MSC had resulted in the release of chemokines and cytokines, including IL-1. Because MSC are primed by inflammatory cytokines, it is likely that the retinal microenvironment produced by optic nerve crush and MSC themselves would be responsible for "licensing" the remaining alive MSC in order to secrete trophic factors that could protect the neurons and/or modulate the local microglia and other retinal glial cells. Recently it was shown that IL-1 and other pro-inflammatory cytokines may support neuronal survival [95–97] and that inflammatory stimulation induced either by lens injury [13,15,98], intravitreal injections of Zymozan [17,99], crystallins [100] or toll-like receptors 2 agonists [101] transforms RGC into a regenerative state, enabling these neurons to survive and grow axons over the inhibitory environment of the injured optic nerve. The inflammatory beneficial effects were associated with the release of oncomodulin by recruited macrophages [16,18] and neutrophils [102], as well as with the modulation of astrocyte-derived CNTF [103], leukemia inhibitory factor (LIF) [19], interleukin-6 (Il-6) [104] and consequent activation of several signaling pathways in the retinal cells. These include Janus kinase/signal transducers and activation of transcription-3 (JAK/STAT3) and phosphatidylinositide 3-kinase/protein kinase B/mammalian target of rapamycin (PI3K/AKT/mTOR) signaling cascades [105,106]. Recent studies targeted these pathways and obtained impressive results on RGC survival and axon regeneration through the optic nerve [10–12]. IL-1β induces phosphorilation of Akt and activation of PI3K/AKT [107–109] and intravitreal injections of this cytokine rescued axotomized RGC from retrograde cell death [110]. These studies introduce a possible neuroprotective role of IL-1β and link ocular inflammation to neuronal survival and regeneration. We speculate that MSC ability to interact with immune cells might direct the complex milieu created by optic nerve damage into a protective environment for RGC, and our results suggest that FGF-2 and IL-1β participate in the trophic and immunomodulatory effect that could promote the activation of signaling cascades such as PI3K/AKT that favor cell survival and regeneration.

Conclusions

We have demonstrated that MSC promote long-term neuroprotection and axon regeneration after optic nerve crush. The prolonged effect, compared to our previous results with BMMC therapy, may be due to a longer permanence of the graft. MSC mechanisms of action may include the upregulation of trophic factors, such as FGF-2, and modulation of neuroinflammation by increasing the expression of cytokines such as IL-1β in the damaged tissue. Further efforts in the understanding of MSC mechanisms of action in the visual system must be made to avoid their application as an empirical therapy, without full awareness of their proper effects in each biological environment [111]. Our results support the therapeutic potential of MSC in the central nervous system, but further studies are necessary to identify additional factors that may be released and the modulated cells, once MSC are injected and persist for a long period of time in damaged neuronal tissue.

Supporting Information

File S1 Figure S1, RGC survival over time. Graphs show the percentage of Tuj1 (A,B) or Brn3a (C,D) positive cells compared to the control (contralateral eyes), at 1.0 mm (A,C) and 3.5 mm (B,D) from the optic disc. Although there is a clear and significant neuroprotective effect of the MSC (asterisks), the percentage of Tuj1- and Brn3a-positive cells decreased at both distances from the optic disc from 16 to 28 days after optic nerve crush. Figure S2, The majority of the cells found in the vitreous body do not express IBA1. (A) Confocal image of an eye section immunostained with a specific antibody to IBA1 (red), 18 weeks after MSC transplantation. (B) Differential interference contrast microscopy image; iron reflection is seen as a dark area in the image. (C) Merged images. IBA1-positive cells were found in the inner retinal layers (arrows). In the vitreous body, the vast majority of nuclei (blue) was not associated with IBA1 expression. Rare IBA1-positive cells were present in the vitreous body (arrowhead). Nuclei were stained with TOPRO3. RPE: retinal pigmented epithelium. Table S1, Number of Tuj1- and Brn3a-positive cells in the retina. Table shows the number of cells per square millimeter of retina, SEM, and the estimated number of cells per retina at 16 and 28 days after injury. Sixteen days after injury, the number of Tuj1-positive cells is 2.7-fold increased in the treated group, whereas the number of Brn3a-positive cells increased 3.8-fold. Twenty-eight days after injury, the number of Tuj1-positive cells increased 2.5-fold in the treated group, whereas the number of Brn3a- positive cells increased 2.2-fold. The number of experiments (n) is indicated at each point. Table S2, Number of axons extending from 0.25 to 2.0 mm from the crush site. Table shows the mean and SEM of axons per nerve at each distance from the crush site at 16 and 28 days after injury. Sixteen days after injury, the number of axons at 1.0 mm from the crush site increased 4.7-fold in the treated group; whereas at 28 days after injury, the number of axons increased 3.0-fold in the treated group. The number of experiments (n) is indicated at each point.

Acknowledgments

We thank Felipe Marins, Fernando Freitas and Suelen Serio for technical assistance and Janet Reid for English language review of the manuscript.

Author Contributions

Conceived and designed the experiments: LAML CZdV FG RMO MFS. Performed the experiments: LAML CZdV AJdSJ GNdS FG ABPdF ALT BDP CT FTM MFS. Analyzed the data: LAML ALT BDP CT FTM MFS. Contributed reagents/materials/analysis tools: RMO MFS. Wrote the paper: LAML RMO MFS.

References

1. Furtado JM, Lansingh VC, Carter MJ, Milanese MF, Pena BN, et al. (2012) Causes of blindness and visual impairment in Latin America. Surv Ophthalmol 57: 149–177.
2. Pirouzmand F (2012) Epidemiological trends of traumatic optic nerve injuries in the largest Canadian adult trauma center. J Craniofac Surg 23: 516–520.
3. Levkovitch-Verbin H, Dardik R, Vander S, Nisgav Y, Kalev-Landoy M, et al. (2006) Experimental glaucoma and optic nerve transection induce simultaneous upregulation of proapoptotic and prosurvival genes. Invest Ophthalmol Vis Sci 47: 2491–2497.
4. Horner PJ, Gage FH (2000) Regenerating the damaged central nervous system. Nature 407: 963–970.
5. Johnson EM Jr, Deckwerth TL (1993) Molecular mechanisms of developmental neuronal death. Annu Rev Neurosci 16: 31–46.
6. Fischer D, He Z, Benowitz LI (2004) Counteracting the Nogo receptor enhances optic nerve regeneration if retinal ganglion cells are in an active growth state. J Neurosci 24: 1646–1651.
7. Lingor P, Teusch N, Schwarz K, Mueller R, Mack H, et al. (2007) Inhibition of Rho kinase (ROCK) increases neurite outgrowth on chondroitin sulphate proteoglycan in vitro and axonal regeneration in the adult optic nerve in vivo. J Neurochem 103: 181–189.
8. Lingor P, Tonges L, Pieper N, Bermel C, Barski E, et al. (2008) ROCK inhibition and CNTF interact on intrinsic signalling pathways and differentially regulate survival and regeneration in retinal ganglion cells. Brain 131: 250–263.
9. Wong EV, David S, Jacob MH, Jay DG (2003) Inactivation of myelin-associated glycoprotein enhances optic nerve regeneration. J Neurosci 23: 3112–3117.
10. Park KK, Liu K, Hu Y, Smith PD, Wang C, et al. (2008) Promoting axon regeneration in the adult CNS by modulation of the PTEN/mTOR pathway. Science 322: 963–966.
11. Smith PD, Sun F, Park KK, Cai B, Wang C, et al. (2009) SOCS3 deletion promotes optic nerve regeneration in vivo. Neuron 64: 617–623.
12. Sun F, Park KK, Belin S, Wang D, Lu T, et al. (2011) Sustained axon regeneration induced by co-deletion of PTEN and SOCS3. Nature 480: 372–375.
13. Fischer D, Pavlidis M, Thanos S (2000) Cataractogenic lens injury prevents traumatic ganglion cell death and promotes axonal regeneration both in vivo and in culture. Invest Ophthalmol Vis Sci 41: 3943–3954.
14. Kurimoto T, Yin Y, Omura K, Gilbert HY, Kim D, et al. (2010) Long-distance axon regeneration in the mature optic nerve: contributions of oncomodulin, cAMP, and pten gene deletion. J Neurosci 30: 15654–15663.
15. Leon S, Yin Y, Nguyen J, Irwin N, Benowitz LI (2000) Lens injury stimulates axon regeneration in the mature rat optic nerve. J Neurosci 20: 4615–4626.
16. Yin Y, Cui Q, Gilbert HY, Yang Y, Yang Z, et al. (2009) Oncomodulin links inflammation to optic nerve regeneration. Proc Natl Acad Sci U S A 106: 19587–19592.
17. Yin Y, Cui Q, Li Y, Irwin N, Fischer D, et al. (2003) Macrophage-derived factors stimulate optic nerve regeneration. J Neurosci 23: 2284–2293.

18. Yin Y, Henzl MT, Lorber B, Nakazawa T, Thomas TT, et al. (2006) Oncomodulin is a macrophage-derived signal for axon regeneration in retinal ganglion cells. Nat Neurosci 9: 843–852.
19. Leibinger M, Muller A, Andreadaki A, Hauk TG, Kirsch M, et al. (2009) Neuroprotective and axon growth-promoting effects following inflammatory stimulation on mature retinal ganglion cells in mice depend on ciliary neurotrophic factor and leukemia inhibitory factor. J Neurosci 29: 14334–14341.
20. Muller A, Hauk TG, Leibinger M, Marienfeld R, Fischer D (2009) Exogenous CNTF stimulates axon regeneration of retinal ganglion cells partially via endogenous CNTF. Mol Cell Neurosci 41: 233–246.
21. Moore DL, Blackmore MG, Hu Y, Kaestner KH, Bixby JL, et al. (2009) KLF family members regulate intrinsic axon regeneration ability. Science 326: 298–301.
22. Johnson TV, Bull ND, Hunt DP, Marina N, Tomarev SI, et al. (2010) Neuroprotective effects of intravitreal mesenchymal stem cell transplantation in experimental glaucoma. Invest Ophthalmol Vis Sci 51: 2051–2059.
23. Zaverucha-do-Valle C, Gubert F, Bargas-Rega M, Coronel JL, Mesentier-Louro LA, et al. (2011) Bone marrow mononuclear cells increase retinal ganglion cell survival and axon regeneration in the adult rat. Cell Transplant 20: 391–406.
24. Levkovitch-Verbin H, Sadan O, Vander S, Rosner M, Barhum Y, et al. (2010) Intravitreal injections of neurotrophic factors secreting mesenchymal stem cells are neuroprotective in rat eyes following optic nerve transection. Invest Ophthalmol Vis Sci 51: 6394–6400.
25. de Lima S, Habboub G, Benowitz LI (2012) Combinatorial therapy stimulates long-distance regeneration, target reinnervation, and partial recovery of vision after optic nerve injury in mice. Int Rev Neurobiol 106: 153–172.
26. Parrilla-Reverter G, Agudo M, Sobrado-Calvo P, Salinas-Navarro M, Villegas-Perez MP, et al. (2009) Effects of different neurotrophic factors on the survival of retinal ganglion cells after a complete intraorbital nerve crush injury: a quantitative in vivo study. Exp Eye Res 89: 32–41.
27. Cen LP, Luo JM, Geng Y, Zhang M, Pang CP, et al. (2012) Long-term survival and axonal regeneration of retinal ganglion cells after optic nerve transection and a peripheral nerve graft. Neuroreport 23: 692–697.
28. Crigler L, Robey RC, Asawachaicharn A, Gaupp D, Phinney DG (2006) Human mesenchymal stem cell subpopulations express a variety of neuro-regulatory molecules and promote neuronal cell survival and neuritogenesis. Exp Neurol 198: 54–64.
29. Uccelli A, Pistoia V, Moretta L (2007) Mesenchymal stem cells: a new strategy for immunosuppression? Trends Immunol 28: 219–226.
30. Heile AM, Wallrapp C, Klinge PM, Samii A, Kassem M, et al. (2009) Cerebral transplantation of encapsulated mesenchymal stem cells improves cellular pathology after experimental traumatic brain injury. Neurosci Lett 463: 176–181.
31. Salem HK, Thiemermann C (2010) Mesenchymal stromal cells: current understanding and clinical status. Stem Cells 28: 585–596.
32. Parr AM, Tator CH, Keating A (2007) Bone marrow-derived mesenchymal stromal cells for the repair of central nervous system injury. Bone Marrow Transplant 40: 609–619.
33. Brenneman M, Sharma S, Harting M, Strong R, Cox CS Jr, et al. (2010) Autologous bone marrow mononuclear cells enhance recovery after acute ischemic stroke in young and middle-aged rats. J Cereb Blood Flow Metab 30: 140–149.
34. de Vasconcelos Dos Santos A, da Costa Reis J, Diaz Paredes B, Moraes L, Jasmin, et al. (2010) Therapeutic window for treatment of cortical ischemia with bone marrow-derived cells in rats. Brain Res 1306: 149–158.
35. Giraldi-Guimaraes A, Rezende-Lima M, Bruno FP, Mendez-Otero R (2009) Treatment with bone marrow mononuclear cells induces functional recovery and decreases neurodegeneration after sensorimotor cortical ischemia in rats. Brain Res.
36. Ohtaki H, Ylostalo JH, Foraker JE, Robinson AP, Reger RL, et al. (2008) Stem/progenitor cells from bone marrow decrease neuronal death in global ischemia by modulation of inflammatory/immune responses. Proc Natl Acad Sci U S A 105: 14638–14643.
37. Yoshihara T, Ohta M, Itokazu Y, Matsumoto N, Dezawa M, et al. (2007) Neuroprotective effect of bone marrow-derived mononuclear cells promoting functional recovery from spinal cord injury. J Neurotrauma 24: 1026–1036.
38. Ribeiro-Resende VT, Pimentel-Coelho PM, Mesentier-Louro LA, Mendez RM, Mello-Silva JP, et al. (2009) Trophic activity derived from bone marrow mononuclear cells increases peripheral nerve regeneration by acting on both neuronal and glial cell populations. Neuroscience 159: 540–549.
39. Mesentier-Louro LA, Coronel J, Zaverucha-do-Valle C, Mencalha A, Paredes BD, et al. (2012) Cell therapy modulates expression of Tax1-binding protein 1 and synaptotagmin IV in a model of optic nerve lesion. Invest Ophthalmol Vis Sci 53: 4720–4729.
40. Barbosa da Fonseca LM, Gutfilen B, Rosado de Castro PH, Battistella V, Goldenberg RC, et al. (2010) Migration and homing of bone-marrow mononuclear cells in chronic ischemic stroke after intra-arterial injection. Exp Neurol 221: 122–128.
41. Yanai A, Hafeli UO, Metcalfe AL, Soema P, Addo L, et al. (2012) Focused magnetic stem cell targeting to the retina using superparamagnetic iron oxide nanoparticles. Cell Transplant 21: 1137–1148.
42. Yu S, Tanabe T, Dezawa M, Ishikawa H, Yoshimura N (2006) Effects of bone marrow stromal cell injection in an experimental glaucoma model. Biochem Biophys Res Commun 344: 1071–1079.
43. Li N, Li XR, Yuan JQ (2009) Effects of bone-marrow mesenchymal stem cells transplanted into vitreous cavity of rat injured by ischemia/reperfusion. Graefes Arch Clin Exp Ophthalmol 247: 503–514.
44. Johnson TV, Bull ND, Martin KR (2010) Identification of barriers to retinal engraftment of transplanted stem cells. Invest Ophthalmol Vis Sci 51: 960–970.
45. Jasmin, Torres AL, Nunes HM, Passipieri JA, Jelicks LA, et al. (2011) Optimized labeling of bone marrow mesenchymal cells with superparamagnetic iron oxide nanoparticles and in vivo visualization by magnetic resonance imaging. J Nanobiotechnology 9: 4.
46. Dominici M, Le Blanc K, Mueller I, Slaper-Cortenbach I, Marini F, et al. (2006) Minimal criteria for defining multipotent mesenchymal stromal cells. The International Society for Cellular Therapy position statement. Cytotherapy 8: 315–317.
47. Cui Q, Yip HK, Zhao RC, So KF, Harvey AR (2003) Intraocular elevation of cyclic AMP potentiates ciliary neurotrophic factor-induced regeneration of adult rat retinal ganglion cell axons. Mol Cell Neurosci 22: 49–61.
48. Xiang M, Zhou L, Macke JP, Yoshioka T, Hendry SH, et al. (1995) The Brn-3 family of POU-domain factors: primary structure, binding specificity, and expression in subsets of retinal ganglion cells and somatosensory neurons. J Neurosci 15: 4762–4785.
49. Nadal-Nicolas FM, Jimenez-Lopez M, Salinas-Navarro M, Sobrado-Calvo P, Alburquerque-Bejar JJ, et al. (2012) Whole number, distribution and co-expression of brn3 transcription factors in retinal ganglion cells of adult albino and pigmented rats. PLoS One 7: e49830.
50. Sanchez-Migallon MC, Nadal-Nicolas FM, Jimenez-Lopez M, Sobrado-Calvo P, Vidal-Sanz M, et al. (2011) Brain derived neurotrophic factor maintains Brn3a expression in axotomized rat retinal ganglion cells. Exp Eye Res 92: 260–267.
51. Nadal-Nicolas FM, Jimenez-Lopez M, Sobrado-Calvo P, Nieto-Lopez L, Canovas-Martinez I, et al. (2009) Brn3a as a marker of retinal ganglion cells: qualitative and quantitative time course studies in naive and optic nerve-injured retinas. Invest Ophthalmol Vis Sci 50: 3860–3868.
52. Berkelaar M, Clarke DB, Wang YC, Bray GM, Aguayo AJ (1994) Axotomy results in delayed death and apoptosis of retinal ganglion cells in adult rats. J Neurosci 14: 4368–4374.
53. Magharious M, D'Onofrio PM, Hollander A, Zhu P, Chen J, et al. (2011) Quantitative iTRAQ analysis of retinal ganglion cell degeneration after optic nerve crush. J Proteome Res 10: 3344–3362.
54. Isenmann S, Wahl C, Krajewski S, Reed JC, Bahr M (1997) Up-regulation of Bax protein in degenerating retinal ganglion cells precedes apoptotic cell death after optic nerve lesion in the rat. Eur J Neurosci 9: 1763–1772.
55. Kermer P, Klocker N, Labes M, Thomsen S, Srinivasan A, et al. (1999) Activation of caspase-3 in axotomized rat retinal ganglion cells in vivo. FEBS Lett 453: 361–364.
56. Kermer P, Ankerhold R, Klocker N, Krajewski S, Reed JC, et al. (2000) Caspase-9: involvement in secondary death of axotomized rat retinal ganglion cells in vivo. Brain Res Mol Brain Res 85: 144–150.
57. Bahr M (2000) Live or let die - retinal ganglion cell death and survival during development and in the lesioned adult CNS. Trends Neurosci 23: 483–490.
58. Kikuchi M, Tenneti L, Lipton SA (2000) Role of p38 mitogen-activated protein kinase in axotomy-induced apoptosis of rat retinal ganglion cells. J Neurosci 20: 5037–5044.
59. Benowitz L, Yin Y (2008) Rewiring the injured CNS: lessons from the optic nerve. Exp Neurol 209: 389–398.
60. Levkovitch-Verbin H (2004) Animal models of optic nerve diseases. Eye (Lond) 18: 1066–1074.
61. Smith JN, Calvi LM (2013) Concise review: current concepts in bone marrow microenvironmental regulation of hematopoietic stem and progenitor cells. Stem Cells 31: 1044–1050.
62. Laroni A, Novi G, Kerlero de Rosbo N, Uccelli A (2013) Towards Clinical Application of Mesenchymal Stem Cells for Treatment of Neurological Diseases of the Central Nervous System. J Neuroimmune Pharmacol.
63. Zhao CP, Zhang C, Zhou SN, Xie YM, Wang YH, et al. (2007) Human mesenchymal stromal cells ameliorate the phenotype of SOD1-G93A ALS mice. Cytotherapy 9: 414–426.
64. Uccelli A, Milanese M, Principato MC, Morando S, Bonifacino T, et al. (2012) Intravenous mesenchymal stem cells improve survival and motor function in experimental amyotrophic lateral sclerosis. Mol Med 18: 794–804.
65. Lee JK, Jin HK, Bae JS (2009) Bone marrow-derived mesenchymal stem cells reduce brain amyloid-beta deposition and accelerate the activation of microglia in an acutely induced Alzheimer's disease mouse model. Neurosci Lett 450: 136–141.
66. Lee JK, Jin HK, Endo S, Schuchman EH, Carter JE, et al. (2010) Intracerebral transplantation of bone marrow-derived mesenchymal stem cells reduces amyloid-beta deposition and rescues memory deficits in Alzheimer's disease mice by modulation of immune responses. Stem Cells 28: 329–343.
67. Lu L, Zhao C, Liu Y, Sun X, Duan C, et al. (2005) Therapeutic benefit of TH-engineered mesenchymal stem cells for Parkinson's disease. Brain Res Brain Res Protoc 15: 46–51.

68. Wright KT, El Masri W, Osman A, Chowdhury J, Johnson WE (2011) Concise review: Bone marrow for the treatment of spinal cord injury: mechanisms and clinical applications. Stem Cells 29: 169–178.
69. Li Y, Chen J, Chen XG, Wang L, Gautam SC, et al. (2002) Human marrow stromal cell therapy for stroke in rat: neurotrophins and functional recovery. Neurology 59: 514–523.
70. Rosado-de-Castro PH, Pimentel-Coelho PM, Barbosa da Fonseca LM, de Freitas GR, Mendez-Otero R (2013) The Rise of Cell Therapy Trials for Stroke: Review of Published and Registered Studies. Stem Cells Dev.
71. Zappia E, Casazza S, Pedemonte E, Benvenuto F, Bonanni I, et al. (2005) Mesenchymal stem cells ameliorate experimental autoimmune encephalomyelitis inducing T-cell anergy. Blood 106: 1755–1761.
72. Karussis D, Kassis I, Kurkalli BG, Slavin S (2008) Immunomodulation and neuroprotection with mesenchymal bone marrow stem cells (MSCs): a proposed treatment for multiple sclerosis and other neuroimmunological/neurodegenerative diseases. J Neurol Sci 265: 131–135.
73. Suzuki M, McHugh J, Tork C, Shelley B, Hayes A, et al. (2008) Direct muscle delivery of GDNF with human mesenchymal stem cells improves motor neuron survival and function in a rat model of familial ALS. Mol Ther 16: 2002–2010.
74. Kim H, Kim HY, Choi MR, Hwang S, Nam KH, et al. (2010) Dose-dependent efficacy of ALS-human mesenchymal stem cells transplantation into cisterna magna in SOD1-G93A ALS mice. Neurosci Lett 468: 190–194.
75. Kim YJ, Park HJ, Lee G, Bang OY, Ahn YH, et al. (2009) Neuroprotective effects of human mesenchymal stem cells on dopaminergic neurons through anti-inflammatory action. Glia 57: 13–23.
76. Osaka M, Honmou O, Murakami T, Nonaka T, Houkin K, et al. (2010) Intravenous administration of mesenchymal stem cells derived from bone marrow after contusive spinal cord injury improves functional outcome. Brain Res 1343: 226–235.
77. Akiyama Y, Radtke C, Kocsis JD (2002) Remyelination of the rat spinal cord by transplantation of identified bone marrow stromal cells. J Neurosci 22: 6623–6630.
78. Bai L, Lennon DP, Caplan AI, DeChant A, Hecker J, et al. (2012) Hepatocyte growth factor mediates mesenchymal stem cell-induced recovery in multiple sclerosis models. Nat Neurosci 15: 862–870.
79. Liu R, Zhang Z, Lu Z, Borlongan C, Pan J, et al. (2013) Human umbilical cord stem cells ameliorate experimental autoimmune encephalomyelitis by regulating immunoinflammation and remyelination. Stem Cells Dev 22: 1053–1062.
80. Quertainmont R, Cantinieaux D, Botman O, Sid S, Schoenen J, et al. (2012) Mesenchymal stem cell graft improves recovery after spinal cord injury in adult rats through neurotrophic and pro-angiogenic actions. PLoS One 7: e39500.
81. Hawryluk GW, Mothe A, Wang J, Wang S, Tator C, et al. (2012) An in vivo characterization of trophic factor production following neural precursor cell or bone marrow stromal cell transplantation for spinal cord injury. Stem Cells Dev 21: 2222–2238.
82. Giunti D, Parodi B, Usai C, Vergani L, Casazza S, et al. (2012) Mesenchymal stem cells shape microglia effector functions through the release of CX3CL1. Stem Cells 30: 2044–2053.
83. Lee JK, Schuchman EH, Jin HK, Bae JS (2012) Soluble CCL5 derived from bone marrow-derived mesenchymal stem cells and activated by amyloid beta ameliorates Alzheimer's disease in mice by recruiting bone marrow-induced microglia immune responses. Stem Cells 30: 1544–1555.
84. Perry VH, Walker M (1980) Amacrine cells, displaced amacrine cells and interplexiform cells in the retina of the rat. Proc R Soc Lond B Biol Sci 208: 415–431.
85. Chen X, Katakowski M, Li Y, Lu D, Wang L, et al. (2002) Human bone marrow stromal cell cultures conditioned by traumatic brain tissue extracts: growth factor production. J Neurosci Res 69: 687–691.
86. Chen Q, Long Y, Yuan X, Zou L, Sun J, et al. (2005) Protective effects of bone marrow stromal cell transplantation in injured rodent brain: synthesis of neurotrophic factors. J Neurosci Res 80: 611–619.
87. Dreyfus H, Sahel J, Heidinger V, Mohand-Said S, Guerold B, et al. (1998) Gangliosides and neurotrophic growth factors in the retina. Molecular interactions and applications as neuroprotective agents. Ann N Y Acad Sci 845: 240–252.
88. Di Nicola M, Carlo-Stella C, Magni M, Milanesi M, Longoni PD, et al. (2002) Human bone marrow stromal cells suppress T-lymphocyte proliferation induced by cellular or nonspecific mitogenic stimuli. Blood 99: 3838–3843.
89. Bartholomew A, Sturgeon C, Siatskas M, Ferrer K, McIntosh K, et al. (2002) Mesenchymal stem cells suppress lymphocyte proliferation in vitro and prolong skin graft survival in vivo. Exp Hematol 30: 42–48.
90. Kassis I, Vaknin-Dembinsky A, Karussis D (2011) Bone marrow mesenchymal stem cells: agents of immunomodulation and neuroprotection. Curr Stem Cell Res Ther 6: 63–68.
91. Kassis I, Grigoriadis N, Gowda-Kurkalli B, Mizrachi-Kol R, Ben-Hur T, et al. (2008) Neuroprotection and immunomodulation with mesenchymal stem cells in chronic experimental autoimmune encephalomyelitis. Arch Neurol 65: 753–761.
92. Shi Y, Su J, Roberts AI, Shou P, Rabson AB, et al. (2012) How mesenchymal stem cells interact with tissue immune responses. Trends Immunol 33: 136–143.
93. Ren G, Zhang L, Zhao X, Xu G, Zhang Y, et al. (2008) Mesenchymal stem cell-mediated immunosuppression occurs via concerted action of chemokines and nitric oxide. Cell Stem Cell 2: 141–150.
94. English K (2013) Mechanisms of mesenchymal stromal cell immunomodulation. Immunol Cell Biol 91: 19–26.
95. Tuttolomondo A, Di Raimondo D, di Sciacca R, Pinto A, Licata G (2008) Inflammatory cytokines in acute ischemic stroke. Curr Pharm Des 14: 3574–3589.
96. Petcu EB, Kocher T, Kuhr A, Buga AM, Kloting I, et al. (2008) Mild systemic inflammation has a neuroprotective effect after stroke in rats. Curr Neurovasc Res 5: 214–223.
97. Pickering M, O'Connor JJ (2007) Pro-inflammatory cytokines and their effects in the dentate gyrus. Prog Brain Res 163: 339–354.
98. Lorber B, Berry M, Logan A (2005) Lens injury stimulates adult mouse retinal ganglion cell axon regeneration via both macrophage- and lens-derived factors. Eur J Neurosci 21: 2029–2034.
99. Ahmed Z, Aslam M, Lorber B, Suggate EL, Berry M, et al. (2010) Optic nerve and vitreal inflammation are both RGC neuroprotective but only the latter is RGC axogenic. Neurobiol Dis 37: 441–454.
100. Fischer D, Hauk TG, Muller A, Thanos S (2008) Crystallins of the beta/gamma-superfamily mimic the effects of lens injury and promote axon regeneration. Mol Cell Neurosci 37: 471–479.
101. Hauk TG, Leibinger M, Muller A, Andreadaki A, Knippschild U, et al. (2010) Stimulation of axon regeneration in the mature optic nerve by intravitreal application of the toll-like receptor 2 agonist Pam3Cys. Invest Ophthalmol Vis Sci 51: 459–464.
102. Kurimoto T, Yin Y, Habboub G, Gilbert HY, Li Y, et al. (2013) Neutrophils express oncomodulin and promote optic nerve regeneration. J Neurosci 33: 14816–14824.
103. Muller A, Hauk TG, Fischer D (2007) Astrocyte-derived CNTF switches mature RGCs to a regenerative state following inflammatory stimulation. Brain 130: 3308–3320.
104. Leibinger M, Muller A, Gobrecht P, Diekmann H, Andreadaki A, et al. (2013) Interleukin-6 contributes to CNS axon regeneration upon inflammatory stimulation. Cell Death Dis 4: e609.
105. Leibinger M, Andreadaki A, Diekmann H, Fischer D (2013) Neuronal STAT3 activation is essential for CNTF- and inflammatory stimulation-induced CNS axon regeneration. Cell Death Dis 4: e805.
106. Leibinger M, Andreadaki A, Fischer D (2012) Role of mTOR in neuroprotection and axon regeneration after inflammatory stimulation. Neurobiol Dis 46: 314–324.
107. Kaushik DK, Thounaojam MC, Kumawat KL, Gupta M, Basu A (2013) Interleukin-1beta orchestrates underlying inflammatory responses in microglia via Kruppel-like factor 4. J Neurochem 127: 233–244.
108. Pousset F, Dantzer R, Kelley KW, Parnet P (2000) Interleukin-1 signaling in mouse astrocytes involves Akt: a study with interleukin-4 and IL-10. Eur Cytokine Netw 11: 427–434.
109. Reddy SA, Huang JH, Liao WS (1997) Phosphatidylinositol 3-kinase in interleukin 1 signaling. Physical interaction with the interleukin 1 receptor and requirement in NFkappaB and AP-1 activation. J Biol Chem 272: 29167–29173.
110. Diem R, Hobom M, Grotsch P, Kramer B, Bahr M (2003) Interleukin-1 beta protects neurons via the interleukin-1 (IL-1) receptor-mediated Akt pathway and by IL-1 receptor-independent decrease of transmembrane currents in vivo. Mol Cell Neurosci 22: 487–500.
111. Bianco P, Cao X, Frenette PS, Mao JJ, Robey PG, et al. (2013) The meaning, the sense and the significance: translating the science of mesenchymal stem cells into medicine. Nat Med 19: 35–42.

Investigation of Cross-Species Translatability of Pharmacological MRI in Awake Nonhuman Primate - A Buprenorphine Challenge Study

Stephanie Seah[1,2]*, Abu Bakar Ali Asad[1,2], Richard Baumgartner[3], Dai Feng[3], Donald S. Williams[1], Elaine Manigbas[4], John D. Beaver[4¤a], Torsten Reese[2¤b], Brian Henry[2], Jeffrey L. Evelhoch[1], Chih-Liang Chin[1,2]

1 Imaging, Merck & Co. Inc., West Point, Pennsylvania, United States of America, **2** Translational Medicine Research Centre, MSD, Singapore, Singapore, **3** Biostatistics and Research Decision Sciences, Merck & Co. Inc., Rahway, New Jersey, United States of America, **4** Imaging, Maccine Pte Ltd, Singapore, Singapore

Abstract

Background: Pharmacological MRI (phMRI) is a neuroimaging technique where drug-induced hemodynamic responses can represent a pharmacodynamic biomarker to delineate underlying biological consequences of drug actions. In most preclinical studies, animals are anesthetized during image acquisition to minimize movement. However, it has been demonstrated anesthesia could attenuate basal neuronal activity, which can confound interpretation of drug-induced brain activation patterns. Significant efforts have been made to establish awake imaging in rodents and nonhuman primates (NHP). Whilst various platforms have been developed for imaging awake NHP, comparison and validation of phMRI data as translational biomarkers across species remain to be explored.

Methodology: We have established an awake NHP imaging model that encompasses comprehensive acclimation procedures with a dedicated animal restrainer. Using a cerebral blood volume (CBV)-based phMRI approach, we have determined differential responses of brain activation elicited by the systemic administration of buprenorphine (0.03 mg/kg i.v.), a partial μ-opioid receptor agonist, in the same animal under awake and anesthetized conditions. Additionally, region-of-interest analyses were performed to determine regional drug-induced CBV time-course data and corresponding area-under-curve (AUC) values from brain areas with high density of μ-opioid receptors.

Principal Findings: In awake NHPs, group-level analyses revealed buprenorphine significantly activated brain regions including, thalamus, striatum, frontal and cingulate cortices (paired *t*-test, versus saline vehicle, $p<0.05$, $n=4$). This observation is strikingly consistent with μ-opioid receptor distribution depicted by [6-O-[^{11}C]methyl]buprenorphine ([^{11}C]BPN) positron emission tomography imaging study in baboons. Furthermore, our findings are consistent with previous buprenorphine phMRI studies in humans and conscious rats which collectively demonstrate the cross-species translatability of awake imaging. Conversely, no significant change in activated brain regions was found in the same animals imaged under the anesthetized condition.

Conclusions: Our data highlight the utility and importance of awake NHP imaging as a translational imaging biomarker for drug research.

Editor: Alessandro Gozzi, Italian Institute of Technology, Italy

Funding: This research was funded by Merck & Co. The authors would like to declare that the following individuals are current or former employees of the funder - Stephanie Seah, Abu Bakar Ali Asad, Richard Baumgartner, Dai Feng, Don Williams, Torsten Reese, Brian Henry, Jeff Evelhoch and Chih-Liang Chin. Their roles include study design, data collection and analysis, decision to publish and preparation of the manuscript.

Competing Interests: Merck provided all funds for this work. As mentioned in the financial disclosures, some authors are current or former employees of Merck and may own stock or hold stock options in Merck. Co-authors Elaine Manigbas and John Beaver were employees of Maccine Pte. Ltd.

* Email: stephanie.seah@merck.com

¤a Current address: Translational Imaging, Global Pharmaceutical Research and Development, Abbott Park, Illonois, United States of America
¤b Current address: MR Imaging, CIC biomaGUNE, San Sebastián, Gipuzkoa, Spain

Introduction

Pharmacological MRI (phMRI) is a neuroimaging technique that allows characterization of changes in neural activity following drug challenge. Drug-induced pharmacodynamic responses detected from alterations in blood oxygenation level dependence (BOLD) signals or relative cerebral blood volume/flow (rCBV/rCBF) can provide as imaging biomarkers to delineate the central effect of drug actions [1,2,3,4]. As a result, significant effort has been devoted to implement phMRI as a translational research tool to develop novel CNS compounds, considering that this *in vivo* imaging technique can be performed in both animals [5,6,7,8] and humans [9,10,11,12]. To date, phMRI has been adopted to interrogate several key neurotransmitter systems, and these findings collectively have highlighted the value of phMRI to elucidate neurobiological mechanisms of drug actions and to gain better understanding of human diseases. In most preclinical imaging studies, animals were anesthetized during image acquisition to minimize movements; however, several lines of evidence have shown that the use of anesthesia could attenuate basal neuronal activity and likely confound drug-induced brain activation patterns [13,14,15,16,17,18,19,20]. Therefore, it is critical to establish translational platforms that permit investigation of pharmacological responses of experimental therapeutics in preclinical species, healthy volunteers and eventually in patients. To this end, phMRI in awake animals has been extensively pursued across various species, such as rodents [19,21,22,23] and nonhuman primates (NHPs) [17,18,24,25,26,27,28].

Awake NHP models are particularly attractive for neuroscience research, in light of greater similarities with humans in clinical and pathological characteristics [29]. It has been demonstrated that NHP and human brains share features in neuronal cytoarchitecture [30] and functional connections [31]. Additionally, the activity and distribution of neurotransmitter systems [32,33], drug metabolism and pharmacokinetic responses [34] are more comparable to human in NHP than in rodent. Nonetheless, despite the improved cross-species translatability offered by awake NHP imaging, animal movements during image acquisition can pose as a major obstacle, since excessive motion can lead to image blurring or ghosting artifacts, and higher baseline signal fluctuations that could diminish sensitivity to detect changes of drug-induced phMRI signals. Furthermore, the level of resting state stability could vary significantly among imaging sessions, which can attribute to compromised test-retest reliability and hindrance to conducting longitudinal studies. To circumvent this challenge, several groups have attempted to develop awake NHP imaging paradigms, in which extensive acclimation procedures are often required [17,27,35,36,37]. Animals were trained to remain still and gradually habituate to the actual scanning environment while using a dedicated animal restrainer that affords better securing of the animal's head and/or body, such as a head-post model [35] or non-invasive helmet approaches [27,36]. In addition, improved data acquisition methods [37], use of contrast agent [38] and optimized data analysis strategies [39] have also been explored to enhance phMRI sensitivity. Nonetheless, it will be essential to establish a systematic approach to evaluate phMRI baseline signals attributable to animal movements and thus characterize the utility, or limitation, of these awake imaging platforms.

Buprenorphine is an opioid agonist that has a high affinity to various opioid receptors, such as μ, δ, κ subtypes [40], and it has been used clinically to treat opiate addiction or pain [41,42]. The clinical efficacy of buprenorphine for pain and opiate addiction is thought to be due to partial agonism at μ–opioid receptors and/or antagonism at κ–opioid receptors [41,42]. Previous studies performed by Upadhyay et al. have shown that buprenorphine elicited BOLD responses in humans correspond to brain regions with abundant μ–opioid receptors and modulate brain functional connectivity ascribed to pain-processing circuitry [43]. Interestingly, congruency in the spatial pattern of buprenorphine-induced brain activation between humans and conscious rats was also observed [21]. In light of these studies in both humans and awake rats, a phMRI study of buprenorphine in awake NHP can assess the congruency of imaging endpoints across species, and thereby determine the utility of an awake NHP imaging platform for translational research.

In this study, we sought to investigate differential responses in brain activity in NHP produced by the systemic administration of buprenorphine under awake and anesthetized conditions. We hypothesized that buprenorphine-induced brain activation pattern observed from awake NHP should highlight the known μ-opioid receptor distribution [44,45] and afford investigation of cross-species translatability of awake NHP imaging in conjunction with previous phMRI data obtained from humans and awake rats [21,43].

Toward this goal, we first constructed a dedicated animal restrainer based on a design previously reported by Andersen et al. [35] and then developed an awake NHP training protocol. Each animal received comprehensive training, including incremental sessions in a mock MRI scanner and acclimatization to the actual imaging environment. The effectiveness of training was evaluated via measured circulating cortisol levels and behavioral scores (e.g. rated by the trainer). Consequently, these criteria were used to select animals thought to be most habituated to the scanner environment for subsequent imaging studies. During the imaging phase, resting state BOLD signals were acquired under awake (both test and re-test) and anesthetized conditions to determine resting state baseline stability and reliability, which served as a measure of the effectiveness or limitation of our acclimation procedures. To assess the cross-species translatability of our awake NHP platform, we imaged brain activity induced by buprenorphine infusion (0.03 mg/kg i.v.) using a CBV-based phMRI approach, where an ultrasmall superparamagnetic iron oxide (USPIO) contrast agent was applied to increase sensitivity [46]. Imaging experiments were conducted following a within-subject study design to differentiate the central effect of buprenorphine and saline vehicle in NHPs imaged under both awake and isoflurane-anesthetized conditions. To characterize the regional specificity of drug effect, a group-level and region-of-interest (ROI) data analysis pipeline was implemented based on a standard monkey brain atlas [47], where drug-induced CBV-based signal change time-course data and corresponding area-under-curve (AUC) were derived from selected brain regions with high density of μ–opioid receptors.

Materials and Methods

Ethics Statement

The following experiments were conducted in accordance with the Institutional Animal Care and Use Committee at Merck & Co. The current study, in addition to its protocol, was approved by the Institutional Animal Care and Use Committee at Merck & Co (Permit Number: 11102130610016). No animals were sacrificed for the purpose of this experiment. Trained veterinarians and animal technicians were involved in the care of the animals as well as all the animal procedures performed during this study.

Animals

Adult female cynomolgus monkeys (Macaca fascicularis, PT Prestasi Fauna Nusantara, Indonesia; $n = 12$, age $= 4$ years - 6 years, body weight $= 2$ kg~4 kg) were allocated for this study. Animals were pair housed at the Maccine facility in temperature- (18 °C–26 °C) and humidity-controlled (30%–70%) rooms maintained on a 12:12 light/dark cycle with lights on at 7:00 AM. Mirrors were placed outside the home cage, and cage toys/ manipulative enrichment, such as Kong toys, Flexi keys, were provided and rotated every week. Radios and televisions were also used as supplementary enrichments. Animals were fed with a diet of monkey chow free of animal protein, as well as a controlled amount of fruits or vegetables, offered twice daily. Aside from daily fruit rations, frozen homemade treats (i.e. fruits, raisins, cereals, etc.) were provided once a week. Tap water was offered ad libitum. Prior to the commencement of the study, a complete physical examination, including hematological/blood chemistry analysis, was performed and reviewed by the attending veterinarian.

Awake Training Protocol

Based on previous work done by Andersen et al. [35], a dedicated animal restrainer was constructed, and the animals were habituated to the restrainer and MRI scanner environment for awake imaging. To alleviate stress and minimize movement during awake imaging, each animal was blindfolded and trained in a phased manner, gradually habituated through different training procedures over several months (see Fig. 1; Phase 1a–c). As shown in Figure 1, our training protocol includes *restrainer training*, *mock scanner training* and *head-post surgery and head-restraint tethering training* phases. During each training session, animal's behavioral gestures (e.g. vocalization, excessive movement, head/body turn) were monitored and scored by a trainer. A low cumulative behavioral score at the end of the training was indicative of a well-behaved animal, suitable for the imaging study. Briefly, during Phase 1a: *restrainer training*, animals were trained to remain still in a primate restraining chair for a period of 30 minutes which was gradually prolonged to a steady state of 120 minutes. Upon achieving this requirement, animals were placed in a prone position in a confinement apparatus for 120 minutes to acclimatize to the restrainer environment. Next, animals were gradually exposed to an MRI-compatible restrainer and the duration of the training period increased by 15 minutes weekly until a steady state of 120 minutes was reached. Additionally, to assess the stress level associated with training procedures, cortisol concentrations were also measured using an electrochemiluminescence immunoassay toolkit (ECLIA, Roche Diagnostics, Singapore), in which blood samples (2 mL) were collected prior to placing the animals inside the restrainer tube and 90-minute-post training. Based on the measured cortisol levels and cumulative behavioral scores over the course of Phase 1a, eight animals were selected and progressed to Phase 1b (*mock scanner training*).

In the *mock scanner training* phase, animals were placed in the restrainer in a mock scanner for a 2-hour time period every other day, in order to habituate them to the scanner environment. At the last training session of this phase, cortisol measurements were repeated (pre- and post-training, $n = 8$) to evaluate the effectiveness of acclimation, and the results were compared with a non-trained control cohort ($n = 6$). Finally, in the *head-post surgery and head-restraint tethering* phase for the selected animals, the head-post component of the restrainer was surgically attached to the skull of each subject [35]. Head tethering restraint training started after animals had fully recovered from the surgery and occurred twice a week until the actual imaging study.

Animal Preparation for the Imaging Study

Animals progressed from the training procedures to imaging studies (see Fig. 1), where they were imaged under both awake and anesthetized conditions for the stability and test-retest reliability study of resting state BOLD signal and subsequently the phMRI experiments. For the anesthetized imaging study, animals were sedated with ketamine (10 mg/kg IM) for induction, while ear plugs and eye lubricant were applied to all the animals, prior to bringing them into the scanner room. The animal was then placed on the patient bed of the MRI scanner in a prone position and ventilated by an MRI-compatible ventilator and bellows system (SurgiVet, Dublin, OH). Anesthesia was maintained through inhalation of a mixture of isoflurane (2%) in medical air. Physiological parameters of each animal, including heart rate, SpO_2, $EtCO_2$, and respiration rate were monitored and recorded throughout the imaging session using an MR-compatible Datex-Ohmeda physiological monitoring system (GE Healthcare, WI). The temperature of the animal was measured via a fiber-optic temperature sensor system (OpSens, Quebec, Canada) and recorded periodically throughout the experiment. For the awake imaging study, animals were blindfolded and placed in a sphinx position within the restrainer used during the training procedures.

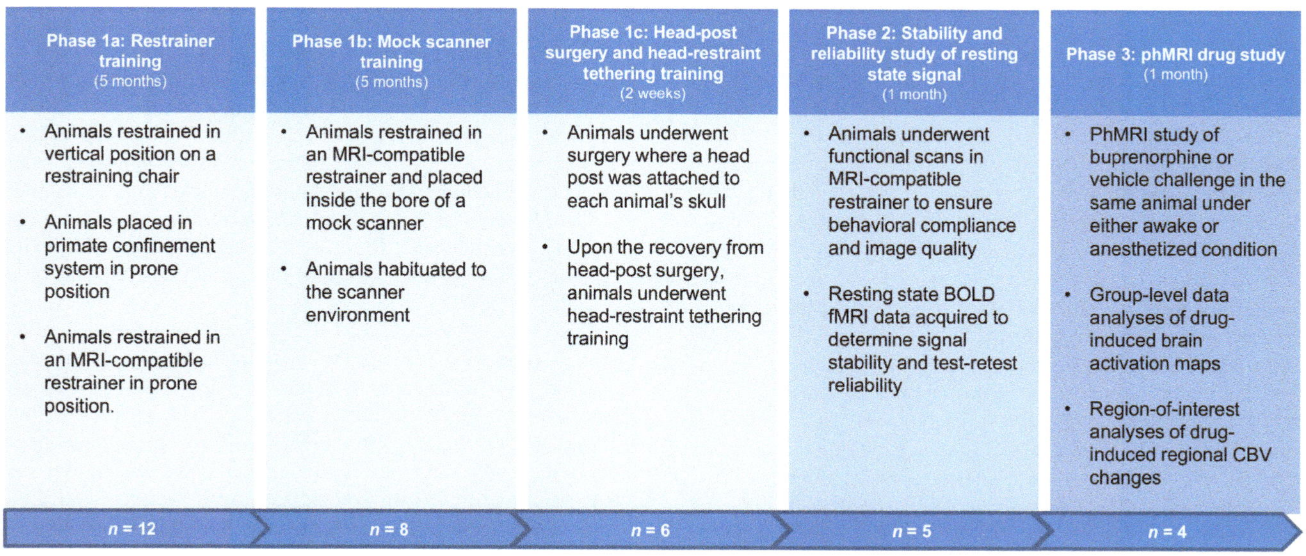

Figure 1. Study protocol of awake imaging in non-human primates. Initial Phase 1a–c focus on the training procedures to reduce animal movement/stress during awake imaging; Phase 2 was the assessment of the stability of resting state signal and its test-retest reliability; Phase 3 was the within-subject pharmacological challenge study, where buprenorphine (0.03 mg/kg i.v.) and vehicle were given to the same animals under awake and anesthetized conditions.

A customized head radiofrequency (RF) coil was securely attached to the head-post of the animal. Also, during each awake imaging session, at least one animal trainer would be assigned to visually monitor the animals.

Evaluation of the Effectiveness or Limitation of Awake Training Protocol

All imaging experiments were conducted on a 3 Tesla TIM Trio MRI scanner (Siemens Medical Solutions, Erlangen, Germany) using a dedicated 8-channel phased-array head coil (RAPID Biomedical GmbH, Germany). Resting state BOLD signal was collected by a single-shot gradient-echo EPI pulse sequence (TR/TE = 3 s/21 ms, in-plane pixel size = 1 mm ×1 mm, slice thickness = 2 mm, and 24 slices with no gap), and 810 imaging volumes (40 minutes in total) were acquired. High resolution brain anatomical images (TR/TE = 700 ms/13 ms, in-plane pixel size = 0.67 mm ×0.67 mm) of individual animals were also acquired in order to co-register with a standard monkey brain atlas [47] for further group-level and ROI analyses. Resting state BOLD signals were acquired from the same animals imaged under anesthetized and awake conditions separately ($n = 5$). Further, to examine the test-retest reliability of resting state BOLD signal during awake imaging, experiments were repeated on a different day. As a result, each animal was imaged three times in total.

Assessment of Cross-species Translatability of Awake NHP

For the phMRI study, selected animals ($n = 4$) underwent four separate sessions (1-week apart to ensure drug washout) on different days (16 scans in total), where a counterbalanced measures design was used to ensure each animal was imaged under different drug challenge (vehicle or buprenorphine) or imaging condition (awake or anesthetized). For each imaging experiment, brain anatomical image and functional datasets were acquired using the same imaging pulse sequences and parameters described above (see *Evaluation of the Effectiveness or Limitation of Awake Training Protocol* section).

To increase the sensitivity of phMRI signals [46], a CBV-based approach using a USPIO contrast agent, 7.5 mg/kg i.v. of Ferumoxytol (AMAG Pharmaceutical, Cambridge MA), was used. A tail vein line was cannulated for the administration of contrast agent and drug, while the indwelling catheter was attached to a saline-filled syringe placed on an infusion pump (Harvard Apparatus, Holliston, MA) located outside the scanner room. All animals were administered intravenously with either 0.03 mg/kg of buprenorphine (Reckitt Benckiser Pharmaceuticals, UK) or saline vehicle. Intramuscular injection of buprenorphine at 0.01 mg/kg or 0.03 mg/kg has been commonly used for analgesia in nonhuman primates [48] and we have adopted the higher dose in the current study. Notably, different doses of buprenorphine were selected in previous phMRI studies in rodent (0.04 mg/kg and 0.1 mg/kg i.v.) or human (0.2 mg/70 kg i.v.) [21,43]. The following imaging protocol was carried out: (i) 5-minute pre-contrast data acquisition, (ii) bolus injection of the contrast agent via the tail vein line (total injection volume = 2 mL), (iii) 10-minute pre-drug baseline acquisition (post-contrast), (iv) infusion of either buprenorphine at 0.03 mg/kg i.v. or saline vehicle (total injection volume = 3 mL) was split into three infusion periods (30 s each) separated by a 1.5-minute interval, in order to minimize potential respiratory suppression related to the buprenorphine injection [43]. Finally, (v) 20-minute period of post-drug imaging acquisition.

Data Analysis

Data analyses were conducted using the FMRIB Software Library (FSL) (http://www.fmrib.ox.au.ul/fls) and in-house Matlab (MathWorks, Natick, MA). First, voxels of the brain were extracted using a brain extraction tool (FSL BET). To characterize the fluctuation of resting state BOLD signals obtained from awake and anesthetized imaging experiments, time-course data of each voxel was derived and expressed as a percentage change relative to the average signal intensity over the entire imaging time period. Then, for each voxel the mean percentage change was calculated by averaging the absolute value of percentage change over time. Consequently, the mean value and standard deviation over the entire brain volume were calculated and reported. Finally, a Bland-Altman plot was used to assess test-retest reliability of awake resting state BOLD signal.

For the phMRI data analysis, FSL was used. Specifically, our data analysis pipeline included the following steps: motion correction (FSL MCFLIRT), brain extraction, spatial smoothing (FWHM = 2 mm) and co-registration to a standard monkey brain atlas [47]. To depict activated brain regions, time-course relative CBV change, ΔrCBV(t), was first calculated from the raw data using a known relationship [46,49],

$$\Delta rCBV(t) = \ln[S_{POST}/S(t)]/\ln[S_{PRE}/S_{POST}] \quad (1)$$

where t is time after drug injection, $S(t)$ is the signal intensity after the drug infusion, S_{POST} is the mean pre-drug baseline signal intensity over the 10-minute period, post contrast agent administration, and S_{PRE} is the mean signal intensity over the 5-minute period, prior to the administration of contrast agent. Then, a general linear model (GLM) was used for the subject-level analysis, where a linear ramp model was used to mimic the infusion response, while the elimination of buprenorphine was based on the known plasma pharmacokinetic of buprenorphine in dogs (brain half-life ~4.5 hr) [50]. Due to the relatively long onset of the ramp function compared to the hemodynamic response function (HRF), the ramp stimulus function in our GLM was not convolved with HRF [43]. To perform unbiased univariate linear regression analysis, nuisance regressors were prepared that account for most of the confounding explanatory variables (EVs), where the mean time-course signals extracted from the ventricles and white matter were included to regress out additional confounds related to physiological noises and/or linear drifts. Further, an in-house Matlab script was written to identify excessive intensity changes (head movement) between imaging time-points, as a de-spiking in the EV. Spike detection was implemented using a median absolute residual variation (MARV) score-based approach [51], while imaging volumes with motion greater than half of a voxel were identified as spikes.

For the group-level and ROI analyses, functional data of each animal was first co-registered to the individual's anatomical images by rigid body translations and rotations and subsequently into a template monkey brain atlas [47] using 12 degrees of freedom affine transformation. These calculated transformation matrix parameters were then applied to the functional dataset and derived statistical maps. Group comparisons were conducted using a mixed-effects paired t-test (FSL FLAME) to determine the group means of the differential effect of vehicle and buprenorphine in both anesthetized and awake animals, threshold at $p<0.05$, in order to identify brain regions affected by the drug or vehicle challenge under awake and anesthetized imaging. In addition, to illustrate the temporal dynamics of rCBV change, time-course data for each imaging condition from selected brain regions were

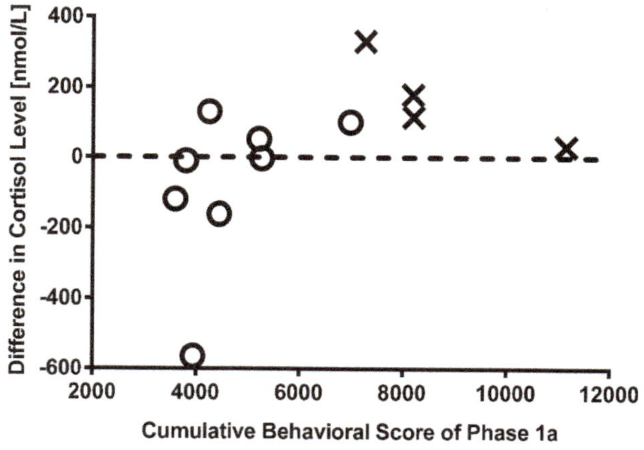

Figure 2. Differences in plasma cortisol concentration and cumulative behavioral scores during Phase 1a used to select animals for Phase 1b. Cumulative behavioral scores over the Phase 1a training obtained from all animals ($n = 12$), in which animals with lower behavioral scores ($n = 8$, 'O') were selected to transition into the Phase 1b study and ones with higher scores were deselected ($n = 4$, '×'). In addition, to assess the stress level during the awake training, plasma cortisol concentrations were measured from these animals at two separate time points (~ one month apart) during this phase, and results indicated that the reduction in cortical level is likely associated with better habituation (i.e. lower behavioral scores).

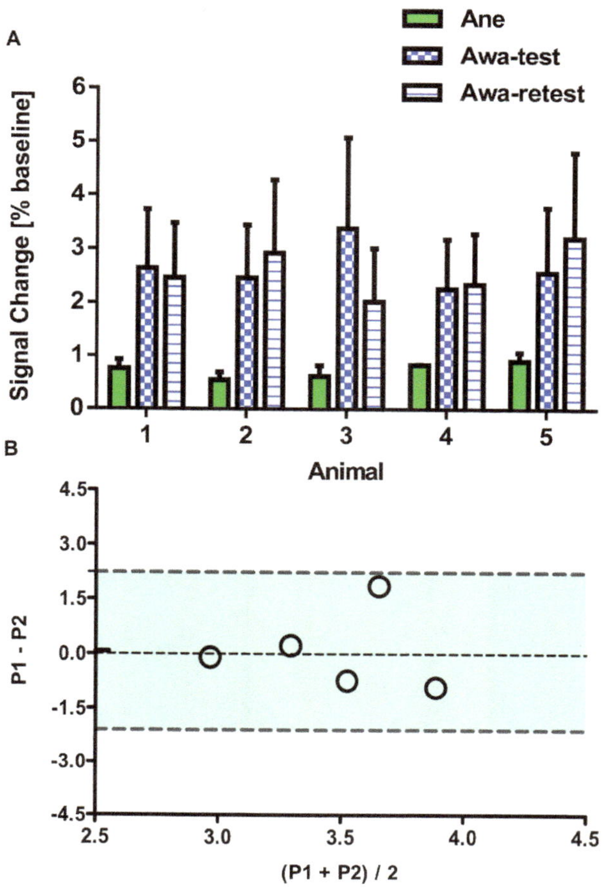

Figure 4. Comparison of resting state stability between anesthetized and awake imaging and test-retest reliability of awake baseline signal. (**A**) Resting state variation of BOLD signal (mean ± SD) obtained from each non-human primate (NHP) imaged under either awake (Awa, test and retest) or anesthetized (Ane) condition. (**B**) Bland-Altman plot for awake imaging data and the dash lines highlight the 95% limits of agreement (P1: represents the first test, P2 represents the retest).

extracted, detrended and plotted. Regional time-course data was calculated by averaging the rCBV change over all the supra-threshold voxels within specific brain regions. Results obtained from the vehicle infusion were exploited to detrend buprenorphine data on a region-by-region basis. Also, ROI analyses of drug-induced ΔrCBV time-course data were performed, in which AUC were obtained from brain regions with high density of μ-opioid receptor such as putamen, caudate, thalamus, cingulate cortex and frontal cortex, where regional AUC values (mean ± SEM) were calculated from all animals treated with either buprenorphine or vehicle and imaged under both anesthetized and awake conditions. Finally, calculated AUC data were subjected to a paired *t*-test (JMP 7.0.1, SAS Institute, Cary NC), with differences considered statistically significant at $p < 0.05$.

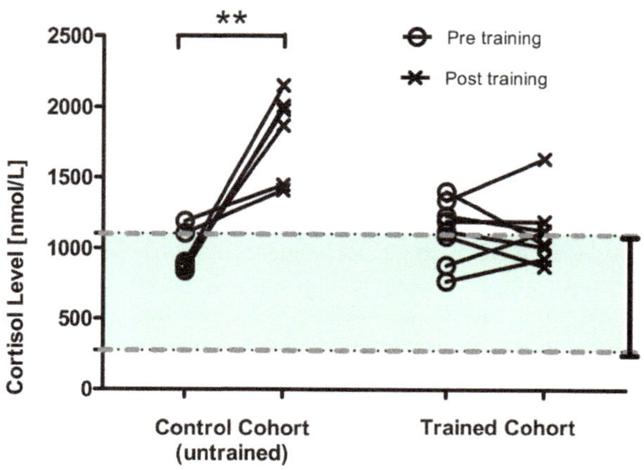

Figure 3. Awake training increased plasma cortisol concentrations in untrained animals, but not in trained animals. Plasma cortisol concentrations measured from the animals ($n = 8$) at prior- and post-90-minute training session during the Phase 1b period. Results indicate that, at the end of training session cortisol levels are significantly elevated in untrained/control animals ($n = 6$), while no significant change was observed in habituated animals (paired *t*-test, **$p < 0.01$). The dash lines highlight the range of normal cortisol concentration observed in cynomolgus monkeys (276 nmol/L to 1104 nmol/L) [52].

Results

Behavioral Scores and Cortisol Levels for Animal Selection

Cumulative behavioral scores obtained from all the animals ($n = 12$) over the entire Phase 1a period are plotted in Figure 2, in which animals with lower overall behavioral scores (better habituated) were selected to transition from Phase 1a to 1b ($n = 8$). These results demonstrate that levels of acclimation can vary within the training cohort, and thereby the selection of desired animals is essential. Within this phase, differences in the cortisol levels measured at two time points (separated by a month) are shown in Figure 2, indicating that elevated cortisol levels are likely observed from animals with higher behavioral scores. To assess the effect of training on stress levels, Figure 3 illustrates the cortisol concentrations obtained from untrained/control animals

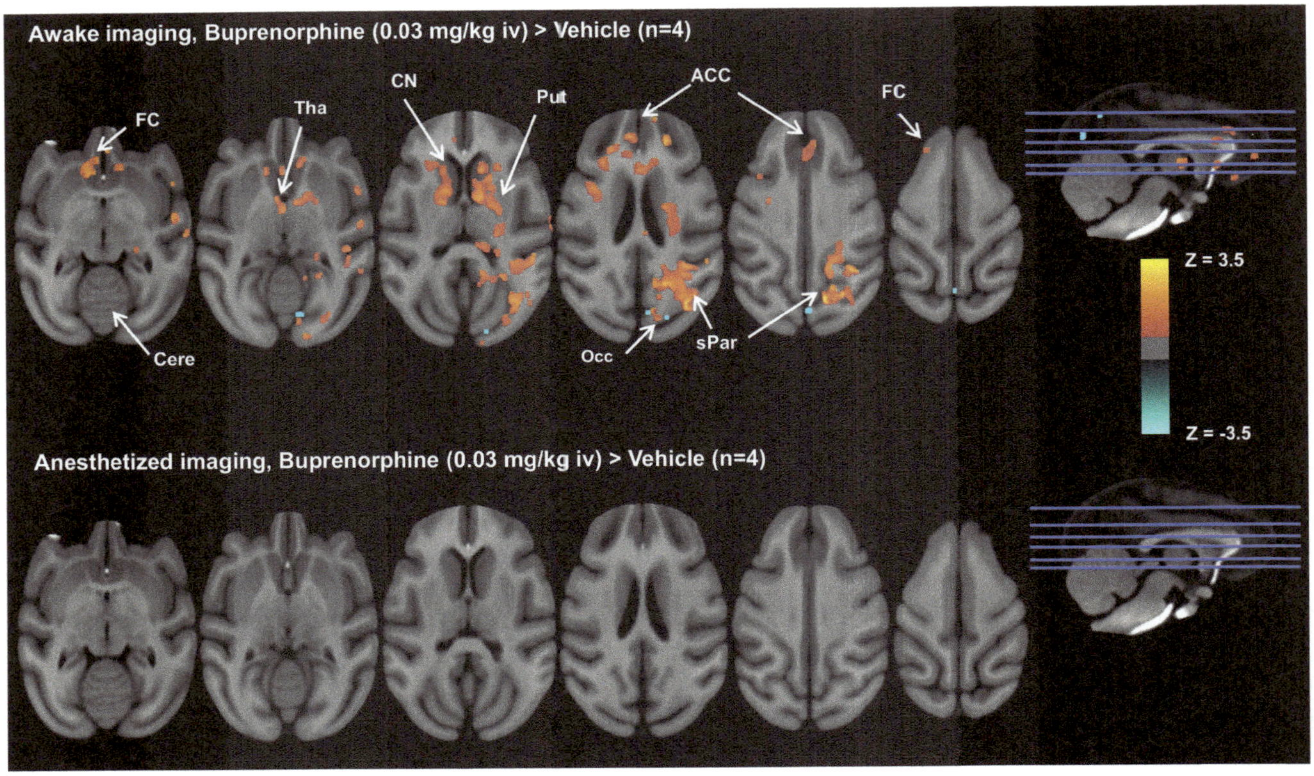

Figure 5. Group comparisons of brain activation patterns between buprenorphine and vehicle under awake and anesthetized imaging. Group comparisons of brain activation patterns showing significant effect of buprenorphine versus vehicle (paired *t*-test, $p<0.05$, $n=4$) under awake and anesthetized imaging. In the awake study, buprenorphine activates brain regions with a high density of μ-opioid receptor, including frontal cortex (FC), thalamus (Tha), anterior cingulate cortices (ACC), caudate nucleus (CN), putamen (Put), and superior parietal lobule (sPar), and limited deactivation was found in occipital cortex (Occ). In contrast, no significant difference in brain activation between buprenorphine and vehicle infusion was observed in anesthetized animals.

($n=6$) as well as our imaging cohort ($n=8$) at pre- and 90-minute-post training session (Phase 1b). As shown, cortisol levels were significantly elevated in untrained animals after they underwent the training session (paired *t*-test, $p<0.01$), while no significant difference was observed in habituated animals. Further, only one from the trained imaging cohort had cortisol concentrations substantially above the previously reported normal range (between 276 nmol/L and 1104 nmol/L) [52]. The lower cortisol level found in the trained cohort implies reduced stress levels in these animals and effective habituation to the restrainer and MRI scanner environment. Finally, two animals were deselected from the cohort due to medical conditions (unrelated to the training), while the remaining six animals were moved forward to Phase 1c.

Effectiveness or Limitation of Awake Training Protocol

Figure 4A shows the percentage variation in resting state baseline signals within the whole brain volume (mean ± SD) from individual animals imaged under awake and anesthetized conditions. Our data indicate that compared to anesthetized imaging, the level of baseline variation was significantly higher (4~5 fold) under the awake condition (paired *t*-test, $p<0.01$). This observation is not unexpected, since there was some animal movement during awake imaging. These findings suggest that a larger change in drug-induced phMRI signals may be needed in order to achieve comparable sensitivity offered by imaging anesthetized animals (i.e. to offset the increased baseline noise). Reasonable test-retest reliability was found from the awake baseline data, considering all the data points were within 95% limits of agreement of the Bland Altman plot (see Fig. 4b). Finally, two animals were deselected from the Phase 3 drug study, due to the increased body weight thus unable to fit into the animal restrainer or the need for repetitive head-post repairs.

Buprenorphine-induced phMRI response under awake and anaesthetized conditions

Figure 5 illustrates group comparisons of brain activation patterns showing significant effect of buprenorphine versus vehicle on rCBV changes (paired t-test, $p<0.05$, $n=4$), while Table 1 lists the results of ROI analyses, including activated brain regions/coordinates, z-statistics, and total percentage activated volumes calculated from the awake study. As shown, under the awake imaging condition, buprenorphine activated brain regions with a high density of μ-opioid receptor including, frontal cortex, thalamus, cingulate cortex, caudate nucleus, putamen, occipital cortex, and superior parietal lobule. Notably, these findings are strikingly consistent with μ-opioid receptor distribution depicted by [6-O-[^{11}C]methyl]buprenorphine ([^{11}C]BPN) positron emission tomography (PET) study in baboons, where the highest [^{11}C]BPN uptakes was observed in striatum (caudate nucleus and putamen) followed by thalamus, cingulate, frontal, parietal, occipital cortices, and then cerebellum [44]. In accordance with the results obtained from the previous study in conscious rodent and human studies [21], similar region-specificity of activated brain structures are also observed in our awake NHP data. Conversely, no significant activation was observed from anesthetized animals (paired *t*-test, vs. vehicle treatment; see Fig. 5B), despite animal

Table 1. Activated brain regions and their volumes induced by buprenorphine infusion derived from the region-of-interest analysis.

Brain Region	Coordinates (X, Y, Z) [mm]	Z-statistics	Activated Volume (percentage) [mm^3]
Cingulate cortex	29.7, 70.0, 25.2	2.52	182.52 (10.80%)
Gyrus rectus	29.5, 61.2, 21.0	2.61	44.39 (11.58%)
Orbital gyrus	26.0, 58.7, 19.5	2.39	2.83 (0.38%)
Caudate Nucleus	35.5, 57.2, 28.0	2.54	224.19 (28.51%)
Putamen	24.2, 57.2, 20.7	2.43	17.84 (2.02%)
Superior frontal gyrus	17.5, 54.5, 35.5	2.51	77.17 (1.46%)
Middle frontal gyrus	17.2, 54.7, 35.0	2.54	11.14 (0.86%)
Precentral gyrus	51.5, 50.5, 23.5	2.51	43.16 (0.79%)
Postcentral gyrus	53.0, 42.0, 25.7	2.66	34.48 (1.79%)
Globus pallidus	37.0, 50.2, 25.0	2.46	27.55 (13.42%)
Internal capsule	36.2, 49.7, 24.7	2.49	23.22 (10.56%)
Amygdala	40.5, 48.2, 12.7	2.50	13.94 (2.37%)
Thalamus	34.5, 48.2, 27.0	2.61	34.48 (3.18%)
Hippocampus	43.2, 43.0, 12.7	2.61	24.06 (4.84%)
Insular cortex	46.7, 42.7, 21.2	2.51	1.09 (0.28%)
Inferior temporal gyrus	48.0, 40.7, 9.5	2.33	0.25 (0.03%)
Superior temporal gyrus	50.2, 31.7, 29.5	2.53	213.33 (6.32%)
Middle temporal gyrus	50.5, 31.0, 29.7	2.61	43.61 (2.89%)
Midbrain	36.2, 39.7, 18.2	2.37	3.28 (0.34%)
Pulvinar nuclei	36.5, 36.2, 27.0	2.43	6.19 (6.14%)
Inferior parietal lobe	38.0, 24.5, 36.7	2.63	120.39 (4.32%)
Superior parietal lobe	36.2, 21.2, 34.5	2.61	72.75 (2.56%)
Superior occipital	37.7, 22.5, 35.0	2.61	87.05 (2.58%)
Lateral occipital	34.2, 12.0, 27.5	2.56	68.58 (3.16%)
Cerebellum	35.5, 19.0, 22.7	2.43	5.77 (0.08%)

Brain regions show differential responses of buprenorphine infusion (0.03 mg/kg i.v.) in awake imaging (vs vehicle, paired *t*-test, $z>2.3$, $n=4$). The *z*-statistic represents the maximum of each brain region with significant difference in rCBV changes between buprenorphine and vehicle treatments, while the coordinates correspond to the location of individual maxima in the standard monkey brain atlas space [47].

physiological parameters (mean ± SEM, $n=4$) being maintained within normal ranges during these experiments (mean heart rate = (119.9±5.1) beats/min, mean SpO_2 =98.8%±0.6%, mean $EtCO_2$ =22.0%±0.4%, and body temperature =36.5 °C±0.1 °C). These results exemplify the undesired anesthetic-drug interactions embedded in the anesthetized animal experiments, while highlighting the need for awake imaging for phMRI studies.

Plots of time-course rCBV changes derived from our ROI analyses are shown in Figure 6, in which activated brain regions identified in the group-level brain activation maps (see Fig. 5) showed significant increases in rCBV following buprenorphine infusion. Buprenorphine produced significant increases in rCBV change (mean ± SD) at frontal cortex (7.3%±0.2%), thalamus (6.5%±0.2%), caudate nucleus (6.2%±0.2%), putamen (5.8%±0.2%), and cingulate cortex (5.1%±0.2%). Of note, it appears that rCBV reached the maximum value around 10-minute-post onset of drug infusion and then maintained at steady state that prolonged over the rest of the imaging period. Area-under-curve of the rCBV time-course data over the entire drug infusion period (AUC), or the above-mentioned steady state period (AUC_{ss}), were calculated and shown in Figure 7. Results depicted that both AUC and AUC_{ss} calculated from thalamus, caudate nucleus, and putamen are significantly higher in buprenorphine-treated awake animals (paired *t*-test, $p<0.05$, vs vehicle), whilst no significant increases in AUC and AUC_{ss} were found in any brain region from the anesthetized study.

Discussion

Previous PET studies in baboons with the opioid receptor radioligand, [^{11}C]BPN revealed high binding activity in striatum, thalamus, cingulate gyrus, frontal cortex, parietal cortex, occipital cortex and cerebellum (in a descending order) [44] and these findings agree well with the known opioid receptor distribution in post-mortem human brain [53]. In this work, we found that buprenorphine infusion in awake, but not anesthetized, NHP produced significant and persistent increase in rCBV at specific brain regions including frontal and cingulate cortices, caudate nucleus, putamen, thalamus, parietal cortex and occipital cortices (see Fig. 5). These activated brain regions are consistent with the binding sites of μ–opioid receptors highlighted in the PET study [44], reflecting the underlying drug actions and subsequent biological responses. Recently, Becerra et al. demonstrated that brain regions activated by buprenorphine in awake rats paralleled that observed in humans, in which buprenorphine elicited BOLD signals in somatosensory and cingulate cortices, insula, striatum,

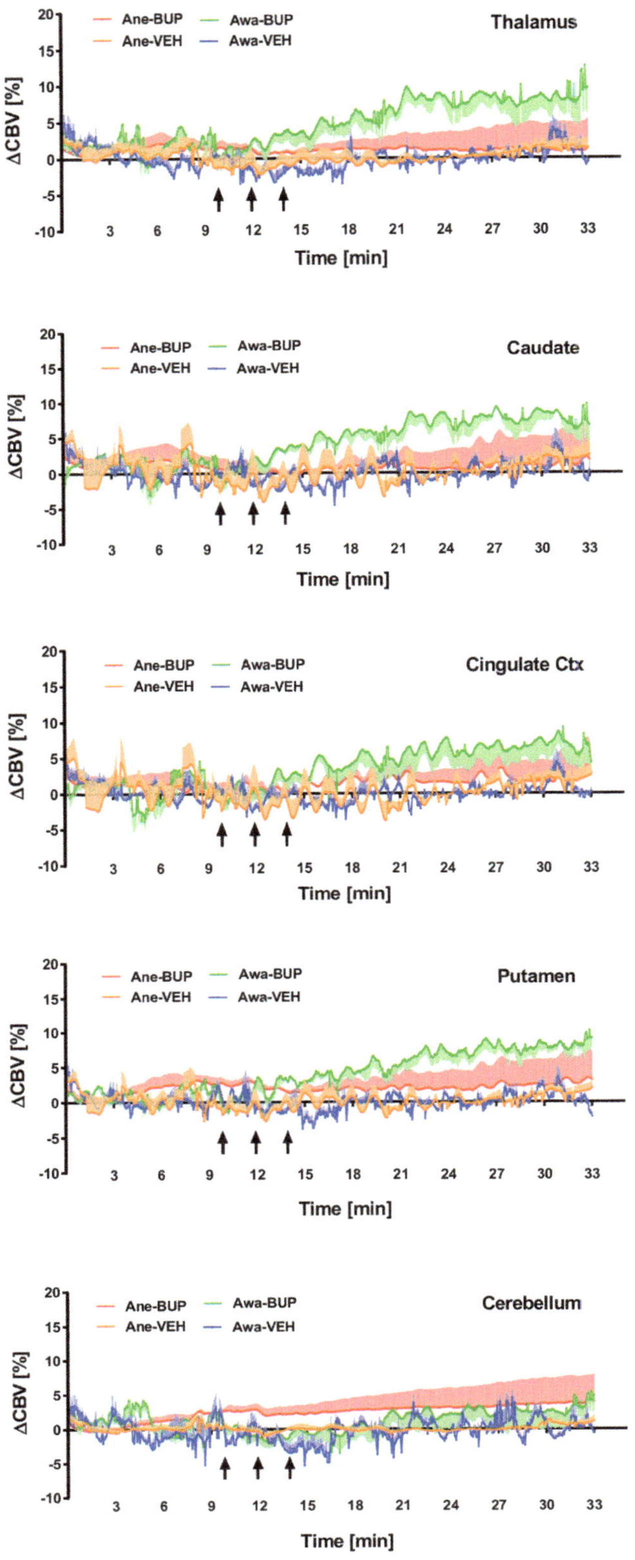

Figure 6. Regional time-course rCBV changes derived from the region-of-interest analysis. Plots of regional time-course rCBV change (mean ± SEM) derived from region-of-interest (ROI) analyses of the imaging cohort ($n = 4$) treated with either buprenorphine (BUP at 0.03 mg/kg i.v.) or vehicle (VEH) and imaged under awake (Awa) or anesthetized (Ane) conditions. The black arrows indicate the three individual dosing time periods (30 s drug infusion separated by 1.5-minute intervals), starting at 10-minute after the contrast agent administration. Results indicated that in awake NHP, buprenorphine infusion produces significant increases in rCBV at brain regions with high density of μ-opioid receptors, but not the area with low concentration of μ-opioid receptors (i.e. cerebellum).

thalamus, periaqueductal gray (PAG), and cerebellum in a dose-dependent manner [21]. Further, in contrast to human data, negative BOLD signals were observed in several brain regions in awake rats and this discrepancy was reconciled with the difference in opioid receptor subtypes and binding affinities between these two species [21]. To examine the congruency of phMRI data across rodent, NHP and humans, it appears that the brain activation patterns obtained from our awake NHP study show greater similarity to human data. For example, very limited deactivation, or decreased rCBV, was found in occipital cortex (see Fig. 5). Also, with the exception of activation in the cerebellum, brain regions activated by buprenorphine in awake NHP are depicted in human data. We attributed inconsistency in cerebellar activation to the difference in drug pharmacokinetic or exposure levels, considering that in the baboon PET study [^{11}C]BPN uptake at cerebellum peaked within 2-minute post tracer injection and eliminated rapidly [44]. Further, unlike previous rodent and human BOLD fMRI studies [21,43], we used a CBV-based approach in the current work. For the CBV-based approach, changes in MRI signal reflect changes in CBV, rather than the concentration of deoxyhemoglobin as in BOLD imaging [54]. While it could depend on the resting state blood volume at specific brain regions, BOLD and CBV contrasts are known to be spatially [54] and temporally [55] coupled. Overall, our data highlight the importance and utility of awake imaging in NHP.

In anesthetized animals, brain activation patterns induced by buprenorphine challenge differ from the previous PET μ–opioid receptor data. In comparison with the vehicle treatment, buprenorphine challenge did not elicit any significant changes in brain activity (see Fig. 5), possibly due to the effect of anesthesia. Also, ROI analyses indicate that the rank order of regional rCBV changes induced by buprenorphine infusion was different between anesthetized and awake imaging (see Fig, 7). For example, in awake NHP the highest rCBV change was found in frontal cortex and followed by thalamus, caudate, putamen, cingulate cortex, and cerebellum, while the rank order (descending) became frontal cortex, cerebellum, putamen, cingulate cortex, thalamus, and caudate under anesthetized imaging. Anesthetic-drug interactions on brain activity has been investigated by several groups [14,16,18,19], and it was concluded that drug-induced brain activation pattern can vary among the anesthetics used. The extent of anesthesia confounds likely pivots on the particular mechanism of action associated with selected anesthetics and test drugs, which might or might not be an issue, depending on the neurotransmitter system investigated. Considering the observed drug-induced activation can result from drug-receptor down-stream biological effects, the use of anesthesia can modulate both direct and indirect neuronal pathways. As such, it is more desirable to perform imaging in preclinical species without anesthesia that enables qualification of imaging biomarkers which represent a closer scenario to that of clinical investigation.

One of the key challenges for awake imaging is to ensure animals remain still during the data acquisition. Significant efforts have been made to establish comprehensive habituation procedures and specialized animal restrainers in order to minimize head and body motion during data acquisition [16,17,24,27,35,37,56,57]. For example, Keliris et al. have developed a sophisticated MRI-compatible training chair and head-post restrainer to image alert monkeys in a natural upright sitting position, and they

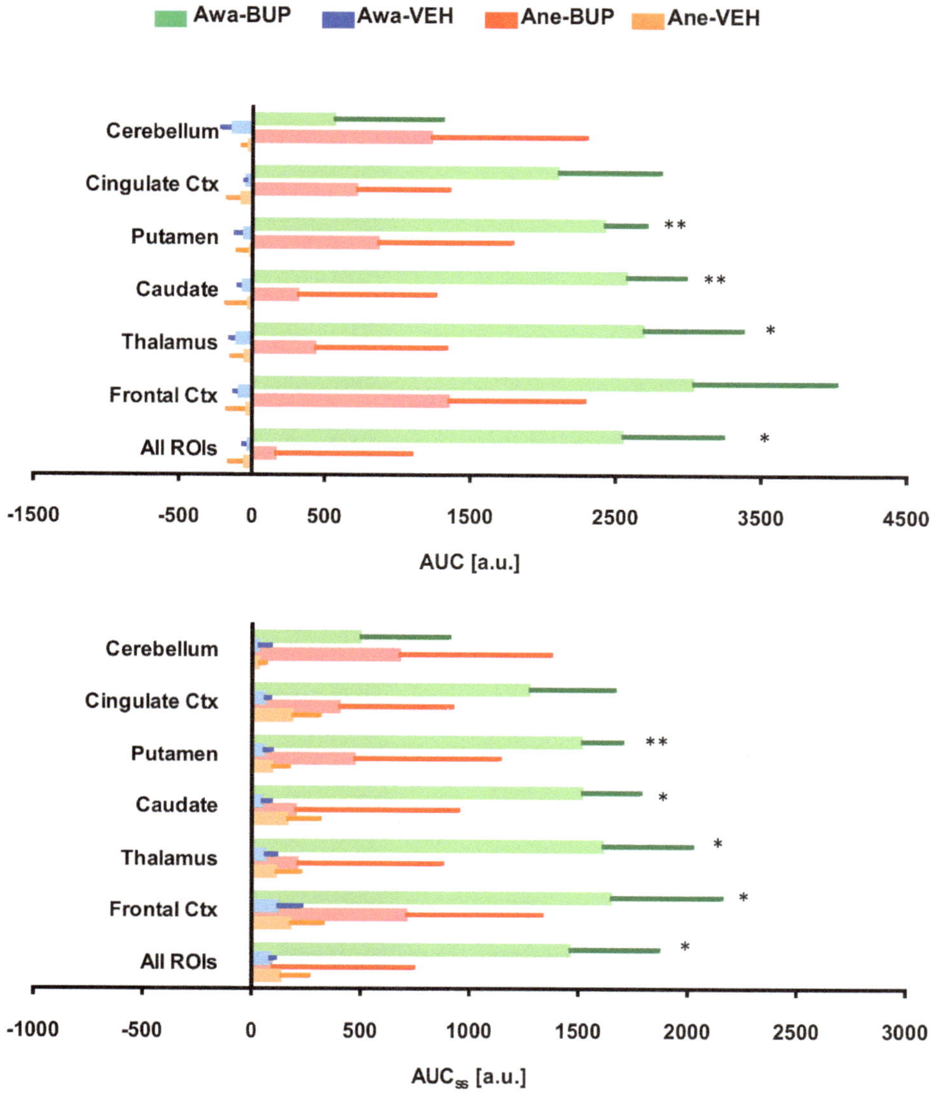

Figure 7. Area-under-curve of regional time-course rCBV change during post-drug infusion derived from the region-of-interest analysis. Results obtained from region-of-interest (ROI) analyses of rCBV time-course data showing the area-under-curve (mean ± SEM) of the entire post-drug infusion period (AUC) or only the steady-state time period (AUC_{ss}). Animals ($n = 4$) were imaged under awake (Awa) or anesthetized (Ane) conditions and treated with either buprenorphine (BUP at 0.03 mg/kg i.v.) or vehicle (VEH). Our data indicated that in awake animals AUC and AUC_{ss} calculated from thalamus, caudate nucleus, and putamen are significantly higher in buprenorphine-treated animals (paired *t*-test, *$p<0.05$, **$p<0.01$ vs vehicle).

found jaw and body movements are the major causes for the fluctuation of fMRI signals [56]. Alternatively, Chen et al. have proposed another approach of integrating an MRI-compatible chair, head-post holder, and volume coil for awake imaging, where in-plane movements can be limited within 80 µm [37]. We have adopted the awake imaging apparatus developed by Andersen et al. [35] and used a custom-made NHP phased-array head coil that can be attached to the head-post for better signal-to-noise ratio (SNR). Without a dedicated NHP MRI scanner [37,56], we have successfully imaged animals in a sphinx position instead. Improved data acquisition and analysis methods have been also developed to enhance the sensitivity to detect targeted drug responses; for example, USPIO imaging contrast agents have been previously exploited to amplify signal changes [36,38] as well as advanced data analysis pipeline for motion correction [39].

To minimize the amount of stress during awake imaging, our study cohort has been trained over several months to acclimatize to the restrainer and scanner environment (see Fig. 1). Some animals showed signs of gradual adaptation to the training, as indicated by the decreased plasma cortisol concentration and behavioral scores (see Fig. 2). This finding is consistent with the results reported by Lee et al. [58], where a weekly decline in cortisol levels was observed in animals receiving chair training for a month. Cortisol levels were also measured in our study, as animals progressed to Phase 1b. We found no significant difference in cortisol concentrations measured at pre- and post- 90-minute training from the trained cohort, whilst in the untrained animals cortisol concentrations elevated significantly (see Fig 3), suggesting that trained animals have been acclimated to the restrainer.

It is noteworthy that in most awake imaging models, a head-post is surgically implanted for the purpose of head fixation. This invasive procedure is however not ideal since the head-post placement requires surgery and can become loose or even detach over time. While this method might be sub-optimal for a longitudinal study, alternative non-invasive approaches have been recently implemented [27,36]. For example, Shrihasam and his colleagues have developed a non-invasive vacuum helmet technique for imaging alert monkeys, and they found that the degrees of translational and rotational head motion during awake imaging are comparable to the same monkey's movements when restrained by a head-post [36]. Likewise, using the expandable foam in combination with a plastic helmet, Murnane et al. have shown the feasibility of imaging conscious monkeys under cocaine challenge without a head-post [27]. There are also disadvantages for this awake imaging approach. For example, awake training is time-consuming and often requires significant effort and resources to habituate the animal. For the current study, it took more than 10 months to complete the awake training protocol and only a sub-group of animals was suitable for the actual imaging study. Although the stress level can be alleviated by extensive training procedures, this factor cannot be completely eliminated.

To develop novel treatments for neurological diseases or psychiatric disorders, PET or single photon emission computed tomography (SPECT) imaging techniques have proved to be useful tools to confirm blood-brain barrier penetration and drug target engagement in the brain, and derived receptor occupancy–drug concentration curves can guide dose selection in clinical development [59,60]. Conversely, biological consequences of drug actions depicted by awake phMRI can offer complimentary pharmacodynamic biomarkers to PET/SPECT imaging. In light of the low success rate associated with the development of novel compounds to treat neurological diseases or psychiatric disorders, phMRI in alert, behaving NHP can serve as a translational imaging platform that affords pharmacodynamic or safety biomarkers, attributed to targeted mechanisms of action. While animal movement and stress during awake imaging increases the noise associated with this approach, the absence of unwanted anesthetic-drug interactions can outweigh efforts needed to overcome these technical hurdles. For the development of CNS compounds, this requirement can be particularly crucial to assess novel experimental therapeutics.

There are limitations for this current study. First, only four animals progressed to the actual imaging experiments and therefore inter-subject variability cannot be properly evaluated. Second, to fully evaluate the utility of this awake phMRI platform, test-retest study of buprenorphine infusion needs to be explored. Third, in the anesthetized imaging study, buprenorphine did not elicit significant changes in rCBV at brain areas with a high density of μ-opioid receptor (see Figure 5). This observation can be attributed to the level of anesthesia used. Previously, Tinker et al. have reported that the percentage volume of minimum alveolar concentration (MAC) of isoflurane in nonhuman primate is 1.28% and the maintaining dose for most applications is around 1.3× MAC (i.e. ~1.7%) [61], whereas 2% isoflurane in medical air was selected to anesthetize animals in our study. In combination with paralytics (e.g. vercuronium or mivacurium) or fentanyl, the feasibility of using a lower level of isoflurane (0.3%~1%) in fMRI studies has been demonstrated [62,63]. However, anesthesia protocols could vary among different studies, depending on the experimental design.

In summary, we have shown that, in awake NHP buprenorphine activated brain regions ascribed to high density of μ-opioid receptors, including caudate nucleus, putamen, thalamus, and cingulate cortex. More importantly, in conjunction with previous buprenorphine phMRI studies in conscious rats and humans, our results establish utility of buprenorphine phMRI across species. Further, based on a standard monkey brain atlas, we have established robust phMRI data and ROI analysis pipeline that allows determination of group-level brain activation patterns. Our results indicated that in the same animal, buprenorphine-induced rCBV changes in awake animals are significantly higher than those obtained under the anesthetized condition. Taken together, our data highlight the utility and importance of awake NHP imaging platform as a translational imaging biomarker for drug research.

Acknowledgments

The authors wish to extend our gratitude to Marie A. Holahan and Fuqiang Zhao for insightful discussion. We would also like to thank Htoon Win, Myoe Lynn and Hamzah Isa for their technical support for this work.

Author Contributions

Conceived and designed the experiments: SS DSW TR BH JLE CLC. Performed the experiments: SS ABMAA EM JDB CLC. Analyzed the data: SS ABMAA RB DF CLC. Wrote the paper: SS ABMAA CLC TR EM.

References

1. Wise RG, Tracey I (2006) The role of fMRI in drug discovery. J Magn Reson Imaging 23: 862–876.
2. Borsook D, Becerra L, Hargreaves R (2006) A role for fMRI in optimizing CNS drug development. Nat Rev Drug Discov 5: 411–424.
3. Leslie RA, James MF (2000) Pharmacological magnetic resonance imaging: a new application for functional MRI. Trends Pharmacol Sci 21: 314–318.
4. Jenkins BG (2012) Pharmacologic magnetic resonance imaging (phMRI): imaging drug action in the brain. Neuroimage 62: 1072–1085.
5. Gozzi A, Schwarz A, Reese T, Bertani S, Crestan V, et al. (2006) Region-specific effects of nicotine on brain activity: a pharmacological MRI study in the drug-naive rat. Neuropsychopharmacology 31: 1690–1703.
6. Mueggler T, Baumann D, Rausch M, Rudin M (2001) Bicuculline-induced brain activation in mice detected by functional magnetic resonance imaging. Magn Reson Med 46: 292–298.
7. Chin CL, Tovcimak AE, Hradil VP, Seifert TR, Hollingsworth PR, et al. (2008) Differential effects of cannabinoid receptor agonists on regional brain activity using pharmacological MRI. Br J Pharmacol 153: 367–379.
8. Chen YC, Galpern WR, Brownell AL, Matthews RT, Bogdanov M, et al. (1997) Detection of dopaminergic neurotransmitter activity using pharmacologic MRI: correlation with PET, microdialysis, and behavioral data. Magn Reson Med 38: 389–398.
9. Schwarz AJ, Becerra L, Upadhyay J, Anderson J, Baumgartner R, et al (2011) A procedural framework for good imaging practice in pharmacological fMRI studies applied to drug development #2: protocol optimization and best practices. Drug Discov Today 16: 671–682.
10. De Simoni S, Schwarz AJ, O'Daly OG, Marquand AF, Brittain C, et al. (2013) Test-retest reliability of the BOLD pharmacological MRI response to ketamine in healthy volunteers. Neuroimage 64: 75–90.
11. Wise RG, Williams P, Tracey I (2004) Using fMRI to quantify the time dependence of remifentanil analgesia in the human brain. Neuropsychopharmacology 29: 626–635.
12. Leppa M, Korvenoja A, Carlson S, Timonen P, Martinkauppi S, et al. (2006) Acute opioid effects on human brain as revealed by functional magnetic resonance imaging. NeuroImage 31: 661–669.
13. Austin VC, Blamire AM, Allers KA, Sharp T, Styles P, et al. (2005) Confounding effects of anesthesia on functional activation in rodent brain: a study of halothane and alpha-chloralose anesthesia. Neuroimage 24: 92–100.
14. Gozzi A, Schwarz A, Crestan V, Bifone A (2008) Drug-anaesthetic interaction in phMRI: the case of the psychotomimetic agent phencyclidine. Magn Reson Imaging 26: 999–1006.
15. Hodkinson DJ, de Groote C, McKie S, Deakin JF, Williams SR (2012) Differential Effects of Anaesthesia on the phMRI Response to Acute Ketamine Challenge. Br J Med Med Res 2: 373–385.
16. Ferris CF, Smerkers B, Kulkarni P, Caffrey M, Afacan O, et al. (2011) Functional magnetic resonance imaging in awake animals. Rev Neurosci 22: 665–674.

17. Liu JV, Hirano Y, Nascimento GC, Stefanovic B, Leopold DA, et al. (2013) fMRI in the awake marmoset: Somatosensory-evoked responses, functional connectivity, and comparison with propofol anesthesia. Neuroimage 78: 186–195.
18. Zhang Z, Andersen AH, Avison MJ, Gerhardt GA, Gash DM (2000) Functional MRI of apomorphine activation of the basal ganglia in awake rhesus monkeys. Brain Res 852: 290–296.
19. Chin CL, Pauly JR, Surber BW, Skoubis PD, McGaraughty S, et al. (2008) Pharmacological MRI in awake rats predicts selective binding of alpha4beta2 nicotinic receptors. Synapse 62: 159–168.
20. Lahti KM, Ferris CF, Li F, Sotak CH, King JA (1999) Comparison of evoked cortical activity in conscious and propofol-anesthetized rats using functional MRI. Magn Reson Med 41: 412–416.
21. Becerra L, Upadhyay J, Chang PC, Bishop J, Anderson J, et al. (2013) Parallel Buprenorphine phMRI Responses in Conscious Rodents and Healthy Human Subjects. J Pharmacol Exp Ther 345: 41–51.
22. Febo M, Segarra AC, Nair G, Schmidt K, Duong TQ, et al. (2005) The neural consequences of repeated cocaine exposure revealed by functional MRI in awake rats. Neuropsychopharmacology 30: 936–943.
23. Baker S, Chin CL, Basso AM, Fox GB, Marek GJ, et al. (2012) Xanomeline modulation of the blood oxygenation level-dependent signal in awake rats: development of pharmacological magnetic resonance imaging as a translatable pharmacodynamic biomarker for central activity and dose selection. J Pharmacol Exp Ther 341: 263–273.
24. Vanduffel W, Fize D, Mandeville JB, Nelissen K, Van Hecke P, et al. (2001) Visual motion processing investigated using contrast agent-enhanced fMRI in awake behaving monkeys. Neuron 32: 565–577.
25. Stefanacci L, Reber P, Costanza J, Wong E, Buxton R, et al. (1998) fMRI of monkey visual cortex. Neuron 20: 1051–1057.
26. Dubowitz DJ, Chen DY, Atkinson DJ, Grieve KL, Gillikin B, et al. (1998) Functional magnetic resonance imaging in macaque cortex. Neuroreport 9: 2213–2218.
27. Murnane KS, Howell LL (2010) Development of an apparatus and methodology for conducting functional magnetic resonance imaging (fMRI) with pharmacological stimuli in conscious rhesus monkeys. J Neurosci Methods 191: 11–20.
28. Mandeville JB, Choi JK, Jarraya B, Rosen BR, Jenkins BG, et al. (2011) FMRI of cocaine self-administration in macaques reveals functional inhibition of basal ganglia. Neuropsychopharmacology 36: 1187–1198.
29. McClure HM (1984) Nonhuman primate models for human disease. Adv Vet Sci Comp Med 28: 267–304.
30. Petrides M, Pandya DN (2002) Comparative cytoarchitectonic analysis of the human and the macaque ventrolateral prefrontal cortex and corticocortical connection patterns in the monkey. Eur J Neurosci 16: 291–310.
31. Nakahara K, Adachi Y, Osada T, Miyashita Y (2007) Exploring the neural basis of cognition: multi-modal links between human fMRI and macaque neurophysiology. Trends Cogn Sci 11: 84–92.
32. Mansour A, Khachaturian H, Lewis ME, Akil H, Watson SJ (1988) Anatomy of CNS opioid receptors. Trends Neurosci 11: 308–314.
33. Smith HR, Beveridge TJ, Porrino LJ (2006) Distribution of norepinephrine transporters in the non-human primate brain. Neuroscience 138: 703–714.
34. Reuning RH, Ashcraft SB, Wiley JN, Morrison BE (1989) Disposition and pharmacokinetics of naltrexone after intravenous and oral administration in rhesus monkeys. Drug Metab Dispos 17: 583–589.
35. Andersen AH, Zhang Z, Barber T, Rayens WS, Zhang J, et al. (2002) Functional MRI studies in awake rhesus monkeys: methodological and analytical strategies. J Neurosci Methods 118: 141–152.
36. Srihasam K, Sullivan K, Savage T, Livingstone MS (2010) Noninvasive functional MRI in alert monkeys. Neuroimage 51: 267–273.
37. Chen G, Wang F, Dillenburger BC, Friedman RM, Chen LM, et al. (2012) Functional magnetic resonance imaging of awake monkeys: some approaches for improving imaging quality. Magn Reson Imaging 30: 36–47.
38. Leite FP, Tsao D, Vanduffel W, Fize D, Sasaki Y, et al. (2002) Repeated fMRI using iron oxide contrast agent in awake, behaving macaques at 3 Tesla. NeuroImage 16: 283–294.
39. Stoewer S, Goense JB, Keliris GA, Bartels A, Logothetis NK, et al. (2011) Realignment strategies for awake-monkey fMRI data. Magn Reson Imaging 29: 1390–1400.
40. Sadee W, Rosenbaum JS, Herz A (1982) Buprenorphine: differential interaction with opiate receptor subtypes in vivo. J Pharmacol Exp Ther 223: 157–162.
41. Heel RC, Brogden RN, Speight TM, Avery GS (1979) Buprenorphine: a review of its pharmacological properties and therapeutic efficacy. Drugs 17: 81–110.
42. Lewis JW (1985) Buprenorphine. Drug Alcohol Depend 14: 363–372.
43. Upadhyay J, Anderson J, Schwarz AJ, Coimbra A, Baumgartner R, et al. (2011) Imaging Drugs with and without Clinical Analgesic Efficacy. Neuropsychopharmacology 36: 2659–2673.
44. Galynker I, Schlyer DJ, Dewey SL, Fowler JS, Logan J, et al. (1996) Opioid Receptor Imaging and Displacement Studies with [6-O-[11C]methyl] Buprenorphine in Baboon Brain. Nuclear Medicine & Biology 23: 325–331.
45. Greenwald MK, Johanson CE, Moody DE, Woods JH, Kilbourn MR, et al. (2003) Effects of buprenorphine maintenance dose on mu-opioid receptor availability, plasma concentrations, and antagonist blockade in heroin-dependent volunteers. Neuropsychopharmacology 28: 2000–2009.
46. Mandeville JB, Marota JJ, Kosofsky BE, Keltner JR, Weissleder R, et al. (1998) Dynamic functional imaging of relative cerebral blood volume during rat forepaw stimulation. Magn Reson Med 39: 615–624.
47. Frey S, Pandya DN, Chakravarty MM, Bailey L, Petrides M, et al. (2011) An MRI based average macaque monkey stereotaxic atlas and space (MNI monkey space). Neuroimage 55: 1435–1442.
48. Nunamaker EA, Halliday LC, Moody DE, Fang WB, Lindeblad M, et al. (2013) Pharmacokinetics of 2 formulations of buprenorphine in macaques (Macaca mulatta and Macaca fascicularis). J Am Assoc Lab Anim Sci 52: 48–56.
49. Wu EX, Tang H, Jensen JH (2004) Applications of ultrasmall superparamagnetic iron oxide contrast agents in the MR study of animal models. NMR Biomed 17: 478–483.
50. Andaluz A, Moll X, Abellan R, Ventura R, Carbo M, et al. (2009) Pharmacokinetics of buprenorphine after intravenous administration of clinical doses to dogs. Vet J 181: 299–304.
51. Jenkinson M, Beckmann CF, Behrens TE, Woolrich MW, Smith SM (2011) Fsl. Neuroimage.
52. Thrall M, Weiser G, Allison R, Campbell T, editors (2012) Veterinary hematology and clinical chemistry 2ed: John Wiely & Sons, Inc.
53. Pfeiffer A, Pasi A, Mehraein P, Herz A (1982) Opiate receptor binding sites in human brain. Brain Res 248: 87–96.
54. Mandeville JB, Marota JJ (1999) Vascular filters of functional MRI: spatial localization using BOLD and CBV contrast. Magn Reson Med 42: 591–598.
55. Shen Q, Ren H, Duong TQ (2008) CBF, BOLD, CBV, and CMRO(2) fMRI signal temporal dynamics at 500-msec resolution. J Magn Reson Imaging 27: 599–606.
56. Keliris GA, Shmuel A, Ku SP, Pfeuffer J, Oeltermann A, et al. (2007) Robust controlled functional MRI in alert monkeys at high magnetic field: effects of jaw and body movements. Neuroimage 36: 550–570.
57. Pinsk MA, Moore T, Richter MC, Gross CG, Kastner S (2005) Methods for functional magnetic resonance imaging in normal and lesioned behaving monkeys. J Neurosci Methods 143: 179–195.
58. Lee JI, Shin JS, Lee JE, Jung WY, Lee G, et al. (2012) Changes of N/L ratio and cortisol levels associated with experimental training in untrained rhesus macaques. J Med Primatol 42: 10–14.
59. Wong DF, Tauscher J, Grunder G (2009) The role of imaging in proof of concept for CNS drug discovery and development. Neuropsychopharmacology 34: 187–203.
60. Hargreaves RJ (2008) The role of molecular imaging in drug discovery and development. Clin Pharmacol Ther 83: 349–353.
61. Fish R, Danneman PJ, Brown M, Karas A (2011) Anesthesia and Analgesia in Laboratory Animals. Elsevier Science: 350.
62. Logothetis NK, Pauls J, Augath M, Trinath T, Oeltermann A (2001) Neurophysiological investigation of the basis of the fMRI signal. Nature 412: 150–157.
63. Wey HY, Li J, Szabo CA, Fox PT, Leland MM, et al. (2010) BOLD fMRI of visual and somatosensory-motor stimulations in baboons. Neuroimage 52: 1420–1427.

15

Identifying Predictors of Early Growth Response and Adverse Radiation Effects of Vestibular Schwannomas to Radiosurgery

Soroush Larjani[1]*, Eric Monsalves[1], Houman Pebdani[1], Boris Krischek[1], Fred Gentili[1], Michael Cusimano[2], Normand Laperriere[3], Caroline Hayhurst[4], Gelareh Zadeh[1]*

1 Department of Neurosurgery, University Health Network, Toronto, Canada, **2** Department of Neurosurgery, St. Michael's Hospital, Toronto, Canada, **3** Radiation Oncology Program, Princess Margaret Hospital, Toronto, Canada, **4** Department of Neurosurgery, The Walton Centre, Liverpool, United Kingdom

Abstract

Purpose: To determine whether pre-treatment growth rate of vestibular schwannomas (VS) predict response to radiosurgery.

Methods: A retrospective review of a prospectively maintained database of all VS patients treated with 12Gy prescription dose between September 2005 and June 2011 at our institution using the Leksell Model 4C Gamma Knife Unit was conducted. Patients who had a minimum of 12-months clinical and radiological assessment before and after radiosurgery were included in this study. Tumor growth rates were calculated using specific growth rate (SGR). Tumor volumes were measured on FIESTA-MRI scans using ITK-SNAP v2.2.

Results: Following radiosurgery, twenty-seven (42.9%) patients showed a significant decrease in volume after one year, twenty-nine (46.0%) stabilized, and seven (11.1%) continued to grow. There was no correlation between VS pre-treatment SGRs with post-treatment SGRs ($p = 0.34$), and incidence of adverse radiation effects (ARE). The reduction in tumors' SGRs after radiosurgery was proportional to pre-treatment SGRs, although this correlation was not statistically significant ($p = 0.19$). Analysis of risk factors revealed a positive correlation between post-treatment SGRs and incidence of non-auditory complications, most of which were attributed to ARE ($p = 0.047$).

Conclusion: Pre-treatment growth rate of VS does not predict tumor response to radiosurgery or incidence of ARE. VS with higher SGRs post-radiosurgery are more likely to experience ARE.

Editor: Kevin Robert Kozak, University of Wisconsin School of Medicine and Public Health, United States of America

Funding: The authors have no funding or support to report.

Competing Interests: The authors have declared that no competing interests exist.

* Email: Soroush.Larjani@gmail.com (SL); Gelareh.Zadeh@uhn.ca (GZ)

Introduction

Vestibular Schwanommas (VS) account for approximately 10% of all intracranial tumors [1,2]. Stereotactic radiosurgery (SRS) is an accepted treatment option for VS that are less than approximately 3 centimeters in diameter. SRS effectively controls VS growth in more than 93% of cases [1,2]. It also eliminates the high risk of irreversible cranial and facial nerve injury, and treatment-related morbidity that is associated with microsurgery. Nevertheless, SRS has associated ARE, such as radiation-induced cranial nerve and brain stem injury [3,4]. In order to decrease the rate of adverse radiation effects (ARE), SRS prescription doses have steadily declined while attempting to maintain tumor control [1,2]. Currently, the optimal recommended prescription dose is between 12–13Gy, where stable disease is achieved at a high rate, and the incidence of ARE is reduced to a minimum [1,3–5].

One factor that has received little attention is whether the pre-treatment growth rate of VS can predict tumor response to radiosurgery, as well as the incidence of SRS complications or ARE. In other central nervous system tumor types, such as glioblastoma, pre-treatment tumor growth rate has been demonstrated to be a predictor of response to radiation therapy [6]. Majority of this research has focused on gliomas where biomathematical models have been developed that utilize a tumor's pre-treatment growth rate to predict response to radiation therapy [6]. In this study we focused on determining whether pre-treatment growth rate of VS can predict the early or short term response to SRS and/or serve as a predictor of ARE.

Methods and Materials

This retrospective study was approved by the Research Ethics Board at University Health Network. This was a retrospective study where patients were fully de-identified/anonymized.

Patients

We retrospectively reviewed a prospectively maintained database of all VS cases treated at our institution with SRS between December 2005 and June 2011. A total of 258 patients with VS were treated at our institution with Leksell Model 4C Gamma Knife (Elekta Instrument, Atlanta, GA). At our institution, radiosurgery is indicated when there is documented evidence of tumor growth within 12 months of the first magnetic resonance imaging (MRI) scan, or when there is a strong patient preference for intervention. All patients were treated with a prescription dose of 12Gy. Treatments were planned using stereotactic CT and stereotactic contrast-enhanced 1.5-mm section T1 and T2 MRI sequences. All patients had standard clinical and radiological assessment 12 months prior to radiosurgery, and 3 months, 6 months, and 12 months after radiosurgery, and then yearly thereafter.

Patients who did not have a minimum of two pre-treatment and/or two post-treatment MRIs that were at least 12 months apart were excluded; this criteria was required in order for us to calculate the radiological growth rates of tumors before and after radiosurgery. In addition, patients who did not have appropriate and/or complete clinical assessment pre- and post-radiosurgery were excluded. We also excluded patients with tumors that underwent pseudoprogression following treatment. Pseudoprogression is the transient increase in tumor volume followed by stability or regression that commonly occurs after radiosurgery [3]. In specific, we defined pseudoprogression as an increase of more than 20% in the first year after radiosurgery, with tumor stabilization or regression within 24 months.

Volumetric Measurements

In this study we evaluated tumor size and growth rate using volumetric measurements. ITK-SNAP v2.2 (University of Pennsylvania, Philadelphia, PA), which is a validated and reliable software for medical image segmentation, was used to examine axial MRI scans, and perform volumetric measurements [7]. The semi-automatic segmentation function was used with 1.5-mm section FIESTA MRI images for volumetric measurements. Manual contouring was used for post-semi-automatic segmentation processing, and for MRI images where differentiation of tumor mass from surrounding tissues was difficult. Two independent trained research assistants were used to delineate the tumor edge, and define image voxels as tumor and non-tumorous, after which measurements of tumor volume were calculated. Subsequently the measurements were verified by a neuroradiologist blinded to the previous measurements who used the same software setup for volumetry. All image reviewers were blinded to the time point of imaging with respect to treatment.

Tumor Growth Rate Measurement

In order to study the relationship between pre-treatment and post-treatment tumor growth rates, patients who had clinical and radiological assessment at least 12 months before and after SRS were selected. Typically, patients had only one radiological assessment prior to radiosurgery, and that was performed 12 months prior to the operation in accordance with the 'wait and scan' policy. Tumor volumes were measured using axial FIESTA MRI scans obtained on appropriate dates, and were recorded in cubic centimeters. Tumor growth rates before and after SRS were calculated using the specific growth rate (SGR) formula: $SGR = \ln(V_2/V_1)/(t_2-t_1)x100\%$, where V_2 and V_1 equaled treatment volume and tumor volume 12 months before treatment, respectively, with t_2 and t_1 equaling corresponding time points. When calculating post-treatment SGRs, V_2 and V_1 equaled tumor volume 12 months post-treatment and treatment volume, respectively, with corresponding time points t_2 and t_1. SGRs were expressed as percent change per annum [8]. Significant growth after radiosurgery was defined as any volumetric growth greater than 20% over a 12-month period [3,4,9]. Tumor regression was defined as an annual volumetric decline of 20%. Annual volumetric changes between −20% and +20% was defined as stable disease; volumetric changes within ±20% are insignificant volumetric progressions or involutions. In a previous study we identified patients that had pseudoprogression [3]. Therefore these patients were excluded from this study to prevent bias in our results.

Radiation Parameters

The dosimetric parameters for SRS were collected and listed in Table 1.

Adverse Radiation Effects

The following clinical symptoms reported after radiosurgery were recorded as ARE: impaired balance, trigeminal neuropathy, facial nerve dysfunction, tinnitus, and hydrocephalus. For the purposes of this study we only collected reports of new symptoms and not ongoing symptoms that would have existed prior to SRS treatment. We were unable to include auditory complications due to incomplete auditory clinical follow-up in this cohort of patients.

Statistical analysis

Linear regression was used to assess the relation of pre-treatment SGR with post-treatment SGR and the extent of reduction in tumor growth rate after radiosurgery. To investigate the relation between age on date of treatment and SGRs, patients were categorized into two groups based on a cut-off age, and tested for correlation; cut-off ages tested were 60, 65, and 70. Independent sample t-test was used for comparison between two independent groups. One-way ANOVA was used for multiple independent group comparisons. Univariate analysis was used to evaluate risk factors in predicting tumor response and post-treatment complications, and to study the relation between the following variables: pre-treatment SGR, post-treatment SGR, ARE, treatment tumor volume, age, sex, and radiation parameters. For all tests, p values ≤0.05 were considered significant. All analyses were performed with IBM SPSS version 20.0 (SPSS, Chicago, IL, USA).

Results

Patient characteristics

Of the 258 VS patients treated with SRS between December 2005 and June 2011, 84 had complete clinical and radiological follow-up for at least 12 months before and after treatment, and therefore qualified for inclusion in this study; this inclusion criteria was necessary to allow us to calculate the tumor growth rates before and after SRS. Of the 84 patients, six patients were further excluded for having bilateral VS with neurofibromatosis type II. Ten other patients were excluded because of having either MRI scans with either poor resolution or greater than 3 millimeters thickness slice scans, which prevented accurate volumetric measurements. Five other patients were excluded as their tumors

Table 1. Analysis Variables and Univariate Analysis.

		Post-treatment SGR		Reduction in SGR after radiosurgery	
Radiation Characteristics	**Median (range)**	**Regression coefficient**	***p***	**Regression coefficient**	***p***
Treatment time (min)	35.20(11.55–79.48)	0.15	0.25	−0.02	0.91
Dose Rate (Gy/min)	2.47(1.80–3.22)	−0.25	0.056	0.18	0.18
CI RTOG[4]	1.31 (1.06–1.86)	−0.03	0.83	0.10	0.48
Gradient Index	2.81 (2.42–4.03)	0.18	0.17	−0.23	0.46
Homogeneity index	2.00 (1.85–2.50)	0.13	0.35	−0.06	0.65
Volume receiving 100% dose (%)	99.12 (96.40–99.88)	0.12	0.38	−0.04	0.79
Target volume receiving 95% dose(%)	99.78 (98.34–99.99)	0.13	0.36	−0.08	0.58
Min dose (Gy)	10.08 (7.00–16.08)	−0.21	0.13	0.15	0.28
Max dose (Gy)	24.00 (22.22–30.10)	−0.09	0.49	0.09	0.51
Mean dose (Gy)	17.12 (15.61–19.37)	−0.13	0.15	0.28	0.08
Volume of 12Gy isodose (cm3)	1.67 (0.14–11.09)	−0.05	0.71	−0.01	0.93
Prescription isodose (%)	50 (40–54)	0.11	0.44	−0.10	0.46
Number of Isocentres	11 (2–22)	−0.01	0.93	0.04	0.79

underwent pseudoprogression following treatment. In sum, a total of 63 patients with unilateral sporadic VS were included in this retrospective study. Twenty-eight (44.4%) patients were males and thirty-five (55.6%) were females. The median radiological and clinical follow-up after radiosurgery was 32 months (range, 12–72 months). The median age at treatment date was 64 years (range, 26–83 years). Twenty-eight patients (44.4%) had left-sided VS. The median tumor volume treated was 1.54 cm^3 (range, 0.14–10.84 cm^3).

Tumor Growth Rate Characteristics

The median VS growth rates in the 12-month period before and after SRS were 55.3% (range, 2.6–172.8%) and −16.1% (range, −141.4–56.6%), respectively. Prior to radiosurgery, fifty-three (84.1%) VS had a significant growth over a 12-month period; their median pre-treatment SGR was 65.9%, and the median post-treatment SGR was -15.8%. One year following radiosurgery, twenty-seven VS (42.9%) showed a decrease in volume, twenty-nine (46.0%) stabilized, and seven (11.1%) continued to grow. Of the tumors that continued to grow, no stabilization or regression was evident at 24 months and therefore the continued growth was not explained by pseudoprogression. Radiosurgery was concluded to have failed in suppressing tumor growth in these patients. The average growth rate at 12 months post-radiosurgery for these tumors was 43.97%. Salvage microsurgical intervention was offered based on presence of symptoms secondary to mass effect or cranial nerve deficits caused by the growing tumors. Only one of the seven (1.6%) patients required salvage microsurgical resection because of symptomatic tumor growth. The pre-treatment growth rates for tumors that continued to grow after radiosurgery were highly variable, and were comparable to those that did not show growth following radiosurgery (i.e. tumor stabilization).

Predictive factors associated with pre- and post-treatment growth rate

No significant correlation was found between pre-treatment or post-treatment tumor growth rates with any of the following factors that we investigated: tumor volume, patients' gender, or age at time of treatment (Table 2). To further investigate the relation between age on date of treatment and SGRs, patients were categorized into two groups based on a cut-off age, and tested for correlation; cut-off ages tested were 60, 65, and 70. No significant correlation was found between age groups and pre-treatment and post-treatment SGRs (Table 3).

Pre-treatment growth rate as predictor of treatment response

Linear regression between pre-treatment and post-treatment SGRs revealed no significant correlation (p = 0.34) (Figure 1a). However, we graphically observed that the growth rates of tumors reduced after radiosurgery in proportion to the tumors' initial pre-treatment growth rates (Figure 1b), although this relation was not statistically significant ($R^2 = 0.899$, $p = 0.19$). We were then interested to see if VS can be categorized into clinically relevant subgroups based on their pre-treatment or post-treatment SGRs. We categorized tumors based on their response to SRS into three groups called regression, stable disease, and growth, using different cut-off values (Table 4), and attempted to see whether the pre-treatment growth rates between these groups significantly differ. We defined 'regression' as a decline in volume of more than the cut-off value, 'growth' as an increase in tumor volume of more than the cut-off value, and 'stable disease' as any volumetric change between 'regression' and 'growth'. The cut-off values, although arbitrary, were chosen such that they could potentially be practically applied in a clincal setting. When we compared the the three groups, there was no significant difference between their pre-treatment growth rates (Table 4).

We also categorized tumors based on their pre-treatment growth rate into slow, medium, and fast growing tumors (called Group I, II, and III, respectively), and attempted to see whether the post-treatment growth rates significantly differ between these groups. We repeated the categorization using different cut-off values. The cut-off values were derived by converting changes in tumors' extrameatal diameter (10, 15, and 20%) that are commonly used in clinical practice, to volumetric changes by making the crude assumption that tumors are spherical; this conversion is commonly used in clinical practice. After categoriz-

Table 2. Correlation between tumor volume, sex, and age, with pre-treatment and post-treatment SGRs.

	Pre-treatment tumor SGR		Post-treatment tumor SGR	
	Regression Coefficient	*p*	Regression Coefficient	*p*
Tumor volume	0.014	0.92	0.033	0.80
Sex	0.112	0.11	0.206	0.36
Age on date of treatment	0.055	0.67	0.006	0.96

ing the tumors into the aforementioned three groups, we compared their post-treatment SGRs; however, they did not significantly differ from each other (Table 4).

Radiation Parameters

Univariate analysis of various dosimetry parameters examined (Table 1) showed no significant correlation with either post-treatment SGR or the extent of reduction in growth rate after radiosurgery.

Adverse radiation effects

Of the 63 patients, twenty (31.7%) experienced some form of new onset complication after SRS that persisted in the time span of the study (Table 5). Of the seven patients whose tumor grew significantly after radiosurgery, only two (3.2%) experienced complications – one patient experienced facial weakness, while the other experienced facial spasms and imbalance. In these two cases, the complications may have been either due to tumor growth or ARE. In all other patients with tumors that did not exhibit significant growth, we attributed complications to ARE. The other 18 (28.5%) patients who experienced ARE had tumors that either stabilized or regressed after radiosurgery. Univariate analysis of risk factors revealed a significant positive relation between post-treatment SGRs and incidence of ARE (Table 5). Patients who experienced ARE had higher post-treatment growth rates than those who did not develop ARE. On multivariate analysis, no new factors were identified to be of significance.

Discussion

SRS has proven to be a highly effective treatment for VS [1,10,11]. Nevertheless, a percentage of VS are resistant to radiosurgery, and continue to grow after treatment. There are currently no known factors that can predict which VS will fail to respond to radiosurgery. The traditional thinking has been that the rate of growth of a VS is a predictor of response to radiosurgery, and based on literature from other CNS tumors it is argued that a faster growing VS will respond more favorably to treatment [12]. We therefore sought to examine whether growth rate of VS prior to radiosurgery is a predictor of treatment response and alteration in tumor growth rate in a one year follow-up period following SRS.

The terminology used in the literature to define tumor size, growth, and control is highly variable, limiting our ability to compare results of radiosurgery between different institutions. Most institutions use a linear measurement for assessing VS size, which is then used to determine suitability for SRS and response to treatment. However linear measurements fail to accurately determine the actual tumor volume [10,13,14]. Volumetric measurements are by far a more reliable and accurate method for assessing three dimensional changes of tumor volume and tumor growth versus linear measurements. However, volumetric measurements are time consuming, which make their integration into clinical practice difficult.

There is currently no standardized system for reporting VS tumor growth rates [2], and as a consequence reports on natural history of VS are highly variable [10,12,15,16]. Battaglia et al. conducted a retrospective study to assess the true effect of 12–13Gy radiation on VS by comparing the growth behavior of tumors with and without radiosurgery [15]. This group concluded that there is no significant difference between the growth patterns of untreated and radiosurgically treated VS particularly for small-sized tumors. However, Battaglia et al. used the Jackler staging system, which is a two-dimensional method, to determine tumor size, which does not measure the actual three-dimensional change in tumor volume.

In our study we used volumetric measurements to accurately quantify tumor growth. We also used a previously agreed upon definition of significant growth to define tumor control and tumor growth, which is any volumetric change greater than 20% as a significant change in tumor size [13]. Based on this definition the tumor control rate was 89% in the first year following SRS. We

Table 3. Independent samples t-test for pre-treatment and post-treatment SGRs, with SGRs classified into two groups based on cut-off age values.

Cut-off age	No. (%)	Pre-treatment SGR *p* value	Post-treatment SGR *p* value
<60	24 (38.1)	0.56	0.72
>60	39 (61.9)		
<65	34 (54.0)	0.83	0.99
>65	29 (46.0)		
<70	50 (79.4)	0.75	0.36
>70	13 (20.6)		

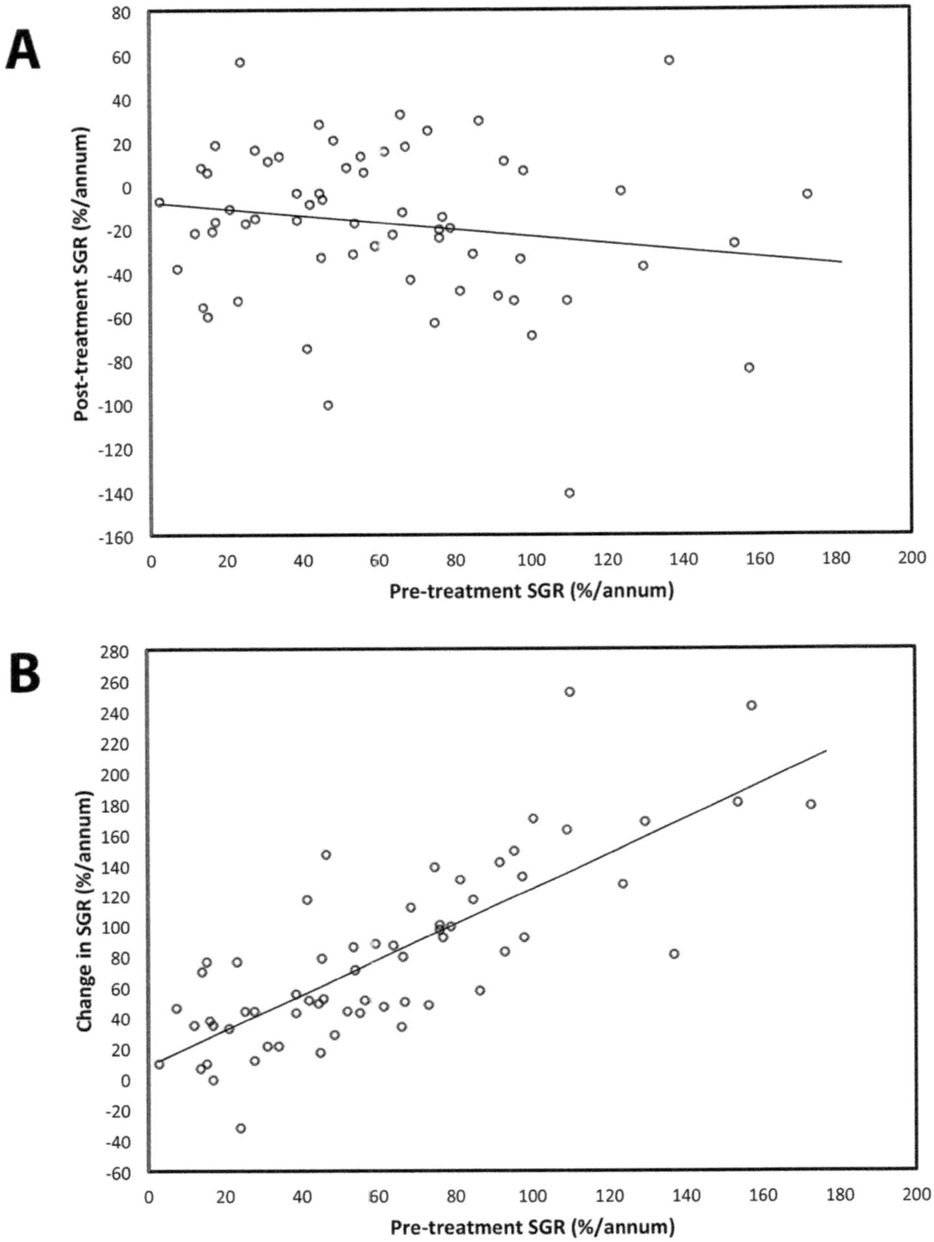

Figure 1. Correlation between pre-treatment SGRs with post-treatment SGRs, and reduction in SGRs after radiosurgery.

were able to demonstrate that regardless of tumor volume most VS respond favorably to 12–13Gy of radiation, and in following SRS have a steep decline in tumor growth rate. Furthermore, we found that the pre-treatment growth rates for tumors that continue to grow after radiosurgery are comparable to those that responded favorably to radiation and showed a decrease in growth. In other words there was no correlation between post-SRS continued growth and pre-treatment growth rate of VS. Tumors that continue growth after radiosurgery are most likely resistant to radiation because of varying intrinsic molecular properties [17]. It is important to acknowledge that in this study we examined the early changes in growth rates of VS following radiosurgery, and the results seen in early regression following treatment are not a unified concept and not necessarily directly correlated with long-term outcome. It is also important to note that increase in tumor volume following radiosurgery can be be due to either tumor cell proliferation or release of cytokines and inflammatory response following treatment, which the latter will not necessarily correlate to tumor progression or growth; however currently the two processes are indistinguishable clinically and radiologically.

We also observed a non-statistically significant but compelling correlation between pre-treatment growth rate and change in growth rate after radiosurgery. We found that the change/reduction in the growth rates of most VS after radiosurgery was proportional to their initial pre-treatment growth rates; for instance, tumors with high growth rates before treatment had the greatest reduction in growth rate after radiosurgery, and tumors with initially low growth rates had the least reduction. The most obvious explanation for this finding is that in short-term, SRS halts tumor growth regardless of how fast the tumor is initially

Table 4. a) Pre-treatment growth rates vs. post-treatment growth rate groups

Post-treatment growth rate	No. (%)	Median pre-treatment growth rate %/annum (range)	*p* value
10% cut-off value			
Regression	36 (57.1)	65.22 (7.37–157.60)	0.84
Control	12 (19.0)	45.00 (2.63–172.76)	
Growth	15 (23.9)	55.31 (17.10–136.87)	
15% cut-off value			
Regression	33 (52.4)	63.98 (7.37–157.60)	0.77
Control	19 (30.2)	45.45 (2.63–172.76)	
Growth	11 (17.4)	61.56 (17.10–136.87)	
20% cut-off value			
Regression	26 (41.3)	71.63 (7.37–157.60)	0.21
Control	30 (47.6)	45.00 (2.63–172.76)	
Growth	7 (11.1)	65.90 (24.16–136.87)	
33% cut-of value			
Regression	17 (27.0)	81.53 (7.37–157.60)	0.20
Control	44 (69.8)	52.56 (2.63–172.76)	
Growth	2 (3.2)	80.52 (24.16–136.87)	

b) Pre-treatment growth rates vs. post-treatment growth rate groups

	Change in diameter (%/annum)	Change in volume (%/annum)	No. (%)	*p* value
First Test				
Group I	<10	<33	17 (27.0)	0.66
Group II	10–15	33–52	12 (19.0)	
Group III	>15	>52	34 (54.0)	
Second Test				
Group I	<10	<33	17 (27.0)	0.19
Group II	10–20	33–73	23 (36.5)	
Group III	>20	>73	23 (36.5)	
Third Test				
Group I	<15	<52	29 (46.0)	0.17
Group II	15–20	52–73	11 (17.5)	
Group III	>20	>73	23 (36.5)	

growing prior to radiosurgery, rather than causing cell death. Consequently, because fast growing tumors have high number of dividng cells, we see the greatest change in growth rate for tumors that have higher growth rates before radiosurgery. Furthermore, because SRS stops tumor growth irrespective of the initial growth rate, it suggests that at least in short-term, fast and slow growing

Table 5. Univariate analysis for ARE.

ARE	No. (%)	Pre-treatment SGR	Post-treatment SGR	Age at treatment
		p value	*p* value	*p* value
Impaired balance	17 (27.0)	0.13	0.19	0.48
Tinnitus	8 (12.7)	0.74	0.23	0.62
Facial numbness	6 (9.5)	0.68	0.61	0.49
Facial palsy	3 (4.8)	0.48	0.59	0.64
Hydrocephalus	1 (1.6)	0.20	0.13	0.38
Adverse Event	20 (31.7)	0.63	0.047*	0.96

* Statistically significant.

tumors respond similarly to radiosurgery. These results are conflicting with the traditional thinking discussed earlier. It is therefore important for similar studies with larger sample sizes to be conducted to further explore and validate our findings on the response of fast and slow growing tumors to radiosurgery.

Furthermore, factors predicting the incidence of ARE are invaluable for clinical decision-making, and more importantly patient counseling. Numerous studies have focused on identifying such factors, and considerable attention has been given to treatment volume as a potential predictor [4,5,18,19]. Tumors of large volume require a greater mass to be irradiated, which theoretically increases the amount of surrounding non-tumorous tissue exposed to radiation. Therefore it has been commonly hypothesized that VS with large volumes are more likely to be associated with ARE. In agreement with this theory, Friedman et al. found a significant correlation between treatment volume and incidence of ARE [19]. More recently, our group demonstrated that patients with VS larger than 5 cm^3 are significantly more likely to develop ARE after radiosurgery [4]. Pre-treatment tumor growth has previously been speculated to be related to the incidence of ARE; Beegle et al. demonstrated that tumor growth before radiosurgery is a significant predictor of ARE. In this study we found no correlation between the two variables [18]. However, we did find that there is a significant correlation between tumors that continue to grow post-treatment and the incidence of non-auditory ARE. However, we are limited in this study by the small sample size and in particular with the number of patients that experienced complications following SRS. Therefore, ongoing multi-institutional studies with larger cohorts that are better powered and include longer patient follow-up are needed to more comprehensively study the relation between growth of VS and their response to radiosurgery, and incidence of ARE.

Conclusion

Traditionally the rate of tumor growth prior to SRS has been considered to be a predictor of response to SRS and possibly ARE. In this study we found that the natural history of VS, most notably tumor growth, and target volume, do not serve as reliable predictors for response to radiosurgery in the early period following treatment. However, our systematic study of change in tumor growth rates demonstrates that VS growing at faster rates have greatest change in growth rate following radiosurgery. We also observed that patients with tumors that continue to grow at significant rates after radiosurgery are more likely to experience post-treatment ARE. Notably, VS that continue to grow following SRS have variable pre-treatment growth rates.

Author Contributions

Conceived and designed the experiments: SL GZ. Performed the experiments: SL HP EM BK CH. Analyzed the data: SL HP EM BK CH GZ. Contributed reagents/materials/analysis tools: MC FG NL GZ. Wrote the paper: SL EM HP BK CH GZ.

References

1. Foote KD, Friedman WA, Buatti JM, Meeks SL, Bova FJ, et al. (2000) Analysis of risk factors associated with radiosurgery for vestibular schwannoma. J Neurosurg 95(3):440–449.
2. Linskey ME, Flickinger JC, Lunsford LD (1993) Cranial nerve length predicts the risk of delayed facial and trigeminal neuropathies after acoustic tumor stereotactic radiosurgery. Int J Radiat Oncol Biol Phys 25(2):227–233.
3. Hayhurst C, Zadeh G (2011) Tumor pseudoprogression following radiosurgery for vestibular schwannoma. Neuro Oncol 14(1):87–92.
4. Hayhurst C, Monsalves E, Bernstein M, Gentili F, Heydarian M, et al (2012) Predicting nonauditory adverse radiation effects following radiosurgery for vestibular schwannoma: A Volume and Dosimetric Analysis. Int J Radiat Oncol Biol Phys 82(5):2041–2046.
5. Ganz JC, Reda WA, Abdelkarim K (2009) Adverse radiation effects after Gamma Knife Surgery in relation to dose and volume. Acta Neurochir 151(1):9–19.
6. Rockne R, Rockhill JK, Mrugala M, Spence AM, Kalet I, et al (2010) Predicting the efficacy of radiotherapy in individual glioblastoma patients in vivo: a mathematical modeling approach. Phys Med Biol 55(12):3271–3285.
7. Yushkevich PA, Piven J, Hazlett HC, Smith RG, Ho S, et al (2006) User-guided 3D active contour segmentation of anatomical structures: Significantly improved efficiency and reliability. NeuroImage 31(3):1116–1128.
8. Mehrara E, Forssell-Aronsson E, Ahlman H, Bernhardt P (2007) Specific growth rate versus doubling time for quantitative characterization of tumor growth rate. Cancer Res 67(8):3970–3975.
9. Plotkin SR, Halpin C, Blakeley JO, Slattery WH 3rd, Welling DB, et al (2009) Suggested response criteria for phase II antitumor drug studies for neurofibromatosis type 2 related vestibular schwannoma. Journal of Neuro-Oncology 93(1):61–77.
10. Mohyuddin A, Vokurka EA, Evans DGR, Ramsden RT, Jackson A (2003) Is clinical growth index a reliable predictor of tumour growth in vestibular schwannomas? Clin Otolaryngol 28: 85–90.
11. Timmer FCA, Mulder JJS, Hanssens PE, van Overbeeke JJ, Donders RT, et al (2011) Gamma knife radiosurgery for vestibular schwannomas: Identification of predictors for continued tumor growth and the influence of documented tumor growth preceding radiation treatment. Laryngoscope 121: 1834–1838.
12. van de Langenberg R, de Bondt BJ, Nelemans PJ, Dohmen AJC, Baumert BG, et al. (2011) Predictors of volumetric growth and auditory deterioration in vestibular schwannomas followed in a wait and scan policy. Otol Neurotol 32(2):338–344.
13. van de Langenberg R, de Bondt BJ, Nelemans PJ, Baumert BG, Stokroos RJ (2009) Follow-up assessment of vestibular schwannomas: volume quantification versus two-dimensional measurements. Neuroradiol J 51(8):517–524.
14. Varughese JK, Wentzel-Larsen T, Vassbotn F, Moen G, Lund-Johansen M (2010) Analysis of vestibular schwannoma size in multiple dimensions: a comparative cohort study of different measurement techniques. Clin Otolaryngol 35: 97–103.
15. Battaglia A, Mastrodimos B, Cueva R (2006) Comparison of growth patterns of acoustic neuromas with and without radiosurgery. Otol Neurotol 27(5):705–712.
16. Timmer FCA, Hanssens PEJ, van Haren AE, et al (2011) Follow-up after gamma knife radiosurgery for vestibular schwannomas: Volumetric and axial control rates. Laryngoscope 121(7):1359–1366.
17. Archibald DJ, Neff BA, Voss SG, Splinter PL, Driscoll CL, et al (2010) B7-H1 expression in vestibular schwannomas. Otol Neurotol 31(6):991–997.
18. Beegle RD, Friedman WA, Bova FJ (2007) Effect of treatment plan quality on outcomes after radiosurgery for vestibular schwannoma. J Neurosurg 107(5):913–916.
19. Friedman WA, Bradshaw P, Myers A, Bova FJ (2006) Linear accelerator radiosurgery for vestibular schwannomas. J Neurosurg 105(5):657–661.

IV t-PA Influences Infarct Volume in Minor Stroke

Kersten Villringer[1]*, Ulrike Grittner[2], Lars-Arne Schaafs[1], Christian H. Nolte[3], Heinrich Audebert[3], Jochen B. Fiebach[1]

1 Academic Neuroradiology, Department of Neurology and Center for Stroke Research, Charité, Berlin, Germany, **2** Department for Biostatistics and Clinical Epidemiology and Center for Stroke Research, Charité, Berlin, Germany, **3** Department of Neurology and Center for Stroke Research, Charité, Berlin, Germany

Abstract

Background: There is an ongoing debate whether stroke patients presenting with minor or moderate symptoms benefit from thrombolysis. Up until now, stroke severity on admission is typically measured with the NIHSS, and subsequently used for treatment decision.

Hypothesis: Acute MRI lesion volume assessment can aid in therapy decision for iv-tPA in minor stroke.

Methods: We analysed 164 patients with NIHSS 0–7 from a prospective stroke MRI registry, the 1000+ study (clinicaltrials.org NCT00715533). Patients were examined in a 3 T MRI scanner and either received (n = 62) or did not receive thrombolysis (n = 102). DWI (diffusion weighted imaging) and PI (perfusion imaging) at admission were evaluated for diffusion - perfusion mismatch. Our primary outcome parameter was final lesion volume, defined by lesion volume on day 6 FLAIR images.

Results: The association between t-PA and FLAIR lesion volume on day 6 was significantly different for patients with smaller DWI volume compared to patients with larger DWI volume (interaction between DWI and t-PA: $p = 0.021$). Baseline DWI lesion volume was dichotomized at the median (0.7 ml): final lesion volume at day 6 was larger in patients with large baseline DWI volumes without t-PA treatment (median difference 3, IQR −0.4–9.3 ml). Conversely, in patients with larger baseline DWI volumes final lesion volumes were smaller after t-PA treatment (median difference 0, IQR −4.1–5 ml). However, this did not translate into a significant difference in the mRS at day 90 ($p = 0.577$).

Conclusion: Though this study is only hypothesis generating considering the number of cases, we believe that the size of DWI lesion volume may support therapy decision in patients with minor stroke.

Trial Registration: Clinicaltrials.org NCT00715533

Editor: Hooman Kamel, Weill Cornell Medical College, United States of America

Funding: The study was supported by the Federal Ministry of Education and Research via the grant Center for Stroke Research Berlin (01 EO 0801). The funders had no role in study design, data collection and analysis, decision to publish, or preparation of the manuscript.

Competing Interests: KV reports that receiving consulting fees by Bayer Schering and JBF reports receiving consulting, lecture and advisory board fees by BMS, Siemens, Perceptive, Synarc, BioImaging Technologies, Novartis, Wyeth, Pfizer, Boehringer Ingelheim, Lundbeck and Sygnis.

* Email: kersten.villringer@charite.de

Introduction

Thrombolysis has become standard therapy in the treatment of acute ischemic stroke and is used within a time frame of ≤ 4.5 hours in Europe since ECASS 3 [1]. However, uncertainty remains when it comes to treating patients with minor stroke or rapidly improving symptoms, especially considering the side effects of t-PA with an increased risk of intracerebral or extracranial haemorrhages [2].

Moreover, there is disagreement regarding the outcome in minor stroke patients with reports of excellent outcome at 3 months follow-up without any intervention [3] but also poor outcome reported in nearly one third when withholding thrombolysis [4,5].

MRI has been suggested to identify patients with minor stroke as well as point out those who might suffer a recurrent stroke and might therefore benefit from thrombolysis. Rajajee et al. [6] and others [7] found vessel pathology to be predictive for recurrent stroke in transient ischemic attacks (TIA) and minor stroke patients as well as for outcome. Vessel pathology was also associated with clinically beneficial treatment effects. However, the included patients showed signs of moderate to severe stroke in an extended time window of <9 hours from symptom onset to treatment [8].

This leaves minor stroke patients who show no vessel pathology but are considered as possibly benefitting from thrombolysis.

CONSORT
TRANSPARENT REPORTING of TRIALS

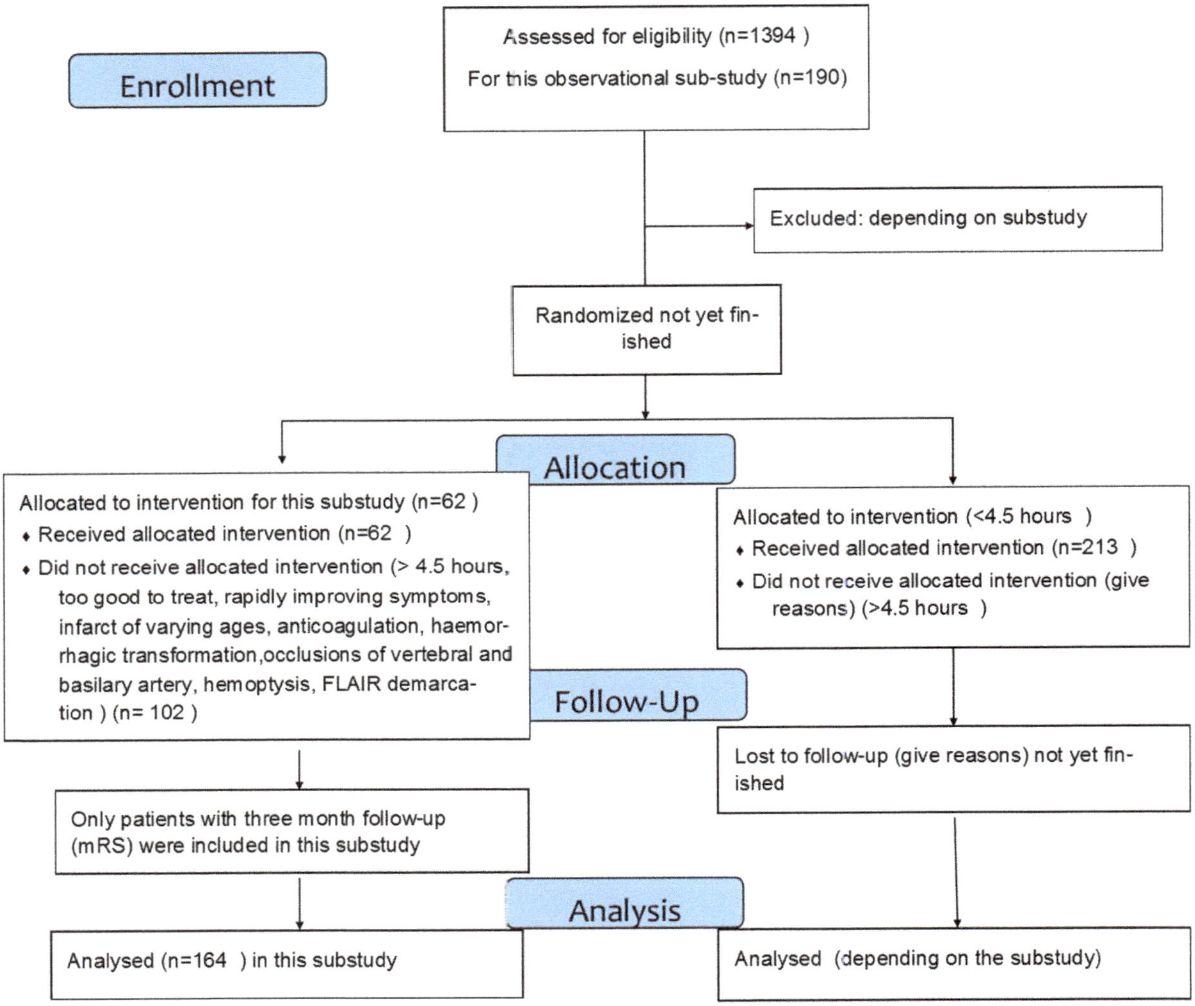

Figure 1. CONSORT 2010 Flow Diagram.

It also has been shown that a mismatch volume of more than 10 ml is predictive of lesion progression and early neurological deterioration [9], though, perfusion imaging cannot always be obtained for instance due to renal failure.

Furthermore, to save time, especially at the end of the mandated time window it might be necessary to shorten the MRI imaging protocol to haemorrhage sensitive sequences (T2*) and diffusion weighted imaging (DWI).

Therefore, we aimed to evaluate the potential of DWI at admission in patients with low/moderate NIHSS in facilitating therapy decision towards thrombolysis by comparing minor stroke patients who did and did not receive t-PA.

Patients and Methods

The protocol for this trial and supporting CONSORT checklist are available as supporting information; see Checklist S1, Protocol S1 and Figure 1.

From 11/2008 until 6/2012 we included 190 patients with ischemic stroke from the observational 1000+ study, registered at clinicaltrials.org NCT00715533.

Ethics statement

Written informed consent was obtained from all patients. The study design (1000+ study) was approved by the ethics committee of the Charité - Universitätsmedizin, Berlin (EA4/026/08).

Table 1. Patients characteristics.

n = 164	NIHSS 0–7 iv t-PA	NIHSS 0–7 non iv t-PA	p[a]
n	**62**	**102**	
gender (female) n (%)	26 (41.9%)	38 (37.3%)	0.621
age (years)	71 (63–77)	70 (62–78)	0.888
onset – MRI (minutes)	105 (79–147)	233 (122–382)	<0.001
DWI (ml)	0.8 (0.3–3.8)	0.7 (0.2–2.3)	0.279
relMTT (ml)	12.0 (0.3–60.2)	6.4 (0.0–35.9)	0.220
MM volume (ml)	7.1 (−0.1–49.8)	3.5 (−0.1–34.2)	0.545
MM ratio	3.1 (0.0–24.6)	3.7 (0.0–16.7)	0.939
FLAIR day6 (ml)	3.2 (0.7–7.0) (n = 46)	2.3 (0.6–8.9) (n = 72)	0.623
mRS day 90	1 (0–2) (n = 62)	1 (0–2) (n = 102)	0.577
NIHSS day1	4 (2–5) (n = 62)	2 (1–4) (n = 102)	0.002
NIHSS day6	1 (0–2) (n = 51)	1 (0–2) (n = 88)	0.57

[a]Mann - Whitney for differences in thrombolysis versus non intravenous (iv) t-PA
Age, onset, volumes, NIHSS, mRS are given as median, interquartile range (IQR)
iv t-PA = intravenous tissue plasminogen activator, ml = millilitre, MM = mismatch

MRI Examination

Data acquisition was performed on a 3 Tesla MRI scanner (Tim Trio, Siemens AG, Erlangen, Germany). The imaging protocol included a diffusion weighted imaging (DWI) (TR/TE/FOV/matrix: 7600 ms/93 ms/230 mm/192×192, slice thickness 2.5 mm, b = 1000 s/mm^2, 6 different directions), bolus – track perfusion imaging (PI) (TR/TE/flip angle/FOV/matrix: 1390 ms/29 ms/60°/230 mm/128×128, slice thickness 5 mm), a fluid-attenuated inversion recovery sequence (FLAIR) (TR/TE/TI/flip angle/FOV/matrix: 8000 ms/100 ms/2370.5 ms/130°/220 mm/256×256, slice thickness 5 mm) and a 3 dimensional time-of-flight magnetic resonance angiography (MRA) (TR/TE/flip angle/field of view/slice thickness: 22 ms/3.9 ms/20°/162*200/0.7 mm). For the perfusion measurements a bolus of 5 ml Gadovist was administered, followed by a saline flush both at a flow rate of 5 ml/s.

Postprocessing of perfusion images was performed with the Siemens standard software package resulting in regional cerebral blood flow (rCBF), regional cerebral blood volume (rCBV) and mean time-to-peak (MTT) maps with the latter used for further analysis. Regions of interests (ROI) were manually drawn on DWI, MTT – maps and FLAIR day 6 images. Lesion volumes were calculated from ROIs, acute absolute mismatch volume (MTT volume – DWI volume) and mismatch ratio (MTT volume/DWI volume) were assessed.

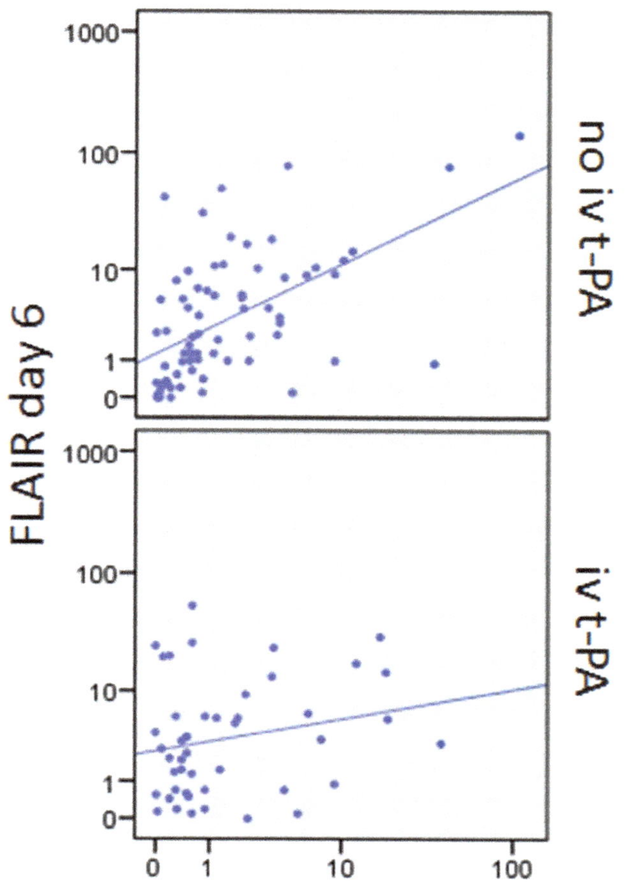

Figure 2. Association between DWI volume day 1 and FLAIR volume day 6.

Statistical analysis

All continuous variables were checked for normal distribution (histogram check, absolute skewness-value <1) before using parametric tests. Otherwise non-parametric statistical tests were applied or the variables were transformed before analysis to reduce skewness in distribution. The Mann-Whitney test was employed to compare differences between groups for quantitative non-normally distributed outcomes. To assess differential treatment ((iv) t-PA) effects for patients with different DWI volume on admission with regard to FLAIR volume on day 6, a regression analysis was performed using log-transformed values for lesion volumes with log-transformed FLAIR volume as outcome. Log-transformation was performed to overcome the skewed distributions. A regression analysis was also used to evaluate the association between vessel status and FLAIR volumes on day 6. A level of $\alpha = 0.05$ was considered significant. No adjustment for multiple testing was applied.

Table 2. Linear regression analysis for FLAIR day 6 (log-tranformed) (n = 118, adjusted $r^2 = 0.23$).

	β (se)	p
constant	0.35 (0.10)	0.001
NIHSS day 1 (log-transformed)	0.20 (0.13)	0.113
DWI volume (log-transformed)	0.64 (0.13)	<0.001
iv t-PA (versus non iv t-PA)	0.001 (0.13)	0.997
Interaction t-PA*DWI volume	−0.44 (0.19)	0.021
Vessel status (reference: no pathology)		
occlusion	0.01 (0.14)	0.928
stenosis	−0.13 (0.16)	0.416

For exploratory purposes we used a median split of 0.7 ml to assess the effect of thrombolysis on DWI and FLAIR volumes. All statistical analyses were performed using SPSS version 20.

Results

The inclusion criteria for this study were as follows:

Visible lesions on DWI at admission, since it could be demonstrated that only 4 out of 299 patients with negative DWI images had perfusion deficits, indicating ischemia [10]. Further criteria were time interval between symptom onset and MRI examination ≤9 hours in view of interventional studies like AXIS or DIAS III/IV, as well as mild to moderate stroke with NIHSS up to 7 [11,12] with or without t-PA therapy.

One-hundred-and-sixty-four out of 190 patients with minor/moderate stroke were considered for further analysis.

The reasons for exclusion were incomplete examinations (n = 7), faulty entry to database (n = 5), unknown symptom onset (n = 5), onset>9 hours (n = 4), mechanical thrombus extraction (n = 2), no visible DWI lesion (n = 1), one haemorrhage and one patient with postictal edema.

The reasons for patients within the time window of less than 4.5 hours (n = 50) for not receiving t-PA were as follows:

Rapidly improving symptoms (n = 24), patients considered "too good" to treat (n = 6), infarcts of varying ages (n = 4), oral anticoagulation (n = 3), haemorrhagic transformation (n = 1), one patient had occlusions of both vertebral arteries and the basilary artery, one had a clear demarcation on FLAIR and the last one had haemoptysis. In 9 patients no further information on the reasons for exclusion from t-PA therapy could be obtained.

Detailed patient characteristics are given in table 1.

There were no significant differences in baseline variables between patients treated with iv t-PA and those not treated, with the exception of time between onset and MRI examination with shorter delays in treated patients, median:105 minutes (IQR 79–145 minutes) compared to 233 minutes (IQR 122–380 minutes) in untreated patients ($p<0.001$). There was also a difference in NIHSS values at admission: median NIHSS 4 (IQR 2–5) in iv t-PA treated patients compared to 2 (IQR 1–4) in the non iv t-PA group ($p = 0.002$). No significant difference for mRS at 3 months follow-up was found between groups (median 1 (IQR 0–2)) ($p = 0.577$).

Though no significant differences between the median DWI volume at admission and FLAIR volume on day 6 could be demonstrated, the regression analysis showed a significant interaction of DWI volume and thrombolysis on FLAIR day 6 volumes as outcome parameter ($p = 0.021$) (figure 2, table 2) indicating differential treatment effects for those with smaller DWI volumes compared to those with larger DWI volumes. To further explore this result we performed a median split [13] at 0.7 ml baseline DWI volume and compared infarct growth in patients who received t-PA and in those who did not (table 3). The largest increase in lesion volume was found in those patients with large admission DWI volumes who did not receive t-PA (median difference: 3.01 ml, IQR: −0.35–9.28 ml). The smallest lesion growth could be detected in patients with large DWI volume who received t-PA (median difference: 0 ml, IQR −4.10–5.00 ml) (figure 3, 4). No significant interaction between vessel status at baseline and outcome could be demonstrated for either groups (iv t-PA treated and untreated) ($p = 0.928$). Analysing both groups separately those patients with occlusions, not receiving iv t-PA showed a tendency towards larger FLAIR day 6 volumes compared to patients with no vessel pathology. Contrary, in patients with vessel occlusion treated with iv t-PA FLAIR volumes on day 6 tended to be smaller compared to those without vessel pathology.

Table 3. Lesion volume changes of DWI volume and FLAIR day 6 by DWI volume categories and t-PA therapy.

	low DWI volume (<0.7 ml)		high DWI volume (≥0.7 ml)	
	iv t-PA (n = 25)	non iv t-PA (n = 32)	iv t-PA (n = 21)	non iv t-PA (n = 40)
DWI volume (ml) median, interquartile range	0.32 (0.15–0.50)	0.18 (0.04–0.48)	3.60 (1.55–10.70)	2.25 (1.10–4.70)
FLAIR volume day 6 (ml) median, interquartile range	2.1 (0.58–4.92)	0.74 (0.20–2.33)	5.50 (0.80–11.35)	5.85 (2.02–12.03)
Difference FLAIR volume day 6/DWI volume (ml) median, interquartile range	1.90 (0.33–4.77)	0.39 (0.04–2.15)	0.00 (−4.10–5.00)	3.01 (−0.35–9.28)

iv = intravenous, n = number, ml = millilitre.

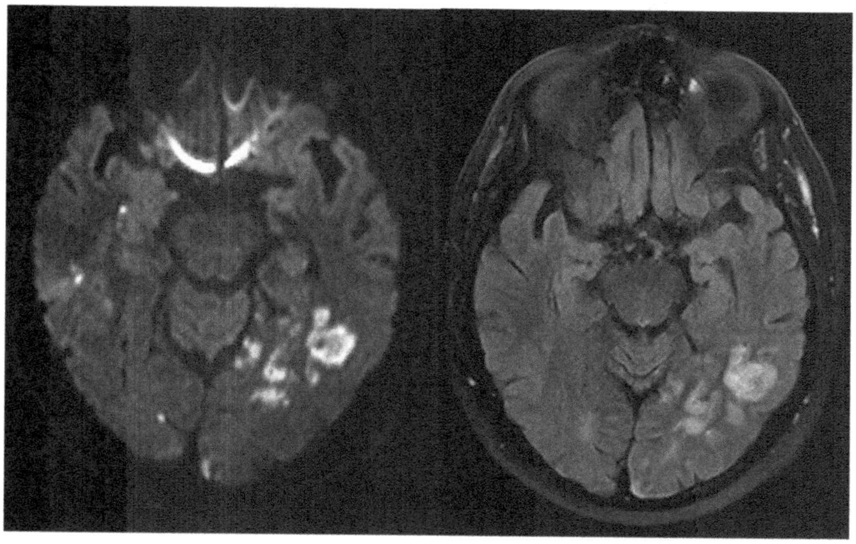

Figure 3. Lesion volume development in minor/moderate stroke after iv t-PA.

Discussion

In this pilot study we found a significant association between infarct volume changes and thrombolytic treatment. Treatment effect in terms of smaller infarct growth was stronger in patients with larger DWI volumes compared to those with smaller DWI volumes. This argues for baseline DWI volume as useful parameter in assisting therapy decision towards or against thrombolysis in minor stroke patients.

There is still considerable uncertainty regarding therapy decision resting upon clinical scales like the NIHSS alone. Many attempts have been undertaken to assess non-isolated symptoms as defining variables in minor stroke (NIHSS ≤6) [14], different combinations of NIHSS items and cut-offs [15] or defining key symptoms like language impairment and distal paresis, which may justify the use of thrombolysis [16].

There have also been many efforts to establish imaging variables capable of predicting deficit and severity of disability due to stroke, therefore aiding therapy decisions. Among those the most common imaging parameter is the perfusion – diffusion mismatch to detect potentially salvageable tissue. Recently, for minor stroke, a volume of mismatch above 10 ml was found to be associated with infarct growth and neurological deterioration [9]. However, there are often situations which impede or even prevent the application of contrast media as well as technical problems like motion artefacts complicating the analysis of perfusion maps. In more severe stroke, there is evidence, that mismatch severity may be relevant for selecting patients suitable for thrombolytic treatment [17] with a mismatch ratio of 2.6 proving the highest

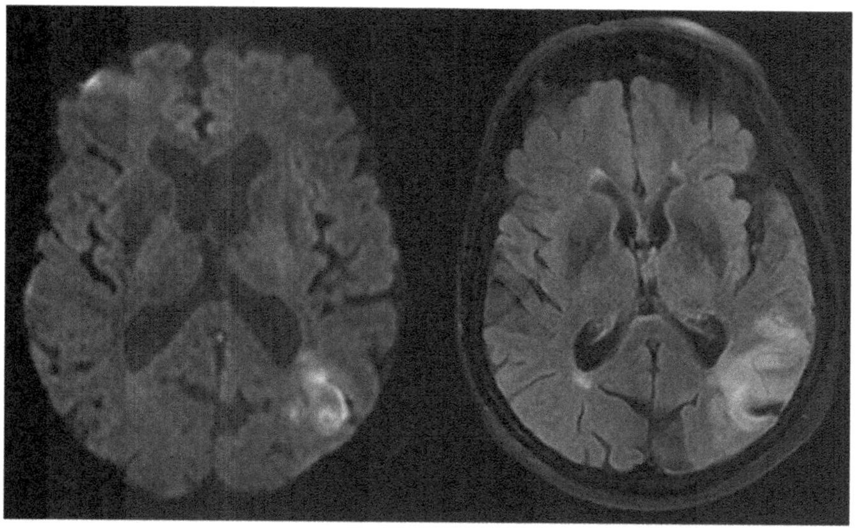

Figure 4. Lesion volume development in minor/moderate stroke without therapy.

sensitivity (90%) and specificity (83%) [18]. In minor stroke this observation was not yet established, but may also apply.

Other studies describe correlations between acute DWI and PI lesion volumes and acute and chronic stroke scales [19–21] with the most powerful predictive parameter for recanalisation being baseline NIHSS score <15 and lower absolute TPP. Furthermore baseline DWI lesion volume was described to be highly correlated with final infarct size ($p<0.0001$) on day 60 [22].

Another strong relationship was reported between infarct extent and location providing a good estimate of neurological deficit within 3 months of stroke onset [23]. However, for the acute/ subacute phase further evidence is required.

The association between the extent of infarct growth and outcome in patients with moderate/severe stroke symptoms has already been proven [24], as well as the contribution of vessel abnormalities [7]. Though, no attempts have been made to assess the prediction of DWI baseline infarct volume on outcome in t-PA treated and untreated minor stroke patients.

As a novel finding in our study, infarct growth was attenuated by thrombolysis in patients with larger DWI infarcts. However, within our small cohort the median mRS at day 90 did not differ significantly in treated and untreated patients, hence, no clear prediction regarding long term outcome can be drawn. Likewise, Urra et al., in a study cohort of 203 patients did not find significant differences in mRS on day 90, but did find a decrease in the mRS in the ordinal regression analysis [25] indicating an improved long term outcome too.

The lack of a significant difference in long term outcome may also be explained by the limited capacity of the mRS in depicting post stroke disorders like fatigue, depression [26] or cognitive problems. These symptoms may be just as likely in low NIHSS stroke patients and can considerably influence quality of life. Hence, other instruments assessing quality of life are required in minor stroke patients [27].

We found no association between vessel status and outcome, but untreated minor stroke patients with vessel occlusions showed, at least for the short term, an increase in infarct volume compared to iv t-PA treated patients, therefore pointing to the effect of thrombolysis. This observation is shared by others [22,28], however, in cohorts of more severe stroke patients compared to our study cohort.

The limitation of our study is clearly the small number of patients, indicating that this study is underpowered to sufficiently predict long term outcome and thus may be considered as only hypothesis generating. Using a median split of baseline DWI volume at 0.7 ml seems to be arbitrary at the moment, however, in dichotomizing the data the influential effect of t-PA treatment could be illustrated. Though, using this method a loss or overestimation of effect size and power in case of bivariate relationships or analysis of independent variables must be kept in mind [13]. Moreover, the extended time window of up to 9 hours after symptom onset may negatively affect lesion volume evolution. This may account for the large increase in large DWI lesion volumes in untreated patients. Another source of bias represents the decision for t-PA treatment based upon clinical reasons alone. Thus, further prospective studies to support or reject our results are required.

Conclusions

The size of baseline DWI infarct volumes can support therapy decision for iv t-PA in minor stroke, in addition to findings of perfusion imaging and NIHSS score. Though, regarding the number of cases, this study must be considered as only hypothesis generating.

Supporting Information

Checklist S1 CONSORT checklist.

Protocol S1 Trial protocol.

Acknowledgments

We thank Ian Wellwood, Ivana Galinovich and Anna Kufner for critical revision of the manuscript and providing advice.

Author Contributions

Conceived and designed the experiments: KV L-AS JBF. Performed the experiments: KV. Analyzed the data: KV UG. Wrote the paper: KV UG CHN HA JBF.

References

1. Hacke W, Kaste M, Bluhmki E, Brozman M, Dávalos A, et al. (2008) Thrombolysis with alteplase 3 to 4·5 hours after acute ischemic stroke. N Engl J Med 359: 1317–1329.
2. National Institute of Neurological Disorders and Stroke rt-PA Stroke Study Group (1995) Tissue plasminogen activator for acute ischemic stroke. N Engl J Med 333: 1581–1587.
3. Nedeltchev K, Schwegler B, Haefeli T, Brekenfeld C, Gralla J, et al. (2007) Outcome of stroke with mild or rapidly improving symptoms. Stroke 38: 2531–2535.
4. Smith EE, Abdullah AR, Petkovska I, Rosenthal E, Koroshetz WJ, et al. (2005) Poor outcomes in patients who do not receive intravenous tissue plasminogen activator because of mild or improving ischemic stroke. Stroke 36: 2497–2499.
5. Barber PA, Zhan J, Demchuk AM, Hill MD, Buchan AM (2001) Why are stroke patients excluded from TPA therapy? An analysis of patient eligibility. Neurology 56: 1015–1020.
6. Rajajee V, Kidwell C, Starkman S, Ovbiagele B, Alger JR, et al. (2006) Early MRI and outcomes of untreated patients with mild or improving ischemic stroke. Neurology 67: 980–984.
7. Coutts SB, Modi J, Patel SK, Demchuk AM, Goyal M, et al; Calgary Stroke Program (2012) CT/CT Angiography and MRI findings predict recurrent stroke after transient ischemic attack and minor stroke. Result of the prospective CATCH study. Stroke 43: 1013–1017.
8. Fiebach JB, Al-Rawi Y, Wintermark M, Furlan AJ, Rowley HA, et al. (2012) Vascular occlusion enables selecting acute ischemic stroke patients for treatment with desmoteplase. Stroke 43: 1561–1566.
9. Asdaghi N, Hill MD, Coulter JI, Butcher KS, Modi J, et al. (2013) Perfusion MR predicts outcome in high-risk transient ischemic attack/minor stroke: a derivation-validation study. Stroke 44: 2486–2492.
10. Kim JT, Park MS, Kim MK, Cho KH (2011) Minor Stroke with total mismatch after acute MCA occlusion. J Neuroimaging 21: 399–402.
11. Hacke W, Albers G, Al-Rawi Y, Bogousslavsky J, Davalos A, et al. (2005) The desmoteplase in acute ischemic stroke trial (DIAS). A phase II MRI-based 9-hour window acute stroke thrombolysis trial with intravenous desmoteplase. Stroke 36: 66–73.
12. Roquer J, Rodriguez-Campello A, Cuadrado-Godia E, Vivanco-Hidalgo M, Jiménez-Conde J, et al. (2010) Acute brain MRI-DWI patterns and stroke recurrence after mild-moderate stroke. J Neurol 257: 947–953.
13. MacCullum RC, Zhang S, Preacher KJ, Rucker DD (2002) On the practice of dichotomization of quantitative variables. Psychol Methods 7: 19–40.
14. Leira EC, Ludwig BR, Gurol E, Torner JC, Adams HP (2012) The types of neurological deficits might not justify withholding treatment in patients with low total National Institutes of Health Stroke Scale scores. Stroke 43: 782–786.
15. Fischer U, Baumgartner A, Arnold M, Nedeltchev K, Gralla J, et al. (2010) What is a minor stroke? Stroke 41: 661–666.
16. Wendt M, Tütüncü S, Fiebach JB, Schweitz JF, Audebert HJ, et al. (2013) Preclusion of ischemic stroke patients from iv-tPA treatment for mild symptoms should not be based on low NIHSS scores. J Stroke Cerebrovasc Dis 22: 550–553.
17. Warach S, Al-Rawi Y, Furlan AJ, Fiebach JB, Wintermark M, et al. (2012) Refinement of the magnetic resonance diffusion-perfusion mismatch concept for thrombolytic patient selection: insights from the desmoteplase in acute stroke trials. Stroke 43: 2313–2318.

18. Kakuda W, Lansberg MG, Thijs VN, Kemp SM, Bammer R, et al. (2008) Optimal definition for PWI/DWI mismatch in acute ischemic stroke patients. J Cereb Blood Flow Metab 28: 887–891.
19. Kimura K, Sakamoto Y, Iguchi Y, Shibazaki K (2011) Serial changes in ischemic lesion volume and neurological recovery after t-PA therapy. J Neurol Sci 304: 35–39.
20. Baird AE, Lövblad KO, Dashe JF, Connor A, Burzynski C, et al. (2000) Clinical correlations of diffusion and perfusion lesion volumes in acute ischemic stroke. Cerebrovasc Dis 10: 441–448.
21. Lövblad KO, Baird AE, Schlaug G, Benfield A, Siewert B, et al. (1997) Ischemic lesion volumes in acute stroke by diffusion-weighted magnetic resonance imaging correlate with clinical outcome. Ann Neurol 42: 164–170.
22. Hermier M, Nighoghossian N, Adeleine P, Berthezène Y, Derex L, et al. (2003) Early magnetic resonance imaging prediction of arterial recanalization and late infarct volume in acute carotid artery stroke. J Cereb Blood Flow Metab 23: 240–248.
23. Phan GP, Chen J, Donnan G, Srikanth V, Wood A, et al. (2010) Development of a new tool to correlate stroke outcome with infarct topography: A proof-of-concept study. Neuroimage 49: 127–133.
24. Barrett KM, Ding YH, Wagner DP, Kallmes DF, Johnston KC, et al. (2009) Change in diffusion-weighted imaging infarct volume predicts neurologic outcome at 90 days. Results of the acute stroke accurate prediction (ASAP) trial serial imaging substudy. Stroke 40: 2422–2427.
25. Urra X, Ariño H, Llull L, Amaro S, Obach V, et al. (2013) The outcome of patients with mild stroke improves after treatment with systemic thrombolysis. PloS one 8: e59420. doi:10.1371/journal.pone.0059420
26. Schwab-Malek S, Vatankhah B, Bogdahn U, Horn M, Audebert HJ (2010) Depressive symptoms and quality of life after thrombolysis in stroke: the TEMPIS study. J Neurol 257: 1848–1854.
27. Schepers VPM, Ketelaar M, Visser-Meily JMA, Dekker J, Lindeman E (2008) Responsiveness of functional health status measures frequently used in stroke research. Disabil Rehabil 28: 1035–1040.
28. Jansen O, Schellinger P, Fiebach JB, Hacke W, Sartor K (1999) Early recanalisation in acute ischaemic stroke saves tissue at risk defined by MRI. Lancet 353: 2036–2037.

Comparison of ^{99m}Tc-3PRGD2 Integrin Receptor Imaging with ^{99m}Tc-MDP Bone Scan in Diagnosis of Bone Metastasis in Patients with Lung Cancer

Weibing Miao[1]*, Shan Zheng[1], Haojie Dai[2], Feng Wang[3], Xiaona Jin[4], Zhaohui Zhu[4]*, Bing Jia[5]

1 Department of Nuclear Medicine, the 1st Affiliated Hospital of Fujian Medical University, Fuzhou, China, **2** Department of Nuclear Medicine, Beijing Tongren Hospital, Beijing, China, **3** Department of Nuclear Medicine, the 1st Affiliated Hospital of Nanjing Medical University, Nanjing, China, **4** Department of Nuclear Medicine, Peking Union Medical College Hospital, Chinese Academy of Medical Sciences and Peking Union Medical College, Beijing, China, **5** Medical Isotopes Research Center, Peking University, Beijing, China

Abstract

Purpose: ^{99m}Tc-3PRGD2, a promising tracer targeting integrin receptor, may serve as a novel tumor-specific agent for single photon emission computed tomography (SPECT). A multi-center study was prospectively designed to evaluate the diagnostic accuracy of ^{99m}Tc-3PRGD2 imaging for bone metastasis in patients with lung cancer in comparison with the conventional ^{99m}Tc-MDP bone scan.

Methods: The patients underwent whole-body scan and chest tomography successively at both 1 h and 4 h after intravenous injection of 11.1 MBq/Kg ^{99m}Tc-3PRGD2. ^{99m}Tc-MDP whole-body bone scan was routinely performed within 1 week for comparison. Three experienced nuclear medicine physicians blindly read the ^{99m}Tc-3PRGD2 and ^{99m}Tc-MDP images. The final diagnosis was established based on the comprehensive assessment of all available data.

Results: A total of 44 patients (29 male, 59±10 years old) with suspected lung cancer were recruited from 4 centers. Eighty-nine bone lesions in 18 patients were diagnosed as metastases and 23 bone lesions in 9 patients were benign. In a lesion-based analysis, ^{99m}Tc-3PRGD2 imaging demonstrated a sensitivity, specificity, and accuracy of 92.1%, 91.3%, and 92.0%, respectively. The corresponding diagnostic values for ^{99m}Tc-MDP bone scan were 87.6%, 60.9%, and 82.1%, respectively in the same patients. ^{99m}Tc-MDP bone scan had better contrast in most lesions, whereas the ^{99m}Tc-3PRGD2 imaging seemed to be more effective to exclude pseudo-positive lesions and detect bone metastases without osteogenesis.

Conclusion: ^{99m}Tc-3PRGD2 is a novel tumor-specific agent based on SPECT technology with a promising value in diagnosis of bone metastasis in patients with lung cancer.

Trial Registration: ClinicalTrials.gov NCT01737112

Editor: Adriano Angelucci, University of L'Aquila, Italy

Funding: This work was financially supported, in part, by the Fujian Provincial Natural Science Foundation (2010J01154), the Capital Special Project for Featured Clinical Application (Z111107058811096), the National Natural Science Foundation of China (NSFC) projects (81171369, 81171370, 81271614, 81071189, 81000625, 30900373, 30930030, 30870728, and 30870725), the Outstanding Youth Fund (81125011), a "973" project (2011CB707703), and grants from the Ministry of Science and Technology of China (2011YQ030114 and 2012ZX09102301-018). The funders had no role in study design, data collection and analysis, decision to publish, or preparation of the manuscript.

Competing Interests: The authors have declared that no competing interests exist.

* Email: miaoweibing@126.com (WM); zhuzhh@pumch.cn (ZZ)

Introduction

Lung cancer is one of the most fatal diseases worldwide. Early diagnosis and accurate evaluation of bone metastasis of lung cancer are essential for therapeutic planning and relapse monitoring [1–3]. Bone scan using ^{99m}Tc-MDP as the tracer is applied to detect bone metastasis. However, its diagnostic value is limited because of the low specificity.

Integrin is mainly involved in the cell-cell and cell-matrix interactions. Integrin $\alpha_v\beta_3$, an important member of the integrin family, is highly relevant to neoplastic angiogenesis, invasion, and metastasis. It is not expressed at all or expressed at a very low level on the quiescent endothelium and other normal tissues [4–8]. Therefore, the integrin $\alpha_v\beta_3$ receptor may be a promising target in the diagnosis, evaluation, and treatment of malignancies [9–12], serving as a tumor-specific agent for single photon emission computed tomography (SPECT).

The tri-peptide sequence of arginine-glycine-aspartic acid (RGD), especially in the cyclic form, has shown high affinity in binding with the receptors of integrin $\alpha_v\beta_3$. Some radiolabeled cyclic RGD monomer peptides, such as ^{18}F-Galacto-RGD, ^{18}F-

Table 1. The recruited patient number and SPECT systems of the 4 centers.

Centers	Recruited patients	SPECT system
The 1st Affiliated Hospital of Fujian Medical University, Fuzhou	21	GE Infinia Hawkeye
Beijing Tongren Hospital, Beijing	11	GE Infinia Hawkeye4
The 1st Affiliated Hospital of Nanjing Medical University, Nanjing	8	Siemens Symbia T6
Peking Union Medical College Hospital, Beijing (The organizing center)	4	Philips Precedence 16

AH111585, and ^{99m}Tc-NC100692, have thus been translated into clinical use and showed potential in the detection of breast and lung cancers [13–20]. ^{99m}Tc-HYNIC-3PEG$_4$-E[c(RGDfK)$_2$] (^{99m}Tc-3PRGD2 in short) is a new cyclic RGD dimmer peptide separated by three PEGs. It shows much higher affinity to integrin $\alpha_v\beta_3$, which enables its higher tumor accumulation than the prior RGD monomer tracers [21–27]. As a SPECT tracer, it is cost-effective and broadly available. Most importantly, it may serve as a novel SPECT tracer specific for the detection of malignant tumors.

In a prior study, we have preliminarily demonstrated that ^{99m}Tc-3PRGD2 imaging at 1 h after injection was sensitive for the detection of lung cancer [28]. This prospective multi-center study was designed to investigate the value of ^{99m}Tc-3PRGD2 as compared with ^{99m}Tc-MDP in the assessment of bone metastasis of lung cancer.

Materials and Methods

The protocol for this trial and supporting CONSORT checklist are available as supporting information; see Checklist S1 and Protocol S1.

Patients

A total of 44 patients (29 males and 15 females; aged from 41 to 76 years old, mean age ±SD, 59.2±9.7) with suspected lung lesions were recruited from 4 centers in China from Feb. 2011 to Jan. 2014, and their definite pathological diagnoses were obtained (Table 1). This study had been approved by the Institute Review Board of Peking Union Medical College Hospital, Chinese Academy of Medical Sciences & Peking Union Medical College firstly and then by each center, including the 1st Affiliated Hospital of Fujian Medical University, Beijing Tongren Hospital and the 1st Affiliated Hospital of Nanjing Medical University. It was part of the clinical trial registered online at NIH ClinicalTrial.gov (NCT01737112). The main reason for the delay in registering the study was to protect the idea of the study. The authors confirm that all ongoing and related trials for this drug/intervention are registered. All the participants provided their written informed consent to participate in this study, and the records were saved by each center. All the patients were identified with suspected primary lung cancer in accordance with the findings of computed tomography (CT) performed within 2 weeks. The "standard of truth" for diagnosis of the lung lesions was based on histopathological findings of surgery or fine needle or bronchoscopic biopsy, and for that of bone lesions was based on the comprehensive analysis of the outcome. The diagnosis of all the bone lesions was confirmed from at least 2 imaging modalities (SPECT/CT/MRI/^{18}F-FDG PET-CT) and 6-month follow-up (Table 2). Patients' clinical records were also taken into consideration. Consensus reading of ^{99m}Tc-3PRGD2 and ^{99m}Tc-MDP images was performed on the same workstation by three experienced nuclear medicine physicians.

Radiopharmaceutical preparation

The kit for preparation of ^{99m}Tc-3PRGD2 was supplied by the Medical Isotopes Research Center, Peking University. Synthesis of the labeling precursor, kit preparation, and ^{99m}Tc-labeling were previously described [27]. ^{99m}Tc-MDP was supplied by the Atom

Table 2. Flowchart of the study.

RESEARCH PROCESS	V1	V2	V3	V4(Surgery)	V5(Follow-up)
Window period		Less than two weeks interval to V4	Less than one week interval to V2		once every 3–6 months
Inclusion/Exclusion criteria	X				
Signed Informed Consent Form	X				
Medical history/Concomitant diseases	X				
CT, MRI, PET/CT	X				
Tumor markers and other laboratory tests	X				
^{99m}Tc-3PRGD$_2$ SPECT		X			
^{99m}Tc-MDP whole body scan			X		
Adverse events		X			
Surgical records and pathology results				X	
Preserved specimens				X	
Subsequent treatment and follow-up					X

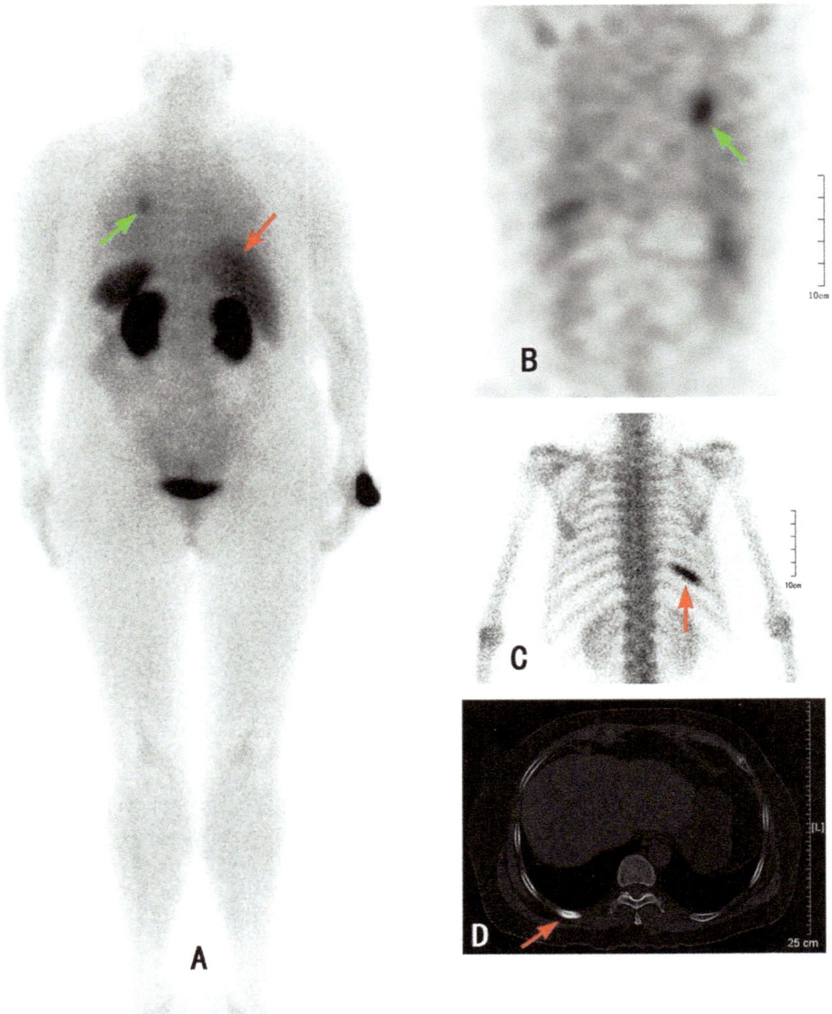

Figure 1. Comparison of ^{99m}Tc-3PRGD2 SPECT, ^{99m}Tc-MDP bone scan (posterior), and CT scan in a 62 year-old woman with left upper lung adenocarcinoma (green arrow) and costal metastasis (red arrow). A: ^{99m}Tc -3PRGD2 WB(+), B: ^{99m}Tc -3PRGD2 SPECT (+), C: ^{99m}Tc -MDP bone scan (+), D: CT (+). WB: whole body.

High-tech Company of China. The radiochemical purity was > 95%.

Imaging protocol

All the scanners were dual-head gamma-cameras, using low-energy high-resolution collimators and a 20% energy window centered on 140 keV. After intravenous injection of 11.1 MBq/kg ^{99m}Tc-3PRGD2, whole body planar scan (10 cm/min) and chest SPECT imaging (zoom ×1, 30 sec/frame/6°) were performed at dual time-points of 1 h and 4 h (^{99m}Tc have a half life of 6 h). ^{99m}Tc-MDP whole body images were acquired at a scan speed of 10 cm/min within 1 week before or after ^{99m}Tc-3PRGD2 imaging.

Image and statistical analyses

Visual image analysis was completed through consensus reading by 3 experienced nuclear medicine physicians blind to the history and pathological diagnosis. All the bone lesions were evaluated lesion by lesion on both whole-body scan and thoracic SPECT images. The image quality, number of lesions, and diagnosis (benign or malignant) were documented.

The sensitivity, specificity, accuracy, positive predictive value (PPV), and negative predictive value (NPV) were employed to determine the efficacy of ^{99m}Tc-3PRGD2 imaging for the diagnosis of bone metastases. The corresponding parameters of ^{99m}Tc-MDP were also calculated for comparison. Chi square test (χ^2 test) was used to make comparison of the rates of different samples, with $P<0.05$ considered significant by using SPSS 15.0 software package.

Results

Among the 44 recruited patients, 38 were confirmed to have pulmonary malignancy, including adenocarcinoma (n = 18), squamous cell carcinoma (n = 13), small cell lung cancer (n = 3), adenosquamous carcinoma (n = 1), metastatic adenocarcinoma (n = 2), and metastatic melanoma (n = 1); 6 were diagnosed with benign lesions, including inflammatory pseudo-tumor (n = 2), granuloma of tuberculosis (n = 2), and fungal infection (n = 2).

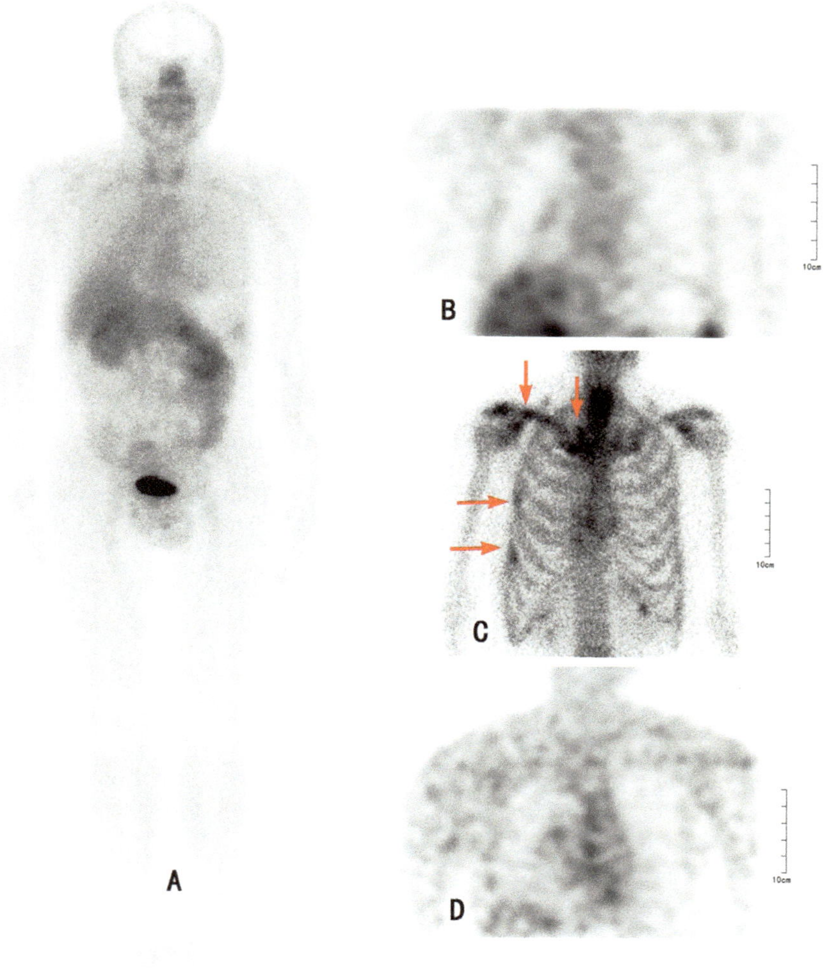

Figure 2. Comparison of ^{99m}Tc-3PRGD2 SPECT, ^{99m}Tc -MDP bone scan, and ^{18}F-FDG PET in a 60 year-old patient with a recent fall-down trauma. The^{99m}Tc -MDP bone scan was positive (red arrows), whereas both ^{99m}Tc-3PRGD2 SPECT and ^{18}F-FDG PET were negative. A: ^{99m}Tc-3PRGD2 WB (-), B: ^{99m}Tc-3PRGD2 SPECT (−), C: ^{99m}Tc-MDP bone scan (+), D: ^{18}F-FDG PET (−). WB: whole body.

In the 44 recruited patients, 27 were found with bone lesions. According to the comprehensive assessment, 18 patients were diagnosed with bone metastasis and 9 with benign bone lesion (Fig. 1–4). In the lesion-based analysis of the 27 patients, 112 bone lesions were detected in total, among which 89 were diagnosed as bone metastasis and 23 were benign lesions. The diagnostic efficacy for the assessment of bone metastasis was compared among the 1-h and 4-h ^{99m}Tc-3PRGD2 imaging and the ^{99m}Tc-MDP whole-body scan (Table 3).

Comparison between the 1-h and 4-h ^{99m}Tc-3PRGD2 imaging in evaluation of bone metastasis

The 4-h ^{99m}Tc-3PRGD2 images showed more prominent uptake in the bone marrow and bowels than the 1-h images, which caused difficulties in identifying bone lesions, especially in the vertebral and pelvic regions (Fig. 3 and 4). According to the lesion-based analysis, the 1-h ^{99m}Tc-3PRGD2 imaging revealed more bone lesions than the 4-h imaging. Both false positive and false negative lesions were more common in the 4-h imaging than in the 1-h imaging. On the 1-h images, there were 2 false positive lesions located in thoracic vertebra (n = 2); whereas on the 4-h images, except for the above-mentioned 2 false positive lesions, there were 4 more false positive lesions in the ribs. Seven false negative lesions occurred in the ribs (n = 5), lumbar vertebra (n = 1), and ilium (n = 1) on the 1-h images; whereas on the 4-h images there were totally 22 false negative lesions, including in the ribs (n = 12), lumbar vertebra (n = 6), ilium (n = 2), and other sites (n = 2).

The sensitivity, accuracy and NPV of the 1-h imaging were 92.1%, 92.0% and 75.0% respectively. These values remarkably decreased to 75.3%, 75.0% and 43.6% on the 4-h imaging ($P <$ 0.05) (Table 3). The specificity and PPV had no significant difference between the 1-h imaging and the 4-h imaging.

Comparison between the 1-h/4-h ^{99m}Tc-3PRGD2 imaging and the ^{99m}Tc-MDP scan

The sensitivity of 1-h 99mTc-3PRGD2 imaging was 92.1% for detection of bone metastasis, and there was no statistical difference between the 1-h 99mTc-3PRGD2 imaging and 99mTc-MDP bone scan (P>0.05). Although ^{99m}Tc-3PRGD2 imaging failed to spot some small lesions as found on ^{99m}Tc-MDP scintigraphy

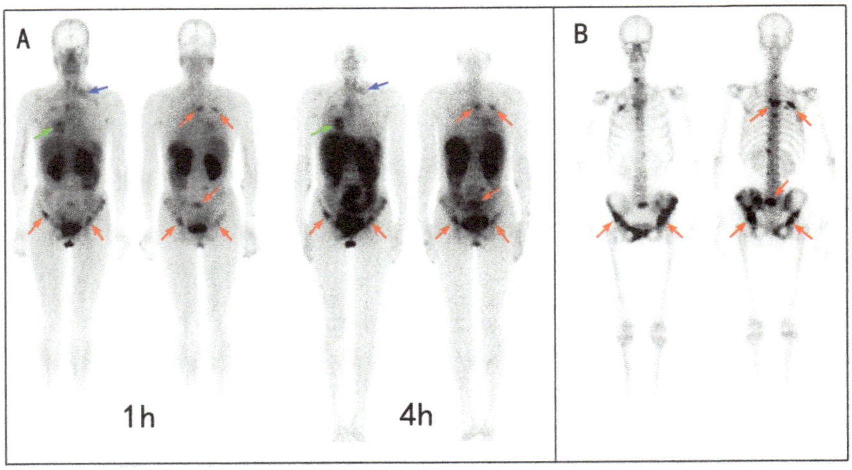

Figure 3. Comparison of ^{99m}Tc-3PRGD2 integrin receptor imaging with ^{99m}Tc-MDP bone scan in a patient with multiple bone metastases. A: The ^{99m}Tc-3PRGD2 imaging showed the lung cancer (green arrow), lymph node metastases (blue arrow), and bone metastases (red arrow) at the same time. The 1-h imaging is better than the 4-h imaging because of the relatively lower background in bone marrow, liver, and spleen. B. ^{99m}Tc-MDP bone scan demonstrated better contrast, facilitating the detection of small bone lesions. However, ^{99m}Tc-MDP accumulated for the bone repair with limited specificity, whereas ^{99m}Tc-3PRGD2 targeted the metastatic tumor directly.

(Fig. 3), it also revealed some lesions undetectable on ^{99m}Tc-MDP scintigraphy (Fig. 4). Moreover, the specificity, accuracy, and PPV were 91.3%, 92.0%, and 97.6%, respectively for the 1-h ^{99m}Tc-3PRGD2 imaging, significantly higher than those for the ^{99m}Tc-MDP bone scan ($P<0.05$). However, the 4-h ^{99m}Tc-3PRGD2 imaging showed significantly lower sensitivity (75.3%) than the ^{99m}Tc-MDP bone scan ($P<0.05$), whereas no significant difference was found between the two methods in the specificity, accuracy, PPV, and NPV (Table 3).

Discussion

Integrin $\alpha_v\beta_3$, an important receptor in the integrin family, is highly relevant to neoplastic angiogenesis. Integrin $\alpha_v\beta_3$ is highly expressed in neovascular endothelium and many kinds of tumor cells; in contrast, it is rarely found in normal tissues and quiescent endothelium. This characteristic makes it an important target in the diagnosis and treatment of malignancies [9–11]. ^{99m}Tc-3PRGD2, a novel radiolabeled RGD-based peptide targeting integrin $\alpha_v\beta_3$ receptor, has recently been translated into clinical application [28]. Compared to the previous RGD-based tracers

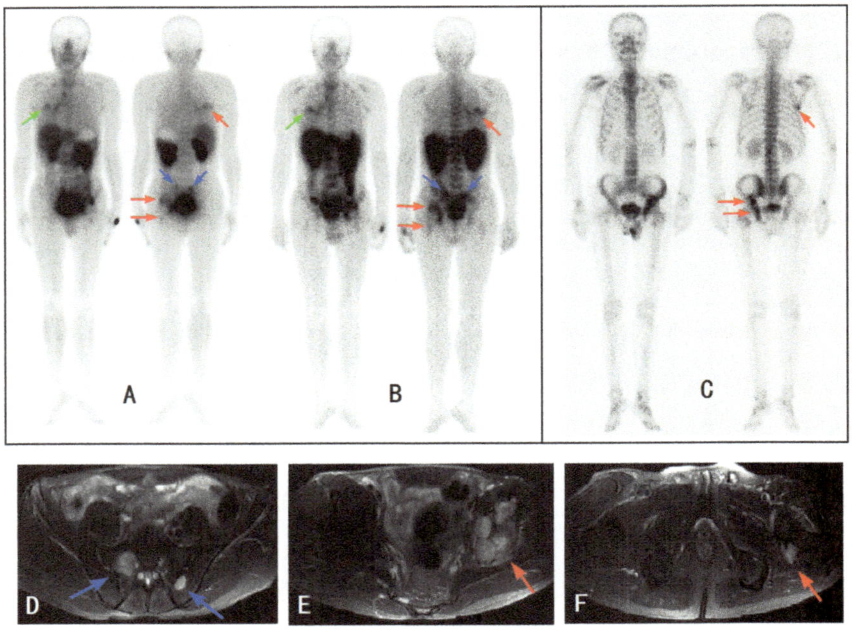

Figure 4. A 48 year-old man with right lung adenocarcinoma (green arrow) and multiple bone metastases (red and blue arrows). ^{99m}Tc-3PRGD2 scans showed two more bone metastases (blue arrows) than the ^{99m}Tc-MDP bone scan. The lesions were confirmed by MRI (lower row). A: 1-h ^{99m}Tc-3PRGD2, B: 4-h ^{99m}Tc-3PRGD2, C: ^{99m}Tc-MDP, D–F: MRI.

Table 3. Comparison of the diagnostic efficacy of ^{99m}Tc-3PRGD2 integrin receptor imaging and ^{99m}Tc-MDP bone scan for bone metastasis.

	Sensitivity	Specificity	Accuracy	PPV	NPV
1-h RGD	**92.1%(82/89)**	**91.3%(21/23)**	**92.0%(103/112)**	**97.6%(82/84)**	**75.0%(21/28)**
4-h RGD	**75.3%(67/89)**	**73.9%(17/23)**	**75.0%(84/112)**	**91.8%(67/73)**	**43.6%(17/39)**
MDP	**87.6%(78/89)**	**60.9%(14/23)**	**82.1%(92/112)**	**89.7%(78/87)**	**56.0%(14/25)**
a	0.989	5.855	4.793	4.503	2.126
X^2 b	4.501	0.890	1.697	0.211	0.939
c	9.269	1.362	11.687	1.678	6.550
a	0.320	**0.016**	**0.029**	**0.034**	0.145
P b	0.034	0.345	0.193	0.646	0.332
c	**0.002**	0.243	**0.001**	0.195	**0.010**

a:1-h RGD vs. MDP.
b:4-h RGD vs. MDP.
c:1-h vs. 4-h RGD.
PPV: positive predictive value; NPV: negative predictive value; RGD: ^{99m}Tc-3PRGD2 imaging; MDP: ^{99m}Tc-MDP bone scan.

such as ^{18}F-Galacto-RGD, ^{18}F-AH111585, and ^{99m}Tc-NC100692, the RGD dimmer structure of ^{99m}Tc-3PRGD2 has significantly enhanced binding affinity to integrin $\alpha_v\beta_3$, resulting in higher and prominent accumulation in tumors [21–27]. Moreover, ^{99m}Tc-3PRGD2 is a SPECT tracer that is more cost-effective and can be more widely applied in clinical practice. A recent multi-center study has revealed the importance of ^{99m}Tc-3PRGD2 in diagnosis of lung cancer [28]. As a further interest, this study compared ^{99m}Tc-3PRGD2 imaging with ^{99m}Tc-MDP bone scan in diagnosis of bone metastasis. To the best of our knowledge, it is the first integrin receptor imaging study focused on the evaluation of bone metastasis.

^{99m}Tc-MDP whole body scan has been widely used in the detection of bone metastasis with high sensitivity but poor specificity. ^{99m}Tc-3PRGD2 can specifically bind to integrin $\alpha_v\beta_3$ receptor in tumor angiogenesis and various types of tumor cells as well [26,27], offering a promising radio-labeled tracer that can compensate the insufficiency of ^{99m}Tc-MDP bone scan in the diagnosis of bone metastasis. This study showed that the 1-h ^{99m}Tc-3PRGD2 imaging had higher specificity, accuracy and PPV than ^{99m}Tc-MDP bone scan in diagnosing bone metastasis of lung cancer. However, integrin avb3 is also expressed on osteoclasts and osteoblasts. This may associate with the false positive and false negative conditions in the patients, although much less than those in the ^{99m}Tc-MDP bone scans. In this study, false positive lesions mainly occurred in thoracic vertebra and were later diagnosed as degenerative changes via comprehensive analysis of CT, MRI, and follow-ups. As known already, some kinds of inflammation can also have neo-vasculature [29,30] and may cause ^{99m}Tc-3PRGD2 accumulation. The false negative lesions occurred most frequently in ribs and lumbar vertebra. The main reason was the moderate to intense ^{99m}Tc-3PRGD2 accumulation in the liver, spleen, bowel, and kidneys. The physiological distribution might make the mild-uptake lesions undetectable on the planar images. However, some of the lesions could be found on the SPECT images. On the other hand, ^{99m}Tc-3PRGD2 is a receptor tracer targeting the tumor cells directly. Therefore, ^{99m}Tc-3PRGD2 imaging may detect some bone metastases undetectable via the ^{99m}Tc-MDP bone scan when no obvious osteogenesis or osteolytic changes exist (Fig. 4).

The sensitivity, accuracy, and NPV were remarkably higher on the 1-h ^{99m}Tc-3PRGD2 imaging when compared to those on the 4-h imaging. There were several probable reasons. First, the blood pool background of the 1-h images was low enough. The elimination of ^{99m}Tc-3PRGD2 in blood pool was rather fast. Jia B. et al discovered that the ^{99m}Tc-3PRGD2 in blood circulation became very low even at 15 minutes [27]. Second, the uptake of the bone marrow and the bowel was higher at 4 h than those at 1 h. The detection of bone lesions was thus more difficult when imaged at 4 h, especially in the lumbar vertebra and pelvic regions. Third, the ^{99m}Tc-3PRGD2 uptake in the bone lesions was similar or even relatively decreased at 4 h in this group of patients. Therefore, the 1-h ^{99m}Tc-3PRGD2 imaging was usually enough for the detection of bone metastasis, whereas performing another imaging at 4 h was time-consuming and inconvenient with few aids to the diagnosis.

There are some limitations of this study. First, it is a challenge to diagnose bone metastasis without pathological confirmation of each lesion. In this study, we employed the comprehensive analysis of all available data as the gold standard; whereas the readers assessed the lesions blind to the other data. Second, the data came from 4 different centers with different SPECT system, resulting in unavoidable variation in images. However, this study was designed prospectively in a way that all SPECT systems met the quality control and the studies strictly followed the same protocol. All the images passed the quality control before a centralized reading. The third limitation of this study is the relatively small number of patients. Further studies involving more patients are suggested, as the current results preliminarily indicate the value of ^{99m}Tc-3PRGD2 imaging as a promising tool to compensate the limited specificity of ^{99m}Tc-MDP bone scan. Based on the findings in this study and as an interest in further clarifying the value of ^{99m}Tc-3PRGD2 imaging, ^{99m}Tc-3PRGD2 imaging may be employed for early assessment of therapeutic response of bone metastasis to compensate the limitation of the conventional imaging methods, including ^{99m}Tc-MDP bone scan, CT, and MRI.

In conclusion, this multi-center study indicates that the 1-h ^{99m}Tc-3PRGD2 imaging has higher specificity, accuracy, and PPV than the ^{99m}Tc-MDP whole body scan in diagnosis of bone metastasis, meriting further studies with more patients. Moreover, the 1-h ^{99m}Tc-3PRGD2 imaging is better than the 4-h imaging and is usually enough for the detection of bone metastasis in patients with lung cancer.

Supporting Information

Checklist S1 CONSORT checklist for the trial.

Protocol S1 Protocol for the trial.

Author Contributions

Conceived and designed the experiments: WM HD FW ZZ. Performed the experiments: WM SZ XJ HD FW. Analyzed the data: WM SZ XJ HD FW ZZ. Contributed reagents/materials/analysis tools: BJ. Wrote the paper: WM ZZ SZ.

References

1. Goldstraw P, Crowley J, Chansky K, Giroux DJ, Groome PA, et al. (2007) The IASLC Lung Cancer Staging Project: proposals for the revision of the TNM stage groupings in the forthcoming (seventh) edition of the TNM Classification of malignant tumours. J Thorac Oncol 2: 706–14.
2. Higgins MJ, Ettinger DS (2009) Chemotherapy for lung cancer: the state of the art in 2009. Expert Rev Anticancer Ther 9: 1365–78.
3. Nishino M, Jackman DM, Hatabu H, Jänne PA, Johnson BE, et al. (2011) Imaging of lung cancer in the era of molecular medicine. Acad Radiol 18: 424–36.
4. Hood JD, Cheresh DA (2002) Role of integrins in cell invasion and migration. Nat Rev Cancer 2: 91–100.
5. Brooks PC, Clark RA, Cheresh DA (1994) Requirement of vascular integrin alphav beta3 for angiogenesis. Science 264: 569–71.
6. Ruoslahti E (2002) Specialization of tumour vasculature. Nat Rev Cancer 2: 83–90.
7. Sengupta S, Chattopadhyay N, Mitra A, Ray S, Dasgupta S, et al. (2001) Role of αvβ3 integrin receptors in breast tumor. J Exp Clin Cancer Res 20: 585–90.
8. Zitzmann S, Ehemann V, Schwab M (2002) Arginine-Glycine-Aspartic acid (RGD)-peptide binds to both tumor and tumor endothelial cells in vivo. Cancer Res 62: 5139–43.
9. Costouros NG, Diehn FE, Libutti SK (2002) Molecular imaging of tumor angiogenesis. J Cell Biochem (Suppl) 39: 72–8.
10. Liu S, Robinson SP, Edwards DS (2005) Radiolabeled integrin αvβ3 antagonists as radiopharmaceuticals for tumor radiotherapy. Topics in Current Chem 252: 117–53.
11. Haubner R, Wester HJ (2004) Radiolabeled tracers for imaging of tumor angiogenesis and evaluation of anti-angiogenic therapies. Curr Pharm Des 10: 1439–55.
12. Pasqualini R, Koivunen E, Ruoslahti E (1997) Alpha v integrins as receptors for tumor targeting by circulating ligands. Nat Biotechnol 15: 542–6.
13. Haubner R, Weber WA, Beer AJ, Vabuliene E, Reim D, et al. (2005) Noninvasive visualization of the activated αVβ3 integrin in cancer patients by positron emission tomography and [18F] Galacto-RGD. PLOS Med 2: 244–52.
14. Haubner R, Wester HJ, Weber WA, Mang C, Ziegler SI, et al. (2001) Noninvasive imaging of αvβ3 integrin expression using 18F-labeled RGD-containing glycopeptide and positron emission tomography. Cancer Research 61: 1781–5.
15. Beer AJ, Haubner R, Goebel M, Luderschmidt S, Spilker ME, et al. (2005) Biodistribution and pharmacokinetics of the αvβ3-selective tracer 18F-Galacto-RGD in cancer patients. J Nucl Med 46: 1333–41.
16. Beer AJ, Haubner R, Sarbia M, Goebel M, Luderschmidt S, et al. (2006) Positron emission tomography using [18F]Galacto-RGD identifies the level of integrin αVβ3 expression in man. Clin Cancer Res 12: 3942–9.
17. McParland BJ, Miller MP, Spinks TJ, Kenny LM, Osman S, et al. (2008) The biodistribution and radiation dosimetry of the Arg-Gly-Asp peptide 18F-AH111585 in healthy volunteers. J Nucl Med 49: 1664–7.
18. Kenny LM, Coombes RC, Oulie I, Contractor KB, Miller M, et al. (2008) Phase I trial of the positron-emitting Arg-Gly-Asp peptide radioligand 18F-AH111585 in breast cancer patients. J Nucl Med 49: 879–86.
19. Bach-Gansmo T, Danielsson R, Saracco A, Wilczek B, Bogsrud TV, et al. (2006) Integrin receptor imaging of breast cancer: a proof-of-concept study to evaluate 99mTc-NC100692. J Nucl Med 47: 1434–9.
20. Axelsson R, Bach-Gansmo T, Castell-Conesa J, McParland BJ; Study Group (2010) An open-label, multi-center, phase 2a study to assess the feasibility of imaging metastases in late-stage cancer patients with the αVβ3-selective angiogenesis imaging agent 99mTc-NC100692. Acta Radiol 51: 40–6.
21. Liu Z, Niu G, Shi J, Liu S, Wang F, et al. (2009) (68)Ga-labeled cyclic RGD dimers with Gly3 and PEG4 linkers: promising agents for tumor integrin alphavbeta3 PET imaging. Eur J Nucl Med Mol Imaging 36: 947–57.
22. Liu Z, Liu S, Wang F, Liu S, Chen X (2009) Noninvasive imaging of tumor integrin expression using (18)F-labeled RGD dimer peptide with PEG (4) linkers. Eur J Nucl Med Mol Imaging 36: 1296–307.
23. Shi J, Wang L, Kim YS, Zhai S, Jia B, et al. (2009) 99mTcO(MAG2-3G3-dimer): a new integrin alpha(v)beta(3)- targeted SPECT radiotracer with high tumor uptake and favorable pharmacokinetics. Eur J Nucl Med Mol Imaging 36: 1874–84.
24. Wang L, Shi J, Kim YS, Zhai S, Jia B, et al. (2009) Improving tumor-targeting capability and pharmacokinetics of (99m)Tc-labeled cyclic RGD dimers with PEG(4) linkers. Mol Pharm 6: 231–45.
25. Shi J, Kim YS, Chakraborty S, Jia B, Wang F, et al. (2009) 2-Mercaptoacetylglycylglycyl (MAG2) as a bifunctional chelator for 99mTc-labeling of cyclic RGD dimers: effect of technetium chelate on tumor uptake and pharmacokinetics. Bioconjugate Chem 20: 1559–68.
26. Liu Z, Jia B, Shi J, Jin X, Zhao H, et al. (2010) Tumor uptake of the RGD dimeric probe 99mTc-G3-2P4-RGD2 is correlated with integrin αVβ3 expressed on both tumor cells and neovasculature. Bioconjug Chem 21: 548–55.
27. Jia B, Liu Z, Zhu Z, Shi J, Jin X, et al. (2011) Blood clearance kinetics, biodistribution, and radiation dosimetry of a kit-formulated integrin αVβ3-selective radiotracer 99mTc-3PRGD2 in non-human primates. Mol Imaging Biol 13: 730–6.
28. Zhu Z, Miao W, Li Q, Dai H, Ma Q, et al. (2012) 99mTc-3PRGD2 for integrin receptor imaging of lung cancer: a multi-center study. J Nucl Med 53: 716–22.
29. Pichler BJ, Kneilling M, Haubner R, Braumüller H, Schwaiger M, et al. (2005) Imaging of delayed-type hypersensitivity reaction by PET and 18FGalacto-RGD. J Nucl Med 46: 184–9.
30. McDonald DM, Choyke PL (2003) Imaging of angiogenesis: From microscope to clinic. Nature Medicine 9: 713–25.

MR Quantification of Total Liver Fat in Patients with Impaired Glucose Tolerance and Healthy Subjects

Zhi Dong[1,¶], Yanji Luo[1,¶], Zhongwei Zhang[2], Huasong Cai[1], Yanbing Li[3], Tao Chan[4], Ling Wu[5], Zi-Ping Li[1*], Shi-Ting Feng[1*]

1 Department of Radiology, The First Affiliated Hospital of Sun Yat-Sen University, Guangzhou, China, **2** Department of Radiology, The University of Texas Southwestern Medical Center, Dallas, Texas, United States of America, **3** Department of Endocrinology and Diabetes Center, The First Affiliated Hospital of Sun Yat-sen University, Guangzhou, China, **4** Medical Imaging Department, Union Hospital, Hong Kong, **5** Department of Radiology, Kiang Wu Hospital, Macao

Abstract

Objective: To explore the correlations between liver fat content and clinical index in patients with impaired glucose tolerance (IGT) and healthy subjects.

Materials and Methods: 56 subjects were enrolled and each of them underwent upper-abdominal MRI examination that involved a T1 VIBE Dixon sequence. 14 was clinically diagnosed with IGT (collectively as IGT group) while 42 showed normal glucose tolerance,(collectively as NGT group). NGT group was further divided into NGTFat (BMI≥25, 18 subjects) and NGTLean (BMI<25, 24 subjects). The total liver fat contents was measured and compared with clinical findings and laboratory results in order to determine statistical correlations between these parameters. Differences among IGT, NGTFat and NGTLean groups were evaluated.

Results: For all the subjects, fat volume fractions (FVFs) ranged from 4.2% to 24.2%, positive correlations was observed with BMI, waist hip ratio(WHR), low density lipoprotein(LDL), fasting plasma insulin(FPI), homeostasis model assessment insulin resistance (HOMA-IR) and homeostasis model assessment β(HOMAβ). FVFs of IGT group (p = 0.004) and NGTFat group (p = 0.006) were significantly higher than those of NGTLean group.

Conclusions: People with higher BMI, WHR and LDL levels tend to have higher liver fat content. Patients with BMI≥25 are more likely to develop IGT. Patients with higher FVF showed higher resistance to insulin, thus obtained a higher risk of developing type 2 diabetes mellitus.

Editor: Melania Manco, Scientific Directorate, Bambino Hospital, Italy

Funding: This work was funded by National Natural Science Foundation of China (81000626), Natural Science Foundation of Guangdong Province (S2013010016004), Zhujiang Scientific and Technological New Star Foundation (2012J2200084), and the Fundamental Research Funds for the Central Universities (10ykpy11). The funders had no role in study design, data collection and analysis, decision to publish, or preparation of the manuscript.

Competing Interests: The authors have declared that no competing interests exist.

* Email: fst1977@163.com (STF); liziping163@163.com (ZL)

These authors contributed equally to this work.

¶ ZD and YJL are co-first authors on this work

Introduction

Ectopic fat deposition is commonly seen in many diseases, especially in metabolic disorders, such as obesity, insulin resistance, and other components of metabolic syndrome. It plays an important role in the development and progression of nonalcoholic fatty liver disease (NAFLD) [1–3]. It is thought to have direct positive impact on the increasing rate of obesity and NAFLD prevalence across the world [4]. According to some researchers, about 10~20% patients with NAFLD are affected by the progressive form of NAFLD, otherwise known as nonalcoholic steatohepatitis (NASH) where 20~30% of patients with NASH will develop cirrhosis and end-stage liver disease [5–7].

Liver fat content is an essential indicator for the progression of NAFLD [8]. So far, many techniques and methods have been developed for diagnosing fatty liver disease and quantifying liver fat content. This can be achieved by techniques such as liver biopsy/pathology, computed tomography (CT) scanning, ultrasound, and magnetic resonance imaging (MRI). However, all these techniques have various shortcomings. For example, the gold standard for assessing fat content in liver, biopsy/pathology, is invasive and subjective to sampling error [9–12]. CT can only be used to detect the existence of fat but not to measure the total amount of the fat content. Furthermore, the accumulative radiation exposure from repeated CT scans can be harmful which limits its role in evaluating disease progression during long term follow up. In comparison, Magnetic resonance (MR) spectroscopy has been widely-applied and can provide accurate evaluation of hepatic fat content, however, it is time consuming and evaluation only limits to part of the liver [13–15].

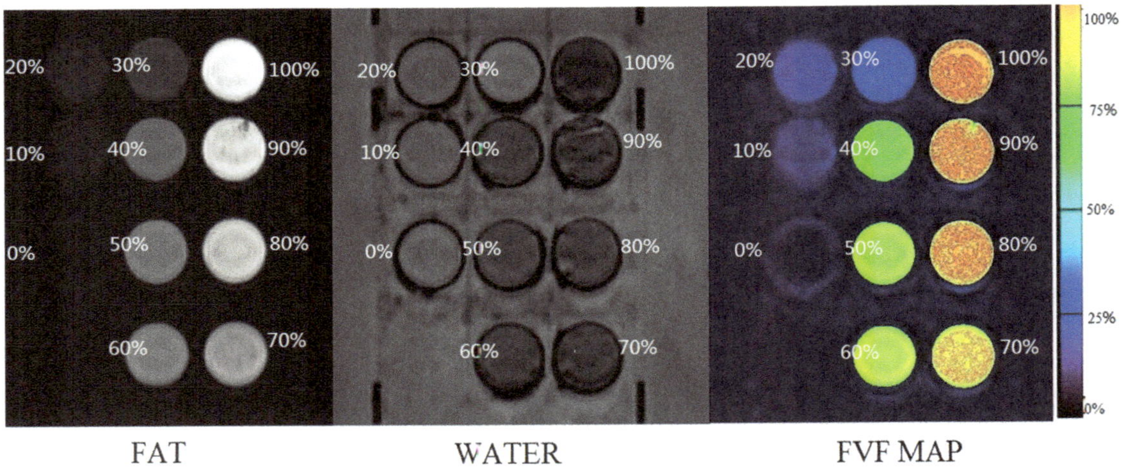

Figure 1. Results of phantom experiment. The bottle on the lower left side is filled with pure water (fat content: 0%), and the upper right one is filled with 100% peanut oil, while others have fat content ranging from 10% to 90% in sequence. In the fat phase image, the higher the fat content is, the higher signal intensity can be seen. But in water phase, the signal intensity of each bottle turned opposite to that of fat phase. The fat volume fraction (FVF) map demonstrates clear differences for different amounts of fat and water through the change of color.

MR technique for quantifying fat content is based on chemical shift imaging. It is one of the most promising techniques due to its non-invasive, radiation-free and easy-to-perform characteristics [14,16]. Dixon technique is a two-point chemical shift-based fat-water separation method described by Dixon in 1984 [17]. It acquires two images with different echo times (TE) to separate the fat signals from the water signals in the same voxel (in-phase and out-of-phase). Pure fat image and water image are obtained by the following equation:

$$W = \frac{SIP + SOP}{2}$$

$$F = \frac{SIP - SOP}{2}$$

(W: water phase; F: fat phase; SIP: signal of in-phase; SOP: signal of out-of-phase).

With this technique, the map of fat deposition in the liver can be displayed, and the fat content across the entire liver can be measured.

Clinical and laboratory parameters such as body mass index (BMI), waist hip ratio (WHR), serum triglycerides (TG), and low density lipoprotein (LDL) levels are thought to be related to extent of fat accumulation in liver [18,19]. Accurate fat quantification of the entire liver, and the investigations of the relationship between liver fat content and clinical parameters may provide information for future clinical interventions. This study aims to validate the use of Dixon technique in total liver fat content quantification, as well as to explore the correlations between liver fat content and clinical paremeters in both healthy subjects and those with impaired glucose tolerance.

Materials and Methods

Ethic statement

The study was conducted in accordance with ethical guidelines for human research, the Health Insurance Portability and Accountability Act (HIPAA) and was approved by the research ethical committee of The First Affiliated Hospital of Sun Yat-sen University. Written informed consent was obtained from all patients, and legal guardian if the patients were younger than 18 years old. Permission was obtained from the hospital for the publications of medical images seen in the Figures.

Phantom validation

We first evaluated the accuracy of the fat-quantifying technique with some fat-water phantoms. Homogeneous emulsions consisting of vegetable (peanut) oil and distilled water were prepared in 50 ml bottles, with fat volume fractions (FVF) of 0%, 10%, 20%, 30%, 40%, 50%, 60%, 70%, 80%, 90%, 100%, using a magnetic stirrer hotplate heated to 50°C. Agar gel (2% by weight) and dioctyl sulfosuccinate sodium salt (15 mmol/L) were added in each bottle to stabilize the emulsions (Figure 1) [20]. All the bottles were placed in a water tank with a temperature of 37°C (mimic the temperature of normal human body).

MR images were obtained using a 3-Tesla whole-body human MRI scanner (SIEMENS 3.0T MAGNETOM Verio). A head coil was used and T1 volumetric interpolated breath-hold examination (VIBE) Dixon sequence was applied with the following parameters: TE, 2.5 ms, 3.7 ms; TR, 5.62 ms; flip angle, 5°; receiver bandwidth, ±504.0 kHz; slice thickness, 3.0 mm. Four images of the phantoms were generated, including in-phase and out-of-phase, as well as fat and water phase images.

Subjects and clinical data

Fifty-six subjects were enrolled in the study. Oral glucose tolerance test was conducted subjects were divided into either impaired glucose tolerance (IGT) group or normal glucose tolerance (NGT) group accordingly. 14 were clinically diagnosed with impaired glucose tolerance (2 males, 12 females, age range 47~58 years old, average age was 53 years old) and 42 with normal glucose tolerance (18 males, 24 females, age range 43~57

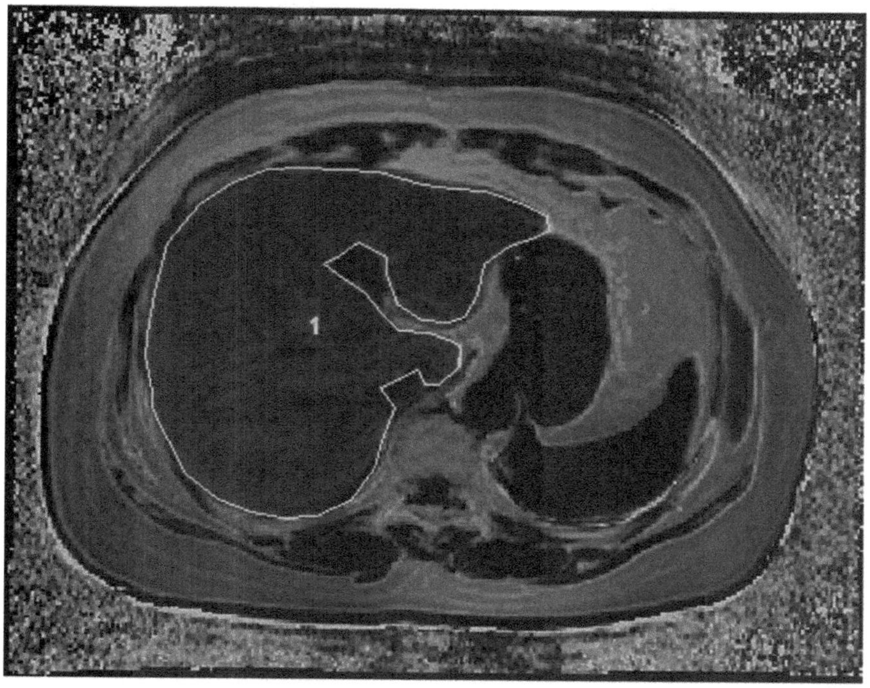

Figure 2. Irregular-shaped Regions of Interest (ROI) (1) covering the entire liver was placed in 21 consecutive slices (max-area centered) on the fat volume fraction (FVF) map of a typical patient. The average FVF in the ROI was recorded.

years old, average age 50 years old). Other clinical parameters and laboratory tests were also measured: BMI, WHR, body fat content (BFC), total cholesterol (CHOL), TG, LDL, fasting plasma insulin (FPI), homeostasis model assessment IR (HOMA-IR), homeostasis model assessmentβ (HOMAβ). NGT group was further divided into two groups according to BMI: NGTFat group, BMI >25 (the upper-limit in healthy people), 18 subjects (BMI: 26.6±1.4); NGTLean group, BMI <25, 24 subjects (BMI: 23.0±1.4). The BMI of all 14 patients in IGT group were higher than 25(BMI: 28.0±2.2).

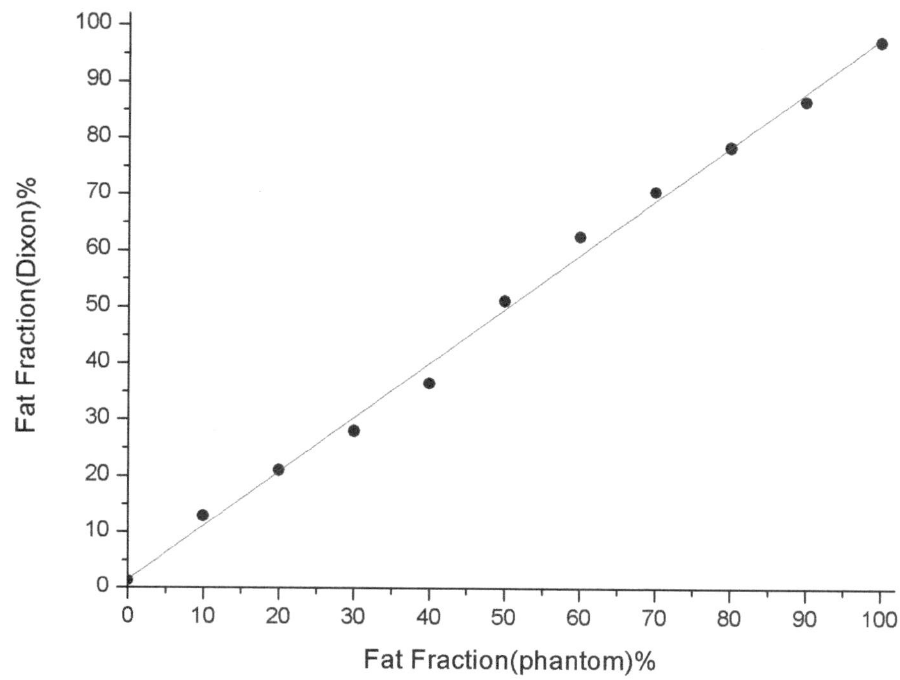

Figure 3. Correlation of actual fat volume fraction (FVF) of the water/fat phantoms against the mean fat fraction computed from Dixon technique. The best-fit-line was displayed. ($r2 = 0.994$, $p = 0.000$).

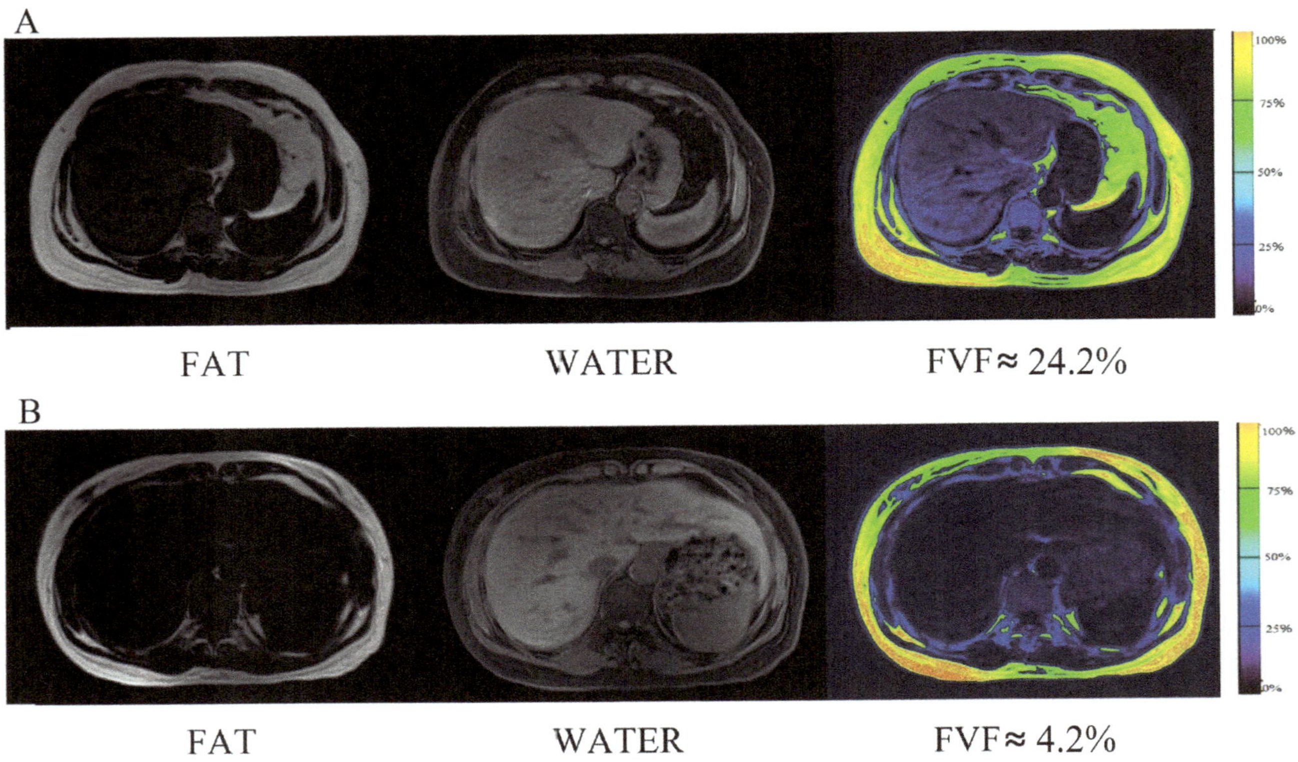

Figure 4. FVF maps of two typical subjects from IGT group (A) and NGTLean group (B). A: a 58 years old female who was diagnosed as IGT (BMI = 31.85), with a mean FVF of 24.23%. The fat phase and FVF map demonstrated that the deposition of fat is homogeneous. B: a 50 years old female (BMI = 23.13) with a mean FVF of 4.15%. The color of the liver in case B is much darker than that in case A, indicating a lower fat content.

Each subject underwent an upper-abdominal MRI examination that involved an initial set of localizer images and then a T1 VIBE Dixon sequence. The imaging parameters were the same as those in the phantom study, with TE of 2.5/3.7 ms and TR of 5.47 ms. All the subjects were imaged in supine position and carefully instructed to breath hold during end inspiration to ensure consistency amongst subjects. Four images, in-phase, out-of-phase, fat-phase and water-phase, were obtained at the same time within a single breath-hold for each patient.

MR Image post processing and analysis

Fat volume fraction (FVF) map was generated by combining the MR images obtained during both fat-phase and water-phase of each subject. This was done by using a newly designed plug-in algorithm created under MATLAB platform (MATLAB r2011b,

Table 1. Correlations between the liver FVF values and clinical parameters in all subjects as determined by Spearman correlation test.[a,b]

Variables	Correlation Coefficient	*P*
BMI	0.595	0.004
BFC	−0.024	0.915
WHR	0.432	0.045
CHOL	0.352	0.108
TG	0.689	0.019
LDL	0.455	0.033
FPI	0.886	0.019
HOMA-IR	0.886	0.019
HOMAβ	0.943	0.005

[a]FVFs have positive correlation with BMI, WHR, TG, LDL, FPI, HOMA-IR and HOMAβ, while BFC and CHOL were found to have no statistical correlation with liver fat content.

[b]FVF, fat volume fraction; BMI, body mass index; BFC, body fat content; WHR, waist hip rate; CHOL, cholesterol; TG, triglyceride; LDL, low density lipoprotein; FPI, fasting plasma insulin; HOMA-IR, homeostasis model assessment insulin resistance; HOMAβ, homeostasis model assessmentβ.

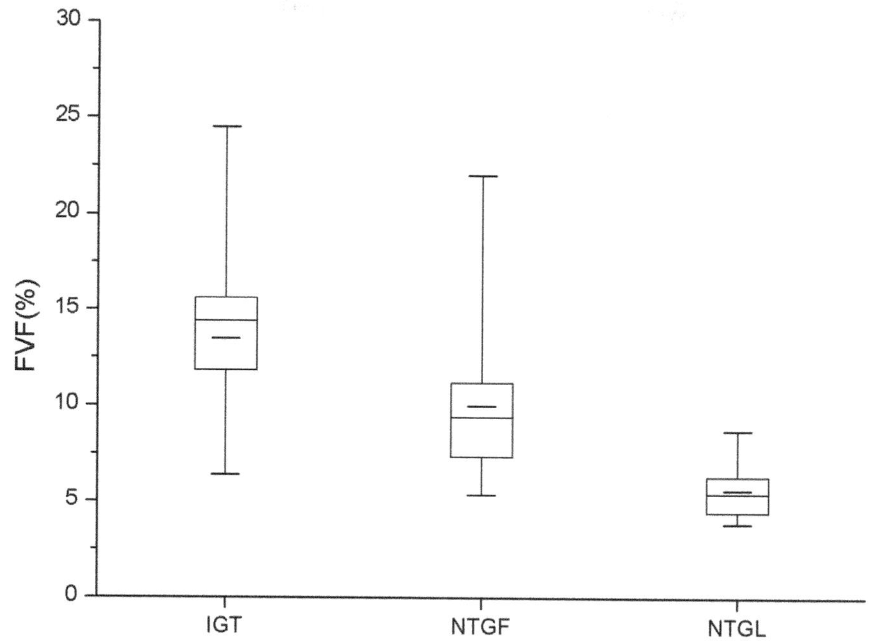

Figure 5. Boxplots of FVF values for the IFT, NGTFat and NGTLean groups. Significant differences was found between IGT group and NGTLean group (p = 0.004), as well as the NGTFat group and NGTLean group (p = 0.006). But there was no significant difference between IGT group and NGTFat group (p = 0.359).

MathWorks, America), using the following equation:

$$FVF = \frac{F}{W+F} \times 100\%$$

(FVF: fat volume fraction; F: fat volume; W: water volume).

In phantom study, two trained radiologists manually traced a round-shaped region of interest (ROI) on each bottle, and recorded the results of FVFs. The diameter of ROI is 3 cm, the size of the transverse section of the bottles. Average FVFs of each bottle were acquired.

In vivo study, two trained radiologists manually placed an irregular-shaped ROI covering the entire liver in 21 consecutive slices (max-area centered) of each patient (Figure 2). The mean FVF in the ROI of each subject was recorded.

Statistical analysis

FVF values were calculated using the Dixon technique and compared to true FVFs in the phantom experiment using linear correlation. In vivo study, statistical correlations between FVFs and results of clinical and laboratory tests were determined by using the Spearman's rank correlation. The difference in FVF between three groups was evaluated using the Wilcoxon test. A p value lower than 0.05 was considered as statistically significant. All the analyses were performed in SPSS (SPSS, Version 13.0, Chicago, IL, USA).

Results

Phantom study

Figure 1 summarizes the results from the phantom study. The bottle on the lower left side is filled will pure water (fat content: 0%), and the upper right one is filled with 100% peanut oil. Others contain fat content ranging from 10% to 90%. During the fat phase image, higher fat content was associated with a higher signal intensity. The opposite was observed during the water phase image where higher fat content was associated with a lower signal intensity. FVF map demonstrated different amounts of water/fat in the emulsions ranging from 0% to 100% with changing color. A graph comparing the actual FVF against fat fraction calculated by Dixon technique also showed excellent correlation (Figure 3, $r2 = 0.994$, $p = 0.000$)). This result indicates that Dixon technique is applicable for measuring the actual fat content of the liver.

In vivo results

For each subject, FVF maps were generated from the source images of both fat phase and water phase. Figure 4 shows the FVF maps of two typical subjects from IGT group (A) and NGTLean group (B) respectively. The darker color of the liver seen in Figure 4B indicates lower fat content in NGTLean group when compared to the IGT group as seen in Figure 4A. Furthermore, in both fat phase image and FVF map (Fig. 4A), the distribution of fat in liver in people with metabolic disorders tended to be homogeneous, which is different from fat accumulation caused by inflammation [21].

For all the subjects, FVFs ranged from 4.2% to 24.2%, and had positive correlation with BMI ($p = 0.004$), WHR ($p = 0.045$), TG ($p = 0.019$), LDL ($p = 0.033$), FPI ($p = 0.019$), HOMA-IR ($p = 0.019$) and HOMAβ ($p = 0.005$) (Table 1, Spearman's rank correlation). For IGT group, FVFs positively correlated with FPI ($p = 0.019$), HOMA-IR ($p = 0.019$), HOMAβ ($p = 0.005$), while the FVFs of healthy groups did not show significant correlation with any of these clinical parameters.

FVFs of IGT group were significantly different from those of NGTLean group ($p = 0.004$), but no significant difference was found between IGT group and NGTFat group ($p > 0.05$). FVFs of NGTLean group were also significantly different from those of NGTFat group ($p = 0.006$) (Figure 5).

Discussion

The amount of the liver fat content is essential in monitoring the progression of NAFLD and it acts as a potential indicator of underlying metabolic disorders [22]. Unlike MR spectroscopy, Dixon technique provides us with separate fat and water phase images within a single breath-hold. Dxion technique is easier to perform than MRS; and the image analysis is also more straightforward. Liver fat content measurement and detection using Dixon technique have been reported in previous studies [23–27]. For example, D'Assignies, G. et al. have evaluated the ability of MRS, Dixon technique and diffusion-weighted MR imaging (DWI) to detect liver steatosis using histopathology as a reference [23]. They have also evaluated the correlations between fat fraction (FF) measured by MRS, Dixon technique and clinical parameters such as LDL and cholesterol concentrations, which showed consistent result with our study. However, their study mainly focuses on the sensitivity, specificity and accuracy in diagnosis of liver steatosis for three different noninvasive MR techniques, MRS, Dixon technique and DWI. In another study, Houchun H. Hu and colleagues have demonstrated a strong potential for IDEAL technique (Iterative Decomposition with Echo Asymmetry and Least squares estimation, a modified Dixon technique) as a liver fat quantification tool and a valuable method for obesity research [24]. However, in the studies mentioned above, only a small oval- or square-shaped ROI on the liver was studied, hence could not appropriately evaluate the total amount of the liver fat content.

In this study, from the separate fat and water phase images, a 3D voxel-wise fat fraction map of the entire abdomen was generated which showed the spatial pattern of ectopic fat, and mean FVF of the entire liver on the map was calculated. For each subject, 21 consecutive slices (max-area centered) of the FVF map was used to generate the liver ROI, and the mean value was recorded to stand for the FVF of this subject. Proved to be dependable by the phantom study, FVFs obtained via the Dixon technique is found to approximately equate to the actual fat content throughout the liver. The spatial information of the liver fat is also readily available (Fig. 1 and Fig. 4).

Under normal circumstance, liver plays an important role in the lipid metabolism. It is involved in free fatty acid uptake from the blood to synthesize TG, essential in the lipoprotein transportation by combining different types of lipids with lipid-carrying protein. When the efficiency of TG synthesis exceeds the transporting capacity of lipoproteins, TG and other types of lipids accumulates in the liver, resulting in fatty liver, or otherwise known as, ectopic fat deposition [1,2]. Unlike fat accumulation resulted from inflammation [21], people with metabolic disorders tend to have homogeneous fat deposition, and this is demonstrated in the FVF maps. Fat accumulation caused by acute hepatitis, for instance, demonstrates focal fat content from local hepatocyte necrosis and proliferation of fibrous connective tissue. However, fat accumulation due to metabolism disorders is a systematic process, and has no region-specific predisposition. Therefore, the possible cause of liver fat deposition may be diagnosed based on the pattern of fat distribution seen in FVF map.

In our study, it was found that FVFs have positive correlations with many clinical and laboratory results such as BMI, WHR, TG and LDL, which are consistent with some previous reports [18,19]. Besides, FVFs in IGT group is significantly higher than those of NGTLean group, while there is no significant difference seen between IGT group and NGTFat group. This indicates that fat people (BMI≥25) tend to have a higher fat content in liver due to increased burden on the liver from high free fatty acids in the blood. When the burden overwhelms the ability of processing fatty acids in liver, the fat will gradually accumulate in liver and this deposition may cause fatty liver diseases. In addition, high serum free fatty acid will slow down the utilization of glucose and stimulate the secretion of insulin. This leads to increased insulin resistance over time, which may eventually progress into IGT. Thus it is possible that the subjects of NGTFat group are at higher risk of developing IGT than people with normal BMI. This can be further supported by the lack of significant differences seen in lier fat content between the IGT and NGTFat subjects where BMIs of subjects in both groups were greater than 25.

On the other hand, we have found that liver fat content did not statistically correlate with BFC. One possible explanation is that high BFC does not equate to high viscera fat content, and the latter contributes much more to the liver fat content than BFC. Instead, WHR provided better reflection regarding the fat distribution of the body. People with high WHR have more fat deposition around the abdomen and in the viscera. Therefore, the higher WHR, the higher viscera fat deposition, and the higher the fat content in liver, as well.

This study also demonstrated that liver fat content has a positive correlation with FPI, HOMA-IR and HOMAβ. That means people with higher liver fat content tend to have higher FPI, HOMA-IR and HOMAβ levels. FPI reflects the body's sensitivity to insulin. Higher FPI is associated with lower insulin sensitivity. HOMA-IR can be calculated from FPI, which reflects insulin resistance. Thus, our results may indicate that people with high HOMA-IR levels are more resistant to insulin. Insulin resistance is recognized as a main risk factor for many metabolic disorders, and it especially increases the probability to develop type 2 diabetes [28]. In our study, FVFs of IGT group was positively correlated with FPI and HOMA-IR. In other words, IGT patients with higher FVFs are more resistant to insulin, and may have a higher risk to develop type 2 diabetes mellitus. Therefore, fat content quantification using Dixon technique has its value as a prognostic tool for IGT patients.

To summarize, this study has verified an accurate, noninvasive and easy-to-perform method based on Dixon technique to quantify the fat content across the entire liver. FVF calculated with the technique reflects the actual liver fat content. The significant correlations of FVF with some other clinical parameters indicate further investigations are necessary for the epidemiology and pathophysiology of NAFLD as well as other metabolism disorders.

Acknowledgments

This work was funded by National Natural Science Foundation of China (81000626), Natural Science Foundation of Guangdong Province (S2013010016004), Zhujiang Scientific and Technological New Star Foundation (2012J2200084), and the Fundamental Research Funds for the Central Universities (10ykpy11).

Author Contributions

Conceived and designed the experiments: ZL STF. Performed the experiments: HSC ZD YJL TC LW ZWZ. Analyzed the data: ZD YJL. Contributed reagents/materials/analysis tools: HSC TC LW. Contributed to the writing of the manuscript: ZD YJL ZL STF HSC YBL TC LW ZWZ.

References

1. Clark JM (2006) The epidemiology of nonalcoholic fatty liver disease in adults. Journal of Clinical Gastroenterology 40: S5–10.
2. Kotronen A, Peltonen M, Hakkarainen A, Sevastianova K, Bergholm R, et al. (2009) Prediction of non-alcoholic fatty liver disease and liver fat using metabolic and genetic factors. Gastroenterology 137: 865–72.
3. Marchesini G, Bugianesi E, Forlani G, Cerrelli F, Lenzi M, et al. (2003) Nonalcoholic fatty liver, steatohepatitis, and the metabolic syndrome. Hepatology 37: 917–23.
4. Vernon G, Baranova A, Younossi ZM (2011) Systematic review: the epidemiology and natural history of non-alcoholic fatty liver disease and non-alcoholic steatohepatitis in adults. Alimentary Pharmacology and herapeutics 34: 274–85.
5. Bacon BR, Farahvash MJ, Janney CG, Neuschwander-Tetri BA (1994) Nonalcoholic steatohepatitis: an expanding clinical entity. Gastroenterology 107: 1103–9.
6. Angulo P (2002) Nonalcoholic fatty liver disease. N Engl J Med 346: 1221–31.
7. Wieckowska A, McCullough AJ, Feldstein AE (2007) Noninvasive diagnosis and monitoring of nonalcoholic steatohepatitis: present and future. Hepatology 46: 582–9.
8. Ligabue G, Besutti G, Scaglioni R, Stentarelli C, Guaraldi G (2013) MR quantitative biomarkers of non-alcoholic fatty liver disease: technical evolutions and future trends. Quant Imaging Med Surg 3: 192–5.
9. Fernández-Salazar L, Velayos B, Aller R, Lozano F, Garrote JA (2011) Percutaneous liver biopsy: patients' point of view. Scand J Gastroenterol 46: 727–31.
10. El-Badry AM, Breitenstein S, Jochum W, Washington K, Paradis V, et al. (2009) Assessment of hepatic steatosis by expert pathologists: the end of a gold standard. Ann Surg 250: 691–7.
11. Bedossa P, Dargère D, Paradis V (2003) Sampling variability of liver fibrosis in chronic hepatitis C Hepatology 38: 1449–57.
12. Ratziu V, Charlotte F, Heurtier A, Gombert S, Giral P, et al. (2005) Sampling variability of liver biopsy in nonalcoholic fatty liver disease. Gastroenterology 128: 1898–906.
13. Bydder M, Yokoo T, Hamilton G, Middleton MS, Chavez AD, et al. (2008) Relaxation effects in the quantification of fat using gradient echo imaging. Magn Reson Imaging 26: 347–59.
14. Guiu B, Petit JM, Loffroy R, Ben Salem D, Aho S, et al. (2009) Quantification of liver fat content: comparison of triple-echo chemical shift gradient-echo imaging and in vivo proton MR spectroscopy. Radiology 250: 95–102.
15. Reeder SB, Robson PM, Yu H, Shimakawa A, Hines CD, et al. (2009) Quantification of hepatic steatosis with MRI: the effects of accurate fat spectral modeling. J Magn Reson Imaging 29: 1332–9.
16. Meisamy S, Hines CD, Hamilton G, Sirlin CB, McKenzie CA, et al. (2011) Quantification of hepatic steatosis with T1-independent, T2-corrected MR imaging with spectral modeling of fat: blinded comparison with MR spectroscopy. Radiology 258: 767–75.
17. Dixon WT (1984) Simple proton spectroscopic imaging. Radiology 153: 189–194.
18. Petta S, Amato MC, Di Marco V, Cammà C, Pizzolanti G, et al. (2012) Visceral adiposity index is associated with significant fibrosis in patients with non-alcoholic fatty liver disease. Aliment Pharmacol Ther 35: 238–47.
19. Monteiro PA, Mota J, Silveira LS, Cayres SU, Antunes BdM, et al. (2013) Morphological and metabolic determinants of nonalcoholic fatty liver disease in obese youth: a pilot study. BMC Res Notes 6: 89.
20. Bernard CP, Liney GP, Manton DJ, Turnbull LW, Langton CM (2008) Comparison of Fat Quantification Methods: A Phantom Study at 3.0T. Journal of magnetic resonance imaging 27: 192–7.
21. Kammen BF, Pacharn P, Thoeni RF, Lu Y, Qayyum A, et al. (2001) Focal fatty infiltration of the liver: analysis of prevalence and CT findings in children and young adults. Am J Roentgenol 177: 1035–9.
22. Reeder SB, Cruite I, Hamilton G, Sirlin CB (2011) Quantitative assessment of liver fat with magnetic resonance imaging and spectroscopy. J Magn Reson Imaging 34: 729–49.
23. D'Assignies G, Martin R, Abdesslem K, Luigi L, Miguel C, et al. (2009) Noninvasive quantitation of human liver steatosis using magnetic resonance and bioassay methods. Eur. Radiol 19: 2033–40.
24. Hu HH, Kim HW, Nayak KS, Goran MI (2010) Comparison of fat–water MRI and single-voxel MRS in the assessment of hepatic and pancreatic fat fractions in humans. Obesity (Silver Spring) 18: 841–7.
25. Leporq B, Ratiney H, Pilleul F, Beuf O (2013) Liver fat volume fraction quantification with fat and water T1 and T2* estimation and accounting for NMR multiple components in patients with chronic liver disease at 1.5 and 3.0 T. Eur Radiol 23: 2175–86.
26. Yokoo T, Shiehmorteza M, Hamilton G, Wolfson T, Schroeder ME, et al. (2011) Estimation of hepatic proton-density fat fraction by using MR imaging at 3.0 T. Radiology 258: 749–59.
27. Yokoo T, Bydder M, Hamilton G, Middleton MS, Gamst AC, et al. (2009) Nonalcoholic fatty liver disease: diagnostic and fat grading accuracy of low-flip-angle multiecho gradient-recalled-echo MR imaging at 1.5 T. Radiology 251: 67–6.
28. Cusi K (2009) Nonalcoholic fatty liver disease in type 2 diabetes mellitus. Curr Opin Endocrinol Diabetes Obes 16: 141–9.

Stochastic Tracking of Infection in a CF Lung

Sara Zarei[1]*, Ali Mirtar[2], Forest Rohwer[3], Peter Salamon[4]

1 Computational Science Research Center, San Diego State University, San Diego, California, United States of America, **2** Electrical and Computer Eng. Dep/University of California San Diego, San Diego, California, United States of America, **3** Department of Biology, San Diego State University, San Diego, California, United States of America, **4** Department of Mathematics and Statistics, San Diego State University, San Diego, California, United States of America

Abstract

Magnetic Resonance Imaging (MRI) and Computed Tomography (CT) scan are the two ubiquitous imaging sources that physicians use to diagnose patients with Cystic Fibrosis (CF) or any other Chronic Obstructive Pulmonary Disease (COPD). Unfortunately the cost constraints limit the frequent usage of these medical imaging procedures. In addition, even though both CT scan and MRI provide mesoscopic details of a lung, in order to obtain microscopic information a very high resolution is required. Neither MRI nor CT scans provide micro level information about the location of infection in a binary tree structure the binary tree structure of the human lung. In this paper we present an algorithm that enhances the current imaging results by providing estimated micro level information concerning the location of the infection. The estimate is based on a calculation of the distribution of possible mucus blockages consistent with available information using an offline Metropolis-Hastings algorithm in combination with a real-time interpolation scheme. When supplemented with growth rates for the pockets of mucus, the algorithm can also be used to estimate how lung functionality as manifested in spirometric tests will change in patients with CF or COPD.

Editor: Wayne Iwan Lee Davies, University of Western Australia, Australia

Funding: This material is based upon work supported by the National Institutes of Health under Grant no. 56586B. The funders had no role in study design, data collection and analysis, decision to publish, or preparation of the manuscript.

Competing Interests: The authors have declared that no competing interests exist.

* Email: sara.zarei@alumni.ucsd.edu

Introduction

Patients with chronic obstructive pulmonary disease (COPD) or cystic fibrosis (CF) have chronic lung inflammation which causes airflow limitation and the scarring of lung tissues. Their airways are generally inflamed and produce excess amounts of mucus that impair the flow of air into and out of their lungs.

Our hypothesis is that the scarring, and ultimate remodeling of a CF lung is mostly due to the contact between the lung lining and the mucus. Inflammatory cytokines induce scars in lung tissue [1]. This contact between mucous biofilm and lung tissue facilitates virulent microbes that also play a role in remodeling a CF lung. In comparison with a normal lung, the airway fluids of CF patients contain large amounts of neutrophils as a result of the inflammatory response [2]. Thus our hypothesis is that mucus accumulation is primarily responsible for damage to the lung and therefore tracking its propagation is a crucial task for better diagnosis and treatment.

Spirometry, the measurement of a patient's breathing, is the standard clinical tool for monitoring lung disease. The two most common spirometric indicators are the forced expiratory volume in one second, FEV_1, and the forced vital capacity, FVC. FEV_1 measures the volume of air that can forcibly be blown out in one second while FVC measures the volume of air that can forcibly be blown out after a full inspiration maneuver. Although these tests provide a global measure of airflow obstruction and restriction, they do not give detailed information about the location of mucus blockage. Additional information is available from the repeated imaging of CF patients' lungs. This is usually in the form of chest x-ray, computed tomography (CT) or magnetic resonance imaging (MRI). Despite the fact that CT is an optimal morphological assessment of CF lung changes, the associated exposure to ionizing radiation is a serious obstacle. Therefore, MRI might be the appropriate method for imaging CF patient's lungs [3,4].

MRI was first introduced as an alternative imaging tool for patients with CF in 1987 [5]. There are numerous methods for the analysis of chest MRI. Theilmann et al. proposed a new MRI imaging method that can spatially locate the pockets of infection and measure the amount of mucus located within each pocket. This information is obtained with a resolution of approximately 1.0 cm^3 [6]. This resolution is equivalent to the last 10 generations of airways combined. Despite the accuracy level of MRI images, they do not contain any micro-level information on smaller airways. Hence the precise location of infection cannot be obtained from the MRI data.

There have been research studies on mesoscopic modeling of Cystic Fibrosis [7]. Such studies however did not address the micro level information about mucus propagation through the airways. The goal of this research is to provide the clinician with an algorithm that can track the location and propagation of mucus in a CF patient's lungs. Tracking the growth, or shrinkage of these pockets can be correlated to the efficacy of different treatment regimens on each pocket. Assuming further progress in metagenomic and transcriptomic analyses of sputum samples, tracking may allow also correlating the growth or shrinkage of these pockets and the composition of the local microbial community structure within the pocket.

The central tool introduced in the present article for tracking pockets of inflammation is based on using our airflow model [8] in reverse, i.e., as the main ingredient in an inverse problem. Our airflow model can calculate the flow and the total resistance corresponding to a given distribution of mucus obstructions in respiratory airways. The solution of the inverse problem is achieved by randomly sampling the many possible mucus configurations consistent with the current information regarding a patient. Many micro-scale distributions match any observed MRI and spirometric data. The fortuitous finding in the calculations described below is that a large majority of the possible distributions fall within narrow ranges of certain parameters such as which generations of airways contain how much mucus. Can we be certain of these most likely locations being the actual mucus distribution? The fact that most of the distributions consistent with the spirometric and MRI data have these features makes them a good bet while not giving us certainty that any *one* configuration is of this form. In fact, however, repeated MRI measurements separated by small challenges such as coughing or even just taking a few deep breaths reveal that mucus inside the lungs of CF patients show small but discernible movements in response to such challenges. Given this dynamic picture, the possibility that all of the configurations of mucus would avoid the configurations that can be realized the largest number of ways is extremely unlikely. We describe below how to construct such distributions that best represent the state of airways corresponding to the patients lung functionality test values (FEV_1 and FVC) and any available MRI or CT data. We use a maximum entropy approach to construct such estimates by sampling all consistent distributions and choosing the one that can be realized the largest number of ways. We find that the predicted microscopic distribution of mucus is generally sharply peaked, allowing us to estimate the distribution of mucus as the one that appears the most frequently in our simulation. The entire computation process can take a long time and would require enormous computational space to run the simulation for the entire 2^{23} airways in a lung. However after running the simulation once for a patient, we can store most of the data so the next simulations only take a few minutes to complete.

Given the micro-scale distribution obtained from our inverse problem, we can use our physiological model [9] to predict the growth and propagation of this distribution, thereby predicting the progression of the disease. This second model requires a rate for the growth of the mucus volume at each location. Currently only one overall average growth rate is available, a growth rate that was estimated based on a forty year CF population average [9]. Predictions of this model with the average growth rate can nonetheless be compared to actual observed disease progression between exacerbations. For predictions during exacerbations, a database of treatment and community specific growth rates are needed and in-principle available from multiple MRI and metagenomic/transcriptomic analyses. Two such datasets allow the extraction of pocket specific growth rates and corresponding linear extrapolation for the mucus volume in each pocket. This can at least lengthen the times between imaging sessions.

Methods

Inverse Problem Using Metropolis-Hastings Algorithm

Our algorithm uses CF patients' spirometry test values of FVC, FEV_1 and any available mucus distribution data from CT scans or MRI as its input. It then identifies the distribution of mucus obstructed bronchioles throughout different airway generations. The model assumes the lung airways to be binary branching trees [10] extending over 23 generations from the bronchus down to the alveoli. It further assumes a fractal structure [11–13] for the parameters of the binary airway tree.

Considering the fact that there are 2^{23} bronchioles in a human lung, there are astronomically many possible configurations for a certain amount of mucus distributed in an airway tree, even given the mucus in each voxel. In fact many of these configurations will result in the same FEV_1 and FVC values. Since exhaustive sampling of these configurations is impossible, we use the Metropolis-Hastings Markov chain Monte Carlo algorithm to sample a few hundred million and base our estimates on such a sample. The goal of this section is to introduce this method.

Our algorithm proceeds from an assumed amount of mucus to be distributed into the 2^{23} airways. It starts from a random distribution and obtains an unbiased sample of configurations satisfying certain requirements. These requirements are implemented as soft constraints via an energy function

$$E=(\alpha)(\text{Calculated FEV}_1-\text{Patient FEV}_1)^2+ (1-\alpha)(\text{Calculated FVC}-\text{Patient FVC})^2 \quad (1)$$

where (α) and $(1-\alpha)$ are weight factors. In our algorithm we set $\alpha=0.5$. The energy function is used as a way to force the sampling to stay near values with low energy, i.e. configurations with approximately correct spirometric readings.

We then examine successive samples by performing a random walk on the space of mucus configurations. Each move in our random walk reallocates the location of some of the mucus. The resulting distribution of mucus configurations turns out to be sharply peaked in certain natural parameters, a fact exploited by our algorithm.

The Metropolis algorithm is a widely used procedure for sampling a sequence from a specified distribution on a large finite set. It describes equilibrium for systems whose configurations have probability proportional to the Boltzmann factor ($e^{-E/T}$). This is a weighting factor which determines the relative probability that the system will be found in a particular configuration at energy E when the temperature of the environment is T [14]. We used a constant temperature, $T=1$, making the probability of a configuration with energy E proportional to $\exp(-E)$.

The following steps describe the Metropolis algorithm [15].

- Initiate the sampling from an arbitrary configuration A, with known energy E_A.
- Define a new neighbor configuration B from configuration A.
- Calculate the new configuration energy, E_B. This trial move is then either accepted or rejected according to the following simple probabilistic rule.
- If $E_B<E_A$ we accept the new configuration.
- if $E_B>E_A$, we may accept configuration B with the following probability.

$$p=e^{-(E_B-E_A)/T} \quad (2)$$

- Repeat until sufficient number of configurations have been collected.

To apply the Metropolis algorithm to our model, we need to define neighboring configurations. Our definition moves a certain amount of mucus between a few chosen bronchioles. This keeps the energy re-evaluation step computationally cheap and, provided we allow such rearrangement between all types of airways, we avoid the problems created by local minima. This assures that the system settles into and stays near the lowest energy configurations as the simulation proceeds [16].

Two-Dimensional Probability Density Function Estimation (PDFE-2D) of Mucus Obstructions

Imaging provides us with the data that corresponds to the spatial location of infection pockets and the amount of mucus within each pocket. Both MRI and CT images can have various resolutions and our approach is scalable to any resolution. For concreteness below we work with a resolution of 1 cm^3 and refer to this smallest volume as a voxel - a volume element.

Since on average the total lung capacity of an adult human is about 6 liters [17], an image will have about 6000 voxels. Using the binary tree structure of the lung airway, we set these voxels at the end of the 13th generation to approximately match the number of these elements to the number of subtrees that remain. Since $2^{13} = 8192 \approx 6000$, we can identify the mucus in the voxel with the mucus in the subtree of $2^{23-13} = 2^{10}$ bronchioles terminating in the alveoli. Thus each voxel in our lung model represents a binary tree structure that has a total of 10 bifurcations, from generation 13 to 23, with a known total amount of mucus obtained from imaging data.

Using a three-dimensional model of the human airway tree that was developed by [18], we are able to map each MRI or CT scan voxel into our lung model's voxels with their corresponding mucus content. The main task of our algorithm is to locate the infection in the airway tree structure of a CF lung. To achieve this goal, we use two summary features for each voxel: (1) the percent of alveoli that are accessible, i.e., not totally blocked and (2) the total resistance to flow from the alveoli to the 13th generation brochiole bronchiole assigned to the voxel. These two microscopic features correspond loosely to the spirometric indicators FVC and FEV_1, respectively.

In order for us to calculate each voxel's resistance and the percent of accessible alveoli (for simplicity, we refer to this as the AA%), we first have to define how mucus is distributed in a voxel's binary tree structure. There is an astronomical number of configurations for filling a binary tree of 10 generations with a given amount of mucus. Approximately, it is given by $(2^{10})^{M/m}$ where M is the total mucus volume and m is the volume of the smallest bronchiole. Thus even at this level, we used Metropolis-Hastings to sample many mucus configurations, recording the values of AA% and resistance for each configuration. We set the amount of mucus within each voxel and calculate the distribution of AA% and resistance: our PDFE-2D distribution.

Hence if a voxel contains 5% mucus, the first step is randomly filling up the voxel's airway tree with the specified mucus amount. Then using the Metropolis algorithm, at each state we move only a fraction of the mucus within a bronchiole that is equivalent to the smallest bronchiole's volume in a lung airway tree. We refer to this as the "unit volume". Once a unit volume is moved to a different location, the corresponding voxel's parameters (AA% and resistance) are recalculated.

In order to expedite the computational process; Dulcinea computing clusters from the Computational Science Research Center at San Diego State University were used for collecting almost 54 million samples. The Dulcinea computing clusters contains 12 workstations each with Dual-Quad Xeon central processing unit (CPU) (E5520 2.27GHz) and Dual Tesla graphic processing unit (GPU) (M1060) which provides the total of 96 CPU cores. The cluster system utilizes 3GB of memory per CPU core for nodes 1 to 10 and utilizes 6GB of memory per CPU core for nodes 11 and 12. After obtaining these samples the probability distributions for different amount of mucus are calculated. Figure 1A to Figure 1D illustrate the probability density function for (5%, 30%, 65%, and 75%) mucus respectively. As shown in Figure 1A, when there is only 5% mucus in a voxel, the most likely configuration has 86% of its alveoli accessible and the voxel's resistance increases by a factor of almost 1.1. When the mucus level reaches almost 30% there are only 27% accessible alveoli and the voxel resistance is almost 2.2 times a healthy voxel with no mucus. On the other hand in Figure 1C and 1D the number of accessible alveoli value approaches zero while the resistance value reaches infinity. This refers to a case that a voxel is almost completely filled with mucus to an extent that no more air can pass through and therefore blocks all the corresponding alveoli at the end of the branching tree.

Figure 2 displays the maximum likelihood combinations of AA% and resistance ratio for different amount of mucus in a voxel. As the mucus reaches almost 60% of the available airway volume in the voxel, there is no remaining access to the alveoli and as a result there is no gas exchange taking place in that particular part of the airway tree. After collecting these distributions, the model can initiate the prediction steps as well as providing the microlevel information about the location of obstructed bronchioles. We will discuss each outcome in the next two sections. Please note that all data underlying the findings of this section have been discussed in the manuscript. Other than the massive computing power needed to produce the findings in Figure 1 and Figure 2, all the relevant data have been shared.

Results

Micro-Level Information on Obstructed Bronchioles

In order to spatially locate each bronchiole in a human airway tree we used Kitaoka et al.'s three-dimensional model [18]. Once we receive the imaging data for each voxel, we need to map the values to our model's voxel using spatial location coordinates. Next we use the probability density function that we found in the previous section to determine the corresponding voxel parameters, AA% and resistance ratio, sampled according to the PDFE-2D distributions. The model randomly select a combination of percent accessible alveoli and resistance for each voxel in a way that the total resistance and number of accessible alveoli from these voxels provide the same value as the patient's FEV_1 and FVC. There is a complex calculation taking place in parallel to obtain the rate of flow (FEV_1) from the total resistance of all the voxels. To find the distribution of voxel parameters we use the Metropolis algorithm to focus the Markov chain to sample many configurations meeting our constraints. This is achieved by choosing the configuration energy provided in Eq(1).

At this stage we have mapped the voxels from imaging data into our model in a way that the total rate of airflow and the accessible alveoli of the lung model resemble the corresponding patient's FEV_1 and FVC values respectively. Once the current state of a CF lung is implemented we can obtain clinically useful information, such as mucus distribution within each voxel or predicted future states of each voxel and associated FEV_1 and FVC values as described in the next section.

Figure 3 displays the flowchart of this process. As shown in this flowchart, once we have all the voxels' parameters, we can select certain voxels for further analysis. We again apply the Metropolis algorithm on the selected voxel in order to visualize the distribution of mucus in its airway tree structure. For the chosen voxel, we have its mucus volume, its resistance and its AA%. We randomly fill out the voxels' airway tree to reach their

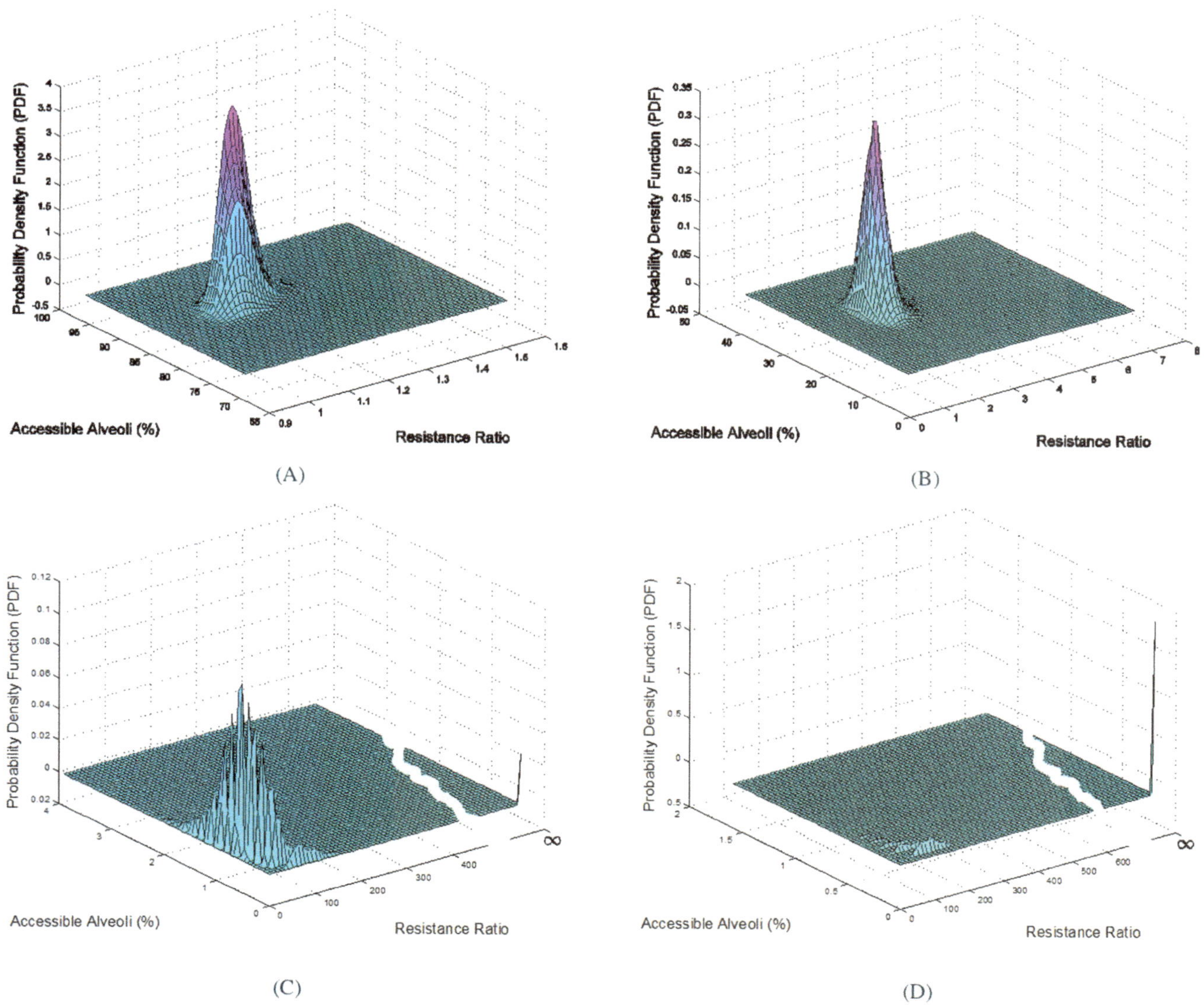

Figure 1. Probability density function for different percent volume of mucus in a small voxel of the lung. (A) 5%, **(B)** 30%, **(C)** 65% **and (D)** 75% Each voxel represents a subtree from generation 13 to 23 of the binary tree structure of lung. The x-axis is the corresponding airflow resistance and the y-axis shows the percent accessible alveoli.

corresponding mucus volume. At each iteration the new resistance and AA% are collected. To move to the neighbor configuration we move a unit volume of mucus in a bronchiole to keep the total mucus volume of the voxel fixed. The state energy we use for this step is as follows:

$$E = (\alpha)(\text{Resistance of the current state} - \text{Target voxel's resistance})^2 + (1-\alpha)(\text{AA\% of the current state} - \text{Target voxel's AA\%})^2 \quad (3)$$

where $\alpha = 0.5$. After we obtained enough samples we constructed the corresponding mucus distribution for the selected voxels. Figures 4 displays two examples of the mucus distribution for voxels that contained (5%) and (30%) mucus. As shown in these figures, as the percent mucus increases, the dominantly filled generation moves to bigger bronchioles. The y axis repressnts represents % normalized mucus where:

$$\text{Normalized mucus in generation n} = \frac{\left(\frac{\text{Mucus Volume in generation } n}{\text{Total mucus volume in voxel}}\right)}{\left(\frac{\text{Airway volume in generation } n}{\text{Total airway volume in voxel}}\right)} \quad (4)$$

Predicting future values of FEV_1 and FVC

In this section we use the mucus distribution and growth model presented in [9] to make predictions about the lung functionality of a CF patient. As can be seen in Figure 5 we use the imaging voxels' data and the constant mucus growth rate from [9], or, if available, infection and treatment specific growth rates specific to each voxel to predict the mucus growth in each pocket of infection. The model again resorts to the Monte Carlo method to randomly select the AA% and resistance from our model described in the

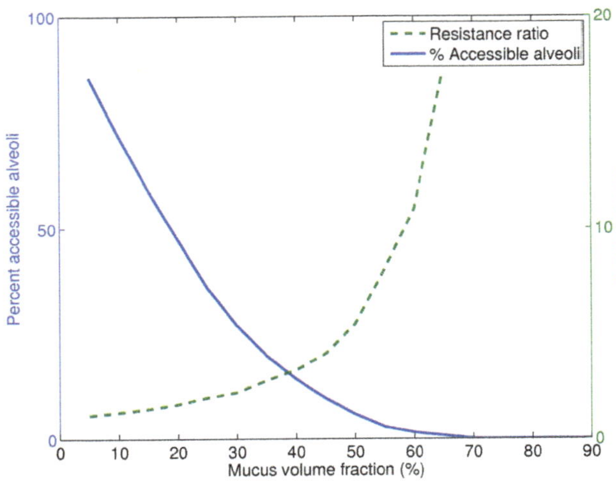

Figure 2. Maximum likelihood of percent of accessible alveoli AA% and airflow resistance for a given mucus volume fraction inside a voxel. The x-axis is mucus volume% and the two y-axes show the most probable combination of the airflow resistance ratio and percent of accessible alveoli. The resistance value increases as the mucus amount rises. Number of accessible alveoli decreases as the mucus volume grows, which leads to a lower lung functionality test value or FVC value.

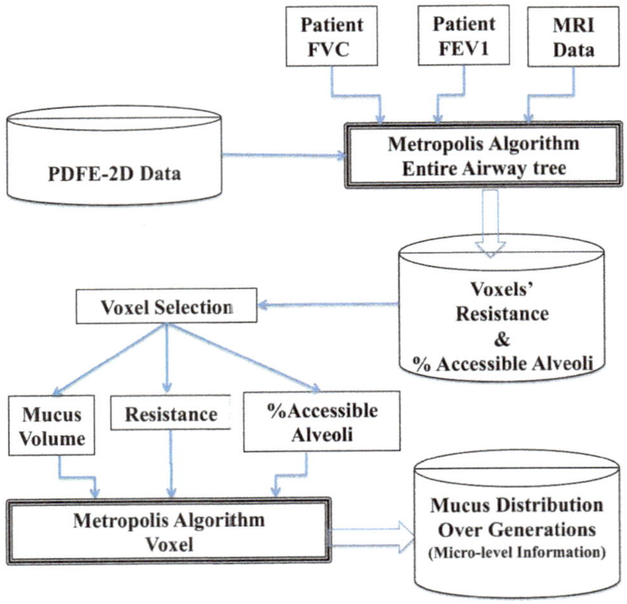

Figure 3. Generating the Micro-level information on obstructed bronchioles. This flowchart shows how the algorithm produces the mucus distribution of a selected voxel. Using the lung functionality test values: FEV1 and FVC and the data obtained from MRI lung imaging we can obtain the corresponding mucus distributions among the different generations of lung.

PDFE-2D section and calculates the new FEV_1 and FVC at each iteration and stores their values. After collecting enough samples we can predict the FEV_1 and FVC distributions for a patient after the indicated time period. For example, Figure 6 displays the probability density function of the predicted FEV_1 and FVC. As shown in the figure it is predicted that FEV_1 and FVC of our CF patient are approximately 61% and 78% respectively.

This method can even be applied to follow a patient's progress with out fewer imaging tests. Since most CF patients take spirometry test more often than any imaging tests, we can use our model without recourse to imaging data. This time the model takes only the FEV_1 and the FVC values of a patient as input. After applying the Metropolis algorithm (using additional rearrangements of mucus between voxels) the model can still provide an estimate of the distribution of mucus throughout the airway tree. This can be propagated using the constant any hypothetical growth rates to predict the next spirometric test. We have created a Matlab GUI version of the algorithm; its sample output is shown in Figures 7, 8 and 9.

Since the mean mucus growth rate was estimated based on years of data from many CF patients, such predictions should work reasonably well for a patient between exacerbations. Our model can also be used to predict the progression during exacerbations, albeit with voxel specific growth rates informed by much more data than we currently possess. Using one mean mucus growth rate is a shortcoming not of our algorithm but rather of the paucity of data to which our predictions have been applied. There is every indication that soon we will have reasonable metagenomic [19–22] and metabolomic [23] tools to assess the microbial composition present in a CF lung and will be able to infer growth rates that are specific to the community composition as well as the antibiotic administered. Entering voxel specific growth rates based on more information than we at present possess and using our program to test predictions can move our understanding of the patient's state to a new and quantitative level.

We can improve the accuracy level of the model by extending the resolution of our PDFE-2D distributions. The current PDFEs were constructed with 5% bins as described in PDFE-2D model section.

Discussion

With current research studies about cystic fibrosis, CF treatment is poised for great strides. Non-genetic treatments such as Ivacaftor (trade name Kalydeco, developed as VX-770) only works on patients with a certain mutation of cystic fibrosis which accounts for 4–5% of cystic fibrosis cases [24].

While an eventual cure for the disease by replacement of the defective gene is likely, we expect such treatment not to be available anytime soon. Rather we anticipate that new observational tools such as metagenomics, transcriptomics, metabolomics and MRI imaging coupled with our modeling approach will give the clinician unprecedented ability to follow and treat the disease. The models will provide quantitative predictions of responses to various drug regimens and prescribe adaptively implemented optimal controls for treatment. Predicting the impact of mucus growth on lung functionality will correlate the current stage of the disease with how infection has been propagating throughout different generations of lung. This will enable the physician with a tool to track this propagation of infection.

The various sub-models required here will soon be informed by data characterizing the microbial communities present. Such data comes from metagenomic and transcriptomics analyses of sputum samples and metabolomic analyses of exhaled air. In our current model we predict the dynamic distribution of mucus in a CF lung in the absence of treatment as a stepping stone for eventually eventual treatment and microbial community specific modeling of the treatment response.

According to a research study done by Willner et al. [25] microbial diversity in a CF lung is much higher than suggested by culturing alone. They were able to characterize the diversity of

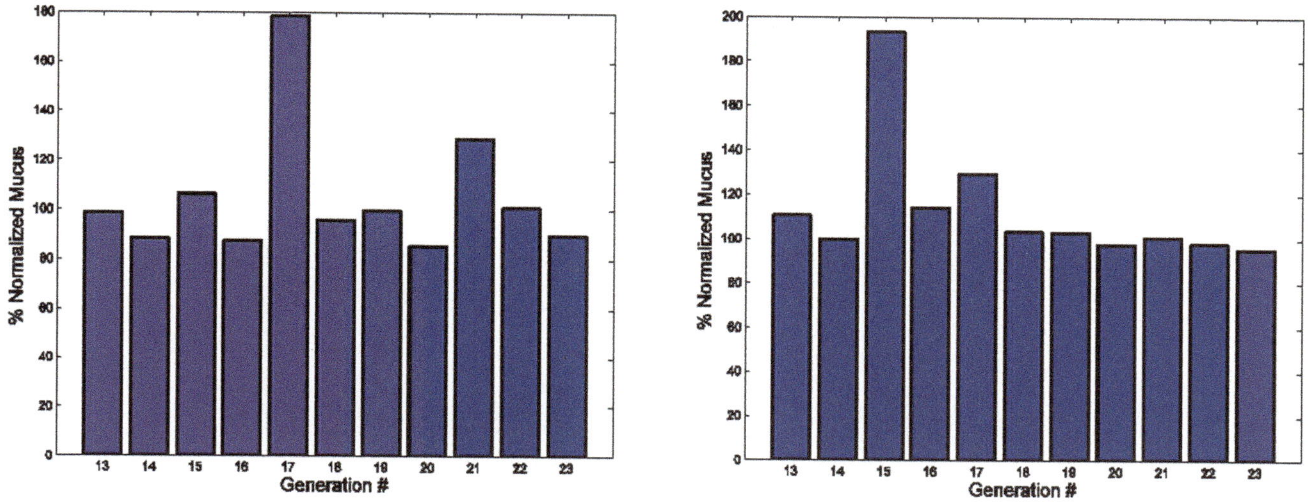

(A) (B)

Figure 4. Mucus distribution among different generations of lung for two selected voxels. Figure (A) represents a voxel with 5% mucus volume that has 78% accessible alveoli: AA and resistance ratio of 1.22. Figure (B) repsresents represents a voxel with 30% mucus that has 19.45% AA and resistance ratio of 4.2. The x-axis is the generation number of the corresponding bronchioles in the selected voxel. The y-axis shows the normalized mucus present, which is equal to the ratio of the mucus amount in a generation to the total mucus volume in a voxel, divided by the ratio of the air volume in that generation to the total voxel volume.

microbial communities in tissue sections from anatomically distinct regions of the CF lung. Their result indicated that microbial communities in the Cystic Fibrosis lung are spatially heterogeneous.This Spatial heterogeneity will cause regional differences in microbial biomass and antibiotic resistance. The next version of the model, can use their results to adjust the parameters according to the microbial communities found and the treatment administered (e.g., timing of antibiotic administration, types of antibiotics, steroids, etc). The present model should be taken as a proof-of-concept step toward that goal. This will provide an opportunity for the researcher, and eventually the clinician, to access a framework for accurate quantitative predictions.

Our methods are completely scalable – the 1.0 cm^3 for the size of one voxel was for illustration. Any resolution scale however forces estimation of the distribution on spatial scales below this resolution. Since estimation of the distribution on finer spatial scales would perforce need the solution of an inverse problem with many possible solutions and since the movement of mucus hinted that the "right answer" would in any case not be a unique distribution, we were led naturally to using Monte Carlo

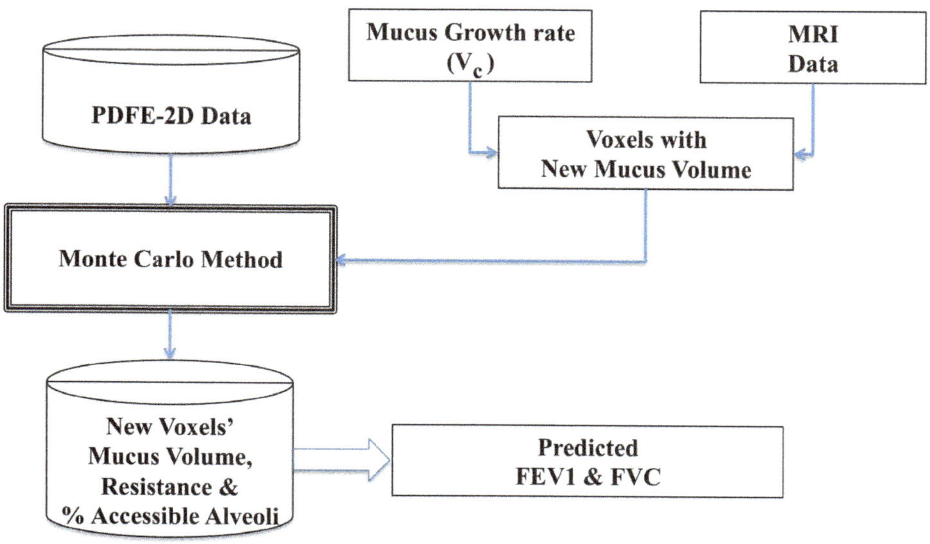

Figure 5. FEV_1 and FVC values predictions predicted from the lung model. This flowchart illustrates the process of how our lung model predicts the FVC and FEV_1 of a CF patient given the previous mucus content of each voxel along with a mucus growth rate.

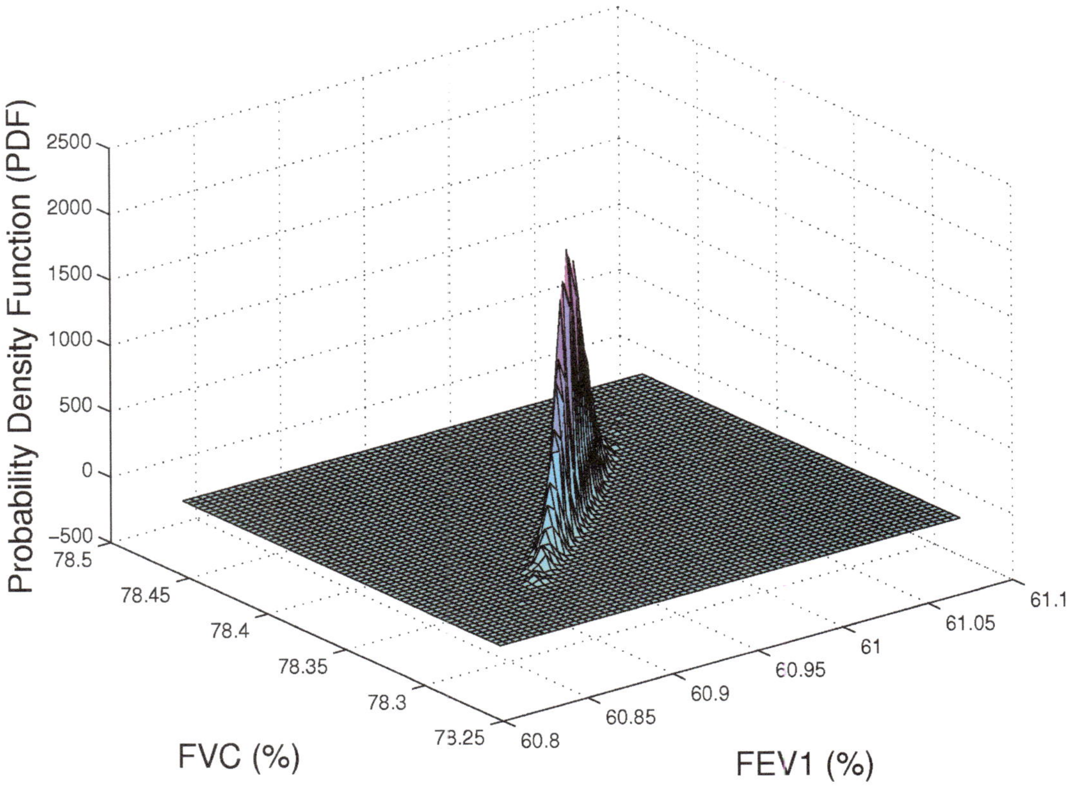

Figure 6. FEV_1 and FVC probability density function estimation. The x-axis shows the predicted FEV_1 values and the y-axis is the predicted FVC values for a hypothetical the synthetic lung example described in the text.

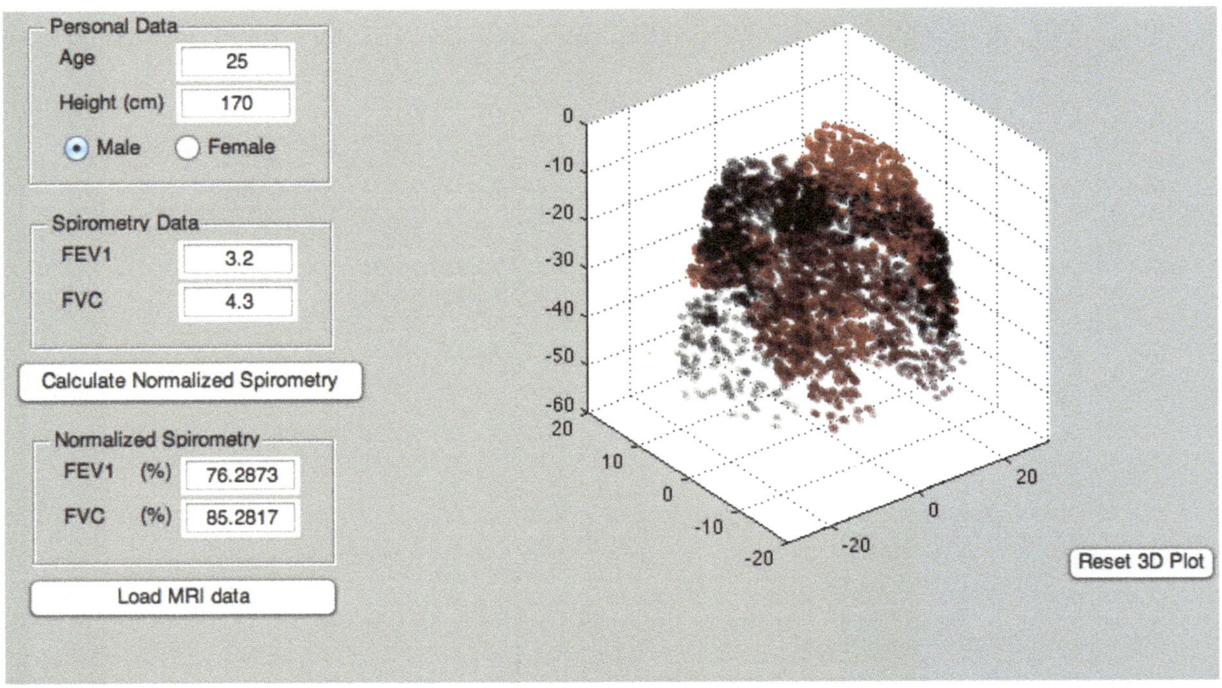

Figure 7. In this window user can enter the input parameters: patient's age, height, sex and Imaging data. The Model displays a 3D-lung that contains all the MRI/CT scan voxels.

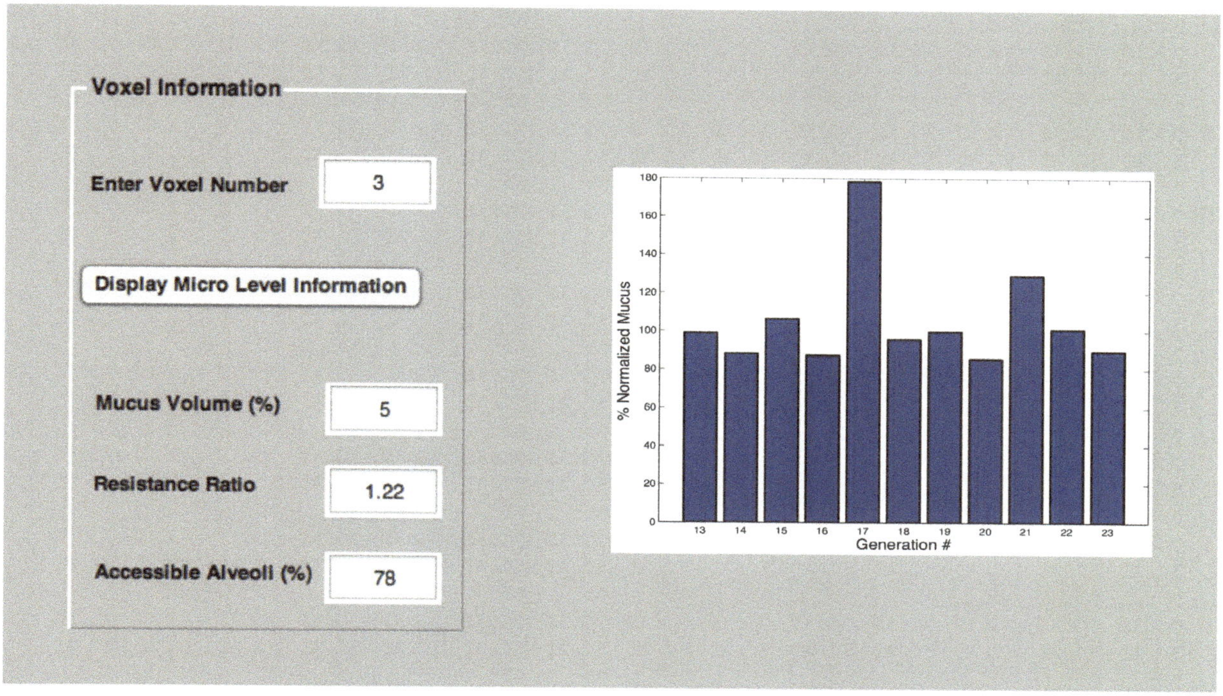

Figure 8. This window shows the mucus distribution among generations. The user selects a voxel and the model displays its corresponding parameters along with the micro-level information.

estimation methods for the most likely distribution and the corresponding spirometric observables. The resulting models and algorithms form a clinically useful tool with which to reassess the various simplest possible sub-models and assumptions used in our work so far. These models can play a crucial role in future treatments of the disease.

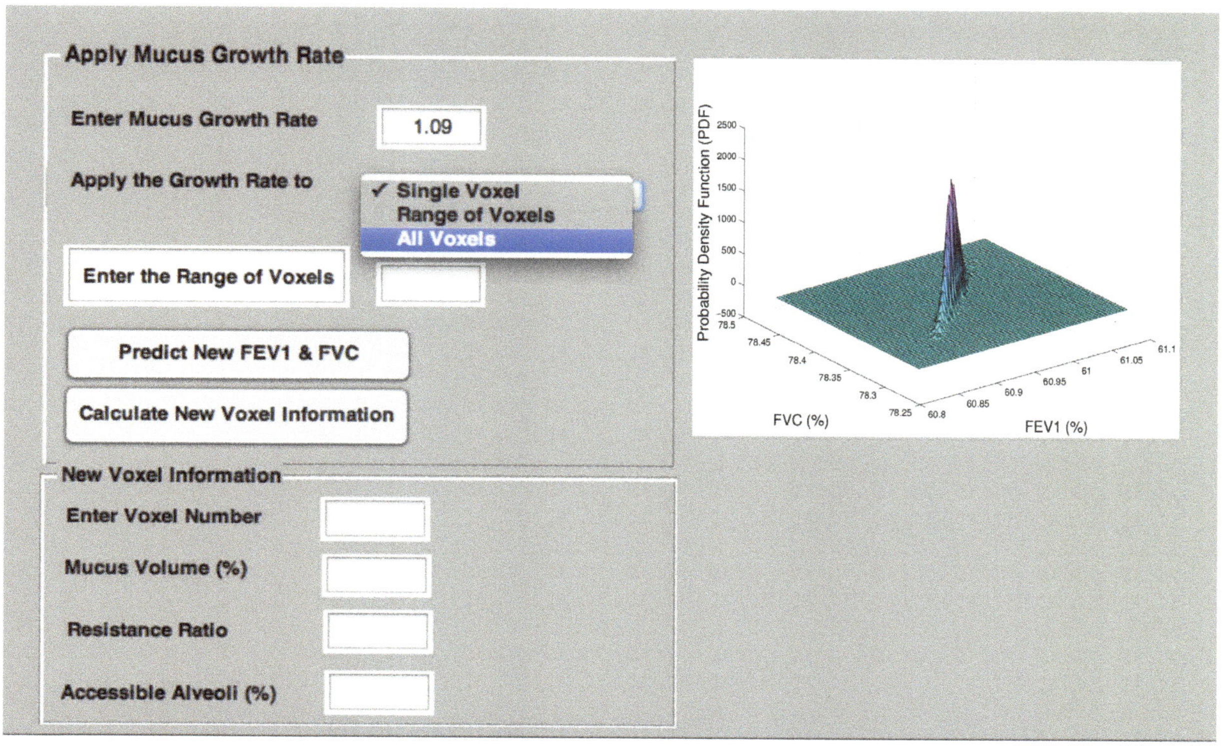

Figure 9. This window provides the user with a probability density function of the predicted FEV_1 and FVC. User can enter a specific mucus growth rate for different voxels and the new FEV_1 and FVC will be calculated.

Supporting Information

File S1 The supporting file Psudo.pdf contains the psudo code of the algorithms and models mentioned in this manuscript.

Acknowledgments

This material is based upon work supported by the National Institutes of Health under Grant no. 56586B.

The funders had no role in study design, data collection and analysis, decision to publish, or preparation of the manuscript.

Author Contributions

Conceived and designed the experiments: SZ AM FR PS. Performed the experiments: SZ AM FR PS. Analyzed the data: SZ AM FR PS. Contributed reagents/materials/analysis tools: SZ AM FR PS. Wrote the paper: SZ AM FR PS.

References

1. Tirouvanziam R (2006) Neutrophilic inflammation as a major determinant in the progression of cystic fibrosis. Drug News Perspect 19: 609–614.
2. Koehler DR, Downey GP, Sweezey NB, Tanswell AK, Hu J (2004) Lung inflammation as a therapeutic target in cystic fibrosis. Amer J of Resp Cell and Mol Biol 31: 377–381.
3. Eichinger M, Puderbach M, Heussel CP, Kauczor HU (2006) Mri in mucoviscidosis (cystic fibrosis). Radiologe, German 46 (4): 275–276.
4. Hopkins SR, Levin DL, Emami K, Kadlecek S, Yu J, et al. (2007) Advances in magnetic resonance imaging of lung physiology. J of App Physiol 102 (3): 1244–1254.
5. Fiel SB, Friedman AC, Caroline DF, Radecki PD, Faerber E, et al. (1987) Magnetic resonance imaging in young adults with cystic fibrosis. Chest 91: 181–184.
6. Theilmann RJ, Arai TJ, Samiee A, Dubowitz DJ, Hopkins SR, et al. (2009) Quantitative mri measurement of lung density must account for the change in t(2) (*) with lung inflation. J of MRI 30: 527–534.
7. Voit EO (2014) Mesoscopic modeling as a starting point for computational analyses of cystic fibrosis as a systemic disease. Biochim et Biophy Acta 1844 (1): 258–270.
8. Zarei S, Mirtar A, Andresen B, Salamon P (2013) Modeling the airflow in a lung with cystic fibrosis. J of Non-Equil Thermodyn 38 (2): 119–140.
9. Zarei S, Mirtar A, Rohwer F, Conrad DJ, Theilmann RJ, et al. (2012) Mucus distribution model in a lung with cystic fibrosis. J of Comp and Math Meth in Med.
10. Weibel ER (1991) Design of airways and blood vessels considered as branching trees. Lung: Sci Found 1: 1061–1071.
11. Altemeier WA, McKinney S, Glenny RW (2005) A fractal analysis of the radial distribution of bronchial capillaries around large airways. J of App Physiol 98: 850–855.
12. Glenny RW, Bernard SL, Robertson HT (2000) Pulmonary blood flow remains fractal down to the level of gas exchange. J of App Physiol 89: 742–748.
13. West BJ (1990) Physiology in fractal dimensions: error tolerance. Anna of Biomed Engi 18 (2): 135–149.
14. Richey M (2010) The evolution of markov chain monte carlo methods. Amer Math Mon 117 (5): 383–413.
15. Saeta PN (2004). The metropolis algorithm: Statistical systems and simulated annealing. URL http://saeta.physics.hmc.edu/courses/p170/Metropolis.pdf.
16. Salamon P, Sibani P, Frost R (2002) Facts, Conjecture, and Improvements for Simulated Annealing. Philadelphia: Society for Industrial and Applied Mathematics.
17. Marieb E, Hoehn K (2010) Human Anatomy and Physiology. Prentice Hall PTR. 8th ED.
18. Kitaoka H, Suk B (1997) Branching design of the bronchial tree based on a diameter-flow relationship. J of App Physiol 82: 968–976.
19. Willner D, Furlan M, Haynes M, Schmieder R, Angly FE, et al. (2009) Metagenomic analysis of respiratory tract dna viral communities in cystic fibrosis and non-cystic fibrosis individuals. PLoS One 4 (10): e7370.
20. Lim YW, Evangelista JS, Schmieder R, Bailey B, Haynes M, et al. (2014) Clinical insights from metagenomic analysis of sputum samples from patients with cystic fibrosis. J of Clin Microbi 52 (2): 425–437.
21. Lim YW, Schmieder R, Haynes M, Furlan M, Matthews TD, et al. (2013) Mechanistic model of rothia mucilaginosa adaptation toward persistence in the cf lung, based on a genome reconstructed from metagenomic data. PloS one 8 (5): e64285.
22. Lim YW, Schmiederb R, Haynesa M, Willnerd D, Furlana M, et al. (2013) Metagenomics and metatranscriptomics: Windows on cf-associated viral and microbial communities. J of Cystic Fibrosis 12 (2): 154–164.
23. Whiteson KL, Meinardi S, Lim YW, Schmieder R, Maughan H, et al. (2014) Breath gas metabolites and bacterial metagenomes from cystic fibrosis airways indicate active ph neutral 2, 3-butanedione fermentation. ISME J.
24. McPhail G, Clancy J (2013) Ivacaftor: The first therapy acting on the primary cause of cystic fibrosis. Drugs of today 49: 253–260.
25. Willner D, Furlan M, Haynes M, Schmieder R, Lim YW, et al. (2011) Spatial distribution of microbial communities in the cystic fibrosis lung. ISME J 6: 471–747.

Consensus between Pipelines in Structural Brain Networks

Christopher S. Parker[1,2]*, Fani Deligianni[2], M. Jorge Cardoso[1], Pankaj Daga[1], Marc Modat[1], Michael Dayan[2,4], Chris A. Clark[2], Sebastien Ourselin[1,3]❡, Jonathan D. Clayden[2]❡

1 Centre for Medical Image Computing, University College London, London, United Kingdom, **2** Imaging and Biophysics Unit, UCL Institute of Child Health, London, United Kingdom, **3** Dementia Research Centre, University College London, London, United Kingdom, **4** Department of Radiology, Weill Cornell Medical College, New York, New York, United States of America

Abstract

Structural brain networks may be reconstructed from diffusion MRI tractography data and have great potential to further our understanding of the topological organisation of brain structure in health and disease. Network reconstruction is complex and involves a series of processesing methods including anatomical parcellation, registration, fiber orientation estimation and whole-brain fiber tractography. Methodological choices at each stage can affect the anatomical accuracy and graph theoretical properties of the reconstructed networks, meaning applying different combinations in a network reconstruction pipeline may produce substantially different networks. Furthermore, the choice of which connections are considered important is unclear. In this study, we assessed the similarity between structural networks obtained using two independent state-of-the-art reconstruction pipelines. We aimed to quantify network similarity and identify the core connections emerging most robustly in both pipelines. Similarity of network connections was compared between pipelines employing different atlases by merging parcels to a common and equivalent node scale. We found a high agreement between the networks across a range of fiber density thresholds. In addition, we identified a robust core of highly connected regions coinciding with a peak in similarity across network density thresholds, and replicated these results with atlases at different node scales. The binary network properties of these core connections were similar between pipelines but showed some differences in atlases across node scales. This study demonstrates the utility of applying multiple structural network reconstrution pipelines to diffusion data in order to identify the most important connections for further study.

Editor: Yong Liu, Chinese Academy of Sciences & National Laboratory of Pattern Recognition, China

Funding: FD and JDC were supported by the EPSRC (EP/J016292/1). PD was funded by EPSRC-CRUK Comprehensive Cancer Imaging Centre of UCL and KCL (grant number C1519AO). SO and MJC were supported by both the EPSRC (EP/H046410/1) and the CBRC Strategic Investment Award (Ref. 168). SO receives funding from the EPSRC (EP/H046410/1, EP/J020990/1, EP/K005278), the MRC (MR/J01107X/1), the EU-FP7 project VPH-DARE@IT (FP7-ICT-2011-9-601055), the NIHR Biomedical Research Unit (Dementia) at UCL and the National Institute for Health Research University College London Hospitals Biomedical Research Centre (NIHR BRC UCLH/UCL High Impact Initiative). MM is supported by the UCL Leonard Wolfson Experimental Neurology Centre. The Dementia Research Centre is an Alzheimers Research Trust Co-ordinating centre and has also received equipment founded by the Alzheimers Research Trust. The funders had no role in study design, data collection and analysis, decision to publish, or preparation of the manuscript.

Competing Interests: The authors have declared that no competing interests exist.

* Email: christopher.parker.10@ucl.ac.uk

❡ These authors contributed equally to this work.

Introduction

Studying brain structural networks using diffusion MRI tractography has recently become a popular research topic in neuroscience [1]. In this field the research aim is to quantify connectivity between grey matter regions via white matter pathways *in vivo*, on a global scale, in order to understand the topological organisation of brain structure and to relate this to aspects of neurological health and disease. The structural topology may be analysed by characterising the brain as a graph, whereby sets of network nodes, representing grey matter regions, transfer information between one another via network edges, representing connecting axonal pathways.

It has been suggested that the organisation of the structural network may reflect neurological phenotype. For example, network metrics such as clustering coefficient and pathlength have been related to the effect of age [2], gender [3] and IQ [4]. In addition, network alterations have been observed in neurological diseases such as Alzheimer's disease [5,6], epilepsy [7,8] and schizophrenia [9–11], meaning such metrics may become useful as topological biomarkers of brain integrity or pathology. However, reconstructing brain network nodes and edges is both a conceptual and practical challenge and there is little agreement between studies of how exactly these should be defined.

Nodes of the brain network, which represent spatially distinct regions of grey matter, may be defined using different parcellation schemes and scales. A common parcellation technique has been to warp the structural image to an anatomical template, such as the AAL atlas [12], where the grey matter regions have been manually labelled in a single representative subject [4,9,11,13]. Alternative warping strategies have been applied; for example, those utilising cortical shape and curvature information [14], or multiple template propagations [15]. In addition, different templates may be used to generate different parcellation schemes. Most parcellations used in whole-brain structural network studies have been relatively coarse, with around 100 brain regions. Because of the uncertainty concerning where to place region boundaries, some studies have divided parcellated regions into smaller pseuodorandom patches [16,17], or performed network analysis across a range of parcellation scales [18–20]. Regions defined in structural space must then be accurately warped to diffusion space in order to estimate the inter-regional connectivity, and a number of registration schemes are available.

Edges of the structural brain network, which represent white matter tracts between two grey matter regions, are frequently quantified based on the number of connecting fibers. As such, the issue of which fiber model, initialisation and tracking technique to use arises. The diffusion tensor model [21], combined with deterministic tracking, is a common technique for reconstructing network edges [14,22–24]. Multiple fibers may be represented using multiple diffusion tensors, the orientation distribution function (ODF) [25], multi-compartment models [26] and the fiber orientation distribution (FOD) [27]. The ball and sticks multi-compartment model is one example of a popular fiber model employed to track through multiple fiber populations in structural network studies [3,28]. In contrast to multi-compartment models, the FOD representation assumes an identical signal response for each fiber population and does not employ model fitting. Deterministic tracking determines inter-regional connectivity by following the dominant fiber orientation whereas probabilistic tracking samples directions from a distribution of orientations to produce a connectivity distribution.

In networks obtained using probabilistic tractography, a continuous measure of connectivity is generated which reflects (to some degree) the probability of connection between all brain regions. A probability threshold may then be applied to produce a binary network, where connections are either absent or present [29]. However, assigning importance to connections is a challenge and the choice of threshold affects the occurance of false positive and negative connections, resulting in a trade-off between sensitivity and specificity of the connections [30,31]. Thresholding also has an intrinsic impact on the network topological measures [32].

Given the complexity and number of steps involved in network reconstruction from the raw diffusion MRI images, it is important to provide an assessment of consensus in networks obtained from alternative reconstruction pipelines which vary not in just one or two components but in the entire reconstruction pipeline (i.e the parcellation, registration and fiber model). This would also enable some assessment of the potential impact in swapping and substituting individual components of the reconstruction.

In this study, we assessed the convergence of structural connectivity networks obtained from two alternative pipelines across a range of network density thresholds, by merging alternative parcellations to a common and equivalent node scale. This allowed us to investigate similarity between independent network reconstructions on a connection-wise basis and to identify the underlying brain connections occuring most robustly in both pipelines. Our results suggest it may be useful to apply multiple pipelines to obtain structural brain networks from diffusion data and to employ the comparison framework described here to identify the most important connections.

Methods

Ethics statement

Informed written consent was obtained from all subjects participating in this study. Processes for consenting and image acquisition were approved by the UCL Research Ethics Committee.

Subjects and image acquisition

Twenty-eight young healthy adult subjects (16 male, mean age $\pm$ s.d. 28.5 $\pm$ 3.9 years) participated in this study. Subjects had no brain abnormalities at the time of scanning, as determined by examination of their structural scan by an expert radiologist. Two T1-weighted images of $1 \times 1 \times 1$ mm resolution were acquired sequentially with a 3D Fast Low-Angle Shot (FLASH) sequence (176 contiguous sagittal slices, 256×224 mm FOV, TR = 11 ms, TE = 4.94 ms and α = 15°) on a 1.5T Siemens Avanto MRI scanner at Great Ormond Street Hospital, London. A diffusion-weighted echo planar sequence (TR = 7300 ms, TE = 81 ms) with 60 noncollinear diffusion directions (b = 1000 s/mm^2) was used to acquire diffusion-weighted images of $2.5 \times 2.5 \times 2.5$ mm and three un-weighted images (b = 0 images). The diffusion-weighted sequence was repeated three times for each subject in a single scanning session.

Image preprocessing

DICOM images were converted into NIfTI format using TractoR [33] and the brain was extracted from all images using FSL's brain extraction tool [34]. In order to increase the signal to noise ratio of the structural image, the two acquired T1-weighted images were registered and averaged in Freesurfer v5.1.0 [35]. The diffusion-weighted volumes were corrected for eddy-current induced distortions by affine registration to an unweighted reference image using the diffusion-specific FSL FDT algorithm [36].

We chose to compare two alternative state-of-the-art reconstruction pipelines (these two pipelines will hereafter be referred to as P1 and P2, Fig 1). Both reconstructions had similar capabilities but varied with respect to the details of the cortical parcellation, registration and probabilistic fiber model method.

Cortical parcellation

To define network nodes, the cortical grey matter of the averaged T1-weighted image was parcellated into regions using automated software. **P1.** NiftySeg was used to parcellate the structural image into 44 cortical regions (22 per hemisphere), as defined by the Hammers Atlas [37]. The parcellation algorithm first labels brain regions by propagating a set of manually labelled T1-weighted images to the structural image [38,39]. The LoAd tissue segmentation algorithm was then applied to the structural image to obtain the cortical grey matter of the parcellated regions [40]. **P2.** Freesurfer was used to parcellate the structural image into 68 cortical regions (34 per hemisphere), as defined by the Desikan-Killiany Atlas [41]. The parcellation algorithm assigns a neuroanatomical label to each location on a cortical surface model of the image, based on probabilistic information from a manually labeled training set [42].

Native and common node scale parcellations

The pipelines employed atlases with a different number of brain regions, preventing a direct connection-wise comparison between them. Therefore, parcels in the native atlases were merged to a common node scale (Fig. 2). The number of merges was the minimum required to give correspondence between the atlases and

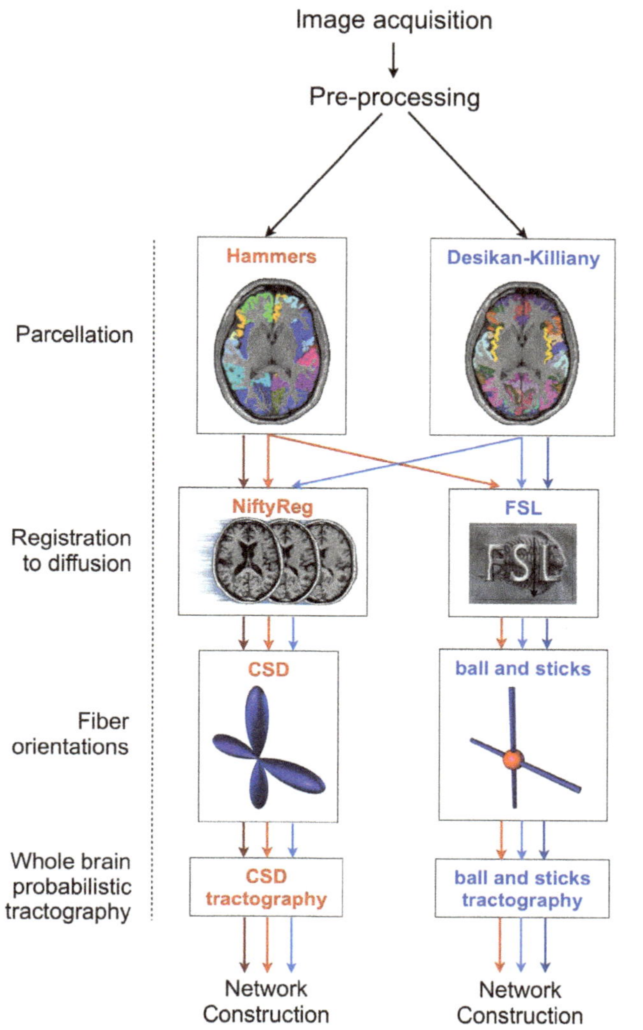

Figure 1. Summary of network reconstruction stages applied to structural and diffusion images for P1 and P2. The pipeline stages are shown on the left and the alternative implementations of the methods are shown inside the boxes. Arrows indicate the passage of merged (dark arrows) and native (light arrows) atlases through the pipeline stages (red and blue refer to Hammers and Desikan-Killiany atlases, respectively). Nodes were defined by registration of the cortical parcels to diffusion space. Edges were defined by performing tractography from the parcel boundary through the fiber orientations. Note that the whole-brain probabilistic tractography methods differed only in relation to the recommended settings for the software used to track through the fiber orientations. The network construction stage calculated the connecting fiber density between all cortical parcel pairs across the entire cerebral cortex and was identical for both pipelines. Applying these stagesto the merged and native atlases resulted in comparisons between pipelines at three node scales; the merged atlas scale (34 nodes, dark arrows), Hammers atlas scale (44 nodes, light red arrows) and Desikan-Killiany scale (68 nodes, light blue arrows). We also applied the registration and whole-brain tractography pipelines to the AAL atlas (not shown).

resulted in 34 brain regions (17 per hemisphere). Parcels in the Desikan-Killiany atlas (P2) were merged across the entire cortex based on anatomical correspondence to their equivalent Hammers atlas (P1) parcels. For example, the pars opercularis, pars orbitalis and pars triangularis parcels in the native Desikan-Killiany atlas corresponded to the inferior frontal gyrus parcel in the native Hammers atlas and therefore in both of the merged atlases. The Desikan-Killiany and Hammers atlases differed fundamentally in temporal lobe regions, meaning an equivalent merging of parcels could not be found. Therefore, the temporal lobe is itself considered as a single node in both merged parcellations (Fig. 2 and 3). The merging process did not result in identical parcellations. The remaining differences in common scale parcellations were due to alternative border criteria as well as alternative parcellation algorithms. Therefore, in addition to the native Desikan-Killiany and Hammers atlases, we also obtained the two merged 34 node scale versions of each atlas for each subject (Fig. 3).

Each common scale parcellation was registered to diffusion space (as described below) using the registration implementation for the corresponding pipeline (e.g. following the P1 registration-tractography for the merged P1 parcellation). We also applied the paired registration-tractography implementation from each pipeline to both of the native atlases. We further tested the robustness of our results by applying each registration-tractography implementation to the Automated Anatomical Labelling (AAL) Atlas parcellation [12], which had cortical 78 regions.

Registration of cortical parcels to diffusion space

The structural and diffusion-weighted images were co-registered in order to define the cortical parcels of interest in diffusion space. The registration field was determined as follows. An affine registration was used to register the first $b=0$ image to the averaged T1-weighted image. The T1-weighted image was then non-linearly registered to the $b=0$ image using the inverse of the transformation acquired in the previous stage as a starting transformation. The transformation field was retained and applied to the cortical parcellation to transform parcels to diffusion space. The categorical nature of the labels was preserved through a nearest neighbour resampling scheme. **P1**. NiftyReg was used to perform the linear and non-linear registrations using the default settings [39,43]. NiftyReg used normalised mutual information to calculate image similarity and a bending energy regularisation with cubic B-spline parameterisation for the non-linear warping. **P2**. The linear and non-linear registration was performed by FSL FLIRT and FNIRT, respectively [36]. Normalised cross correlation and sum-of-squared difference was used to calculate image similarity for the linear and non-linear warping stages, respectively. The membrane energy was used to regulate the non-linear warp field which was parameterised as a cubic B-spline scheme.

Fiber orientations

The orientations of fiber bundles at each voxel were inferred using one of two methods. **P1**. Constrained spherical deconvolution (CSD) was applied to estimate the underlying fibre orientation distributions (FOD) in each voxel, using MRTrix [44]. CSD assumes that the observed diffusion signal is a convolution of fiber orientations and a diffusion signal response function, meaning the fiber orientations may be extracted by spherical deconvolution of the diffusion signal. The maximum spherical harmonic order for the deconvolution was set to 8. **P2**. A ball and two sticks multi-compartment fiber model was fitted to the diffusion data, using the Bayesian Estimation of Diffusion Parameters Obtained using Sampling Techniques (BEDPOSTX) algorithm in FSL. The BEDPOSTX algorithm uses Markov chain Monte Carlo sampling to estimate the uncertainty in fibre orientations [45].

Probabilistic fiber tractography

The paths of fiber trajectories in the brain were reconstructed by seeding 100 probabilistic fibers from the interior boundary voxels of each cortical parcel. The interior boundary voxels were

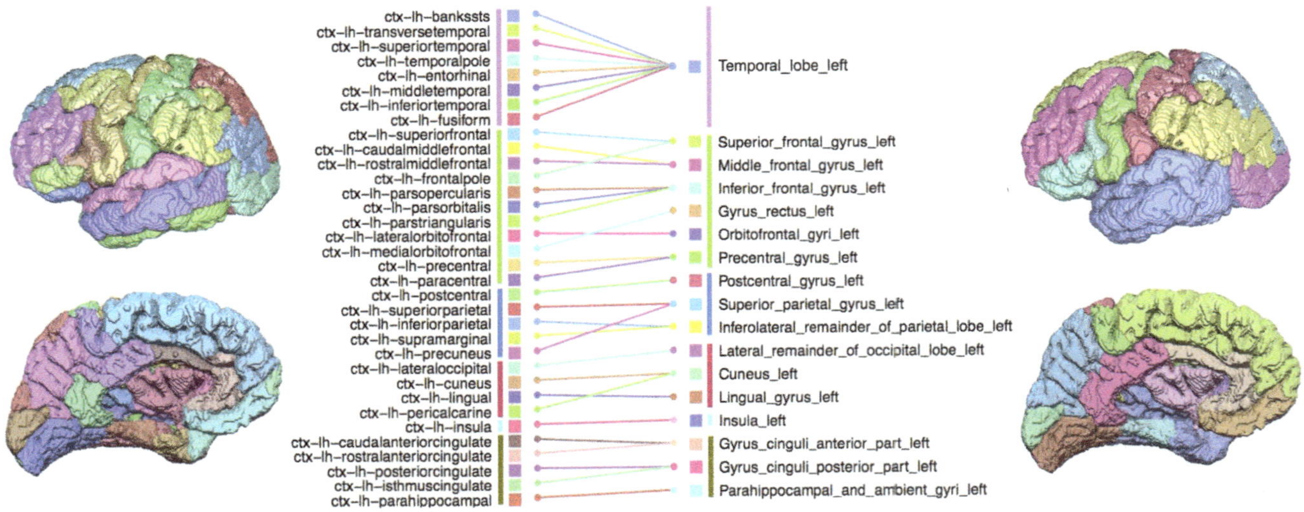

Figure 2. Merging cortical parcels of P2 parcellations. The native scale P2 parcellation (68 parcels) is shown on the left and the merged P2 parcellation (34 parcels) is shown on the right. The merging pattern was identical for both hemispheres and therefore only the left hemisphere is shown. The colour scheme of brain regions is as in Fig. 2. Lines represent merging of native scale parcels (left) to their equivalent common scale parcels (right). Coloured vertical lines correspond to regions in the temporal (purple), frontal (green), parietal (blue), occipital (red), insula (light-blue) or limbic (yellow) lobes. Native scale P1 parcellations (44 nodes) were merged to the common scale parcellation by merging all temporal lobe parcels.

the intersection of the dilated binary cortical parcellation with the fiber propagation mask (defined for each pipeline below). **P1**. Fibers were propagated using the default settings in MRTrix [46]. The sampling interval was 0.2 mm, maximum curvature threshold was 60° and minimum fiber orientation dispersion (FOD) amplitude threshold for tracking through a voxel was 0.1. The propagation mask was defined as the union of white matter, sub-cortical grey matter and ventricle regions from the LoAd tissue segmentation provided by NiftySeg. **P2**. The default settings in FSL ProbTrack algorithm were used to determine the fiber trajectories [26]. The sampling interval was 0.5 mm and stopping criteria meant that fibers terminate if they curve by more than 80°. The propagation mask was defined as the white matter segmentation provided as part of the Freesurfer output, and included white matter, sub-cortical and ventricular regions.

Note that P1 initiates fibers by uniform sampling of boundary voxels with a FOD amplitude greater or equal to 0.2, whereas P2 initiates fibers from the centre of each boundary voxel. Also, P1 terminates fibers if the FOD amplitude is below 0.1. For both pipeline tracking schemes, fibers were terminated immediately after leaving the propagation mask so that their cortical parcel connections could be recorded.

Network construction

Network construction and analysis was performed using the R programming language [47]. Cortical parcels were represented as network nodes and the fiber connections between them as edges. Fibers connected node pairs if their end-point coordinates terminated within two distinct cortical parcels. The connection weight between two cortical nodes was defined as the density of

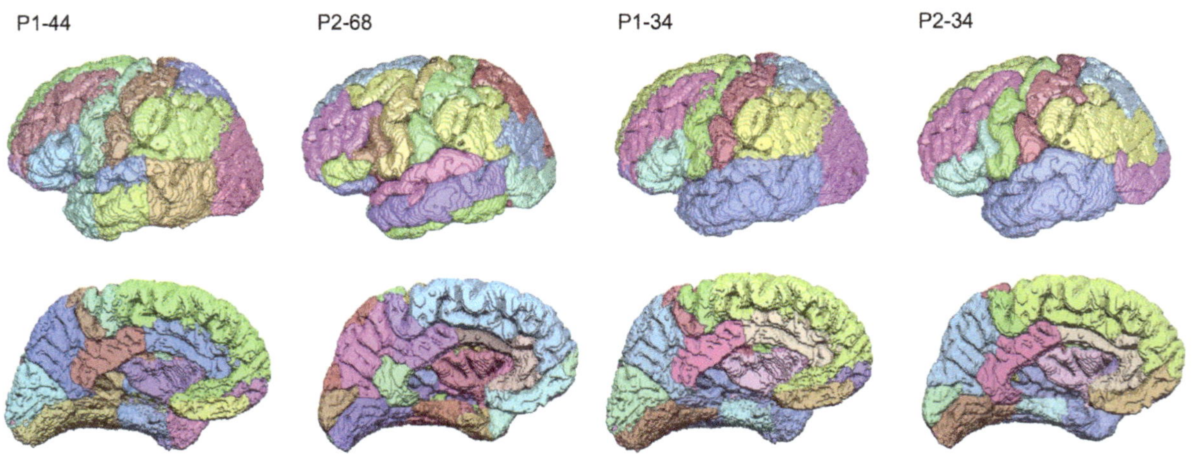

Figure 3. Representative cortical parcellations of P1 and P2 at the native and common node scale. Temporal lobe regions in P1 native scale parcellations (P1-44, far left) were merged, resulting in a lower scale parcellation (P1-34, middle right). Selected regions across the entire cerebral cortex in P2 native scale parcellations (P2-68, middle left) were merged (P2-34, see Fig. 1). This resulted in a common and anatomically equivalent parcellation scale of 34 nodes for both P1 and P2 networks.

connecting fibres (as in [48]), calculated as the sum of connecting fibers divided by the mean volume of the seed (boundary) voxels adjacent to the two parcels (boundary voxels were assigned to the nearest parcel by Euclidean distance). Performing this calculation for all fibers produces an N-by-N undirected matrix of connection weights, where N is the number of nodes in the parcellation (either 34, 44, 68 or 78). The weighted cortical connection matrix was calculated for the repeat diffusion scans of all subjects. The subject mean weighted connection matrices (across the three repeat diffusion scans) were calculated for all subjects by averaging each weight across all scans.

Convergence between alternative pipelines

Convergence between alternative pipelines was investigated in binary networks of equal density. Binary networks were generated by thresholding the subject weighted networks and convergence was quantified for all possible densities in the range [0,1], by selecting the x highest ranked connections in the weighted matrix, for $x = 1 : c$, where c is the total number of possible connections (calculated as $(N^2 - N)/2$). Connections of equal weight (predominantly weights of value 0), were randomly assigned a rank, meaning connections were chosen randomly if the network density threshold intersected connections of equal weight. Convergence was quantified between the pair-wise subject binary networks using the Dice Similarity Coefficient (DC). DC was defined as the proportion of intersecting connections relative to the total number of connections at that density. This measure is identical to the percentage convergence measure of network similarity used in [49] for networks of equal density.

Our investigation was interested in similarity between pipelines independent of network density effects (denser networks have a higher DC by chance). Therefore, at each network density, we computed a one sample t-statistic between the observed DC across all subjects to the expected DC value, using a two-tailed t-test. The expected DC value was equal to the network density, d, as the number of connections expected to agree in two random binary networks ($d.d.c$) was divided by the total number of connections ($d.c$). Our null hypothesis was that similarity between pipelines was equal to that by chance, given the density. The p-value computed from this t-statistic was our estimate of the significance of the similarity. To estimate the dependency of the significance on our sample population, we bootstrapped the subjects 1000 times at each network density. As lower p-values represented higher similarity, we inspected the negative logarithm of the p-value to obtain a global maximum significance and corresponding network density where the binary network similarity was most reliably different from random.

Network properties of the consensus network

The binary networks corresponding to the peak convergence threshold will hereafter be referred to as 'consensus networks' for convenience. The graph theoretical proprerties of the consensus networks were calculated for all subjects using the igraph package [50] in the R programming language. The global properties of characteristic pathlength [51] and global efficiency [52], and the local properties of local efficiency [52], clustering coefficient [53] and assortativity [54], were calculated as described in [55].

Results

Convergence between alternative network reconstructions

The raw weights matrix represents the connecting fiber density between cortical region pairs across the entire cerebral cortex. The connecting fiber density was highly correlated between subject mean networks obtained from alternative reconstructions in terms of both rank and weight (34 nodes: Spearman $\rho = 0.675 \pm 0.06$, Pearson $r = 0.630 \pm 0.061$, 44 nodes: Spearman $\rho = 0.677 \pm 0.076$, Pearson $r = 0.702 \pm 0.085$, 68 nodes: Spearman $\rho = 0.586 \pm 0.095$, Pearson $r = 0.632 \pm 0.085$), confirming that these pipelines had yeilded similar networks.

A general trend of decreasing DC with decreasing network density was observed. The grand mean DC across all subjects and densities was 0.741 ± 0.165, 0.759 ± 0.132 and 0.724 ± 0.135 for the 34, 44 and 68 atlas scales, respectively. At a network density of 1 the DC was 1 as all connections existed in both pipelines. Clearly, the DC should be interpreted in the context of the expected similarity of random networks at the same density (Fig. S1).

The networks were significantly more similar between pipelines than by chance across all density thresholds (Fig. 4). Similarity increased approximately linearly with increasing threshold (corresponding to a decreasing network density), until very high thresholds were reached, where a peak similarity was observed (at network densities between 0.1–0.2, depending on the atlas), after which similarity decreased sharply towards 0. The peak similarity threshold resulted in binary networks that were most highly similar between the pipelines whilst accounting for the expected similarity at this density by chance. The most highly significant similarity was found at densities of 0.196, 0.161 and 0.106 (110, 152 and 242 connections) for node scales of 34, 44 and 68, respectively. The magnitude of the significance was similar between atlases of different scales ($-\log p \sim = 75$) at the peak similarity threshold.

Similar results were obtained using the AAL atlas. The weighted networks were highly correlated between pipelines in terms of rank and weight (Spearman $\rho = 0.703 \pm 0.161$, Pearson $r = 0.692 \pm 0.162$) and the grand mean DC was 0.701 ± 0.114 (Fig. S1). The peak similarity was observed at a density of 0.142 (427 connections), where $-\log p$ was 48.9 (Fig. 4).

The paths of fibers underlying peak convergent connections are shown in Fig. 5. Fibers representing the inter-lobe connections, intra-lobe connections and inter-hemispheric connections are shown for a representative subject reconstructed through the P1 pipeline. By visual inspection, it can be appreciated that the spatial distribution of fibers corresponds with known major anatomical tracts according to previous literature [56]. Major white matter tracts, such as the inferior longitudinal fasciculus, superior longitudinal fasciculus, cingulum and arcuate, were represented by fibers underlying inter-lobe connections. On the other hand, fibers representing intra-lobe connections appeared to be mostly cortical U-fibers.

Network properties of consensus networks

The convergent connections of the consensus networks are summarised in Fig. 6. The connections that agreed between pipelines tended to be similar across subjects. The convergent connections, which had high hemispheric symmetry, were primarily between ipsilateral intra-lobe regions and between bilateral homotopic regions. The left and right insula gyri were the most highly connected nodes in the consensus network.

The density of the consensus networks decreased when comparing lower to higher node scales atlases, whereas the number of connections increased. The graph theoretical metrics of global pathlength, clustering coefficient, global efficiency, local efficiency and assortativity, which were calculated for all consensus networks, are shown in Table 1. Graph theoretical properties of the consensus networks were similar between pipelines employing

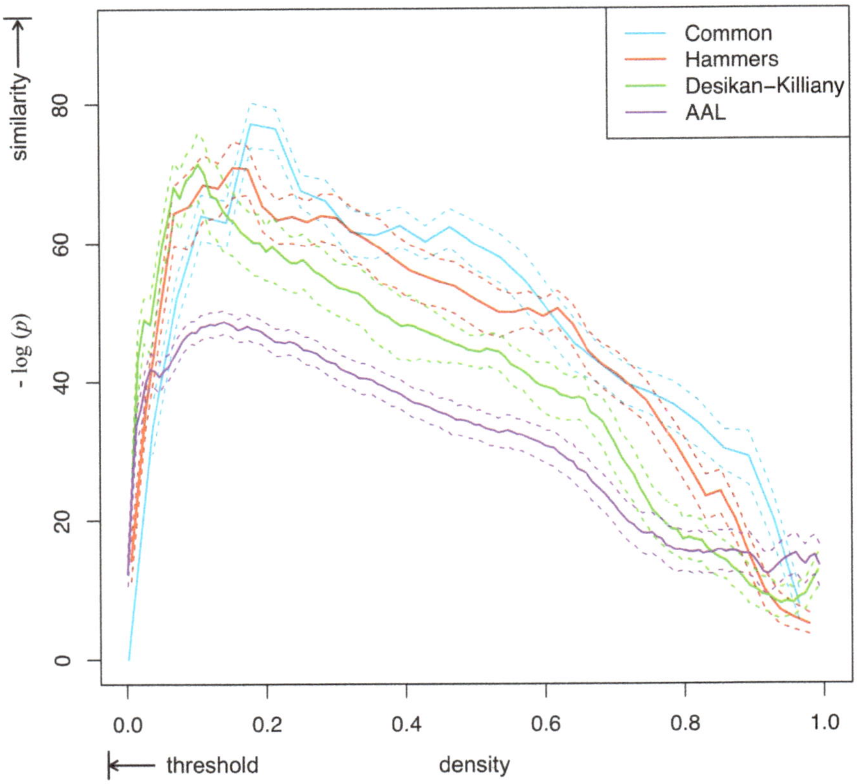

Figure 4. Similarity between P1 and P2 networks across density thresholds using atlases at three node scales. Significance of similarity was calculated by comparing the distribution of within-subject DC to the expected DC by chance, given the density of the networks. Shown is the mean negative log p-value of the DC between binary networks thresholded at a given density. The within-subject DC's were bootstrapped to obtain a standard error on the mean (dashed lines). A global peak similarity was found at a density of 0.196, 0.161, 0.106 and 0.142 for the Common (34 nodes), Hammers (44 nodes), Desikan-Killiany (68 nodes) and AAL (78 nodes) atlases, respectively.

atlases at the same node scale, whereas some differences were found in graph theoretical properties between atlases of different node scales. The global pathlength and clustering were not significantly different between pipelines at the same scale but tended to increase and decrease in higher node scale atlases, whereas global efficiency tended to decrease. Assortativity was less stable between pipelines and showed no clear trend with node scale. The AAL atlas consensus networks had a relatively high density considering the number of network nodes in the parcellation, compared to other atlases.

Discussion

In this study, we quantified the convergence of probabilistic structural networks obtained using two independent state-of-the-art reconstruction pipelines over a range of network density

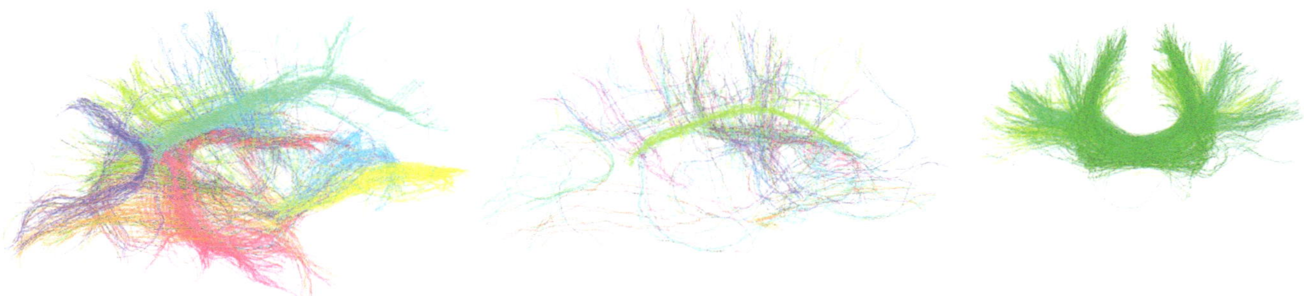

Figure 5. P1 fibers underlying convergent connections in the left hemisphere of a repre-sentative subject. Fibers are coloured by their network connection. (a) Inter-lobe fibers viewed from the medial aspect. (b) Intra-lobe fibers viewed from the medial aspect. (c) Inter-hemispheric fibers shown from the coronal aspect. The paths of fibers underlying convergent inter-lobe connections agrees with that of major anatomical tracts, such as the ILF (orange) and cingulum (green). Convergent intra-lobular connections were mostly represented by short-range cortical U-fibers. Convergent inter-hemispheric fibers travel via the corpus callosum and connected homotopic cortical regions, such as the superior, middle and inferior frontal gyri (green). For visual clarity, a maximum of 200, 50 and 100 fibers from the subset of whole-brain tractography fibers are shown per connection for (a), (b) and (c), respectively. Also, only fibers greater than 7 cm are shown for (a) and (b) and greater than 10 cm for (c).

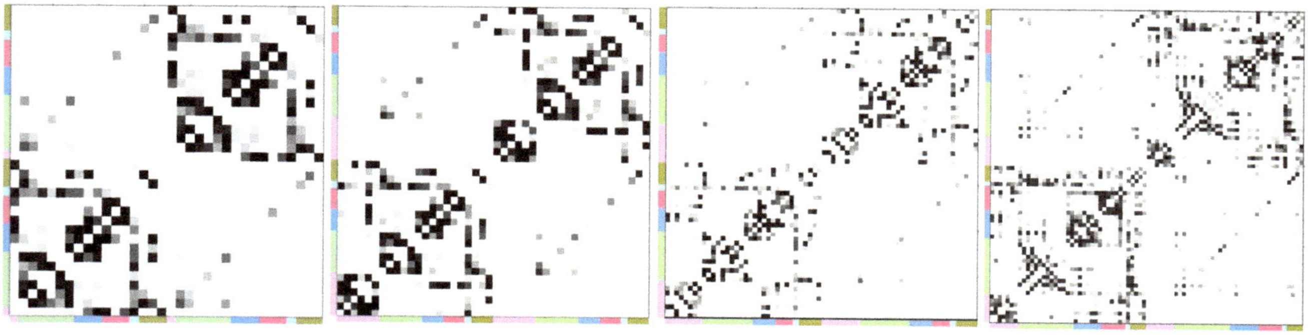

Figure 6. Prevalance of convergent connections across subjects at the peak convergence density. The prevalance is shown for the common (left), Hammers (middle-left), Desikan-Killiany (right-left) and AAL (right) atlases. Convergent connections were defined as the intersection of subject networks thresholded at the peak convergence density obtained from our bootstrap statistical analysis. The node lobe memberships are indicated by the adjacent colour bars, as in Figure 2. Colours represent the temporal (purple), frontal (green), parietal (blue), occipital (red), insula (turquoise) and cingulate (brown) lobes.

thresholds, by merging alternative parcellation schemes to an anatomically equivalent and common node scale. We also replicated our experiment using both the native parcellation scales and an alternative (AAL) parcellation scheme. Our results show there is high agreement between the two alternative reconstruction methods. We observed a global peak convergence corresponding to the brain network that occured most robustly between the two methods. The graph theoretical properties of these 'consensus networks' were highly similar between pipelines employing the same atlas but showed some variation across atlases at different node scales. Fibers representing these networks recovered the majority of major white matter tracts in all atlases, giving us confidence that the network has reasonably high anatomical validity.

Convergence between alternative network reconstructions

Individual components of the structural network reconstruction pipeline can impact on network anatomical accuracy or the network metrics, meaning the combinatorial choice of which complete reconstruction pipeline to employ is of great importance. Previous studies have found that graph theoretical properties of binary structural brain networks, such as hierarchical modularity and small-worldness, were similar across alternative acquisition and parcellation methods (at the same node scale) [57], as well as between alternative connection weighting schemes [31,58]. However, the agreement between completely independent reconstruction methods of similar capability has not been previously addressed. We found that the mean DC across all subjects and densities was significantly higher than by chance for all atlases, meaning that alternative reconstructions yielded connection weights that were ranked similarly across the entire rank profile. We therefore observed a highly significant agreement between structural networks obtained from two independent state-of-the-art reconstruction pipelines for the first time. This is an important finding since it demonstrates agreement between individual network connections as opposed to network topological measures, which may have resulted from a wider array of connection configurations. Furthermore, we can have some confidence that the networks are robust to swapping individual stages between the pipelines to some degree.

A high similarity may be expected given the similar capabilities of the pipelines. High correlation in connection rank profiles is an intrinsic property of probabilistic tractography studies, whereby probabilistic fibers tend to disperse from the true anatomical tracts as they encounter complex fiber architectures or noise in the diffusion data. This leads to densely populated network weights where the connectivity profile of neighbouring nodes is highly correlated. This may be the primary reason for such a high convergence across the entire density range, even at very low density thresholds (Fig. 4). Although highly significant relative to random networks, the similarity of AAL atlas pipelines was lower than the other atlases. This was due to a number of subjects' weighted networks having a relatively high number of non-connected (and therefore randomly ranked) region pairs, leading to a lower convergence across thresholds (Fig. S1).

A global maximum convergence across thresholds was identified and this corresponded to a sparse network with approximately 100–300 connections (network densities of 0.1–0.2), depending on the atlas. We propose that the connections in the consensus network correspond highly with the underlying anatomical substrate compared to other thresholds. Therefore, for studies employing similar network reconstruction methods, we speculate that this is an appropriate threshold to apply to the weighted networks for balancing sensitivity and specificity to true brain connections.

The convergence decreased sharply towards zero when the network density was below the peak convergent density. This may be explained by factors such as the relatively large impact of rank mismatches in connections between pipelines (due to differences in their respective sensitivity) when the number of connetions is low, or a homogenous weight distribution of the highest ranking connections leading to effectively random ranking and lower convergence.

Reus *et. al.* (2013) [30] recently assessed the impact of threshold on the sensitivity and specificity of brain network connections. Using the Desikan-Killiany atlas with 68 nodes, they estimated the number of true positive connections as 420.7 (corresponding to a network density of 18.5%), which is slightly higher than our study. This difference could be explained by their use of a different experimental design, whereby a model of the true positive distribution was fitted to the prevalance distribution calculated across subject binary networks obtained from deterministic tractography. It is interesting to note that while [30] and our study used different pipelines and analysis methods, the estimate of the number of brain connections is of a similar magnitude. The number of connections in the consensus networks was 110, 152 and 242 (corresponding to network densities of 0.196, 0.161 and

Table 1. Graph theoretical properties of peak convergent networks.

Atlas (nodes)	DC	Connections	Density	PL	CC	G.Eff	L Eff	AS
Common (34)	0.71 ± 0.03	110	0.196					
P1				2.39 ± 0.08	0.47 ± 0.02	0.42 ± 0.01	0.71 ± 0.04	0.12 ± 0.09
P2				2.42 ± 0.17	0.47 ± 0.05	0.42 ± 0.03	0.72 ± 0.05	0.04 ± 0.08
Hammers (44)	0.74 ± 0.05	152	0.161					
P1				2.69 ± 0.11	0.48 ± 0.02	0.37 ± 0.02	0.74 ± 0.03	0.10 ± 0.10
P2				2.61 ± 0.11	0.48 ± 0.04	0.38 ± 0.02	0.71 ± 0.03	0.06 ± 0.06
Freesurfer (68)	0.66 ± 0.05	242	0.106					
P1				2.93 ± 0.14	0.41 ± 0.03	0.34 ± 0.02	0.67 ± 0.05	0.12 ± 0.06
P2				2.94 ± 0.18	0.43 ± 0.04	0.34 ± 0.02	0.71 ± 0.04	0.02 ± 0.05
AAL (78)	0.70 ± 0.11	427	0.142					
P1				2.40 ± 0.09	0.45 ± 0.03	0.42 ± 0.02	0.42 ± 0.01	0.11 ± 0.07
P2				2.43 ± 0.04	0.47 ± 0.01	0.41 ± 0.01	0.42 ± 0.01	0.07 ± 0.06

Graph theoretical characteristics of subject binary networks thresholded at the peak convergence density. Shown are the mean ± standard deviation of the graph theoretical properties of Pathlength (PL), Clustering Coefficient (CC), Global Efficiency (G. Eff), Local Efficiency (L. Eff) and Assortativity (AS), across subjects.

0.106) for atlas of node scale 34, 44 and 68, respectively. This trend of an increasing number of connections occuring consistently between pipelines at higher node scales may be expected given the increase in possible region pairs. Similarly, [30] found that the estimated number of true positive connections increased in the Harvard-Oxford atlas, which has 96 nodes.

Other studies have investigated the effect of threshold on anatomical validity of structural networks, by utilising a ground truth for particular sub-components of the network. Li *et. al.* (2012) investigated the effect of threshold on the sensitivity and specificity of structural network connections, using connectvity data derived from post-mortem tract tracing techniques in the macaque brain as a ground truth [31]. The performance of several tractography strategies was assessed by analysing the area under the receiver operating characteristic curve. However, their study was limited to a subset of brain regions due to limited availability of tract tracing data in macaque brain and an optimal threshold for performing network analysis was not reported. Bastiani *et. al.* (2012) used a network 'quality control' technique to analyse the sensitivity and specificity of brain network connections across thresholds for deterministic tractography reconstruction techniques [59]. However, their sensitivity and specificity metrics measured connectivity between sets of regions known to be connected according to *a priori* information and therefore may have had limited applicability to other connections across the network. In contrast to these works, our study utilised information across all brain region pairs and compared two independent pipelines as opposed to performing a more focussed study on individual fiber tractography reconstruction stages.

We found high similarity in graph theoretical propeties of the consensus networks when comparing those derived from the same node scale atlas. This may be expected, given the convergence of connections at the peak convergence density was above 65%, and that the networks had the same connection density, which is known to significantly impact upon the graph theoretical metrics [32]. Despite high similarity across alternative pipelines at the same node scale, some graph theoretical properties were significantly different across node scales. Most notably, the number of connections in the consensus network increased and density of the network decreased in atlases at higher node scales. This could be due to division of connections between multiple parcels at higher node scales due to an increase in the number of possible regional pairs.

We found that the peak convergence density using the AAL atlas was similar to that of the Desikan-Killiany atlas, despite the AAL atlas having a higher node scale. This may be because the AAL atlas uses a fundamentally different type of parcellation scheme and algorithm. While the Desikan-Killiany atlas contains only the grey matter region of the cortex, the AAL atlas represents larger regions which include both grey and white matter. This may have increased the number of robustly occurring cortical connections, as some streamlines, which may otherwise have become truncated before reaching the grey matter of the cortex (due to noise and tissue partial volume effects), intersect these parcels. Furthermore, the AAL segmentation algorithm uses an affine registration between the subject brain and a standard brain from MNI space, meaning subject differences in brain morphology are not considered. Larger parcels and limited ability to account for individual brain variation may have meant single connections became distributed across multiple parcels in the network, leading to a high peak convergence network density compared to the Hammers and Desikan-Killiany atlases (Fig. 4).

With the exception of the AAL atlas, the pathlength and global efficiency tended to increase and decrease, respectively, in consensus networks with increasing node scale atlases. This may due to the lower consensus network densities at higher node scales, resulting in a decrease in the ratio of edges to nodes. Also, clustering coefficient and local efficiency decreased when comparing the consensus networks obtained from the Hammers (44 nodes) to the Desikan-Killiany atlas (68 nodes). Zalesky *et. al.* (2010) examined the effect of node scale on the pathlength and clustering coefficient of networks generated using deterministic tractography and found that an increase and decrease in the pathlength and clustering coefficient metrics, respectively [60]. Their study examined a wide range of node scales (from 82 to 4000 in steps of 500) whereas our study re-affirms these findings at finer node scale increments. However, clustering and local efficiency showed no clear trend with node scale when comparing the Common (34 nodes) and Hammers atlases (44 nodes).

It should be noted that although the observed correspondence of connection fiber paths with known white matter tracts does suggests some degree of anatomical truth to the underlying connections in the consensus networks (Fig. 5), spurious network weights may be included in the consensus networks due to a common bias in the tractography methods. Therefore, although the reconstructed tracts are sensible, they are unlikely to be exhaustive. For example, local tractography techniques may produce shorter fibers than found *in vivo*, as fibers are deflected from the true path due to noise and limited angular resolution. This may have meant connection weights between distant regions were lower than expected. Some network reconstruction methods have accounted for this by penalizing the weighting of shorter inter-regional distances [31]. In addition to the weighting scheme, many other alternative pipelines are available which may result in different convergence results. Therefore, it should be emphasised that we demonstrated agreement between two pipelines out of a large number of possibilities and that our results may not apply to pipelines which employ different parcellation, registration or tractography methods. Finally, the peak convergent threshold described here was derived from a population of healthy individuals and may not represent an appropriate threshold for other clinical populations where connections may have become altered or absent.

Conclusion

High convergence between two independent state-of-the-art structural network reconstruction pipelines was observed on a connection-wise basis for all density thresholds. A sparse 'consensus network', which occured most robustly between the pipelines, was identified in four atlases, and had a density of between 10% and 20% (100–250 connections). We propose that these connections have high anatomical validity compared to other thresholds, which is useful given the inherent difficulty in defining thresholds for brain network studies. The pipeline had relatively little effect on the network properties of the consensus networks, although some relationship with atlas node scale was observed, in agreement with previous studies. When performing structural network analysis, it may be useful to apply multiple pipelines to diffusion-weighted data and to use the comparison framework described here to identify the most important connections.

Supporting Information

Figure S1 Normalised dice similarity coefficient between pipelines across density thresholds for all subjects. The normalised similarity coefficient was calculated by subtracting the expected from the observed dice coefficient at each density. Shown are the the subject normalised dice coefficients (left) and the mean normalised dice coefficient ± standard deviation (right) for pipelines using the Common (top), Hammers (middle-top), Desikan-Killiany (middle-lower) and AAL (lower) atlases. A peak normalised dice coefficient is observed for densities in the region of 0.05–0.20 for all atlases.

Acknowledgments

The authors acknowledge the contributions of Kiran Seunarine who provided guidance in using FSL and MRTrix software and in composing figures.

Author Contributions

Conceived and designed the experiments: CSP JDC SO. Performed the experiments: CSP. Analyzed the data: CSP JDC SO. Contributed reagents/materials/analysis tools: FD MC PD MM MD CAC JDC SO. Wrote the paper: CSP.

References

1. Bullmore E, Sporns O (2009) Complex brain networks: graph theoretical analysis of structural and functional systems. Nat Rev Neurosci 10: 186–198.
2. Duarte-Carvajalino JM, Jahanshad N, Lenglet C, McMahon KL, de Zubicaray GI, et al. (2012) Hierarchical topological network analysis of anatomical human brain connectivity and differences related to sex and kinship. Neuroimage 59: 3784–3804.
3. Gong G, Rosa-Neto P, Carbonell F, Chen ZJ, He Y, et al. (2009) Age-and gender-related differences in the cortical anatomical network. J Neurosci 29: 15684–15693.
4. Li Y, Liu Y, Li J, Qin W, Li K, et al. (2009) Brain anatomical network and intelligence. PLoS Comput Biol 5: e1000395.
5. Lo CY, Wang PN, Chou KH, Wang J, He Y, et al. (2010) Diffusion tensor tractography reveals abnormal topological organization in structural cortical networks in alzheimer's disease. J Neurosci 30: 16876–16885.
6. Shao J, Myers N, Yang Q, Feng J, Plant C, et al. (2012) Prediction of alzheimer's disease using individual structural connectivity networks. Neurobiol Aging 33: 2756–2765.
7. Vaessen MJ, Jansen JF, Vlooswijk MC, Hofman PA, Majoie HM, et al. (2012) White matter network abnormalities are associated with cognitive decline in chronic epilepsy. Cereb Cortex 22: 2139–2147.
8. Zhang Z, Liao W, Chen H, Mantini D, Ding JR, et al. (2011) Altered functional-structural coupling of large-scale brain networks in idiopathic generalized epilepsy. Brain 134: 2912–2928.
9. van den Heuvel MP, Mandl RC, Stam CJ, Kahn RS, Pol HEH (2010) Aberrant frontal and temporal complex network structure in schizophrenia: a graph theoretical analysis. J Neurosci 30: 15915–15926.
10. Zalesky A, Fornito A, Seal ML, Cocchi L, Westin CF, et al. (2011) Disrupted axonal fiber connectivity in schizophrenia. Biol Psychiatr 69: 80–89.
11. Wang Q, Su TP, Zhou Y, Chou KH, Chen IY, et al. (2012) Anatomical insights into disrupted small-world networks in schizophrenia. Neuroimage 59: 1085–1093.
12. Tzourio-Mazoyer N, Landeau B, Papathanassiou D, Crivello F, Etard O, et al. (2002) Automated anatomical labeling of activations in spm using a macroscopic anatomical parcellation of the MNI MRI single-subject brain. Neuroimage 15: 273–289.
13. Gong G, He Y, Concha L, Lebel C, Gross DW, et al. (2009) Mapping anatomical connectivity patterns of human cerebral cortex using in vivo diffusion tensor imaging tractography. Cereb Cortex 19: 524–536.
14. Wen W, Zhu W, He Y, Kochan NA, Reppermund S, et al. (2011) Discrete neuroanatomical networks are associated with specific cognitive abilities in old age. J Neurosci 31: 1204–1212.
15. Robinson EC, Hammers A, Ericsson A, Edwards AD, Rueckert D (2010) Identifying population differences in whole-brain structural networks: a machine learning approach. NeuroImage 50: 910–919.
16. Hagmann P, Kurant M, Gigandet X, Thiran P, Wedeen VJ, et al. (2007) Mapping human whole-brain structural networks with diffusion MRI. PloS One 2: e597.
17. Tymofiyeva O, Hess CP, Ziv E, Tian N, Bonifacio SL, et al. (2012) Towards the baby connectome: mapping the structural connectivity of the newborn brain. PloS One 7: e31029.
18. Hagmann P, Cammoun L, Gigandet X, Meuli R, Honey CJ, et al. (2008) Mapping the structural core of human cerebral cortex. PLoS Biol 6: e159.

19. Hagmann P, Sporns O, Madan N, Cammoun L, Pienaar R, et al. (2010) White matter maturation reshapes structural connectivity in the late developing human brain. Proc Natl Acad Sci 107: 19067–19072.
20. Echtermeyer C, Han CE, Rotarska-Jagiela A, Mohr H, Uhlhaas PJ, et al. (2011) Integrating temporal and spatial scales: human structural network motifs across age and region of interest size. Front Neuroinformatics 5: 10.
21. Basser PJ, Mattiello J, LeBihan D (1994) Estimation of the effective self-diffusion tensor from the NMR spin echo. J Magn Reson Series B 103: 247–54.
22. Shu N, Liu Y, Li J, Li Y, Yu C, et al. (2009) Altered anatomical network in early blindness revealed by diffusion tensor tractography. PLoS One 4: e7228.
23. Hagmann P, Sporns O, Madan N, Cammoun L, Pienaar R, et al. (2010) White matter maturation reshapes structural connectivity in the late developing human brain. Proc Natl Acad Sci 107: 19067–19072.
24. Bai F, Shu N, Yuan Y, Shi Y, Yu H, et al. (2012) Topologically convergent and divergent structural connectivity patterns between patients with remitted geriatric depression and amnestic mild cognitive impairment. J Neurosci 32: 4307–4318.
25. Wedeen VJ, Hagmann P, Tseng WYI, Reese TG, Weisskoff RM (2005) Mapping complex tissue architecture with diffusion spectrum magnetic resonance imaging. Magn Reson Med 54: 1377–1386.
26. Behrens T, Woolrich M, Jenkinson M, Johansen-Berg H, Nunes R, et al. (2003) Characterization and propagation of uncertainty in diffusion-weighted MR imaging. Magn Reson Med 50: 1077–1088.
27. Tournier JD, Calamante F, Gadian DG, Connelly A (2004) Direct estimation of the fiber orientation density function from diffusion-weighted MRI data using spherical deconvolution. NeuroImage 23: 1176–1185.
28. Duarte-Carvajalino JM, Jahanshad N, Lenglet C, McMahon KL, de Zubicaray GI, et al. (2012) Hierarchical topological network analysis of anatomical human brain connectivity and differences related to sex and kinship. Neuroimage 59: 3784–3804.
29. Vaessen M, Hofman P, Tijssen H, Aldenkamp A, Jansen J, et al. (2010) The effect and reproducibility of different clinical DTI gradient sets on small world brain connectivity measures. Neuroimage 51: 1106.
30. de Reus MA, van den Heuvel MP (2013) Estimating false positives and negatives in brain networks. NeuroImage 70: 402–409.
31. Li L, Rilling JK, Preuss TM, Glasser MF, Hu X (2012) The effects of connection reconstruction method on the interregional connectivity of brain networks via diffusion tractography. Hum Brain Mapp 33: 1894–1913.
32. van Wijk BC, Stam CJ, Daffertshofer A (2010) Comparing brain networks of different size and connectivity density using graph theory. PLoS One 5: e13701.
33. Clayden JD, Maniega SM, Storkey AJ, King MD, Bastin ME, et al. (2011) Tractor: Magnetic resonance imaging and tractography with r. J Statistical Software 44: 1–18.
34. Smith SM (2002) Fast robust automated brain extraction. Hum Brain Mapp 17: 143–155.
35. Reuter M, Rosas HD, Fischl B (2010) Highly accurate inverse consistent registration: a robust approach. NeuroImage 53: 1181–96.
36. Jenkinson M, Smith S (2001) A global optimisation method for robust affine registration of brain images. Med Image Anal 5: 143–156.
37. Hammers A, Allom R, Koepp MJ, Free SL, Myers R, et al. (2003) Three-dimensional maximum probability atlas of the human brain, with particular reference to the temporal lobe. Hum Brain Mapp 19: 224–247.
38. Cardoso JM, Leung K, Modat M, Keihaninejad S, Cash D, et al. (2013) STEPS: Similarity and Truth Estimation for Propagated Segmentations and its application to hippocampal segmentation and brain parcelation. Med Image Anal 17: 671–84.
39. Modat M, Ridgway GR, Taylor ZA, Lehmann M, Barnes J, et al. (2010) Fast free-form deformation using graphics processing units. Comput Methods Prog Biomed 98: 278–284.
40. Cardoso MJ, Clarkson MJ, Ridgway GR, Modat M, Fox NC, et al. (2011) Load: A locally adaptive cortical segmentation algorithm. NeuroImage 56: 1386–1397.
41. Desikan RS, Ségonne F, Fischl B, Quinn BT, Dickerson BC, et al. (2006) An automated labeling system for subdividing the human cerebral cortex on MRI scans into gyral based regions of interest. Neuroimage 31: 968–980.
42. Fischl B, van der Kouwe A, Destrieux C, Halgren E, Ségonne F, et al. (2004) Automatically parcellating the human cerebral cortex. Cereb Cortex 14: 11–22.
43. Rueckert D, Sonoda LI, Hayes C, Hill DL, Leach MO, et al. (1999) Nonrigid registration using free-form deformations: application to breast MR images. IEEE Trans Med Imaging 18: 712–21.
44. Tournier JD, Calamante F, Connelly A (2007) Robust determination of the fibre orientation distribution in diffusion MRI: non-negativity constrained super-resolved spherical deconvolution. NeuroImage 35: 1459–1472.
45. Behrens T, Berg HJ, Jbabdi S, Rushworth M, Woolrich M (2007) Probabilistic diffusion tractography with multiple fibre orientations: What can we gain? Neuroimage 34: 144–155.
46. Tournier J, Calamante F, Connelly A (2012) Mrtrix: Diffusion tractography in crossing fiber regions. Int J Imaging Syst Technol 22: 53–66.
47. Team RC (2012). R: a language and environment for statistical computing. vienna: R foundation for statistical computing; 2012. URL http://www.R-project.org/.
48. Cheng H, Wang Y, Sheng J, Sporns O, Kronenberger WG, et al. (2012) Optimization of seed density in DTI tractography for structural networks. J Neurosci Methods 203: 264–272.
49. Gong G, He Y, Chen ZJ, Evans AC (2012) Convergence and divergence of thickness correlations with diffusion connections across the human cerebral cortex. Neuroimage 59: 1239–1248.
50. Csardi G, Nepusz T (2006) The igraph software package for complex network research. InterJournal Complex Systems: 1695.
51. Watts DJ, Strogatz SH (1998) Collective dynamics of 'small-world' networks. Nat 393: 440–442.
52. Latora V, Marchiori M (2001) Efficient behavior of small-world networks. Physical review letters 87: 198701.
53. Newman ME (2003) The structure and function of complex networks. SIAM review 45: 167–256.
54. Newman ME (2002) Assortative mixing in networks. Physical review letters 89: 208701.
55. Rubinov M, Sporns O (2010) Complex network measures of brain connectivity: uses and interpretations. Neuroimage 52: 1059–1069.
56. Catani M, Thiebaut de Schotten M (2008) A diffusion tensor imaging tractography atlas for virtual in vivo dissections. Cortex 44: 1105–1132.
57. Bassett DS, Brown JA, Deshpande V, Carlson JM, Grafton ST (2011) Conserved and variable architecture of human white matter connectivity. Neuroimage 54: 1262–1279.
58. Cheng H, Wang Y, Sheng J, Kronenberger WG, Mathews VP, et al. (2012) Characteristics and variability of structural networks derived from diffusion tensor imaging. NeuroImage 61: 1153–64.
59. Bastiani M, Shah NJ, Goebel R, Roebroeck A (2012) Human cortical connectome reconstruction from diffusion weighted mri: the effect of tractography algorithm. NeuroImage 62: 1732–1749.
60. Zalesky A, Fornito A, Harding IH, Cocchi L, Yücel M, et al. (2010) Whole-brain anatomical networks: does the choice of nodes matter? Neuroimage 50: 970.

Permissions

All chapters in this book were first published in PLOS ONE, by The Public Library of Science; hereby published with permission under the Creative Commons Attribution License or equivalent. Every chapter published in this book has been scrutinized by our experts. Their significance has been extensively debated. The topics covered herein carry significant findings which will fuel the growth of the discipline. They may even be implemented as practical applications or may be referred to as a beginning point for another development.

The contributors of this book come from diverse backgrounds, making this book a truly international effort. This book will bring forth new frontiers with its revolutionizing research information and detailed analysis of the nascent developments around the world.

We would like to thank all the contributing authors for lending their expertise to make the book truly unique. They have played a crucial role in the development of this book. Without their invaluable contributions this book wouldn't have been possible. They have made vital efforts to compile up to date information on the varied aspects of this subject to make this book a valuable addition to the collection of many professionals and students.

This book was conceptualized with the vision of imparting up-to-date information and advanced data in this field. To ensure the same, a matchless editorial board was set up. Every individual on the board went through rigorous rounds of assessment to prove their worth. After which they invested a large part of their time researching and compiling the most relevant data for our readers.

The editorial board has been involved in producing this book since its inception. They have spent rigorous hours researching and exploring the diverse topics which have resulted in the successful publishing of this book. They have passed on their knowledge of decades through this book. To expedite this challenging task, the publisher supported the team at every step. A small team of assistant editors was also appointed to further simplify the editing procedure and attain best results for the readers.

Apart from the editorial board, the designing team has also invested a significant amount of their time in understanding the subject and creating the most relevant covers. They scrutinized every image to scout for the most suitable representation of the subject and create an appropriate cover for the book.

The publishing team has been an ardent support to the editorial, designing and production team. Their endless efforts to recruit the best for this project, has resulted in the accomplishment of this book. They are a veteran in the field of academics and their pool of knowledge is as vast as their experience in printing. Their expertise and guidance has proved useful at every step. Their uncompromising quality standards have made this book an exceptional effort. Their encouragement from time to time has been an inspiration for everyone.

The publisher and the editorial board hope that this book will prove to be a valuable piece of knowledge for researchers, students, practitioners and scholars across the globe.

List of Contributors

Xiaoyu Guo and Ralph Etienne-Cummings
Dept. of Electrical and Computer Engineering, Johns Hopkins University, Baltimore, MD, United States of America

Hyun-Jae Kang
Dept. of Computer Science, Johns Hopkins University, Baltimore, MD, United States of America

Emad M. Boctor
Dept. of Computer Science, Johns Hopkins University, Baltimore, MD, United States of America
Dept. of Radiology, Johns Hopkins University, Baltimore, MD, United States of America

Samantha Huang, Stephanie Rossi and Jyrki Ahveninen
Harvard Medical School, Athinoula A. Martinos Center for Biomedical Imaging, Department of Radiology, Massachusetts General Hospital, Charlestown, Massachusetts, United States of America

Matti Hämä läinen
Harvard Medical School, Athinoula A. Martinos Center for Biomedical Imaging, Department of Radiology, Massachusetts General Hospital, Charlestown, Massachusetts, United States of America
Harvard-MIT Division of Health Sciences and Technology, Cambridge, Massachusetts, United States of America

Kaspar-Josche Streitberger, Jing Guo and Ingolf Sack
Department of Radiology, Charité - Universitätsmedizin Berlin, Berlin, Germany

Martin Reiss-Zimmermann and Karl-Titus Hoffmann
Department of Neuroradiology, Universitätsmedizin Leipzig, Leipzig, Germany

Florian Baptist Freimann
Department of Neurosurgery, Universitätsmedizin Göttingen, Göttingen, Germany

Simon Bayerl
Department of Neurosurgery, Charité - Universitätsmedizin Berlin, Berlin, Germany

Felix Arlt
Department of Neurosurgery, Universitätsmedizin Leipzig, Leipzig, Germany

Jens Wuerfel
Institute of Neuroradiology, Universitätsmedizin Göttingen, Göttingen, Germany
NeuroCure, Charité - Universitätsmedizin Berlin, Berlin, Germany

Jürgen Braun
Institute of Medical Informatics, Charité - Universitätsmedizin Berlin, Berlin, Germany

Kelly Rowe Bijanki, Brendan Hodis, Michael C. Brumm, Emily L. Harlynn and Laurie M. McCormick
Department of Psychiatry, University of Iowa Roy J. and Lucille A. Carver College of Medicine, Iowa City, Iowa, United States of America

William A. Mehan Jr., R. Gilberto González, Bradley R. Buchbinder, John W. Chen, William A. Copen, Rajiv Gupta, Joshua A. Hirsch, George J. Hunter, Scott Hunter, Jason M. Johnson, Hillary R. Kelly, Mykol Larvie, Michael H. Lev, Stuart R. Pomerantz, Otto Rapalino, Sandra Rincon, Javier M. Romero, Pamela W. Schaefer, Vinil Shah
Neuroradiology Division, Massachusetts General Hospital, Harvard Medical School, Boston, Massachusetts, United States of America

Xingyu Zhang, Brett R. Cowan, Avan Suinesiaputra, Alistair A. Young and Pau Medrano-Gracia
Department of Anatomy with Radiology, University of Auckland, Auckland, New Zealand

David A. Bluemke
National Institute of Biomedical Imaging and Bioengineering, Bethesda, Maryland, United States of America

J. Paul Finn and Carissa G. Fonseca
Department of Radiology, University of California Los Angeles, Los Angeles, California, United States of America

Alan H. Kadish and Daniel C. Lee
Feinberg Cardiovascular Research Institute, Northwestern University Feinberg School of Medicine, Chicago, Illinois, United States of America

Joao A. C. Lima
The Donald W. Reynolds Cardiovascular Clinical Research Center, The Johns Hopkins University, Baltimore, Maryland, United States of America

Bratislav Mišić, Zainab Fatima, Nathan Churchill, Michele Korostil, Stephen C. Strother and Anthony R. McIntosh
Rotman Research Institute, Baycrest Centre, Toronto, Ontario, Canada

Mary K. Askren
Department of Radiology, University of Washington, Seattle, Washington, United States of America

Martin Buschkuehl
MIND Research Institute, Irvine, California, United States of America

Bernadine Cimprich
School of Nursing, University of Michigan, Ann Arbor, Michigan, United States of America

Patricia J. Deldin, Susanne Jaeggi, Ethan Kross, Scott Peltier, Patricia A. Reuter-Lorenz and John Jonides
Department of Psychology, University of Michigan, Ann Arbor, Michigan, United States of America

Misook Jung
Department of Psychology, Chungnam University, Daejeon, South Korea

Katherine M. Krpan
Department of Psychology, University of South Carolina, Columbia, South Carolina, United States of America

Marc G. Berman
Department of Psychology, University of South Carolina, Columbia, South Carolina, United States of America
Department of Psychology, University of Chicago, Chicago, Illinois, United States of America

Masaki Katsura, Hiroki Sasaki, Harushi Mori, Akira Kunimatsu and Kuni Ohtomo
Department of Radiology, The University of Tokyo School of Medicine, Tokyo, Japan

Satoshi Hirose and Seiki Konishi
Department of Physiology, The University of Tokyo School of Medicine, Tokyo, Japan
Department of Physiology, Juntendo University School of Medicine, Tokyo, Japan

Koji Jimura
Department of Physiology, The University of Tokyo School of Medicine, Tokyo, Japan
Department of Physiology, Juntendo University School of Medicine, Tokyo, Japan
Precision and Intelligence Laboratory, Tokyo Institute of Technology, Yokohama, Japan

Armelle Viard, Vincent de La Sayette, Béatrice Desgranges and Francis Eustache
Inserm, U1077, Caen, France
Université de Caen Basse-Normandie, UMR-S1077, Caen, France
Ecole Pratique des Hautes Etudes, UMR-S1077, Caen, France
Centre Hospitalier Universitaire, U1077, Caen, France

Pascale Piolino
Université Paris Descartes, Institut de Psychologie, Memory and Cognition Lab, Paris, France
Inserm UMR S894, Centre de Psychiatrie et Neurosciences, Paris, France

Serge Belliard
Inserm, U1077, Caen, France
Université de Caen Basse-Normandie, UMR-S1077, Caen, France
Ecole Pratique des Hautes Etudes, UMR-S1077, Caen, France
Centre Hospitalier Universitaire, U1077, Caen, France
CHU Pontchaillou, Rennes, France

Juan F. P. J. Abascal, Paula Montesinos, Eugenio Marinetto and Javier Pascau
Departamento de Bioingeniería e Ingeniería Aeroespacial, Universidad Carlos III de Madrid, Madrid, Spain
Instituto de Investigación Sanitaria Gregorio Marañón (IiSGM), Madrid, Spain

Manuel Desco
Departamento de Bioingeniería e Ingeniería Aeroespacial, Universidad Carlos III de Madrid, Madrid, Spain
Instituto de Investigación Sanitaria Gregorio Marañón (IiSGM), Madrid, Spain
Centro de Investigación en Red de Salud Mental (CIBERSAM), Madrid, Spain

Owen Phillips and Margherita Di Paola
Clinical and Behavioural Neurology Dept, IRCCS Santa Lucia Foundation, Rome, Italy

Ferdinando Squitieri and Francesca Elifani
IRCSS Neuromed, Pozzilli, Italy

Cristina Sanchez-Castaneda and Umberto Sabatini
Radiology Dept, IRCCS Santa Lucia Foundation, Rome, Italy

Carlo Caltagirone
Clinical and Behavioural Neurology Dept, IRCCS Santa Lucia Foundation, Rome, Italy
Neuroscience Dept, University of Rome "Tor Vergata", Rome, Italy

Sarah H. Baum
Department of Neurobiology and Anatomy, University of Texas Medical School at Houston, Houston, Texas, United States of America
Vanderbilt Brain Institute, Vanderbilt University, Nashville, Tennessee, United States of America

Michael S. Beauchamp
Department of Neurobiology and Anatomy, University of Texas Medical School at Houston, Houston, Texas, United States of America

Louise Alessandra Mesentier-Louro, Camila Zaverucha-do-Valle, Almir Jordão da Silva-Junior,

Gabriel Nascimento-dos-Santos, Fernanda Gubert, Ana Beatriz Padilha de Figueirêdo, Ana

Luiza Torres, Bruno D. Paredes, Rosalia Mendez-Otero and Marcelo F. Santiago
Instituto de Biofísica Carlos Chagas Filho, Universidade Federal do Rio de Janeiro, Rio de Janeiro, Brazi,
Instituto Nacional de Ciência e Tecnologia de Biologia Estrutural e Bioimagem, INBEB, Rio de Janeiro, Brazil

Camila Teixeira
National Center of Structural Biology and Bioimaging (CENABIO), Universidade Federal do Rio de Janeiro, Rio de Janeiro, Brazil

Fernanda Tovar-Moll
National Center of Structural Biology and Bioimaging (CENABIO), Universidade Federal do Rio de Janeiro, Rio de Janeiro, Brazil
D'Or Institute for Research and Education (IDOR), Rio de Janeiro, Brazil
Institute of Biomedical Sciences (ICB), Universidade Federal do Rio de Janeiro, Rio de Janeiro, Brazil

Stephanie Seah, Abu Bakar Ali Asad and Chih-Liang Chin
Imaging, Merck & Co. Inc., West Point, Pennsylvania, United States of America
Translational Medicine Research Centre, MSD, Singapore, Singapore

Richard Baumgartner and Dai Feng
Biostatistics and Research Decision Sciences, Merck & Co. Inc., Rahway, New Jersey, United States of America

Donald S. Williams and Jeffrey L. Evelhoch
Imaging, Merck & Co. Inc., West Point, Pennsylvania, United States of America

Elaine Manigbas and John D. Beaver
Imaging, Maccine Pte Ltd, Singapore, Singapore

Torsten Reese and Brian Henry
Translational Medicine Research Centre, MSD, Singapore, Singapore

Soroush Larjani, Eric Monsalves, Houman Pebdani, Boris Krischek, Fred Gentili and Gelareh Zadeh
Department of Neurosurgery, University Health Network, Toronto, Canada

Michael Cusimano
Department of Neurosurgery, St. Michael's Hospital, Toronto, Canada

Normand Laperriere
Radiation Oncology Program, Princess Margaret Hospital, Toronto, Canada

Caroline Hayhurst
Department of Neurosurgery, The Walton Centre, Liverpool, United Kingdom

Kersten Villringer, Lars-Arne Schaafs and Jochen B. Fiebach
Academic Neuroradiology, Department of Neurology and Center for Stroke Research, Charité, Berlin, Germany

Ulrike Grittner
Department for Biostatistics and Clinical Epidemiology and Center for Stroke Research, Charité, Berlin, Germany

Christian H. Nolte and Heinrich Audebert
Department of Neurology and Center for Stroke Research, Charité, Berlin, Germany

Weibing Miao and Shan Zheng
Department of Nuclear Medicine, the 1st Affiliated Hospital of Fujian Medical University, Fuzhou, China

Haojie Dai
Department of Nuclear Medicine, Beijing Tongren Hospital, Beijing, China

Feng Wang
Department of Nuclear Medicine, the 1st Affiliated Hospital of Nanjing Medical University, Nanjing, China

Xiaona Jin and Zhaohui Zhu
Department of Nuclear Medicine, Peking Union Medical College Hospital, Chinese Academy of Medical Sciences and Peking Union Medical College, Beijing, China

Bing Jia
Medical Isotopes Research Center, Peking University, Beijing, China

Zhi Dong, Yanji Luo, Zi- Ping Li, Shi-Ting Feng and Huasong Cai
Department of Radiology, The First Affiliated Hospital of Sun Yat-Sen University, Guangzhou, China

Zhongwei Zhang
Department of Radiology, The University of Texas Southwestern Medical Center, Dallas, Texas, United States of America

Yanbing Li
Department of Endocrinology and Diabetes Center, The First Affiliated Hospital of Sun Yat-sen University Guangzhou, China

Tao Chan
Medical Imaging Department, Union Hospital, Hong Kong

Ling Wu
Department of Radiology, Kiang Wu Hospital, Macao

Sara Zarei
Computational Science Research Center, San Diego State University, San Diego, California, United States of America

Ali Mirtar
Electrical and Computer Eng. Dep/University of California San Diego, San Diego, California, United States of America

Forest Rohwer
Department of Biology, San Diego State University, San Diego, California, United States of America

Peter Salamon
Department of Mathematics and Statistics, San Diego State University, San Diego, California, United States of America

Christopher S. Parker
Centre for Medical Image Computing, University College London, London, United Kingdom
Imaging and Biophysics Unit, UCL Institute of Child Health, London, United Kingdom

Fani Deligianni, Chris A. Clark and Jonathan D. Clayden
Imaging and Biophysics Unit, UCL Institute of Child Health, London, United Kingdom

M. Jorge Cardoso, Pankaj Daga and Marc Modat
Centre for Medical Image Computing, University College London, London, United Kingdom

Michael Dayan
Imaging and Biophysics Unit, UCL Institute of Child Health, London, United Kingdom
Department of Radiology, Weill Cornell Medical College, New York, New York, United States of America

Sebastien Ourselin
Centre for Medical Image Computing, University College London, London, United Kingdom
Dementia Research Centre, University College London, London, United Kingdom

Index

A
Anterior Thalamic Radiation, 137, 139
Arbitrary Pattern Injection, 1, 3, 11, 13
Arcuate Fasciculus, 131, 137, 139
Audiovisual Speech, 141-143, 145-146, 148-149
Auspis, 1-5, 8-13
Axon Regeneration, 151, 154, 162, 164-166

B
Beam Steering Method, 13
Binary Network, 215, 219
Block-design Localizer, 143
Blood Oxygenation Level Dependence, 167
Bone Marrow, 151-152, 158, 162, 165-166, 195-197
Bone Metastasis, 192-193, 195, 197
Brain Mri, 43, 46, 50, 190
Brain Networks, 26, 66, 71, 75, 85, 215-216, 221, 223-224
Buprenorphine, 167-177

C
Cardiac Cine Mri, 120-121, 128
Cardiac Remodeling, 53, 63
Cardiovascular Disease, 54-55
Cell Therapy, 151-152, 158, 161, 165-166
Central Nervous System, 34, 159, 164-165, 178
Central Neurons, 151
Cerebral Blood Volume, 167, 177, 187
Cf Lung, 206, 208, 210-211, 214
Compressed Sensing, 120-121, 126, 128-129
Computed Tomography, 192, 199, 206
Cystic Fibrosis, 206, 210-211, 214

D
Degeneration, 117-118, 130, 134, 140, 151, 155, 158-159, 161, 165
Diffusion Tensor Imaging, 34, 130-131, 140, 224
Drug-induced Brain, 167-168, 174

E
End Diastole, 54
End Systole, 54

F
Fronto-temporal Interaction, 87, 91, 94-95

G
Gb Tissue, 28
Glioblastoma, 27, 34, 178, 184

H
Hemodynamic Response Function, 89, 105, 145, 170
Huntington's Disease, 130-132, 139-140

I
Inferior Occipital Fasciculus, 131
Intracranial Hemorrhages, 44-45, 48
Intraocular Injections, 153
Ischemic Heart Disease, 53

L
Lateral Prefrontal Cortex, 20, 87, 89-90, 94-95
Left Ventricle, 53, 55, 57, 62, 65
Lung Cancer, 192-194, 196-198

M
Magnetic Resonance Imaging, 25, 27, 39, 42, 52, 54, 65, 85, 97, 102, 120, 129-130, 140-141, 151-153, 176-177, 191, 199, 205-206, 214, 224
Memory Retrieval, 87, 89, 95-96, 99, 102, 119
Mental Illness, 36
Mesenchymal Stem Cells, 151-152, 155, 165-166
Mid-plane Detection, 1, 3, 6, 8
Minor Stroke, 185-186, 189-190
Msc Transplantation, 151, 155-156, 158-159, 161-163
Myocardial Infarction, 53-55, 61-65, 120, 128-129
Myocardium Infarction, 121

N
Neuroimaging, 14-15, 37, 39, 42-43, 52, 66, 68, 72-73, 77, 85, 95-96, 99, 103, 118-119, 132, 167, 190
Neuronal Survival, 151, 163-164
Neuroprotective, 151, 155, 162, 164-166
Neurotransmitter, 168, 174, 176

O
Optic Nerve Crush, 151-156, 158-159, 161-164
Optic Nerve Injury, 151-152, 158, 161-162, 165
Optic-nerve Crush, 153

P
Pipelines, 215-217, 219-223
Plasma Cortisol, 171, 175
Positron Emission Tomography, 67, 96, 167, 198
Pre-treatment Growth Rate, 178, 180, 182-183
Psychophysiological Interaction, 87, 89, 94
Psychotic Depression, 36-42

R
Radiation, 54, 67-68, 80, 131, 137, 139, 178-182, 184, 198-200, 206

S
Semantic Dementia, 98-99, 102, 105, 110, 116-119
Signal-to-noise Ratio, 120, 132, 175
Stochastic Tracking, 206
Structural Brain Networks, 215-216, 221
Superior Temporal Sulcus, 141, 143, 146-147, 149

T
Thrombolysis, 185-191
Transient Ischemic Attacks, 185
Transmitted Signals, 4

U
Ultrasound, 1-13
Ultrasound Pulse, 2-4, 10-11

V
Vessel Pathology, 185, 188
Vitreous Body, 151, 153-159, 161-162, 164

W
Whole-brain Analysis, 141, 143, 145, 147